Clinical Neuroanatomy
for Medical
Students

By the Same Author

Atlas of Clinical Anatomy

Gross Anatomy Dissector

Gross Anatomy: A Review with Questions and Explanations

Clinical and Functional Histology for Medical Students

Neuroanatomy: A Review with Questions and Explanations

Clinical Anatomy for Medical Students, Fourth Edition

Translation:
Clinical Neuroanatomy for Medical Students
Spanish Edition 1982
Editorial Medica Pan Americana S.A.

Clinical Neuroanatomy for Medical Students

Third Edition

Richard S. Snell, M.D., Ph.D.

Emeritus Professor of Anatomy, George Washington University
School of Medicine and Health Sciences, Washington, D.C.

Little, Brown and Company
Boston/Toronto/London

Library of Congress Cataloging-in-Publication Data

Snell, Richard S.
    Clinical neuroanatomy for medical students / Richard S. Snell.—
    3rd ed.
        p.   cm.
    Includes bibliographical references and index.
    ISBN 0-316-80244-1
    1. Neuroanatomy.   2. Nervous system—Diseases.   I. Title.
    [DNLM: 1. Nervous system—anatomy & histology.   WL 101 S671c]
    QM451.S64   1992
    616.8—dc20
    DNLM/DLC
    for Library of Congress   91-44527
                                                     CIP

Second Printing

Printed in the United States of America

KP

To My Students—Past, Present, and Future

Contents

Frontal pole

Longitudinal fissure

Precentral sulcus

Frontal lobe

Precentral gyrus

Central sulcus

Left cerebral hemisphere

Postcentral gyrus

Parietal lobe

Postcentral sulcus

A

Occipital lobe

Occipital pole

Frontal lobe

Longitudinal fissure

Right cerebral hemisphere

Olfactory tract

Optic chiasma

Temporal lobe

Midbrain

Oculomotor nerve

Pons

Pyramid

Cerebellum

Medulla oblongata

Olive

B

Fig. P-1. A. Superior view of the brain.
B. Inferior view of the brain.

Fig. P-2. A. Anterior view of the brain.
B. Posterior view of the brain.

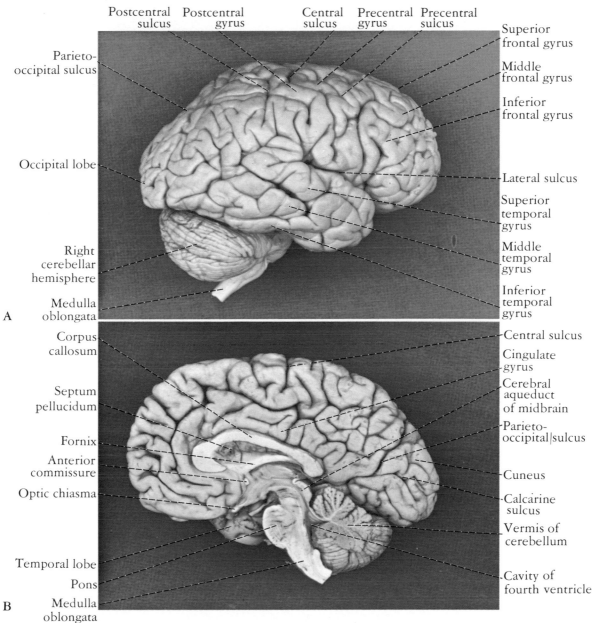

Postcentral sulcus   Postcentral gyrus   Central sulcus   Precentral gyrus   Precentral sulcus

Parieto-occipital sulcus

Occipital lobe

Right cerebellar hemisphere

Medulla oblongata

A

Superior frontal gyrus

Middle frontal gyrus

Inferior frontal gyrus

Lateral sulcus

Superior temporal gyrus

Middle temporal gyrus

Inferior temporal gyrus

Corpus callosum

Septum pellucidum

Fornix

Anterior commissure

Optic chiasma

Temporal lobe

Pons

Medulla oblongata

B

Central sulcus

Cingulate gyrus

Cerebral aqueduct of midbrain

Parieto-occipital sulcus

Cuneus

Calcarine sulcus

Vermis of cerebellum

Cavity of fourth ventricle

Fig. P-3. A. Right lateral view of the brain.
B. Medial view of the right side of the brain follow-ing median sagittal section.

Anterior horn of lateral ventricle

Claustrum

Insula

Lateral sulcus

Corpus callosum

Septum pellucidum

Caudate nucleus

Lentiform nucleus

A

Lateral ventricle

Caudate nucleus
Third ventricle

Lentiform nucleus

Mammillary body

Corpus callosum

Fornix

Medial thalamic nuclei

Lateral thalamic nuclei
Optic nerve

B

Corpus callosum

Choroid plexus in lateral ventricle

Pons

C

Fig. P-4. Coronal sections of the brain passing through (A) the anterior horn of the lateral ventricle, (B) the mammillary bodies, and (C) the pons.

Anterior horn of
lateral ventricle

Internal capsule
(anterior limb)

Genu of internal capsule

Internal capsule
(posterior limb)

Third ventricle

Posterior horn
of lateral ventricle

Genu of corpus callosum

Head of caudate nucleus

Anterior column of fornix

Claustrum

Putamen

Globus pallidus

Lentiform
nucleus

Thalamus

Splenium of
corpus callosum

A

Caudate nucleus

Thalamus

Lentiform nucleus

Internal capsule

Crus cerebri of midbrain

Pons

Medulla oblongata

Corpus callosum

Lateral ventricle

Fornix

Third ventricle

Third ventricle
(inferior part)

Cerebellum

B

Fig. P-5. A. Horizontal section of the cerebrum
showing the lentiform nucleus, the caudate nucleus,
the thalamus, and the internal capsule.
B. Oblique coronal section of the brain.

Trigeminal nerve

Vestibulocochlear nerve

Roots of glossopharyngeal, vagus, and cranial part of accessory nerves

Roots of hypoglossal nerve

Olfactory bulb

Olfactory tract

Optic nerve

Optic chiasma

Optic tract

Oculomotor nerve

Trochlear nerve

Trigeminal nerve

Spinal root of accessory nerve

A

Longitudinal fissure

Uncus

Crus cerebri

Trochlear nerve

Pons

Inferior cerebellar peduncle

Olive

Gyrus rectus

Optic chiasma

Infundibulum

Mammillary body

Posterior perforating substance in floor of interpeduncular fossa

Oculomotor nerve

Groove for basilar artery

Anterior median fissure

Pyramid

B

Fig. P-6. A. Inferior view of the brain showing cranial nerves. The abducent and facial nerves cannot be seen.
B. Enlarged inferior view of the central part of the brain.

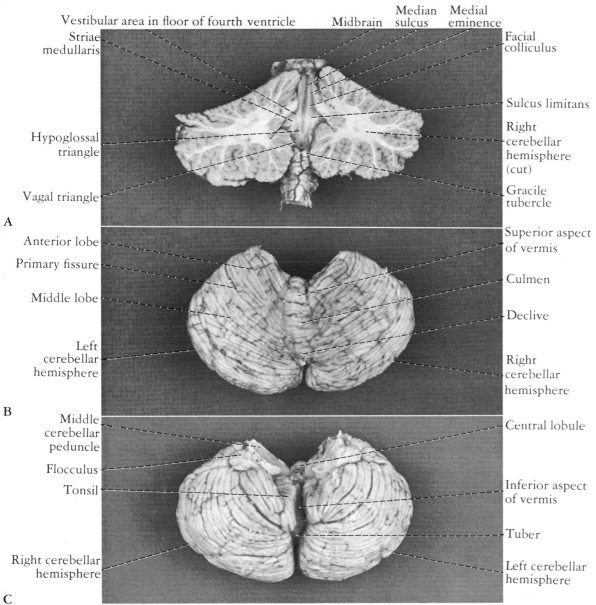

Vestibular area in floor of fourth ventricle   Midbrain   Median sulcus   Medial eminence

Striae medullaris

Hypoglossal triangle

Vagal triangle

A

Facial colliculus

Sulcus limitans

Right cerebellar hemisphere (cut)

Gracile tubercle

Anterior lobe

Primary fissure

Middle lobe

Left cerebellar hemisphere

B

Superior aspect of vermis

Culmen

Declive

Right cerebellar hemisphere

Middle cerebellar peduncle

Flocculus

Tonsil

Right cerebellar hemisphere

C

Central lobule

Inferior aspect of vermis

Tuber

Left cerebellar hemisphere

Fig. P-7. A. Posterior view of the brainstem. The greater part of the cerebellum has been removed to expose the floor of the fourth ventricle.
B. Superior view of the cerebellum showing vermis and right and left cerebellar hemispheres.
C. Inferior view of the cerebellum showing vermis and right and left cerebellar hemispheres.

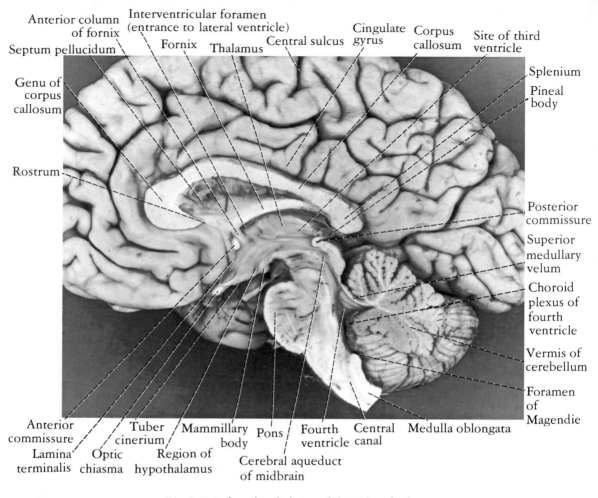

Anterior column of fornix

Interventricular foramen (entrance to lateral ventricle)

Septum pellucidum

Fornix

Thalamus

Central sulcus

Cingulate gyrus

Corpus callosum

Site of third ventricle

Genu of corpus callosum

Splenium

Pineal body

Rostrum

Posterior commissure

Superior medullary velum

Choroid plexus of fourth ventricle

Vermis of cerebellum

Foramen of Magendie

Anterior commissure

Lamina terminalis

Optic chiasma

Tuber cinerium

Region of hypothalamus

Mammillary body

Pons

Cerebral aqueduct of midbrain

Fourth ventricle

Central canal

Medulla oblongata

Fig. P-8. Enlarged medial view of the right side of the brain following median sagittal section, showing the continuity of the central canal, fourth ventricle, cerebral aqueduct, and the third ventricle and entrance into the lateral ventricle through the interventricular foramen.

Preface

Clinical Neuroanatomy for Medical Students continues to be very popular among first and second year students. Dental and allied health students are also increasingly using this book. First year residents in neurology often refer to this text for a quick review before starting their rotation. Again, I wish to thank the many medical students and faculty who have written to me from different medical centers with suggestions to improve this edition.

Physicians have frequently expressed to me their concern about the too detailed neuroanatomy that is still taught to medical students in spite of extensive curricula revisions carried out by medical schools in recent years. The many recommendations in the *General Professional Education of the Physician for the Twenty-first Century (GPEP) Report* stress that medical faculties must limit the amount of factual information that students are expected to memorize. Unfortunately, it is easier to state these recommendations than to carry them out. In my experience, many faculty still continue to fill their lectures with an inordinate amount of detail and lose sight of the fact that a medical stu-

dent is going to be a physician and not a neuroscientist.

The philosophy underlying the preparation of the first edition has not changed in this third edition. It is an attempt to offer the practical aspects of neuroanatomy in a simplified manner. The everyday use of CT scans and MR images in neurological practice has necessitated the introduction of many new examples, together with diagrams explaining the normal anatomy of horizontal brain sections. Again, emphasis has been placed on function where possible, although deep inroads into neurophysiology have been avoided.

To give further emphasis to the importance of basic science to clinical practice, the Clinical Notes section in each chapter has been retained and brought up to date. Clinical Problems requiring a knowledge of neuroanatomy for solution are presented at the end of each chapter. In order that students may self-test their knowledge of basic neuroanatomy, National Board type questions have been included at the end of each chapter. (K type questions have been retained.) ␣␣␣␣␣roanatomical liter␣␣␣

updated to include recent research, should a student wish to acquire a deeper knowledge of an area of interest.

The illustrations have purposely been kept simple, and for the most part they are diagrammatic. Some of the illustrations have been modified, and new ones have been added.

I am most grateful to the following colleagues in the neurosciences who provided me with photographic examples of neuroanatomical material: Dr. Nikolajs Cauna, Emeritus Professor of Anatomy, University of Pittsburgh School of Medicine; Dr. Turlough M. J. Fitzgerald, Professor and Chairman of Anatomy, University College, Galway, Ireland; and Dr. Alan Peters, Professor and Chairman of Anatomy, Boston University School of Medicine.

I am greatly indebted to Dr. David O. Davis of the Department of Radiology at the George Washington University School of Medicine for the loan of radiographs and CT scans that have been reproduced in different sections of this book. I am also grateful to Dr. Gordon Sze of the Department of Radiology at Yale University Medical Center for examples of CT scans and MR images of the brain. I wish to thank Tom McCarthy, Chief Medical Photographer in the Department of Radiology at Yale, for his excellent work in reproducing the radiographs.

As in the past, I wish to express my sincere thanks to Myra Feldman for the earlier preparation of the artwork and to Ira Grunther, AMI, for the very fine new art in this edition.

Finally, to the staff of Little, Brown and Company I once again wish to express my deep gratitude for their continued enthusiasm and support throughout the preparation of this book.

R.S.S.

Clinical Neuroanatomy
for Medical
Students

Chapter 1
Organization of the
Nervous System

The nervous system and the endocrine system control the functions of the body. The nervous system is composed basically of specialized cells, whose function is to receive sensory stimuli and to transmit them to effector organs, whether muscular or glandular (Fig. 1-1). The sensory stimuli that arise either outside or inside the body are correlated within the nervous system, and the efferent impulses are coordinated so that the effector organs work harmoniously together for the well-being of the individual. In addition, the nervous system of higher species has the ability to store sensory information received during past experiences; and this information, when appropriate, is integrated with other nervous impulses and channeled into the common efferent pathway.

CENTRAL AND PERIPHERAL NERVOUS SYSTEMS

The nervous system is divided into two main parts, for purposes of description: the **central nervous system** (Fig. 1-2A), which consists of the brain and spinal cord, and the **peripheral nervous system** (Fig. 1-2B), which consists of the cranial and spinal nerves and their associated ganglia.

In the central nervous system the brain and spinal cord are the main centers where correlation and integration of nervous information occur; therefore, it is not surprising that they are well protected (Fig. 1-3). Both the brain and spinal cord are suspended in fluid, the **cerebrospinal fluid**, and they are further protected by the bones of the skull and the vertebral column.

The central nervous system is composed of large numbers of nerve cells and their processes, which are supported by specialized tissue called **neuroglia** (Fig. 1-4). **Neuron** is the name given to the nerve cell and all its processes. The long processes of a nerve cell are called **axons** or **nerve fibers**.

The interior of the central nervous system is organized into gray and white matter. **Gray matter** consists of nerve cells and the proximal portions of their processes embedded in neuroglia. **White matter** consists of nerve fibers embedded in neuroglia

In the peripheral nervous system the cranial and spinal nerves, which consist of bundles of nerve fi-

Fig. 1-1. The relationship of afferent sensory stimuli to memory bank, correlation and coordinating centers, and common efferent pathway.

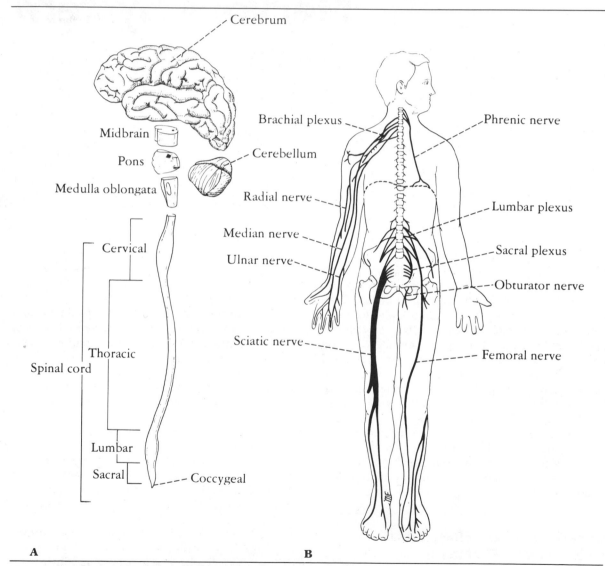

A   **B**

Fig. 1-2. A. The main divisions of the central nervous system.
B. The parts of the peripheral nervous system (the cranial nerves have been omitted).

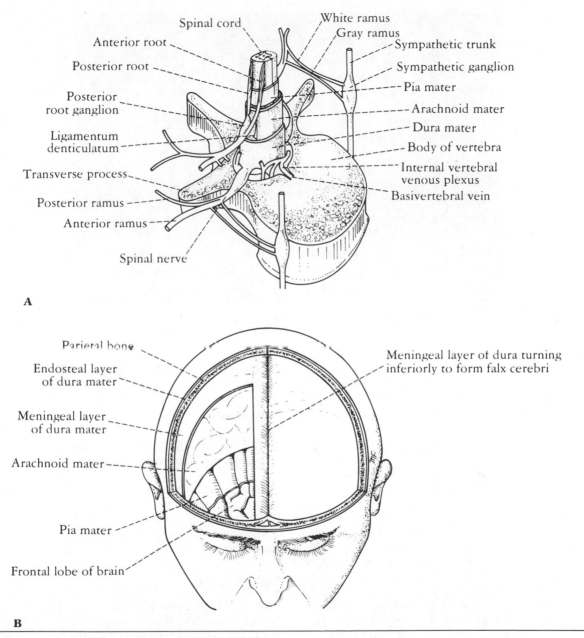

Spinal cord

Anterior root

Posterior root

Posterior
root ganglion

Ligamentum
denticulatum

Transverse process

Posterior ramus

Anterior ramus

Spinal nerve

White ramus

Gray ramus

Sympathetic trunk

Sympathetic ganglion

Pia mater

Arachnoid mater

Dura mater

Body of vertebra

Internal vertebral
venous plexus

Basivertebral vein

A

Parietal bone

Endosteal layer
of dura mater

Meningeal layer
of dura mater

Arachnoid mater

Pia mater

Frontal lobe of brain

Meningeal layer of dura turning
inferiorly to form falx cerebri

B

**Fig. 1-3. A. Protective coverings of spinal cord.
B. Protective coverings of brain.**

Fig. 1-4. Photomicrograph of several large nerve cells with surrounding neuroglia.

bers or axons, conduct information to and from the central nervous system. Although surrounded by fibrous sheaths as they run to different parts of the body, they are relatively unprotected and are commonly damaged by trauma.

Autonomic Nervous System

The autonomic nervous system is the part of the nervous system concerned with the innervation of involuntary structures, such as the heart, smooth muscle, and glands within the body. It is distributed throughout the central and peripheral nervous systems. The autonomic system may be divided into two parts, the **sympathetic** and the **parasympathetic**, and in both parts there are afferent and efferent nerve fibers.

The activities of the sympathetic part of the autonomic system prepare the body for an emergency. It accelerates the heart rate, causes constriction of the peripheral blood vessels, and raises the blood pressure. It brings about a redistribution of the blood, so that blood leaves the areas of the skin and intestine and becomes available to the brain, heart, and skeletal muscle. At the same time it inhibits peristalsis of the intestinal tract and closes the sphincters.

The activities of the parasympathetic part of the autonomic system are aimed at conserving and restoring energy. It slows the heart rate, increases peristalsis of the intestine, increases glandular activity, and opens the sphincters.

MAJOR DIVISIONS OF THE CENTRAL NERVOUS SYSTEM

Before proceeding to a detailed description of the spinal cord and brain, it is essential to understand the main features of these structures and their general relationship to one another. Later, the more intricate parts will be studied in depth.

Spinal Cord

The spinal cord is a grayish-white structure that begins superiorly at the foramen magnum in the skull, where it is continuous with the **medulla oblongata** of the brain (Figs. 1-5 and 1-6). It terminates inferiorly in the adult at the level of the **lower border of the first lumbar vertebra**. In the young child it is relatively longer and ends at the upper border of the third lumbar vertebra. The spinal cord is situated within the **vertebral canal** of the vertebral column and is surrounded by three

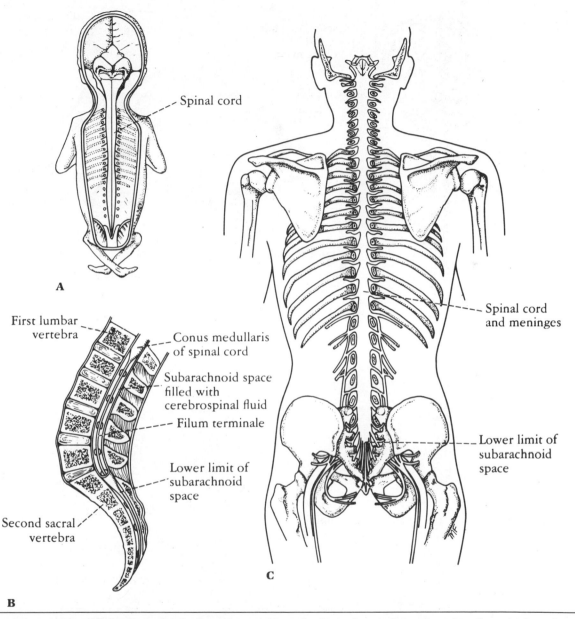

Spinal cord

A

First lumbar vertebra

Conus medullaris of spinal cord

Subarachnoid space filled with cerebrospinal fluid

Filum terminale

Lower limit of subarachnoid space

Second sacral vertebra

B

Spinal cord and meninges

Lower limit of subarachnoid space

C

Fig. 1-5. A. Fetus with brain and spinal cord exposed on the posterior surface. Note that the spinal cord extends the full length of the vertebral column.
B. Sagittal section of vertebral column in adult, showing spinal cord terminating inferiorly at the level of the lower border of the first lumbar vertebra.
C. Adult spinal cord and covering meninges, showing relationship to surrounding structures.

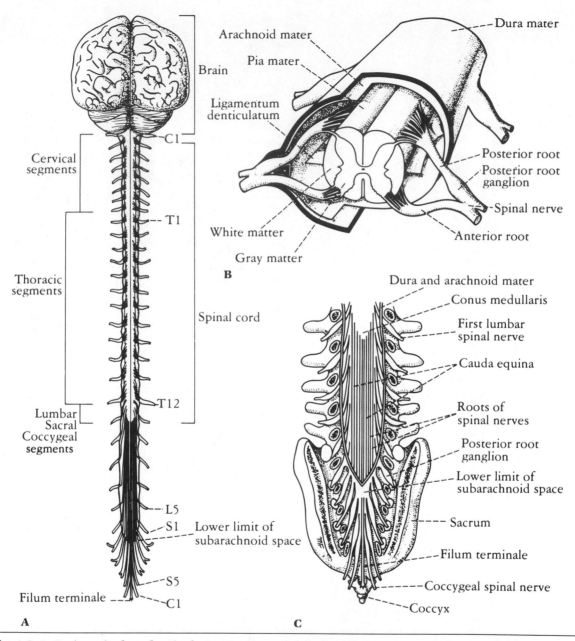

Brain

Arachnoid mater

Pia mater

Dura mater

Ligamentum denticulatum

Cervical segments

C1

Thoracic segments

T1

Spinal cord

Posterior root

Posterior root ganglion

Spinal nerve

Anterior root

White matter

Gray matter

B

Dura and arachnoid mater

Conus medullaris

First lumbar spinal nerve

Cauda equina

Lumbar
Sacral
Coccygeal
segments

T12

Roots of spinal nerves

Posterior root ganglion

Lower limit of subarachnoid space

Sacrum

L5

S1   Lower limit of subarachnoid space

Filum terminale

Coccygeal spinal nerve

S5

Filum terminale — C1

A

Coccyx

C

**Fig. 1-6. A. Brain, spinal cord, spinal nerve roots, and spinal nerves as seen on their posterior aspect.
B. Transverse section through spinal cord in the thoracic region, showing anterior and posterior roots of a spinal nerve and the meninges.
C. Posterior view of lower end of spinal cord and cauda equina, showing their relationship with the lumbar vertebrae, sacrum, and coccyx.**

meninges (Figs. 1-3A and 1-6): the **dura mater**, the **arachnoid mater**, and the **pia mater**. Further protection is provided by the **cerebrospinal fluid**, which surrounds the spinal cord in the **subarachnoid space**.

The spinal cord is roughly cylindrical (Fig. 1-6). However, in the cervical region, where it gives origin to the brachial plexus, and in the lower thoracic and lumbar regions, where it gives origin to the lumbosacral plexus, there are fusiform enlargements, called the **cervical and lumbar enlargements** (Fig. 1-2A). Inferiorly, the spinal cord tapers

off into the **conus medullaris**, from the apex of which a prolongation of the pia mater, the **filum terminale**, descends to attach to the back of the coccyx (Fig. 1-5B). The cord possesses, in the midline anteriorly, a deep longitudinal fissure, the **anterior median fissure**, and, on the posterior surface, a shallow furrow, the **posterior median sulcus** (Fig. 1-7).

Along the entire length of the spinal cord are attached 31 pairs of spinal nerves by the **anterior or motor roots** and the **posterior or sensory roots** (Figs. 1-6 and 1-7). Each root is attached to the

Fig. 1-7. A. Transverse section through lumbar part of spinal cord, oblique view. B. Transverse section through lumbar part of spinal cord, face view, showing anterior and posterior roots of a spinal nerve.

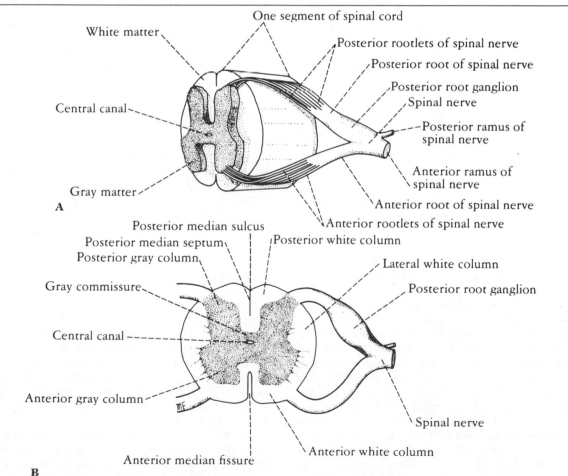

cord by a series of rootlets, which extend the whole length of the corresponding segment of the cord. Each posterior nerve root possesses a **posterior root ganglion**, the cells of which give rise to peripheral and central nerve fibers.

Structure of Spinal Cord

The spinal cord is composed of an inner core of **gray matter**, which is surrounded by an outer covering of **white matter** (Fig. 1-7). The gray matter is seen on cross section as an H-shaped pillar with **anterior and posterior gray columns**, or **horns**, united by a thin **gray commissure** containing the small **central canal**. The white matter, for purposes of description, may be divided into **anterior, lateral, and posterior white columns** (Fig. 1-7). The anterior column on each side lies between the midline and the point of emergence of the anterior nerve roots; the lateral column lies between the emergence of the anterior nerve roots and the entry of the posterior nerve roots; and the posterior column lies between the entry of the posterior nerve roots and the midline.

Brain

The brain lies in the cranial cavity and is continuous with the spinal cord through the foramen magnum (see Figs. 1-6A, 1-8, and 1-10). It is surrounded by three meninges (Fig. 1-9): the **dura mater**, the **arachnoid mater**, and the **pia mater**, and these are continuous with the corresponding meninges of the spinal cord.

The brain is conventionally divided into three major divisions. These are, in ascending order from the spinal cord, the **rhombencephalon** or hindbrain, the **mesencephalon** or midbrain, and the **prosencephalon** or forebrain. The rhombencephalon may be subdivided into the **myelencephalon** or medulla oblongata, the **metencephalon** or pons, and the **cerebellum**. The prosencephalon may also be subdivided into the **diencephalon** (between brain), which is the central part of the forebrain, and the **telencephalon** or cerebrum. The **brainstem** (a collective term for the medulla oblongata, pons, and midbrain) is that part of the brain that remains after the cerebral hemispheres and cerebellum are removed (see Fig. 1-8).

Hindbrain

The hindbrain consists of the medulla oblongata (myelencephalon), the pons (metencephalon), and the cerebellum (Figs. 1-11 and 1-12).

MEDULLA OBLONGATA

The medulla oblongata is conical in shape and connects the pons superiorly to the spinal cord inferiorly (see Figs. 1-8 and 1-11). A **median fissure** is present on the anterior surface of the medulla, and on each side of this fissure is a swelling, called the **pyramid**. Posterior to the pyramids are the **olives**, which are oval elevations produced by the underlying **olivary nuclei**. Posterior to the olives are the **inferior cerebellar peduncles**, which connect the medulla to the cerebellum (Fig. 1-14).

On the posterior surface of the inferior part of the medulla oblongata (Fig. 1-14) are the **gracile** and **cuneate tubercles**, produced by the medially placed underlying **nucleus gracilis** and the laterally placed underlying **nucleus cuneatus**.

PONS

The pons is situated on the anterior surface of the cerebellum, inferior to the midbrain and superior to the medulla oblongata (see Figs. 1-11 and 1-12). It is much greater in anteroposterior and transverse dimensions than the medulla. The pons, or bridge, derives its name from the large number of transverse fibers on its anterior aspect connecting the two cerebellar hemispheres.

CEREBELLUM

The cerebellum lies within the posterior cranial fossa posterior to the pons and the medulla oblongata (see Figs. 1-10 and 1-12). It consists of two hemispheres connected by a median portion, the **vermis**. The cerebellum is connected to the midbrain by the **superior cerebellar peduncles**, to the pons by the **middle cerebellar peduncles**, and to the medulla by the **inferior cerebellar peduncles** (Fig. 1-14).

The surface layer of each cerebellar hemisphere is called the **cortex** and is composed of gray matter (Fig. 1-15). The cerebellar cortex is thrown into

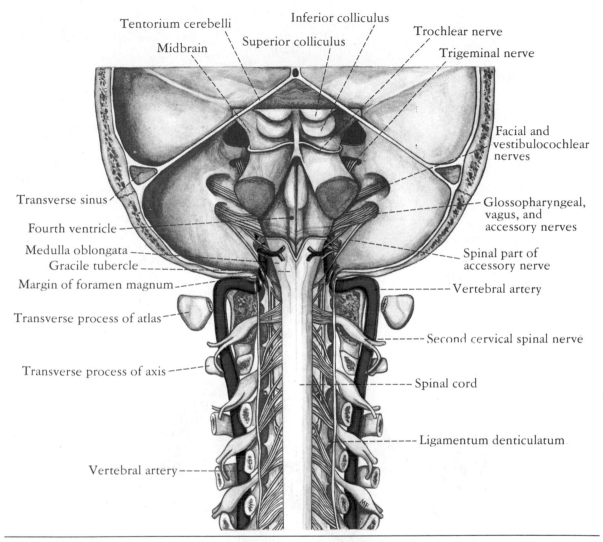

Fig. 1-8. Posterior view of the brainstem after removal of the occipital and parietal bones and the cerebrum, the cerebellum, and the roof of the fourth ventricle. Laminae of the upper cervical vertebrae have also been removed.

Superficial nerves of scalp
Superficial vein of scalp
Skin
Skin
Superficial fascia
Epicranial aponeurosis
Emissary vein
Loose connective tissue
Diploic vein
Pericranium (periosteum)
Superior sagittal sinus
Outer table of parietal bone
Arachnoid granulation
Diploë
Endosteal layer of dura
Inner table of parietal bone
Meningeal layer of dura
Cerebral vein in
subarachnoid space
Arachnoid
Cerebral artery in
subarachnoid space
Pia mater
Inferior sagittal sinus
Cerebral cortex
Falx cerebri

A

Facial and vestibulocochlear nerves
Diploic vein
Great cerebral vein
Superior sagittal sinus
Inferior sagittal sinus
Straight sinus
Falx cerebri
Trochlear nerve
Oculomotor nerve
Trigeminal nerve
Optic nerve
Olfactory bulb
Sphenoparietal
sinus
Tentorium
cerebelli
Glossopharyngeal,
vagus, and
accessory nerves
Hypoglossal nerve
Superior
petrosal sinus
Abducent nerve

B

Fig. 1-9. A. Coronal section of upper part of head showing layers of scalp, sagittal suture of skull, falx cerebri, venous sinuses, arachnoid granulations, emissary veins, and relationship of cerebral blood vessels to subarachnoid space.
B. Interior of skull, showing dura mater and its contained venous sinuses.

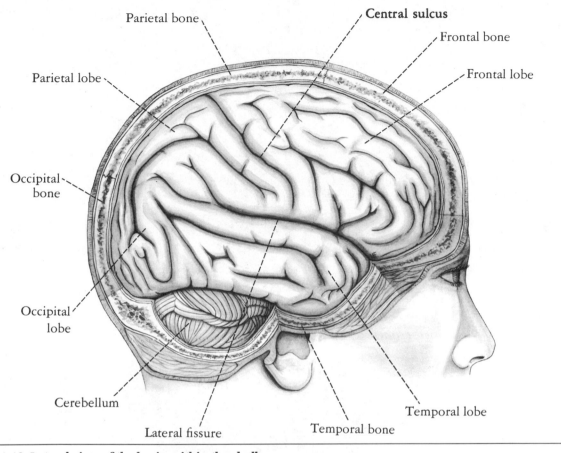

Parietal bone

Central sulcus

Frontal bone

Parietal lobe

Frontal lobe

Occipital bone

Occipital lobe

Cerebellum

Lateral fissure

Temporal bone

Temporal lobe

Fig. 1-10. Lateral view of the brain within the skull.

folds, or folia, separated by closely set transverse fissures. Certain masses of gray matter are found in the interior of the cerebellum, embedded in the white matter; the largest of these is known as the **dentate nucleus** (Fig. 1-14).

The cavity of the hindbrain is the **fourth ventricle** (see Figs. 1-13, 1-14, and 1-15). This is bounded anteriorly by the pons and the medulla oblongata, and posteriorly by the **superior and inferior medullary vela** and the cerebellum. The fourth ventricle is connected superiorly to the third ventricle by the **cerebral aqueduct**, and inferiorly it is continuous with the central canal of the spinal cord (Figs. 1-14 and 1-15). It communicates with the subarachnoid space through three openings in the inferior part of the roof: a median opening and two lateral openings (Figs. 1-14 and 1-15).

Midbrain

The midbrain is the narrow part of the brain that connects the forebrain to the hindbrain (see Figs. 1-2A, 1-13, and 1-16). The narrow cavity of the midbrain is the **cerebral aqueduct**, which connects the third and fourth ventricles (see Fig. 1-13). The **tectum** is that part of the midbrain that lies posterior to the cerebral aqueduct (Fig. 1-17); it has four surface swellings, namely, the **two superior and two inferior colliculi** (Figs. 1-16 and 1-17). The **cerebral peduncles** are situated anterior to the aqueduct (Fig. 1-17). Each peduncle is divided into an anterior part, the **crus cerebri**, and a posterior part, the **tegmentum**, by a pigmented band of gray matter, the **substantia nigra**. A large, ovoid, very vascular mass of cells, the **red nucleus**, easily recognized by its color, is situated

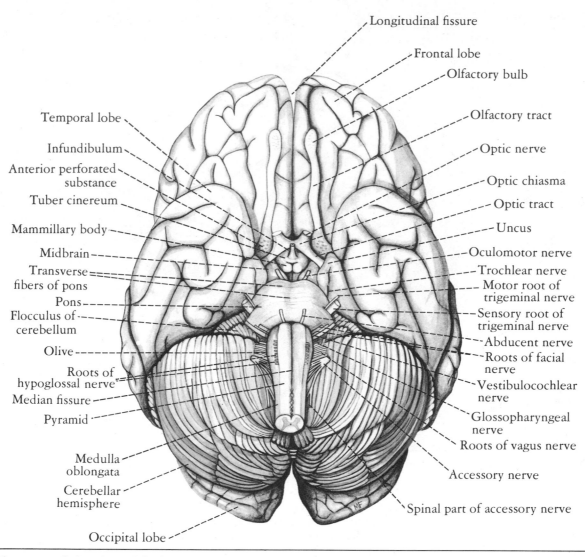

Longitudinal fissure

Frontal lobe

Olfactory bulb

Olfactory tract

Optic nerve

Optic chiasma

Optic tract

Uncus

Oculomotor nerve

Trochlear nerve

Motor root of
trigeminal nerve

Sensory root of
trigeminal nerve

Abducent nerve

Roots of facial
nerve

Vestibulocochlear
nerve

Glossopharyngeal
nerve

Roots of vagus nerve

Accessory nerve

Spinal part of accessory nerve

Temporal lobe

Infundibulum

Anterior perforated
substance

Tuber cinereum

Mammillary body

Midbrain

Transverse
fibers of pons

Pons

Flocculus of
cerebellum

Olive

Roots of
hypoglossal nerve

Median fissure

Pyramid

Medulla
oblongata

Cerebellar
hemisphere

Occipital lobe

Fig. 1-11. Inferior view of the brain.

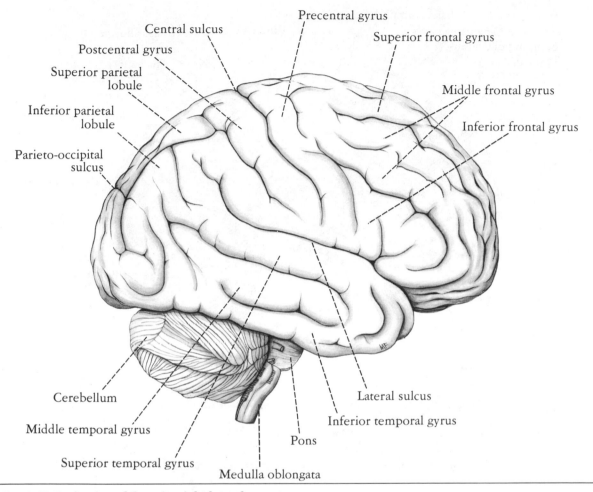

Fig. 1-12. Brain viewed from its right lateral aspect.

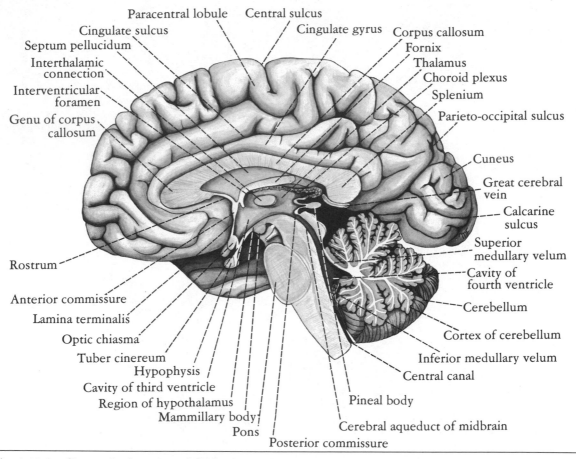

Fig. 1-13. Median sagittal section of the brain to show the third ventricle, the cerebral aqueduct, and the fourth ventricle.

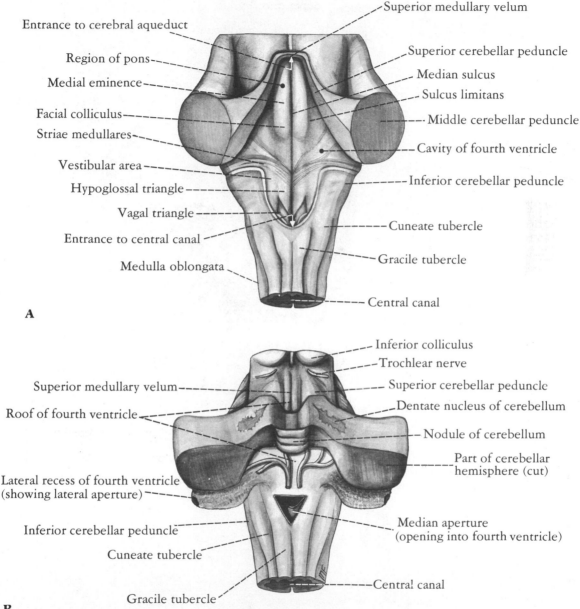

Entrance to cerebral aqueduct

Region of pons

Medial eminence

Facial colliculus

Striae medullares

Vestibular area

Hypoglossal triangle

Vagal triangle

Entrance to central canal

Medulla oblongata

Superior medullary velum

Superior cerebellar peduncle

Median sulcus

Sulcus limitans

Middle cerebellar peduncle

Cavity of fourth ventricle

Inferior cerebellar peduncle

Cuneate tubercle

Gracile tubercle

Central canal

A

Superior medullary velum

Roof of fourth ventricle

Lateral recess of fourth ventricle
(showing lateral aperture)

Inferior cerebellar peduncle

Cuneate tubercle

Gracile tubercle

Inferior colliculus

Trochlear nerve

Superior cerebellar peduncle

Dentate nucleus of cerebellum

Nodule of cerebellum

Part of cerebellar
hemisphere (cut)

Median aperture
(opening into fourth ventricle)

Central canal

B

**Fig. 1-14. A. Posterior view of the pons and the medulla oblongata, showing the cavity of the fourth ventricle. The cerebellum has been removed.
B. Posterior view of the roof of the fourth ventricle after removal of the greater part of the cerebellum.**

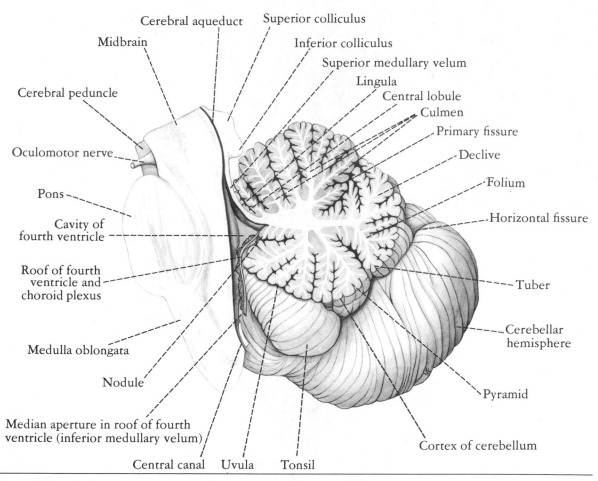

Fig. 1-15. Sagittal section through the brainstem and the cerebellum.

Fig. 1-16. Posterior view of the brainstem showing the two superior and the two inferior colliculi of the tectum of the midbrain.

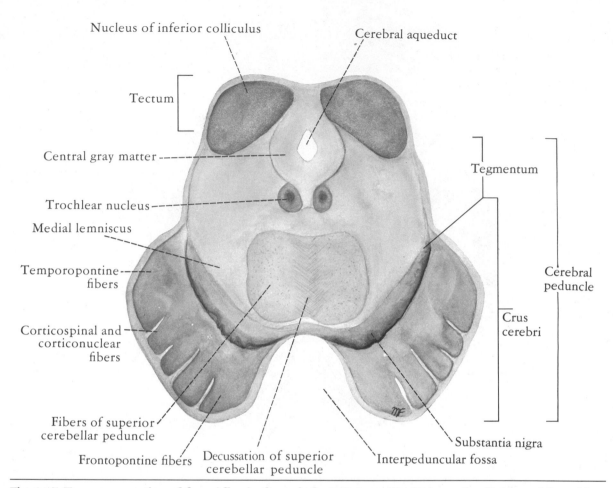

Nucleus of inferior colliculus

Cerebral aqueduct

Tectum

Central gray matter

Tegmentum

Trochlear nucleus

Medial lemniscus

Temporopontine fibers

Cerebral peduncle

Corticospinal and corticonuclear fibers

Crus cerebri

Fibers of superior cerebellar peduncle

Frontopontine fibers

Decussation of superior cerebellar peduncle

Substantia nigra

Interpeduncular fossa

Fig. 1-17. Transverse section of the midbrain through the inferior colliculi shows the division of the midbrain into the tectum and the cerebral peduncles. Note that the cerebral peduncles are subdivided by the substantia nigra into the tegmentum and the crus cerebri.

in the tegmentum on each side at the level of the superior colliculus (see Fig. 12-4).

DIENCEPHALON

The diencephalon is almost completely hidden from the surface of the brain. It consists of a dorsal **thalamus** and a ventral **hypothalamus** (see Figs. 1-13 and 1-16). The thalamus is a large egg-shaped mass of gray matter that lies on either side of the third ventricle. The anterior end of the thalamus forms the posterior boundary of the **interventric-**

ular foramen, the opening between the third and lateral ventricles (see Fig. 1-13). The posterior end of the thalamus is expanded to form a large swelling, the **pulvinar** (see Fig. 1-16).

The hypothalamus forms the lower part of the lateral wall and floor of the third ventricle (see Fig. 1-13). The following structures are found in the floor of the third ventricle, from front to back: the **optic chiasma**, the **tuber cinereum**, the **infundibulum**, the **mammillary bodies**, and the **posterior perforated substance**. The cephalic, or rostral, end of the third ventricle is bounded by a thin sheet, the **lamina terminalis** (see Fig. 1-13).

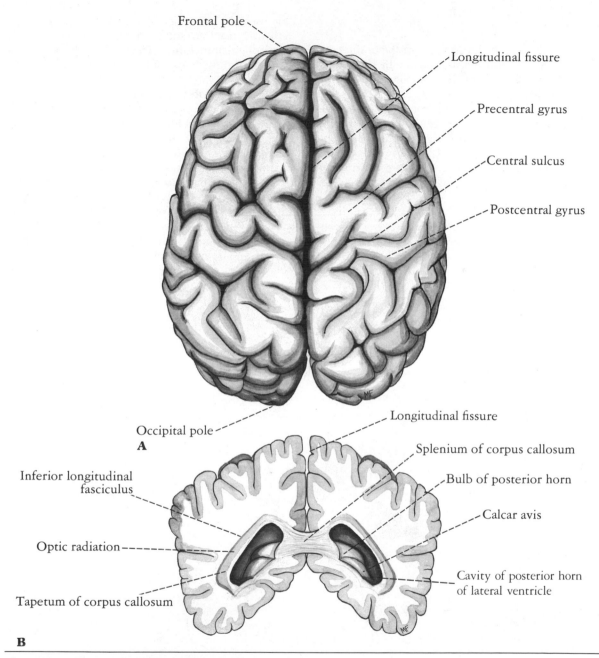

Frontal pole

Longitudinal fissure

Precentral gyrus

Central sulcus

Postcentral gyrus

Occipital pole

A

Longitudinal fissure

Splenium of corpus callosum

Bulb of posterior horn

Calcar avis

Inferior longitudinal fasciculus

Optic radiation

Tapetum of corpus callosum

Cavity of posterior horn of lateral ventricle

B

Fig. 1-18. A. The cerebrum viewed from its superior aspect.
B. Coronal section through the posterior parts of the cerebral hemispheres.

CEREBRUM

The cerebrum, the largest part of the brain, consists of two cerebral hemispheres, which are connected by a mass of white matter called the **corpus callosum** (see Figs. 1-12, 1-13, and 1-18). Each hemisphere extends from the frontal to the occipital bones, superior to the anterior and middle cranial fossae; posteriorly, the cerebrum lies above the tentorium cerebelli (see Fig. 1-9). The hemispheres are separated by a deep cleft, the **longitudinal fissure**, into which projects the **falx cerebri** (see Fig. 1-9).

The surface layer of each hemisphere, the **cortex**, is composed of gray matter. The cerebral cortex is thrown into folds, or **gyri**, separated by fissures, or **sulci** (see Figs. 1-12 and 1-18). The surface area of the cortex is greatly increased by

this means. A number of the large sulci are conveniently used to subdivide the surface of each hemisphere into **lobes** (Fig. 1-19). The lobes are named from the bones of the cranium under which they lie.

The **frontal lobe** is situated anterior to the **central sulcus** and superior to the **lateral sulcus** (Fig. 1-19). The **parietal lobe** is situated posterior to the central sulcus and superior to the lateral sulcus. The **occipital lobe** lies inferior to the **parieto-occipital sulcus**. Inferior to the lateral sulcus is situated the **temporal lobe** (Fig. 1-19). The extreme ends of each hemisphere are often called the **frontal, occipital, and temporal poles**.

Within the hemisphere is a central core of white matter, containing several large masses of gray matter, the **basal nuclei** or **ganglia**. A fan-shaped collection of nerve fibers, termed the **corona ra-**

Fig. 1-19. Cerebral cortex viewed from its right lateral aspect, showing the lobes and large sulci.

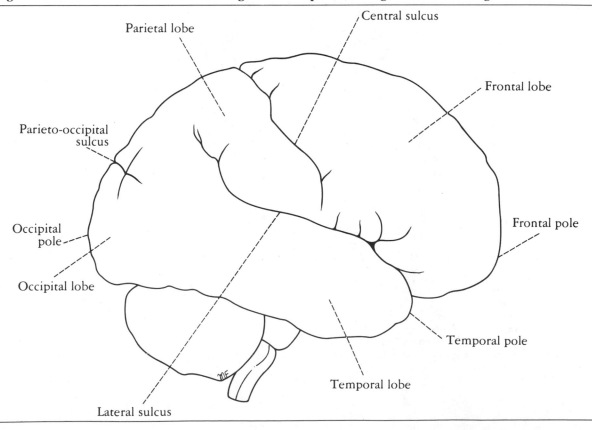

diata (Fig. 1-20), passes in the white matter to and from the cerebral cortex to the brainstem. The corona radiata converges on the basal nuclei and passes between them as the **internal capsule**. The tailed nucleus situated on the medial side of the internal capsule is referred to as the **caudate nucleus** (Figs. 1-21 and 1-22) and the lens-shaped nucleus on the lateral side of the internal capsule is called the **lentiform nucleus**.

The cerebral hemispheres are connected across the midline by bundles of commissural nerve fibers, the largest of which is the **corpus callosum**, referred to previously (Figs. 1-13 and 1-18).

The cavity present within each cerebral hemisphere is called the **lateral ventricle** (Fig. 1-23). The lateral ventricles communicate with the third ventricle through the **interventricular foramina**.

During the process of development, the cerebrum becomes enormously enlarged and overhangs the diencephalon, the midbrain, and the hindbrain. The caudate and lentiform nuclei and the thalamus become situated close together, so that the internal capsule has the caudate nucleus and thalamus on its medial side and the lentiform nucleus on its lateral side (Figs. 1-21 and 1-22).

Fig. 1-20. Right lateral view showing continuity of corona radiata, internal capsule, and crus cerebri of the cerebral peduncles. Note the position of the lentiform nucleus lateral to the internal capsule.

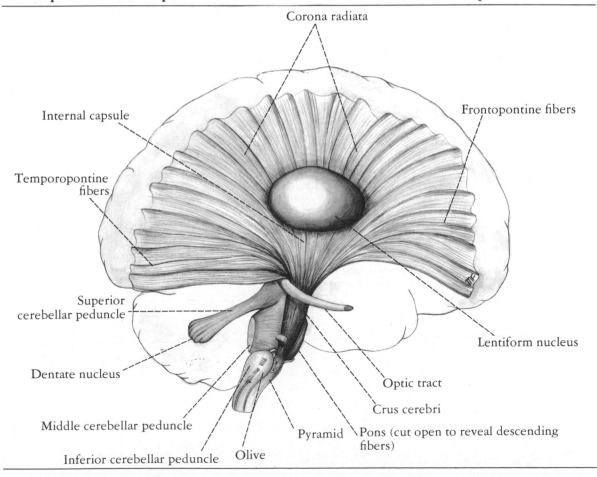

Corona radiata

Internal capsule

Frontopontine fibers

Temporopontine fibers

Superior cerebellar peduncle

Dentate nucleus

Lentiform nucleus

Optic tract

Crus cerebri

Middle cerebellar peduncle

Pyramid

Pons (cut open to reveal descending fibers)

Inferior cerebellar peduncle   Olive

Gray matter of cerebral cortex

Genu of corpus callosum

White matter of cerebrum

Anterior horn of lateral ventricle

Septum pellucidum

Head of caudate nucleus

Anterior column of fornix

Internal capsule
(anterior limb)

Genu of internal capsule

Claustrum

Putamen

Lentiform
nucleus

Third ventricle

Globus
pallidus

Internal capsule
(posterior limb)

Insular cortex

Lateral sulcus

External capsule

Pineal body

Thalamus

Superior colliculus

Tail of caudate
nucleus

Choroid plexus

Inferior colliculus

Posterior horn
of lateral ventricle

Optic radiation

Vermis of cerebellum

Cerebellar hemispheres

Fig. 1-21. Horizontal section of the cerebrum, showing the relationship between the lentiform nucleus, the caudate nucleus, the thalamus, and the internal capsule.

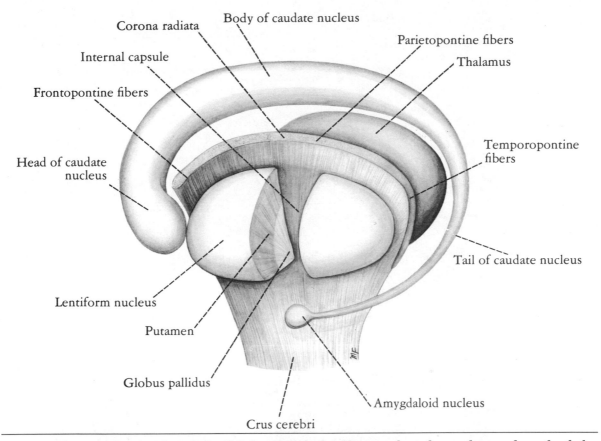

Corona radiata

Body of caudate nucleus

Parietopontine fibers

Internal capsule

Thalamus

Frontopontine fibers

Temporopontine fibers

Head of caudate nucleus

Lentiform nucleus

Tail of caudate nucleus

Putamen

Globus pallidus

Amygdaloid nucleus

Crus cerebri

Fig. 1-22. Diagram showing the relationship between the lentiform nucleus, the caudate nucleus, the thalamus, and the internal capsule, as seen from the left lateral side.

MAJOR DIVISIONS OF THE PERIPHERAL NERVOUS SYSTEM

The peripheral nervous system consists of the cranial and spinal nerves and their associated ganglia.

Cranial and Spinal Nerves

The cranial and spinal nerves are seen on dissection to be cords of grayish-white color made up of bundles of nerve fibers supported by connective tissue.

There are 12 pairs of **cranial nerves** (see Fig. 1-11), which leave the brain and pass through foramina in the skull. There are 31 pairs of **spinal nerves** (see Fig. 1-6), which leave the spinal cord and pass through intervertebral foramina in the vertebral column. The spinal nerves are named according to the regions of the vertebral column with which they are associated: 8 **cervical**, 12 **thoracic**, 5 **lumbar**, 5 **sacral**, and 1 **coccygeal**. Note that there are 8 cervical nerves and only 7 cervical vertebrae and that there is 1 coccygeal nerve and there are 4 coccygeal vertebrae.

Each spinal nerve is connected to the spinal cord by two roots: the **anterior root** and the **posterior root** (Fig. 1-24). The anterior root consists of bundles of nerve fibers carrying nerve impulses away from the central nervous system. Such nerve fibers are called **efferent fibers**. Those efferent fibers that go to skeletal muscles and cause them to con-

Fig. 1-23. A cast of the ventricular cavities of the brain as seen from:
A. Lateral view.
B. Anterior view.
C. Superior view.

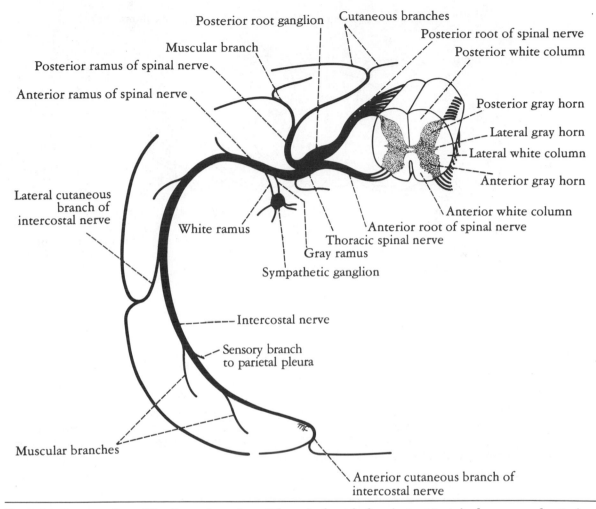

Fig. 1-24. Cross section of the thoracic region of the spinal cord, showing roots, spinal nerve, and anterior and posterior rami and their branches. Note that an intercostal nerve is formed from the anterior rami of T1–11 spinal nerves.

tract are called **motor fibers** (Fig. 1-25). Their cells of origin lie in the anterior gray horn of the spinal cord.

The posterior root consists of bundles of nerve fibers, called **afferent fibers** (Fig. 1-25), that carry nervous impulses to the central nervous system. Because these fibers are concerned with conveying information about sensations of touch, pain, temperature, and vibration, they are called **sensory fibers**. The cell bodies of these nerve fibers are sit-

uated in a swelling on the posterior root called the **posterior root ganglion** (Figs. 1-24 and 1-25).

The spinal nerve roots pass from the spinal cord to the level of their respective intervertebral foramina, where they unite to form a **spinal nerve** (Fig. 1-26). Here the motor and sensory fibers become mixed together, so that a spinal nerve is made up of a mixture of motor and sensory fibers.

Because of the disproportionate growth in length of the vertebral column during development, com-

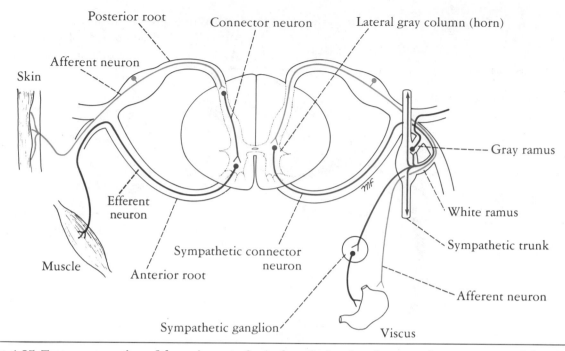

Posterior root

Connector neuron

Lateral gray column (horn)

Afferent neuron

Skin

Gray ramus

Efferent neuron

White ramus

Sympathetic trunk

Muscle

Sympathetic connector neuron

Afferent neuron

Anterior root

Sympathetic ganglion

Viscus

Fig. 1-25. Transverse section of thoracic part of spinal cord, showing the general arrangement of the somatic part of the nervous system (left) compared with the autonomic part of the nervous system (right).

pared with that of the spinal cord, the length of the roots increases progressively from above downward (Fig. 1-26). In the upper cervical region the spinal nerve roots are short and run almost horizontally, but the roots of the lumbar and sacral nerves below the level of the termination of the cord (lower border of the first lumbar vertebra in the adult) form a vertical leash of nerves around the **filum terminale** (Fig. 1-27). Together these lower nerve roots are called the **cauda equina**.

After emerging from the intervertebral foramen, each spinal nerve immediately divides into a large **anterior ramus** and a smaller **posterior ramus**, each containing both motor and sensory fibers (see Fig. 1-24). The posterior ramus passes posteriorly around the vertebral column to supply the muscles and skin of the back. The anterior ramus continues anteriorly to supply the muscles and skin over the antero-lateral body wall, and all the muscles and skin of the limbs.

The anterior rami join one another at the root of the limbs to form complicated **nerve plexuses**

(see Fig. 1-2B). The cervical and brachial plexuses are found at the root of the upper limbs and the **lumbar and sacral plexuses** are found at the root of the lower limbs.

Ganglia

Ganglia may be divided into sensory ganglia of spinal nerves (posterior root ganglia) and cranial nerves, and autonomic ganglia.

SENSORY GANGLIA

Sensory ganglia are fusiform swellings (see Fig. 1-24) situated on the posterior root of each spinal nerve just proximal to the root's junction with a corresponding anterior root. They are referred to as **posterior root ganglia**. Similar ganglia that are also found along the course of cranial nerves V, VII, VIII, IX, and X are called **sensory ganglia** of these nerves.

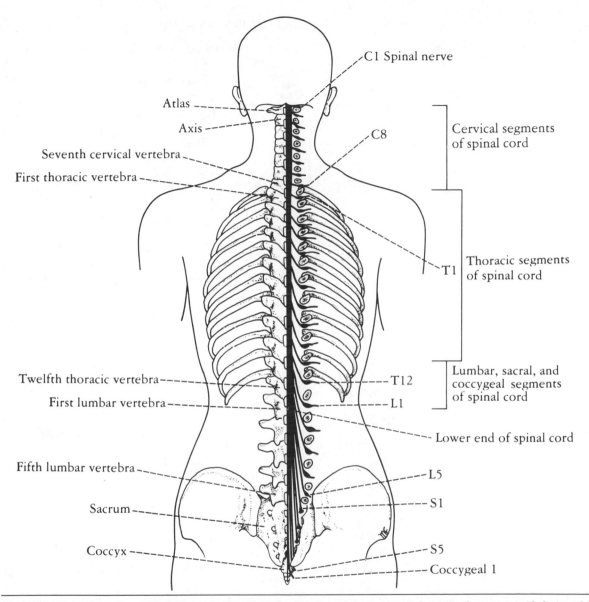

C1 Spinal nerve

Atlas

Axis

C8

Cervical segments of spinal cord

Seventh cervical vertebra

First thoracic vertebra

T1

Thoracic segments of spinal cord

Twelfth thoracic vertebra

T12

First lumbar vertebra

L1

Lumbar, sacral, and coccygeal segments of spinal cord

Lower end of spinal cord

Fifth lumbar vertebra

L5

Sacrum

S1

Coccyx

S5

Coccygeal 1

Fig. 1-26. Posterior view of spinal cord, showing the origins of the roots of the spinal nerves and their relationship to the different vertebrae. On the right, the laminae have been removed to expose the right half of the spinal cord and the nerve roots.

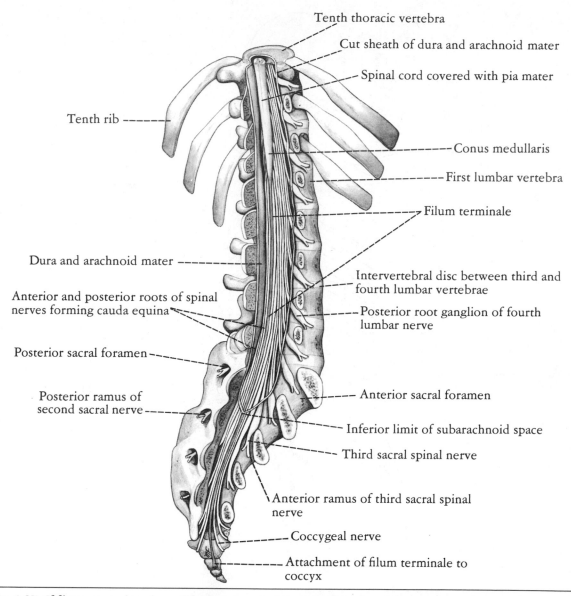

Tenth thoracic vertebra

Cut sheath of dura and arachnoid mater

Spinal cord covered with pia mater

Tenth rib

Conus medullaris

First lumbar vertebra

Filum terminale

Dura and arachnoid mater

Intervertebral disc between third and fourth lumbar vertebrae

Anterior and posterior roots of spinal nerves forming cauda equina

Posterior root ganglion of fourth lumbar nerve

Posterior sacral foramen

Anterior sacral foramen

Posterior ramus of second sacral nerve

Inferior limit of subarachnoid space

Third sacral spinal nerve

Anterior ramus of third sacral spinal nerve

Coccygeal nerve

Attachment of filum terminale to coccyx

Fig. 1-27. Oblique posterior view of the lower end of the spinal cord and the cauda equina. On the right, the laminae have been removed to expose the right half of the spinal cord and the nerve roots.

AUTONOMIC GANGLIA

Autonomic ganglia, which are often irregular in shape, are situated along the course of efferent nerve fibers of the autonomic nervous system. They are found in the paravertebral sympathetic chains (see Figs. 1-24 and 1-25) around the roots of the great visceral arteries in the abdomen and close to, or embedded within, the walls of various viscera.

It is essential that this brief outline of the organization of the nervous system be understood before proceeding further.

CLINICAL NOTES

INJURIES TO THE SPINAL CORD AND BRAIN

The spinal cord and brain are well protected. Both are suspended in fluid, the **cerebrospinal fluid**, and are surrounded by the bones of the vertebral column and skull. Unfortunately, if the forces of violence are sufficiently great these protective structures can be overcome, with consequent damage to the delicate underlying nervous tissue. Moreover, the cranial and spinal nerves and blood vessels are also likely to be injured.

Spinal Cord Injuries

The degree of spinal cord injury at different vertebral levels is governed largely by anatomical factors. In the cervical region, dislocation or fracture dislocation is common, but the large size of the vertebral canal often prevents severe injury to the spinal cord. However, when there is considerable displacement of the bones or bone fragments, the cord is sectioned. Respiration ceases if the lesion occurs above the segmental origin of the phrenic nerves (C3, 4, and 5), since the intercostal muscles and the diaphragm are paralyzed, and death occurs.

In fracture dislocations of the thoracic region, displacement is often considerable and the small size of the vertebral canal results in severe injury to the spinal cord.

In fracture dislocations of the lumbar region, two anatomical facts aid the patient. First, the spinal cord in the adult extends down only as far as the level of the lower border of the first lumbar vertebra (see Fig. 1-27). Second, the large size of the vertebral foramen in this region gives the roots of the cauda equina ample room. Nerve injury may therefore be minimal in this region.

Injury to the spinal cord may produce partial or complete loss of function at the level of the lesion, and partial or complete loss of function of afferent and efferent nerve tracts below the level of the lesion. The symptoms and signs of such injuries will be considered after the detailed structure of the spinal cord has been discussed, and the ascending and descending tracts have been considered in Chapters 20 and 21.

Spinal Nerve Injuries

The intervertebral foramina (Fig. 1-28) transmit the spinal nerves and the small segmental arteries and veins, all of which are embedded in areolar tissue. Each foramen is bounded superiorly and inferiorly by the pedicles of adjacent vertebrae, anteriorly by the lower part of the vertebral body and by the intervertebral disc, and posteriorly by the articular processes and the joint between them. In this situation, the spinal nerve is very vulnerable and may be pressed on or irritated by disease of the surrounding structures. Herniation of the intervertebral disc, fractures of the vertebral bodies, and osteoarthritis involving the joints of the articular processes or the joints between the vertebral bodies may all result in pressure, stretching, or edema of the emerging spinal nerve.

Herniation of the intervertebral discs occurs most commonly in those areas of the vertebral column where a mobile part joins a relatively immobile part, e.g., the cervicothoracic junction and the lumbosacral junction. In these areas the posterior part of the anulus fibrosus of the disc ruptures, and the central nucleus pulposus is forced posteriorly like toothpaste out of a tube. This herniation of the nucleus pulposus may result either in a central protrusion in the midline under the posterior longitudinal ligament of the vertebrae or in a lateral pro-

Fig. 1-28. A. Joints in cervical, thoracic, and lumbar regions of vertebral column.
B. Third lumbar vertebra seen from above, showing relationship between intervertebral disc and cauda equina.
C. Sagittal section through three lumbar vertebrae, showing ligaments and intervertebral discs. Note relationship between emerging spinal nerve in an intervertebral foramen and the intervertebral disc.

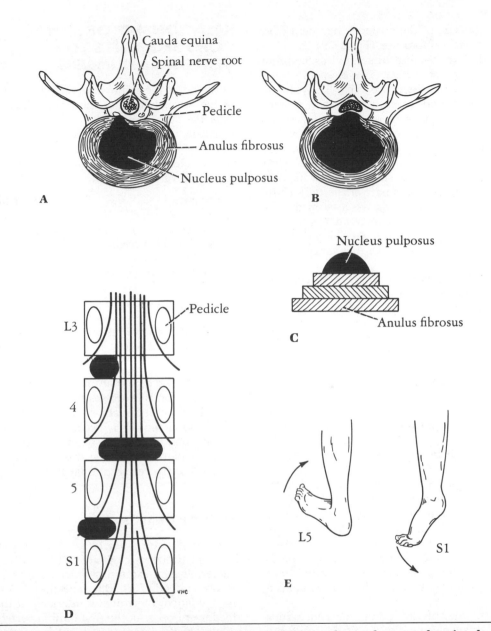

Fig. 1-29. A. Posterolateral rupture of anulus fibrosus, permitting nucleus pulposus to herniate backward and exert pressure on a spinal nerve root or spinal nerve.
B. Posterior rupture of anulus fibrosus, showing nucleus pulposus exerting pressure on spinal nerve roots of cauda equina.
C. Diagrammatic representation of intervertebral disc, showing concentric rings of anulus fibrosus and centrally placed, rounded nucleus pulposus.
D. Diagrammatic representation of posterior view of vertebral bodies in lumbar region, showing relationship that might exist between herniated nucleus pulposus and spinal nerve roots.
E. Pressure on L5 motor nerve root produces weakness of dorsiflexion of ankle joint; pressure on S1 motor nerve root produces weakness of plantar flexion of the ankle joint.

trusion at the side of the posterior ligament close to the intervertebral foramen (Fig. 1-29).

Cervical disc herniations are less common than in the lumbar region. The discs most susceptible to this condition are those between the fifth and sixth and seventh vertebrae. Lateral protrusions cause pressure on a spinal nerve or its roots. Each spinal nerve emerges above the corresponding vertebra; thus, the protrusion of the disc between the fifth and sixth cervical vertebrae may compress the C6 spinal nerve or its roots. Pain is felt near the lower part of the back of the neck and shoulder and along the area in the distribution of the spinal nerve involved. Central protrusions may press on the spinal cord and the anterior spinal artery and involve the various spinal tracts.

Lumbar disc herniations are more common than cervical disc herniations (Fig. 1-29). The discs most usually affected are those between the fourth and fifth lumbar vertebrae and between the fifth lumbar vertebra and the sacrum. In the lumbar region, the roots of the cauda equina run posteriorly over a number of intervertebral discs (Fig. 1-29). A lateral herniation may press on one or two roots and often involves the nerve root going to the intervertebral foramen just below. The nucleus pulposus occasionally herniates directly backward and, if it is a large herniation, the whole cauda equina may be compressed, producing paraplegia.

In lumbar disc herniations, pain is referred down the leg and foot in the distribution of the affected nerve. Since the sensory posterior roots most commonly pressed upon are the fifth lumbar and first sacral, pain is usually felt down the back and lateral side of the leg, radiating to the sole of the foot. This condition is often called **sciatica**. In severe cases there may be paresthesia or actual sensory loss.

Pressure on the anterior motor roots causes muscle weakness. Involvement of the fifth lumbar motor root produces weakness of dorsiflexion of the ankle, while pressure on the first sacral motor root causes weakness of plantar flexion, and the ankle jerk may be diminished or absent (Fig. 1-29).

A large, centrally placed protrusion may give rise to bilateral pain and muscle weakness in both legs. Acute retention of urine may also occur.

RELATIONSHIP OF SPINAL CORD SEGMENTS TO VERTEBRAL NUMBERS

In the adult the spinal cord terminates at the level of the lower border of the first lumbar vertebra; thus the spinal segments do not correspond numerically with the vertebrae that lie at the same level (see Fig. 1-26). The following will help a physician determine which spinal segment is related to a given vertebral body.

Vertebrae	*Spinal Segment*
Cervical vertebrae	Add 1
Upper thoracic vertebrae	Add 2
Lower thoracic vertebrae (7–9)	Add 3
Tenth thoracic vertebra	L1 and 2 cord segments
Eleventh thoracic vertebra	L3 and 4 cord segments
Twelfth thoracic vertebra	L5 cord segment
First lumbar vertebra	Sacral and coccygeal cord segments

It will be seen on examination of a patient's back that the spinous processes lie approximately at the same level as the vertebral bodies. In the lower thoracic region, however, because of the length and extreme obliquity of the spinous processes, it is useful to remember that the tips of the spines lie at the level of the vertebral body below.

Lumbar Puncture

Lumbar puncture may be performed to withdraw a sample of cerebrospinal fluid for microscopic or bacteriological examination, or to inject drugs to combat infection or induce anesthesia. Fortunately, the spinal cord terminates inferiorly at the level of the lower border of the first lumbar vertebra in the adult. (In the infant it may reach inferiorly to the third lumbar vertebra.) The subarachnoid space extends inferiorly as far as the lower border of the second sacral vertebra. The lower lumbar part of the vertebral canal is thus occupied by the subarachnoid space, which contains the lumbar and sacral nerve roots and the filum terminale (the cauda equina). A needle introduced into the subarachnoid space in this region usually pushes the nerve roots to one side without causing damage.

With the patient lying on his side with the vertebral column well flexed, the space between adjoining laminae in the lumbar region is opened to a maximum (Fig. 1-30). An imaginary line joining the highest points on the iliac crests passes over the fourth lumbar spine. Using a careful aseptic technique and local anesthesia, the physician passes the lumbar puncture needle, fitted with a stylet, into the vertebral canal above or below the fourth lumbar spine. The needle will pass through the following anatomical structures before it enters the subarachnoid space: (1) skin, (2) superficial fascia, (3) supraspinous ligament, (4) interspinous ligament, (5) ligamentum flavum, (6) areolar tissue containing the internal vertebral venous plexus, (7) dura mater, and (8) arachnoid mater. The depth to which the needle will have to pass will vary from 1 inch (2.5 cm) or less in a child to as much as 4 inches (10 cm) in an obese adult.

As the stylet is withdrawn, a few drops of blood commonly escape. This usually indicates that the point of the needle is situated in one of the veins of the internal vertebral plexus and has not yet reached the subarachnoid space. If the entering needle should stimulate one of the nerve roots of the cauda equina, the patient will experience a fleeting discomfort in one of the dermatomes or a muscle will twitch, depending on whether a sensory or a motor root was impaled.

The cerebrospinal fluid pressure may be measured by attaching a manometer to the needle. When the patient is in the recumbent position, the **normal pressure is about 60 to 150 mm of water**. The pressure shows oscillations corresponding to the movements of respiration and the arterial pulse.

A block of the subarachnoid space in the vertebral canal, which may be caused by a tumor of the spinal cord or the meninges, may be detected by compressing the internal jugular veins in the neck. This raises the cerebral venous pressure and inhibits the absorption of cerebrospinal fluid in the arachnoid granulations (see p. 346), thus producing a rise in the manometer reading of the cerebrospinal fluid pressure. If this rise fails to occur, the subarachnoid space is blocked and the patient is said to exhibit a positive **Queckenstedt's sign**.

Caudal Anesthesia

Solutions of anesthetics may be injected into the sacral canal through the sacral hiatus. The solutions pass upward in the loose connective tissue and bathe the spinal nerves as they emerge from the dural sheath (Fig. 1-31). Obstetricians use this method of nerve block to relieve the pains of the second stage of labor. The advantage is that when administered by this method the anesthetic does not affect the infant.

Head Injuries

A blow to the head may cause the scalp to be merely bruised; severe blows may cause the scalp to be torn or split. Even if the head is protected by a crash helmet, the brain may be severely damaged without clinical evidence of scalp injury.

Severe blows to the head often result in the skull's changing shape at the point of impact. Small objects may penetrate the skull and produce local laceration of the brain. Larger objects applied with great force may shatter the skull, and fragments of bone are driven into the brain at the site of impact.

In the adult, fractures of the skull are common, but in the young child less so. In the infant, the skull bones are more resilient than in the adult, and they are separated by fibrous sutural ligaments. In the adult the inner table of the skull is particularly brittle. Moreover, the sutural ligaments begin to ossify during middle age.

The type of fracture that occurs in the skull will depend on the age of the patient, the severity of the blow, and the area of the skull receiving the trauma. The **adult skull** may be likened to an eggshell because it possesses a certain limited resilience, beyond which it splinters. A severe, localized blow will produce a local indentation, often accompanied by splintering of the bone. Blows to the vault often result in a series of linear fractures, which radiate out through the thin areas of the bone. The petrous parts of the temporal bones and the occipital crests strongly reinforce the base of the skull and tend to deflect linear fractures.

The **young child's skull** may be likened to a table tennis ball because a localized blow produces a depression without splintering. This common type

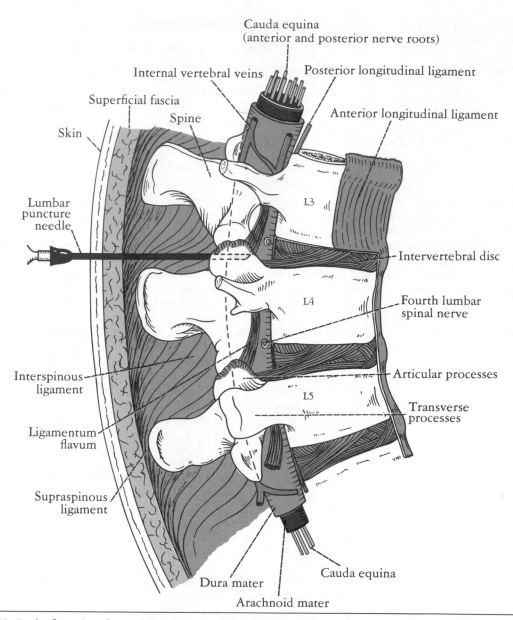

Fig. 1-30. Sagittal section through lumbar part of vertebral column in position of flexion. Note that spines and laminae are well separated in this position, allowing introduction of lumbar puncture needle into subarachnoid space.

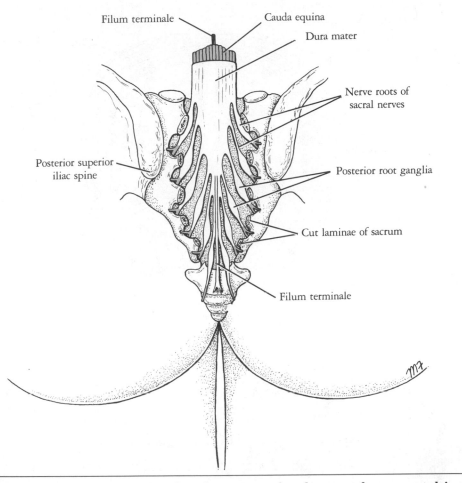

Filum terminale

Cauda equina

Dura mater

Nerve roots of
sacral nerves

Posterior superior
iliac spine

Posterior root ganglia

Cut laminae of sacrum

Filum terminale

Fig. 1-31. Posterior view of sacrum. Laminae have been removed to show sacral nerve roots lying within sacral canal.

of circumscribed lesion is referred to as a "pond" fracture.

Brain Injuries

Brain injuries are produced by displacement and distortion of the neuronal tissues at the moment of impact (Fig. 1-32). The brain, which is incompressible, may be likened to a water-soaked log floating submerged in water. The brain is floating in the cerebrospinal fluid in the subarachnoid space and is capable of a certain amount of anteroposterior and lateral gliding movement. The anteroposterior movement is limited by the attachment of the superior cerebral veins to the superior sagittal sinus. Lateral displacement of the brain is limited by the falx cerebri. The tentorium cerebelli and the falx cerebelli also restrict displacement of the brain.

It follows from these anatomical facts that blows on the front or back of the head lead to displacement of the brain, which may produce severe cerebral damage, stretching and distortion of the brainstem, and stretching and even tearing of the commissures of the brain. Blows to the side of the head produce less cerebral displacement, and the injuries to the brain consequently tend to be

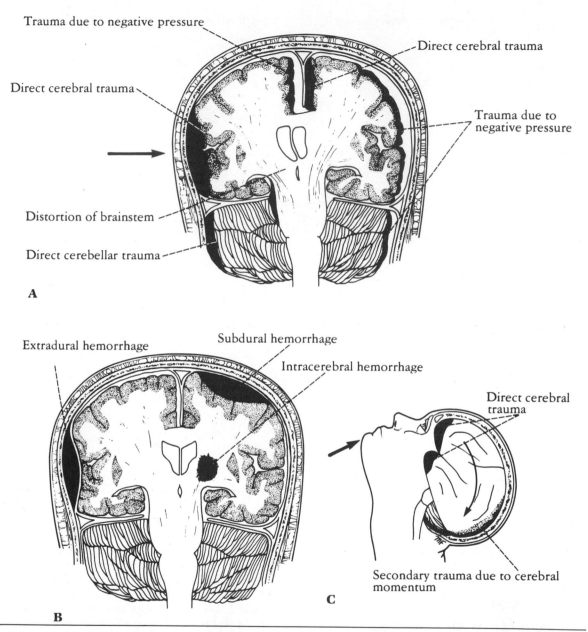

Fig. 1-32. A. Mechanisms of acute cerebral injury when blow is applied to lateral side of the head. B. Varieties of intracranial hemorrhage. C. Mechanism of cerebral trauma following a blow on the chin. The movement of the brain within the skull can also tear the cerebral veins.

less severe. It should be noted, however, that the falx cerebri is a tough structure and may cause considerable damage to the softer brain tissue in cases where there has been a severe blow to the side of the head (Fig. 1-32). Furthermore, it is important to remember that glancing blows to the head may cause considerable rotation of the brain, with shearing strains and distortion of the brain, particularly in areas where further rotation is prevented by bony prominences in the anterior and middle cranial fossae. Brain lacerations are very likely to occur when the brain is forcibly thrown against the sharp edges of bone within the skull—the lesser wings of the sphenoid, for example.

It is interesting to note that when the brain is suddenly given momentum within the skull, the part of the brain that moves away from the skull wall is subjected to diminished pressure, because the cerebrospinal fluid has not had time to accommodate to the brain movement. This results in a suction effect on the brain surface, with rupture of surface blood vessels.

A sudden severe blow to the head, as in an automobile accident, may result in damage to the brain at two sites: (1) at the point of impact, and (2) at the pole of the brain opposite the point of impact, where the brain is thrown against the skull wall. This is referred to as **contrecoup injury**.

The movement of the brain within the skull at the time of head injuries not only is likely to cause avulsion of cranial nerves but commonly leads to rupture of tethering blood vessels. Fortunately, the large arteries found at the base of the brain are tortuous and this, coupled with their strength, explains why they are rarely torn. The thin-walled cortical veins, which drain into the large dural venous sinuses, are very vulnerable and can produce severe subdural or subarachnoid hemorrhage (Fig. 1-32).

Intracranial Hemorrhage

Although the brain is cushioned by the surrounding cerebrospinal fluid in the subarachnoid space, any severe hemorrhage within the relatively rigid skull will ultimately exert pressure on the brain.

Intracranial hemorrhage may result from trauma or cerebral vascular lesions (Fig. 1-32). Four varieties will be considered here: (1) extradural, (2) subdural, (3) subarachnoid, and (4) cerebral.

Extradural hemorrhage results from injuries to the meningeal arteries and veins. The anterior division of the middle meningeal artery is the common artery to be damaged. A comparatively minor blow to the side of the head, resulting in fracture of the skull in the region of the anterior inferior portion of the parietal bone, may sever the artery (Fig. 1-32). The arterial injury is especially likely to occur if the artery enters a bony canal in this region. Bleeding occurs under high pressure and strips up the meningeal layer of dura from the internal surface of the skull. The intracranial pressure rises, and the enlarging blood clot exerts local pressure on the underlying precentral gyrus (motor area). In order to stop the hemorrhage, the torn artery must be ligated or plugged. The burr hole through the skull wall should be placed about 1½ inches (4 cm) above the midpoint of the zygomatic arch.

Subdural hemorrhage results from tearing of the superior cerebral veins where they enter the superior sagittal sinus (Fig. 1-9). The cause is usually a blow on the front or back of the head, resulting in excessive anteroposterior displacement of the brain within the skull. This condition, which is much more common than middle meningeal hemorrhage, can be produced by a sudden minor blow. Once the vein is torn, blood under low pressure begins to accumulate in the potential space between the dura and the arachnoid. In about one-half of the patients the condition is bilateral.

Acute and chronic forms of the clinical condition occur, depending on the speed of accumulation of fluid in the subdural space. For example, if the patient starts to vomit, the venous pressure will rise as the result of a rise in the intrathoracic pressure. Under these circumstances the subdural blood clot will increase rapidly in size and produce acute symptoms. In the chronic form, over a course of several months, the small blood clot will attract fluid by osmosis, so that a hemorrhagic cyst is formed, which gradually expands and produces pressure symptoms. In both forms the blood clot must be removed through burr holes in the skull.

Subarachnoid hemorrhage results from leakage or rupture of a congenital aneurysm on the cerebral arterial circle or, less commonly, from an angioma (tumor of a blood vessel). The symptoms, which are sudden in onset, will include severe headache, stiffness of the neck, and loss of consciousness. The diagnosis is established by performing computed tomography (CT) or magnetic resonance imaging (MRI) or by withdrawing heavily bloodstained cerebrospinal fluid through a lumbar puncture.

Cerebral hemorrhage is generally due to rupture of the thin-walled **lenticulostriate artery** (see Fig. 28-9) (p. 549), a branch of the middle cerebral artery (Fig. 1-32). The hemorrhage involves important descending nerve fibers in the internal capsule and produces hemiplegia on the opposite side of the body. The patient immediately loses consciousness, and the paralysis is evident when consciousness is regained. The diagnosis is established by performing a CT brain scan or an MRI.

Space-Occupying Lesions within the Skull

Space-occupying or expanding lesions within the skull include tumor, hematoma, and abscess. Since the skull is a rigid container of fixed volume these lesions will add to the normal bulk of the intracranial contents.

An expanding lesion is first accommodated by the expulsion of cerebrospinal fluid from the cranial cavity. Later the veins become compressed, interference with the circulation of blood and cerebrospinal fluid begins, and the intracranial pressure starts to rise. The venous congestion results in increased production and diminished absorption of cerebrospinal fluid, the volume of the cerebrospinal fluid begins to rise, and so a vicious circle is established.

The position of the tumor within the brain may have a dramatic effect on the signs and symptoms. For example, a tumor that obstructs the outflow of cerebrospinal fluid or directly presses upon the great veins will cause a rapid increase in intracranial pressure. The signs and symptoms that enable the physician to localize the lesion will depend on the interference with the brain and the degree of destruction of the nervous tissue produced by the lesion. Severe headache, possibly due to the stretching of the dura mater, and vomiting, due to pressure on the brainstem, are common complaints.

A lumbar puncture should **not** be performed in patients with suspected intracranial tumor. The

withdrawal of cerebrospinal fluid may lead to a sudden displacement of the cerebral hemisphere through the notch in the tentorium cerebelli into the posterior cranial fossa (Fig. 1-33) or herniation of the medulla oblongata and cerebellum through the foramen magnum. CT scans or MRIs are now used in making the diagnosis.

Autonomic Nervous System

This part of the nervous system is concerned with the innervation of involuntary structures. Because it is distributed throughout the central and peripheral nervous systems, symptoms of abnormal autonomic function are common to numerous neurological diseases. Primary abnormal function of the autonomic system is rare. In **primary megacolon (Hirschsprung's disease)** there is a complete failure of development of the parasympathetic ganglion cells in the pelvic colon. This congenital defect results in the child's being unable to pass meconium and the abdomen becomes enormously distended. In **primary Raynaud's disease**, in which there is vasospasm of the arterioles of the fingers on exposure to cold, the cause may be hyperactivity of the sympathetic part of the autonomic system. Traumatic damage to the parasympathetic centers in the spinal cord will result in loss of sexual function and of the normal control of the urinary bladder and rectum.

Computed Tomography (CT)

Computed tomography has been introduced for the detection of intracranial lesions. The procedure is quick, safe, and accurate. The total dose of irradiation is no greater than for a conventional skull radiograph.

Computed tomography relies on the same physics as conventional x-rays, in that structures are distinguished from one another by their ability to absorb energy from x-rays. The x-ray tube emits a narrow beam of radiation as it passes in a series of scanning movements through an arc of 180 degrees around the patient's head. The x-rays having passed through the head are collected by a special x-ray detector. The information is fed to a com-

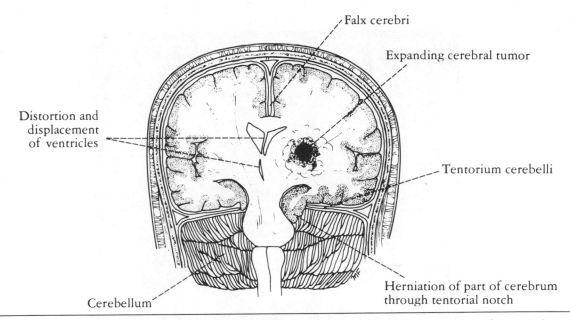

Falx cerebri

Expanding cerebral tumor

Distortion and displacement of ventricles

Tentorium cerebelli

Herniation of part of cerebrum through tentorial notch

Cerebellum

Fig. 1-33. Sudden displacement of cerebral hemispheres through the tentorial notch into the posterior cranial fossa following a lumbar puncture; the cerebral tumor is situated in the right cerebral hemisphere. A CT scan or an MRI should be used rather than a lumbar puncture when investigating a cerebral tumor.

puter that processes the information, which is then displayed as a reconstructed picture on a televisionlike screen. Essentially, the observer sees an image of a thin slice through the head, which may then be photographed for later examination (Fig. 1-34).

The sensitivity is such that small differences in x-ray absorption can be easily displayed. The gray matter of the cerebral cortex, white matter, internal capsule, corpus callosum, ventricles, and subarachnoid spaces can all be recognized. An intravascular iodine-containing medium can be injected, which has recently been found to enhance greatly the contrast between tissues having a different blood flow.

Magnetic Resonance Imaging (MRI)

The technique of magnetic resonance imaging uses the magnetic properties of the hydrogen nucleus excited by radiofrequency radiation transmitted by a coil surrounding the head. The excited hydrogen nuclei emit a signal that is detected as induced electric currents in a receiver coil. The MRI scan is absolutely safe to the patient and, because it provides better differentiation between gray and white matter, its use can be more revealing than a CT scan. The reason for this is that gray matter contains more hydrogen in the form of water than does white matter and the hydrogen atoms are less bound in fat (Fig. 1-35).

CLINICAL PROBLEMS

Answers on Page 583

1. A professor of neurology turned to his students and said, "Before we go around the wards this morning I want you to be absolutely certain that you understand what I mean by the terms: (a) **neuron**, (b) **neuroglia**, (c) **gray matter**, (d) **white matter**, and (e) **cerebrospinal fluid**." Are you sure of the precise meaning of these terms?

2. After examining a 12-year-old boy who had loss of muscular coordination (ataxia), especially of

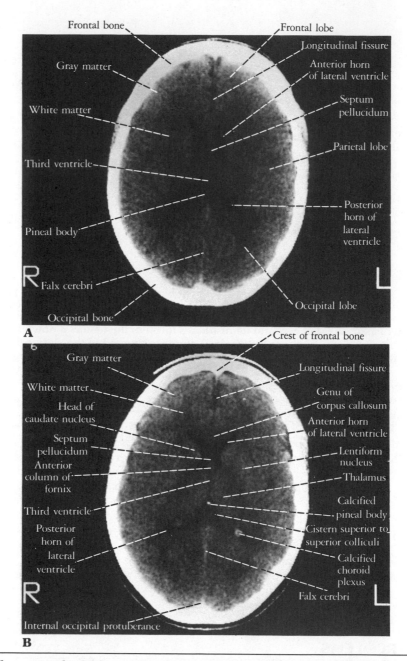

Frontal bone

Gray matter

White matter

Third ventricle

Pineal body

Falx cerebri

Occipital bone

A

Frontal lobe

Longitudinal fissure

Anterior horn of lateral ventricle

Septum pellucidum

Parietal lobe

Posterior horn of lateral ventricle

Occipital lobe

Crest of frontal bone

Gray matter

White matter

Head of caudate nucleus

Septum pellucidum

Anterior column of fornix

Third ventricle

Posterior horn of lateral ventricle

Internal occipital protuberance

B

Longitudinal fissure

Genu of corpus callosum

Anterior horn of lateral ventricle

Lentiform nucleus

Thalamus

Calcified pineal body

Cistern superior to superior colliculi

Calcified choroid plexus

Falx cerebri

Fig. 1-34. Computed tomography (CT) scan showing the structure of the brain. (A) and (B) represent horizontal cuts (axial sections).

Fig. 1-35. Magnetic resonance imaging (MRI) showing the structure of the brain. A. Sagittal. B. Coronal (contrast enhanced). Compare with Figure 1-34. Note the better differentiation between gray and white matter.

the lower limbs, and excessively high longitudinal arches of his feet (pes cavus), a physician made a diagnosis of **Friedreich's ataxia**. The physician explained to a student that this familial hereditary disease results in a steadily progressive degeneration of the posterior and lateral white columns of the spinal cord. What are the posterior and lateral columns of the spinal cord? Where is the white matter in relation to the gray matter in the spinal cord?

3. Familial dysautonomia is a rare disorder that occurs most often in Jewish children. It is characterized by defective lacrimation, excessive sweating (hyperhidrosis), attacks of high blood pressure (hypertension), and raised body temperature (hyperpyrexia). The disease largely affects the autonomic nervous system. Using your knowledge of neuroanatomy, would you say that the autonomic nervous system is a distinctly separate nervous system? Does the autonomic nervous system have afferent as well as efferent nervous pathways?

4. After a laminectomy in the lower cervical region, the dura and arachnoid matter were incised and the spinal cord was seen to be fusiformly enlarged. The neurosurgeon turned to a fourth-year medical student who was watching the operation and asked, "Is the spinal cord of uniform diameter throughout its length?" How would you have answered that question?

5. A 45-year-old woman was examined by her physician and found to have carcinoma of the thyroid gland. Apart from the swelling in the neck, the patient also complained of back pain in the lower thoracic region, with a burning soreness radiating around the right side of her thorax over the tenth intercostal space. Although the back pain was often relieved by changing posture, it was worsened by coughing and sneezing. A lateral radiograph of the thoracic part of the vertebral column revealed a secondary carcinomatous deposit in the tenth thoracic vertebral body. Further physical examination revealed muscular weakness of both legs. Using your knowledge of neuroanatomy, explain the following: (a) the pain in the back, (b) the soreness over the right tenth intercostal space, (c) the muscular weakness of both legs, and (d) which segments of the spinal cord lie at the level of the tenth thoracic vertebral body.

6. A 35-year-old coal miner was crouching down at the mine face to inspect a drilling machine. A large rock suddenly became dislodged from the roof of the mine shaft and struck the miner on the upper part of his back. Examination by a physician showed an obvious forward displacement of the upper thoracic spines on the eighth thoracic spine. What anatomical factors in the thoracic region determine the degree of injury that may occur to the spinal cord?

7. A 20-year-old man with a long history of tuberculosis of the lungs was examined by an orthopedic surgeon because of the sudden development of a humpback (kyphosis). He also had symptoms of a stabbing pain radiating around both sides of his thorax intensified by coughing or sneezing. A diagnosis of tuberculous osteitis of the fifth thoracic vertebra was made, with the collapse of the vertebral body responsible for the kyphosis. Using your knowledge of neuroanatomy, explain why the collapse of the fifth thoracic vertebral body should produce pain in the distribution of the fifth thoracic segmental nerve on both sides.

8. A 50-year-old man woke up one morning with a severe pain near the lower part of the back of the neck and left shoulder. The pain was also referred along the outer side of the left upper arm. Movement of the neck caused an increase in the intensity of the pain, which was also accentuated by coughing. A lateral radiograph of the neck showed a slight narrowing of the space between the fifth and sixth cervical vertebral bodies. An MRI showed disruption of the intervertebral disc between the fifth and sixth cervical vertebrae. State which nerve root was involved, using your knowledge of anatomy. Also state the nature of the disease.

9. A medical student offered to help a fellow student straighten out the bumper of his foreign sports car. He had just finished his course in neuroanatomy and was in poor physical shape. Undaunted, he attempted to lift the end of the bumper while his friend stood on the other end. Suddenly he felt an acute pain in the back that extended down the back and outer side of his right leg. Later he was examined by an orthopedic surgeon, who found that the pain was accentuated by coughing. A lateral radiograph

of the lumbar vertebral column revealed nothing abnormal. An MRI, taken in the sagittal plane, showed a small posterior prolapse of the nucleus pulposus in the disc between the fifth lumbar and the first sacral vertebrae. A diagnosis of herniation of the intervertebral disc between the fifth lumbar and first sacral vertebrae was made. Explain the symptoms of this disease, using your knowledge of neuroanatomy. Which spinal nerve roots were pressed upon?

10. A 5-year-old child was seen in the emergency room and a diagnosis of acute meningitis was made. The resident decided to perform a lumbar puncture in order to confirm the diagnosis. Using your knowledge of neuroanatomy, where would you perform a lumbar puncture? Name, in order, the structures pierced when a lumbar puncture needle is introduced into the subarachnoid space.

11. A young woman, finding herself pregnant, told her friends that she hated the idea of going through the pain of childbirth but she equally detested the thought of having a general anesthetic. Is there a specialized local analgesic technique that will provide painless labor?

12. While crossing the road, a pedestrian was struck on the right side of his head by a passing car. He fell to the ground but did not lose consciousness. After resting for an hour and then getting up, he appeared to be confused and irritable. Later, he staggered and fell to the floor. On questioning, he was seen to be drowsy, and twitching of the lower left half of his face and left arm was noted. A diagnosis of extradural hemorrhage was made. Which artery is likely to have been damaged? What is responsible for the drowsiness and muscle twitching?

13. At the postmortem examination of a 3-year-old boy with hydrocephalus, a tumor was found in the midbrain obstructing the cerebral aqueduct. Using your knowledge of neuroanatomy, explain the site of the cerebral aqueduct and indicate how blockage of this channel could produce hydrocephalus.

14. A 45-year-old woman was examined by a neurologist and found to have an intracranial tumor. She complained of severe headaches, which occurred during the night and early morning. She described the pain as "bursting" in nature, and although at first, six months ago, they were intermittent, they were now more or less continuous. Coughing, stooping, and straining at stool made the pain worse. The pain was accompanied by vomiting on three recent occasions. What is the sequence of events that occurs within the skull as the intracranial pressure rises? Would you perform a routine lumbar puncture on every patient you suspected of having an intracranial tumor?

15. While examining an unconscious 18-year-old man admitted to the emergency room following a motorcycle accident, the neurosurgeon asked the attending medical student what happens to the brain in an accident in which it is suddenly decelerated within the skull. What is the value of wearing a crash helmet?

16. What do you understand by the terms: (a) **contrecoup injury**, (b) **subarachnoid hemorrhage**, (c) **subdural hemorrhage**, and (d) **cerebral hemorrhage**?

17. A well-known professor of medicine started his lecture on expanding intracranial lesions by stating, "The skull and vertebrae provide the central nervous system with a rigid case that communicates with the outside only through the vascular system." Explain this statement, using your knowledge of neuroanatomy.

18. A pediatrician asked a medical student on a ward round how, by a simple physical examination, he would be able to assess the intracranial pressure in a newborn infant. The student was also asked to comment on why the adult skull often responds to trauma in a different way from a young child's skull. How would you respond to these questions?

19. The neurologist, having carefully examined a 5-year-old boy, determined that the child was suffering from a tumor of the cerebellum, and commented that it was probably a medulloblastoma. Where is the cerebellum in relation to other parts of the brain? Where is the cerebellum situated in the skull?

20. A 20-year-old man began to suffer from epilepsy following a severe head injury in an automobile accident. A neurologist determined that he had injured the right frontal lobe of his brain. What is meant by the term *frontal lobe of the brain?*

NATIONAL BOARD TYPE QUESTIONS

Answers on Page 619

IN EACH OF THE FOLLOWING QUESTIONS, ANSWER:
- (a) IF (1) ONLY IS CORRECT
- (b) IF (2) ONLY IS CORRECT
- (c) IF BOTH (1) AND (2) ARE CORRECT, OR
- (d) IF NEITHER (1) NOR (2) IS CORRECT

1. Which of the following statements is (are) correct?
   - (1) The sympathetic part of the autonomic nervous system increases peristalsis of the intestine and opens the sphincters.
   - (2) The function of the parasympathetic part of the autonomic nervous system is aimed at conserving and restoring energy.

2. Which of the following statements is (are) correct in relation to the spinal cord?
   - (1) The cerebrospinal fluid occupies the subarachnoid space and lies between the arachnoid and the dura.
   - (2) The filum terminale is formed by the arachnoid mater.

3. Which of the following statements is (are) correct in relation to the spinal cord?
   - (1) A single segment of the spinal cord is attached to a posterior and an anterior root of a single spinal nerve by a number of rootlets.
   - (2) The internal vertebral venous plexus lies between the pia and the arachnoid.

Select the best response:

4. The following statements concerning the spinal cord are correct **except**:
   - (a) It has an inner core of gray matter and an outer covering of white matter.
   - (b) Inferiorly the cord tapers off to form the conus medullaris.
   - (c) The central canal is situated in the white commissure.
   - (d) The efferent nerve fibers that supply skeletal muscles have their cells of origin in the anterior gray horn.
   - (e) The ligamentum denticulatum anchors the lateral borders of the spinal cord to the dura and arachnoid.

5. The following statements concerning the medulla oblongata are correct **except**:
   - (a) The pyramid is a swelling present on the anterior surface of the medulla on each side of the midline.
   - (b) On the posterior surface of the inferior part of the medulla oblongata are the gracile and cuneate tubercles.
   - (c) The fourth ventricle lies posterior to the upper part of the medulla oblongata.
   - (d) The olives are oval elevations lying posterior to the inferior cerebellar peduncles.
   - (e) The medulla oblongata becomes continuous with the spinal cord at the foramen magnum.

6. The following statements concerning the midbrain are correct **except**:
   - (a) The cerebral aqueduct forms the cavity of the midbrain.
   - (b) The cerebral peduncles are divided by the substantia nigra into the tectum and the crus cerebri.
   - (c) The posterior surface possesses the two superior and two inferior colliculi.
   - (d) The red nuclei are situated in the tegmentum at the level of the superior colliculi.
   - (e) The trochlear nerve can be seen on the posterior surface just inferior to the inferior colliculi.

In the following questions, answer:
- (a) IF (1), (2), AND (3) ONLY ARE CORRECT
- (b) IF (1) AND (3) ONLY ARE CORRECT
- (c) IF (2) AND (4) ONLY ARE CORRECT
- (d) IF (4) ONLY IS CORRECT, OR
- (e) IF ALL ARE CORRECT

7. Which of the following statements is (are) correct concerning the cerebellum?
   - (1) It lies within the posterior cranial fossa.
   - (2) The cerebellar cortex is composed of gray matter.
   - (3) The vermis is the name given to that part joining the cerebellar hemispheres together.
   - (4) The dentate nucleus is a mass of white matter found in each cerebellar hemisphere.

8. Which of the following statements is (are) correct concerning the pons?
   - (1) It forms part of the floor of the fourth ventricle.
   - (2) It lies above the tentorium cerebelli.

(3) It connects the medulla oblongata to the midbrain.

(4) It is connected to the cerebellum by the inferior cerebellar peduncles.

9. Which of the following statements is (are) correct concerning the cerebrum?

(1) The cerebral hemispheres are separated by a deep cleft called the central sulcus.

(2) The lobes are named from the skull bones under which they lie.

(3) The corpus callosum is a mass of gray matter lying within each cerebral hemisphere.

(4) The internal capsule is an important collection of nerve fibers having the caudate nucleus and the thalamus on its medial side and the lentiform nucleus on its lateral side.

10. Which of the following statements is (are) correct concerning the peripheral nervous system?

(1) There are 12 pairs of cranial nerves.

(2) There are 8 pairs of cervical spinal nerves.

(3) A spinal nerve is formed by the union of an anterior and a posterior root in an intervertebral foramen.

(4) A posterior root ganglion contains the cell bodies of sensory nerve fibers entering the spinal cord.

11. Which of the following statements is (are) correct concerning the central nervous system?

(1) A CT brain scan can distinguish between white matter and gray matter.

(2) The lateral ventricles are in direct communication with the fourth ventricle.

(3) An MRI of the brain uses the magnetic properties of the hydrogen nucleus excited by radiofrequency radiation transmitted by a coil surrounding the patient's head.

(4) Following trauma and sudden movement of the brain within the skull, the large arteries at the base of the brain are commonly torn.

12. Which of the following statements is (are) correct concerning the cerebrospinal fluid?

(1) With the patient in the recumbent position, the normal pressure is about 60 to 150 mm of water.

(2) It protects the brain and spinal cord from traumatic injury.

(3) Compressing the internal jugular veins in the neck raises the cerebrospinal fluid pressure.

(4) The cerebrospinal fluid in the central canal of the spinal cord is unable to enter the fourth ventricle.

Match the vertebral levels listed below on the left with the approximate spinal cord segmental levels listed below on the right. Answers may be used more than once.

13. First lumbar vertebra

14. Third thoracic vertebra

15. Fifth cervical vertebra

16. Eighth thoracic vertebra

17. Fourth lumbar vertebra

(a) Sixth cervical spinal cord segment

(b) Sacral and coccygeal cord segments

(c) Fifth thoracic spinal cord segment

(d) Eleventh thoracic spinal cord segment

(e) None of the above

ADDITIONAL READING

Bydder, G. M. et al. Clinical NMR imaging of the brain. *Am. J. Radiol.* 139:215, 1982.

Crosby, E. C., Humphrey, T., and Lauer, E. W. *Correlative Anatomy of the Nervous System.* New York: Macmillan, 1962.

Pernkopf, E. *Atlas of Topographic and Applied Human Anatomy* (3rd ed.). Vol. 1. Baltimore and Munich: Urban & Schwarzenberg, 1989.

Snell, R. S. *Atlas of Clinical Anatomy.* Boston: Little, Brown, 1978.

Snell, R. S. *Clinical Anatomy for Medical Students* (4th ed.). Boston: Little, Brown, 1992.

Sobotta, J. *Atlas of Human Anatomy.* Vol. 1. H. Ferner and J. Staubesand (eds.). Baltimore and Munich: Urban & Schwarzenberg, 1983.

Weisberg, L. A. *Cerebral Computed Tomography: A Text-Atlas.* Philadelphia: Saunders, 1978.

Williams, P. L., Warwick, R., Dyson, M., and Bannister, L. H. (eds.). *Gray's Anatomy* (37th Brit. ed.). Philadelphia: Saunders, 1989.

Chapter 2
The Neuron

Neuron is the name given to the nerve cell and all its processes (Fig. 2-1). Neurons are excitable cells that are specialized for the reception of stimuli and the conduction of the nerve impulse. They vary considerably in size and shape, but each possesses a **cell body** or **perikaryon**, from whose surface project one or more processes called **neurites** (Fig. 2-2). Those neurites responsible for receiving information and conducting it toward the cell body are called **dendrites**. The single long neurite that conducts impulses away from the cell body is called the **axon**. The dendrites and axons are often referred to as **nerve fibers**.

Neurons are found in the brain and spinal cord and in ganglia.

VARIETIES OF NEURONS

Although the size of the cell body of a neuron may be as small as 5 μm or as large as 135 μm in diameter, the processes or neurites may extend over a distance of more than 1 meter. The number, length, and mode of branching of the neurites provide a morphological method for classifying neurons.

Unipolar neurons are those in which the cell body has a single neurite that divides a short distance from the cell body into two branches, one proceeding to some peripheral structure and the other entering the central nervous system (Fig. 2-3). The branches of this single neurite have the structural and functional characteristics of an axon. In this type of neuron the fine terminal branches found at the peripheral end of the axon at the receptor site are often referred to as the dendrites. Examples of this form of neuron are found in the posterior root ganglion.

Bipolar neurons possess an elongated cell body, from each end of which a single neurite emerges (Fig. 2-3). Examples of this type of neuron are found in the retinal bipolar cells and the cells of the sensory cochlear and vestibular ganglia.

Multipolar neurons have a number of neurites arising from the cell body (Fig. 2-3). With the exception of the long process, the axon, the remainder of the neurites are dendrites. Most neurons of the brain and spinal cord are of this type.

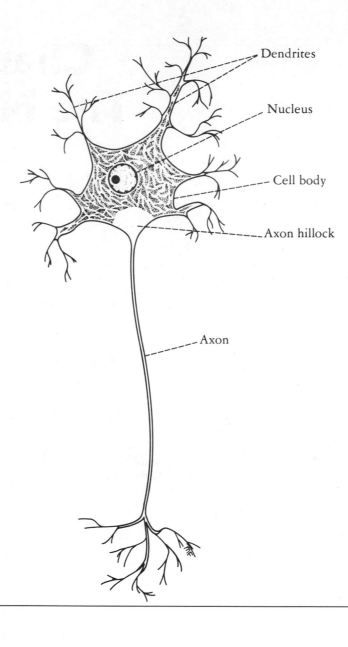

Dendrites

Nucleus

Cell body

Axon hillock

Axon

Fig. 2-1. A neuron.

Fig. 2-2. Photomicrograph of a smear preparation of the spinal cord showing a neuron with its cell body or perikaryon and its processes or neurites.

Neurons may also be classified according to size:

Golgi type I neurons have a long axon that may be 1 meter or more in length in extreme cases (Figs. 2-4, 2-5, and 2-6). The axons of these neurons form the long fiber tracts of the brain and spinal cord and the nerve fibers of peripheral nerves. The pyramidal cells of the cerebral cortex, the Purkinje cells of the cerebellar cortex, and the motor cells of the spinal cord are good examples.

Golgi type II neurons have a short axon that terminates in the neighborhood of the cell body or is entirely absent (Figs. 2-5 and 2-6). They greatly outnumber the Golgi type I neurons. The short dendrites that arise from these neurons give them a star-shaped appearance. These neurons are very numerous in the cerebral and cerebellar cortex and are often inhibitory in function.

STRUCTURE OF THE NEURON

The **nerve cell body**, like that of other cells, consists essentially of a mass of cytoplasm in which a nucleus is embedded (Figs. 2-7 and 2-8); it is bounded externally by a limiting membrane. It is interesting to note that the volume of cytoplasm within the nerve cell body is often far less than the total volume of cytoplasm in the neurites. The cell bodies of the small granular cells of the cerebellar cortex measure about 5 μm in diameter, whereas those of the large anterior horn cells may measure as much as 135 μm in diameter.

The **nucleus*** is commonly centrally located within the cell body and is typically large, rounded, and pale and the fine chromatin granules are widely dispersed (Figs. 2-6 and 2-7). There is usually a single prominent nucleolus, which is concerned with the synthesis of ribonucleic acid (RNA). The large size of the nucleolus probably is due to the high rate of protein synthesis, which is necessary to maintain the protein level in the large cytoplasmic volume that is present in the long neurites as well as in the cell body.

In the female one of the two X chromosomes is compact and is known as the **Barr body**. It is composed of sex chromatin and is situated at the inner surface of the nuclear envelope. The nuclear envelope is double-layered and possesses fine nuclear pores, through which materials can diffuse into and out of the nucleus (Figs. 2-8 and 2-9).

The **cytoplasm** is rich in granular and agranular endoplasmic reticulum (Figs. 2-9 and 2-10) and contains the following organelles and inclusions: (1) Nissl substance, (2) the Golgi apparatus, (3) mitochondria, (4) microfilaments, (5) microtubules, (6) lysosomes, (7) centrioles, and (8) lipofuscin, melanin, glycogen, and lipid.

Nissl substance consists of granules that are distributed throughout the cytoplasm of the cell body, except for the region close to the axon, called the **axon hillock** (Fig. 2-11). The granular mate-

---

*The term *nucleus* used in cytology must not be confused with the term *nucleus* in neuroanatomy, which refers to a discrete group of nerve cell bodies in the central nervous system.

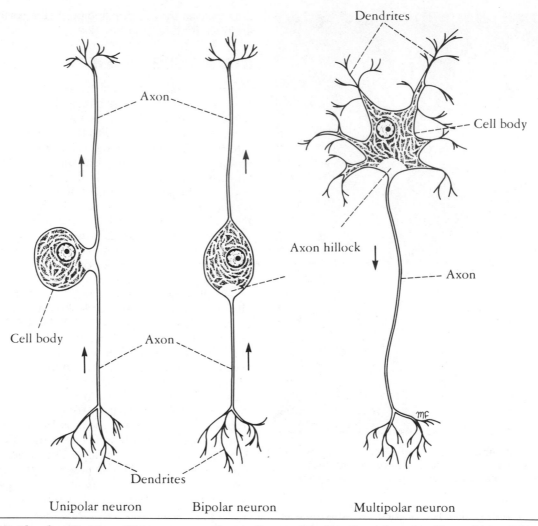

Fig. 2-3. The classification of neurons according to the number, length, and mode of branching of the neurites.

Molecular layer

Dendritic processes of Purkinje cells

Purkinje cell

Granular layer

Fig. 2-4. Photomicrograph of silver-stained section of the cerebellar cortex showing two Purkinje cells. These are examples of Golgi type I neurons.

Golgi type II neurons

Pyramidal cells (Golgi type I neurons)

Golgi type II neurons

Fig. 2-5. Photomicrograph of a silver-stained section of the cerebral cortex. Note the presence of large pyramidal cells, which are examples of Golgi type I neurons, and numerous Golgi type II neurons.

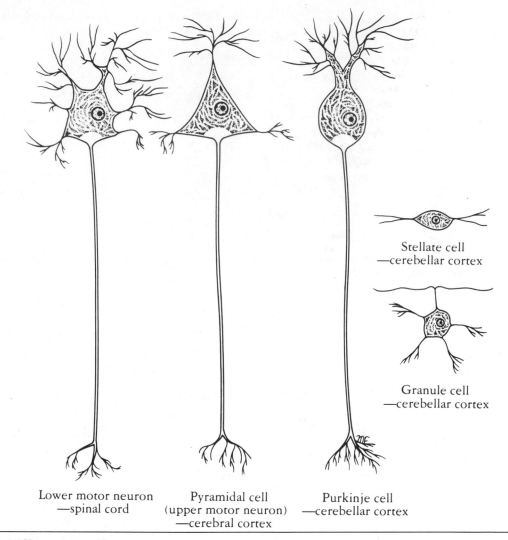

Lower motor neuron
—spinal cord

Pyramidal cell
(upper motor neuron)
—cerebral cortex

Purkinje cell
—cerebellar cortex

Stellate cell
—cerebellar cortex

Granule cell
—cerebellar cortex

Fig. 2-6. Different types of neurons.

Dendrite

Nucleus

Nucleolus

Body of nerve cell

Neuropil

Fig. 2-7. Photomicrograph of section of anterior gray column of spinal cord showing two large motor nerve cells with nuclei. Note the prominent nucleolus in one of the nuclei.

rial also extends into the proximal parts of the dendrites; it is not present in the axon.

Electron micrographs show that the Nissl substance is composed of rough-surfaced endoplasmic reticulum (Fig. 2-12) arranged in the form of broad cisternae stacked one on top of the other. Although many of the ribosomes are attached to the surface of the endoplasmic reticulum, many more lie free in the intervals between the cisternae. Since the ribosomes contain RNA, the Nissl substance is basophilic and can be well demonstrated by staining with toluidine blue or other basic aniline dyes (Fig. 2-11) and using the light microscope.

The Nissl substance is responsible for synthesizing protein, which flows along the dendrites and the axon and replaces the proteins that are broken down during cellular activity. Fatigue or neuronal damage causes the Nissl substance to move and become concentrated at the periphery of the cytoplasm. This phenomenon, which gives the impression that the Nissl substance has disappeared, is known as **chromatolysis**.

The **Golgi apparatus**, when seen with the light microscope after staining with a silver-osmium method, appears as a network of irregular wavy threads around the nucleus. In electron micrographs it appears as clusters of flattened cisternae and small vesicles made up of smooth-surfaced endoplasmic reticulum (Fig. 2-9).

The protein produced by the Nissl substance is transferred to the Golgi apparatus, where it is temporarily stored and where carbohydrate may be added to the protein. The Golgi apparatus is also thought to be active in lysosome production and in the synthesis of cell membranes. The latter function is particularly important in the formation of synaptic vesicles at the axon terminals.

Mitochondria are found scattered throughout the cell body, dendrites, and axons (see Figs. 2-8 and 2-9). They are spherical or rod-shaped. In electron micrographs the walls show a characteristic double membrane (Fig. 2-8). The inner membrane is thrown into folds or cristae that project into the center of the mitochondrion. Mitochondria possess

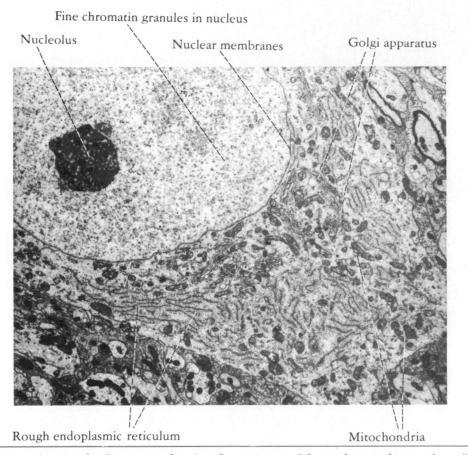

Fig. 2-9. Electron micrograph of a neuron showing the structure of the nucleus and a number of cytoplasmic organelles. (Courtesy Dr. J. M. Kerns.)

Cytoplasm of neuron

Nucleus

Plasma membrane

Nuclear membranes

Rough endoplasmic reticulum

Fig. 2-10. Electron micrograph of a neuron showing nuclear and plasma membranes and cytoplasmic organelles. (Courtesy Dr. J. M. Kerns.)

many enzymes, which are localized chiefly on the inner mitochondrial membrane. These enzymes take part in the tricarboxylic acid cycle and the cytochrome chains of respiration. Mitochondria are therefore important in nerve cells, as in other cells, in the production of energy.

Neurofibrils, as seen with the light microscope, are numerous fibrils running parallel to each other through the cell body into the neurites when the cytoplasm is stained with silver (Fig. 2-13). With the electron microscope, the neurofibrils may be resolved into bundles of **microfilaments,** each filament measuring about 7 nm in diameter (Fig. 2-14). The microfilaments contain actin and myosin and probably assist in cell transport.

Microtubules are revealed with the electron microscope and are similar to those seen in other

types of cells. They measure about 20 to 30 nm in diameter and are found interspersed among the microfilaments (Fig. 2-14). They extend throughout the cell body and its processes. The function of microtubules is believed to be the transport of substances from the cell body to the distal ends of the cell processes.

Cell transport can take place in both directions in the cell body and its processes. It is of two kinds: rapid (100 mm per day) and slow (1 to 3 mm per day). **Rapid transport** carries proteins and other materials including transmitter substances. It is believed that a ratchetlike action using proteins projecting from the surface of the microtubules is involved. The contraction of the microfilaments may assist this process. Separate channels between the microtubules and microfilaments permit the

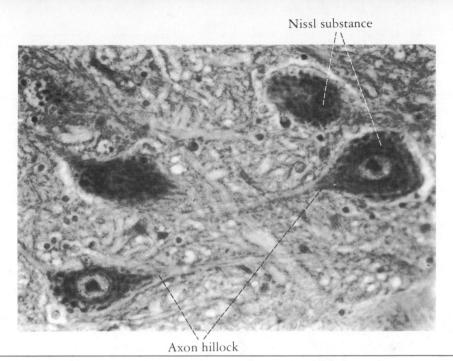

Nissl substance

Axon hillock

Fig. 2-11. Photomicrograph of section of anterior gray column of spinal cord stained with toluidine blue. Note the presence of dark-staining Nissl substance in cytoplasm of four neurons.

Nissl substance

Nissl substance

Fig. 2-12. Electron micrograph of cytoplasm of two neurons showing the structure of Nissl bodies (substance). (Courtesy Dr. J. M. Kerns.)

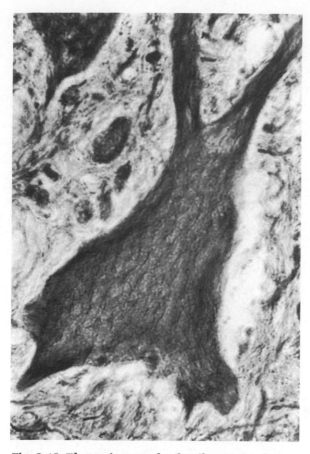

Fig. 2-13. Photomicrograph of a silver-stained section of a neuron. Shows the presence of large numbers of neurofibrils in the cytoplasm of the cell body and the neurites.

flow in both directions. **Slow transport** involves the bulk movement of the cytoplasm and includes the movement of mitochondria and other organelles. The mechanism is unknown.

Lysosomes are membrane-bound vesicles measuring about 8 nm in diameter. They serve the cell by acting as intracellular scavengers and contain hydrolytic enzymes. They are formed by the budding off from the Golgi apparatus. Lysosomes exist in three forms: (1) **primary lysosomes**, which have just been formed, (2) **secondary lysosomes**, which contain partially digested material (myelin figures), and (3) **residual bodies**, in which the enzymes are inactive and which have evolved from digestible materials such as pigment and lipid.

Centrioles are small, paired structures found in immature dividing nerve cells. Each centriole is a hollow cylinder whose wall is made up of bundles of microtubules. They are associated with the formation of the spindle during cell division and in the formation of microtubules. Centrioles are also found in mature nerve cells, where they are believed to be involved in the maintenance of microtubules.

Lipofuscin (pigment material) occurs as yellowish-brown granules within the cytoplasm (Fig. 2-15). It is believed to be formed as the result of lysosomal activity and it represents a harmless metabolic by-product. Lipofuscin accumulates with age.

Melanin granules are found in the cytoplasm of cells in certain parts of the brain (for example, the substantia nigra of the midbrain). Their presence may be related to the catecholamine-synthesizing ability of these neurons whose neurotransmitter is dopamine.

Plasma Membrane

The plasma membrane forms the continuous external boundary of the cell body and its processes and in the neuron it is the site for the initiation and conduction of the nerve impulse (Figs. 2-10 and 2-14). The membrane is about 8 nm thick, too thin to be seen with the light microscope. When viewed under the electron microscope, the plasma membrane appears as two dark lines with a light line between them.

The plasma membrane is composed of an inner and an outer layer of very loosely arranged protein molecules, each layer about 2.5 nm thick, separated by a middle layer of lipid about 3 nm thick. The lipid layer is made up of two rows of phospholipid molecules arranged so that their hydrophobic ends are in contact with each other and their polar ends are in contact with the protein layers. Certain protein molecules lie within the phospholipid layer and span the entire width of the lipid layer. These molecules provide the membrane with hydrophilic channels through which inorganic ions may enter and leave the cell. Carbohydrate molecules are attached to the outside of the plasma membrane and are linked to the proteins or the lipids, forming what is known as the **cell coat**, or **glycocalyx**.

The plasma membrane and the cell coat together form a semipermeable membrane that al-

Microfilaments

Plasma membranes

Microfilaments

Microtubules

A

B

Microtubules

Fig. 2-14. Electron micrograph of dendrites showing the presence of microfilaments and microtubules within their cytoplasm. (Courtesy Dr. J. M. Kerns.)
A. Longitudinal section of two adjacent dendrites.
B. Transverse section of a dendrite.

Lipofuscin granules

Fig. 2-15. Photomicrograph of longitudinal section of posterior root ganglion showing the presence of lipofuscin granules within the cytoplasm of sensory neurons.

lows diffusion of certain ions through it, but restricts others. In the resting state (unstimulated state) the K^+ ions diffuse through the plasma membrane from the cell cytoplasm to the tissue fluid (Fig. 2-16). The permeability of the membrane to K^+ ions is much greater than to the Na^+ ions, so that the passive efflux of K^+ is much greater than the influx of Na^+. This results in a steady potential difference of about 80 mV, which can be measured across the plasma membrane since the inside of the membrane is negative with respect to the outside. This potential is known as the **resting potential**.

Excitation of the Plasma Membrane of the Nerve Cell Body

When the nerve cell is excited (stimulated) by electrical, mechanical, or chemical means, a rapid change in membrane permeability to Na^+ ions takes place and Na^+ ions diffuse through the plasma membrane into the cell cytoplasm from the tissue fluid (Fig. 2-16). This results in the membrane's becoming progressively depolarized. The sudden influx of Na^+ ions followed by the altered polarity produces the so-called **action potential**. This potential is, however, very brief, lasting about 5 msec, for very quickly the increased membrane permeability for Na^+ ions ceases and that for K^+ ions increases, so that the K^+ ions start to flow from the cell cytoplasm and so return the localized area of the cell to the resting state.

Once generated, the action potential spreads over the plasma membrane, away from the site of initiation, and is conducted along neurites as the **nerve impulse**. This impulse is self-propagated and its size and frequency do not alter (Fig. 2-16). Once the nerve impulse has spread over a given region of plasma membrane another action potential cannot be elicited immediately. The duration of this nonexcitable state is referred to as the **refractory period**.

It is important to realize that the greater the strength of the initial stimulus, the larger will be the initial depolarization and the greater the spread into the surrounding areas of the plasma membrane. Should multiple excitatory stimuli be

Resting state (unstimulated state)

Excited state (stimulated state)

Return to resting state

Nerve impulse

Site of summation of multiple stimuli

All-or-none action potentials with transient reversal of polarity

Fig. 2-16. The ionic and electrical changes that occur in a neuron when it is stimulated.

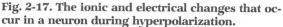

Hyperpolarization

Fig. 2-17. The ionic and electrical changes that occur in a neuron during hyperpolarization.

applied to the surface of a neuron, then the effect can be **summated**. For example, subthreshold stimuli may pass over the surface of the cell body and be summated at the root of the axon and so initiate an action potential.

Inhibitory stimuli are believed to produce their effect by causing an influx of Cl^- ions through the plasma membrane into the neuron, thus producing hyperpolarization and reducing the excitatory state of the cell (Fig. 2-17).

Sodium and Potassium Channels

The so-called sodium and potassium channels, through which physiologists believe the sodium and potassium ions diffuse through the plasma membrane, have not been identified. It is possible that some of the protein molecules that extend through the full thickness of the plasma membrane may serve as channels. Each channel is thought to be controlled by an electrically charged gate that can open or close the channel.

In the nonstimulated state, the gates of the potassium channels are wider open than those of the sodium channels, which are nearly closed. This permits the potassium ions to diffuse out of the cell cytoplasm more readily than the sodium ions can diffuse in. In the stimulated state, the gates of the sodium channels are at first wide open; then the gates of the potassium channels are opened and the gates of the sodium channels are nearly closed again. It is the opening and closing of the sodium and potassium channels that is thought to produce the depolarization and repolarization of the plasma membrane.

THE NERVE CELL PROCESSES

The processes of a nerve cell, often called neurites, may be divided into dendrites and an axon.

The **dendrites** are the short processes of the cell body (Fig. 2-18). Their diameter tapers as they extend from the cell body and they often branch profusely. In many neurons the finer branches bear large numbers of small projections called **dendritic spines**. The cytoplasm of the dendrites closely resembles that of the cell body and contains Nissl granules, mitochondria, microtubules, microfilaments, ribosomes, and agranular endoplasmic reticulum. Dendrites should be regarded merely as extensions of the cell body to increase the surface area for the reception of axons from other neurons. Essentially they conduct the nerve impulse toward the cell body.

Axon is the name given to the longest process of the cell body. It arises from a small conical elevation on the cell body, devoid of Nissl's granules, called the **axon hillock** (Figs. 2-8 and 2-19). Occasionally, an axon arises from the proximal part of a dendrite. An axon tends to have a smooth surface and is uniform in diameter.

Axons tend not to branch close to the cell body; collateral branches may occur along their length. Shortly before their termination, axons commonly branch profusely. The distal ends of the terminal branches of the axons are often enlarged; they are called **terminals** or **boutons terminaux** (Fig. 2-20).

Axons may be very short, as seen in many neurons of the central nervous system, or extremely long, as seen when they extend from a peripheral receptor in the skin of the toe to the spinal cord and thence to the brain.

The diameter of axons varies considerably with different neurons. Those of larger diameter conduct impulses rapidly and those of smaller diameter conduct impulses very slowly.

The plasma membrane bounding the axon is called the **axolemma**. The cytoplasm of the axon is termed the **axoplasm**. Axoplasm differs from the cytoplasm of the cell body in possessing no Nissl granules or Golgi apparatus. The sites for the

Nerve cell body Dendrite   Dendrite   Mitochondria

Neuropil

Microtubules and microfilaments

Axons synapsing on dendrite

A   B

Fig. 2-18. A. Light photomicrograph of a motor neuron in the anterior gray column of the spinal cord, showing the nerve cell body, two dendrites, and the surrounding neuropil.
B. Electron micrograph of a dendrite showing axodendritic synapses. (Courtesy Dr. J. M. Kerns.)

Fig. 2-19. Electron micrograph of longitudinal section of a neuron from the cerebral cortex, showing the detailed structure of the region of the axon hillock and the initial segment of the axon. Note the absence of Nissl substance (rough endoplasmic reticulum) in the axon hillock and the presence of numerous microtubules in the axoplasm. Note also the axon terminals (arrows) forming axoaxonal synapses with the initial segment of the axon. (Courtesy Dr. A. Peters.)

Axon containing large numbers of
presynaptic vesicles

Terminal expansion of axon (bouton terminal)

Axodendritic
synapse

Dendrite

Axodendritic synapses

Fig. 2-20. Electron micrograph showing multiple axodendritic synapses. Note the presence of large numbers of presynaptic vesicles within the axons. (Courtesy Dr. J. M. Kerns.)

production of protein, namely RNA and ribosomes, are absent.

The **initial segment** of the axon is the first 50 to 100 μm after it leaves the axon hillock of the nerve cell body (Fig. 2-19). This is the most excitable part of the axon and is the site at which an action potential originates. It is important to remember that under normal conditions an action potential does not originate on the plasma membrane of the cell body, but always at the initial segment.

It is usual to state that an axon always conducts impulses away from the cell body. The axons of sensory posterior root ganglion cells are an exception; here the long neurite, which is indistinguishable from an axon, carries the impulse toward the cell body. (See unipolar neurons, p. 47.)

Axon Transport

Materials are transported from the cell body to the axon terminals **(orthograde transport)** and to a lesser extent in the opposite direction **(retrograde transport).**

Fast orthograde transport of 100 mm per day refers to the transport of proteins and transmitter substances or their precursors. **Slow orthograde transport** of 1 to 3 mm per day refers to the transport of axoplasm and includes the microfilaments and microtubules.

Retrograde transport explains how the cell bodies of nerve cells respond to changes in the distal end of the axons. Pinocytotic vesicles arising at the axon terminals can be quickly returned to the cell body. Worn-out organelles can be returned to the cell body for breakdown by the lysosomes.

Axon transport is brought about by microtubules assisted by the microfilaments (see p. 56).

Synapses

The nervous system consists of a large number of neurons that are linked together to form functional conducting pathways. Where two neurons come into close proximity and functional interneuronal communication occurs, the site of such communication is referred to as a **synapse*** (Fig. 2-21). Communication at a synapse, under physiological conditions, takes place in one direction only. Synapses occur in a number of forms (Fig. 2-21). The most common type is that which occurs between an axon of one neuron and the dendrite or cell body of the second neuron. As the axon approaches the synapse it may have a terminal expansion (bouton terminal) or it may have a series of expansions (bouton de passage), each of which makes synaptic contact. In other types of synapses the axon synapses on the initial segment of another axon, that is, proximal to where the myelin sheath begins, or there may be synapses between terminal expansions from different neurons. Depending on the site of the synapse, they are often referred to as **axodendritic**, **axosomatic**, or **axoaxonic** (Fig. 2-21).

The manner in which an axon terminates varies considerably in different parts of the nervous system. For example, a single axon may terminate on a single neuron, as in the case of a climbing fiber in the cerebellar cortex ending on a single Purkinje cell; or a single axon may synapse with multiple neurons, as in the case of the parallel fibers of the cerebellar cortex synapsing with multiple Purkinje cells. In the same way, a single neuron may have synaptic junctions with axons of many different neurons. The arrangement of these synapses will determine the means by which a neuron can be stimulated or inhibited. **Synaptic spines**, extensions of the surface of a neuron, form receptive sites for synaptic contact with afferent boutons (Fig. 2-21).

*The definition has come to include the site at which a neuron comes into close proximity with a skeletal muscle cell and functional communication occurs.

Synapses are of two types: chemical and electrical. Most synapses are chemical, in which a chemical substance, the **neurotransmitter**, passes across the narrow space between the cells and becomes attached to a protein molecule in the postsynaptic membrane called the **receptor**. Chemical synapses are either excitatory or inhibitory. Once stimulation or inhibition has taken place, the neurotransmitter is broken down by an enzyme or it is taken up by the presynaptic axon terminal.

Electrical synapses are ordinary gap junctions between two neurons. They permit the spread of activity from one neuron to another and thus ensure that a group of neurons performing an identical function act together. Since there is no chemical transmitter, there is minimal delay in getting the information across between the cells.

Ultrastructure of Chemical Synapses

On examination with the electron microscope, synapses are seen to be areas of structural specialization (Figs. 2-20 and 2-22). The apposed surfaces of the terminal axonal expansion and the neuron are called the **presynaptic** and **postsynaptic membranes**, respectively, and they are separated by a **synaptic cleft** measuring 20 nm wide. The presynaptic and postsynaptic membranes are thickened and the adjacent underlying cytoplasm shows increased density. On the presynaptic side, the dense cytoplasm is broken up into groups and on the postsynaptic side the density often extends into a **subsynaptic web**. **Presynaptic vesicles**, mitochondria, and occasional lysosomes are present in the cytoplasm close to the presynaptic membrane (Fig. 2-22). On the postsynaptic side, the cytoplasm often contains parallel cisternae. The synaptic cleft contains polysaccharides.

The presynaptic terminal contains many small presynaptic vesicles that contain the neurotransmitter. The vesicles fuse with the presynaptic membrane and discharge the neurotransmitter into the synpatic cleft by a process of exocytosis (Fig. 2-23).

When synapses are first formed in the embryo they are recognized as small zones of density separated by a synaptic cleft. Later they mature into well-differentiated structures. The presence of simple, undifferentiated synapses in the postnatal ner-

Axodendritic

A

Axosomatic

B

Axoaxonic

C

Axodendritic or axoaxonic   Axodendritic with dendritic spine   Axoaxonic
D

Fig. 2-21. A, B, C, and D. Different types of chemical synapses.

Axons near termination   Presynaptic vesicles   Dendrite   Terminal expansion of axon

Mitochondria   Synaptic sites   Microtubules interspersed among microfilaments

Fig. 2-22. High-power electron micrograph of axodendritic synapses showing the thickening of the cell membranes at the synaptic sites, presynaptic vesicles, and the presence of mitochondria within the axons near their termination. (Courtesy Dr. J. M. Kerns.)

vous system has led to the suggestion that synapses can be developed as required and possibly undergo atrophy when redundant.

Neurotransmitters at Synapses

The presynaptic vesicles and the mitochondria play a key role in the release of neurotransmitter substances at synapses. The vesicles contain the neurotransmitter substance that is released into the synaptic cleft; the mitochondria provide adenosine triphosphate (ATP) for the synthesis of new transmitter substance.

The majority of neurons produce and release

only one type of transmitter at all their nerve endings. However, a few neurons release an excitor transmitter, such as glutamate, at one synapse and a neuropeptide at another synapse. Different neurons may produce and release different transmitter substances. For example, acetylcholine is widely used by different neurons in the central and peripheral parts of the nervous system, whereas dopamine is released by neurons in the substantia nigra. Glycine, another transmitter, is found principally in synapses in the spinal cord.

The following are chemical substances known to act as neurotransmitters and there are probably many more yet to be discovered: acetylcholine (ACh), norepinephrine, epinephrine, dopamine, gly-

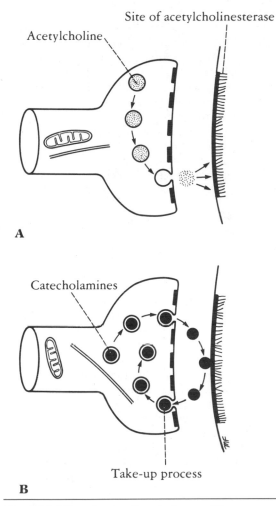

Fig. 2-23. The release of neurotransmitters.
A. Acetylcholine.
B. Catecholamines.

cine, serotonin, gamma-aminobutyric acid (GABA), enkephalins, substance P, and glutamic acid.

ACTION OF NEUROTRANSMITTERS

All neurotransmitters are released from their nerve endings by the arrival of the nerve impulse. Once in the synaptic cleft they achieve their objective by raising or lowering the resting potential of the postsynaptic membrane for a brief period of time.

The receptor proteins on the postsynaptic membrane bind the transmitter substance, thereby increasing the membrane permeability. In the case of excitatory synapses the permeability to most ions is increased, but with inhibitory synapses there is an increase in permeability to chloride ions. At an excitatory synapse the postsynaptic membrane is depolarized, whereas at an inhibitory synapse the postsynaptic membrane is hyperpolarized.

The excitatory and the inhibitory effects on the postsynaptic membrane of the neuron will depend on the summation of the postsynaptic responses at the different synapses. If the overall effect is one of depolarization the neuron will be excited and an action potential will be initiated at the initial segment of the axon and a nerve impulse will travel along the axon. If, on the other hand, the overall effect is one of hyperpolarization the neuron will be inhibited and no nerve impulse will arise.

DISTRIBUTION AND FATE OF NEUROTRANSMITTERS

The distribution of the neurotransmitters varies in different parts of the nervous system. **Acetylcholine** is found at the neuromuscular junction (see p. 133), in autonomic ganglia, and at parasympathetic nerve endings. In the central nervous system, the motor neuron collaterals to the **Renshaw cells** are cholinergic. In the hippocampus, the ascending reticular pathways, and the afferent fibers for the visual and auditory systems, the neurotransmitters are also cholinergic.

Norepinephrine is found at sympathetic nerve endings. In the central nervous system, it is found in high concentration in the hypothalamus. **Dopamine** is found in high concentration in different parts of the central nervous system, for example, in the basal ganglia.

The effect produced by a neurotransmitter is limited by its destruction or reabsorption. For example, in the case of acetylcholine, the effect is limited by the destruction of the transmitter in the synaptic gutter by the enzyme **acetylcholinesterase** (AChE) (Fig. 2-23). However, with the **catecholamines** the effect is limited by the return of the transmitter to the presynaptic nerve ending (Fig. 2-23).

CLINICAL NOTES

GENERAL CONSIDERATIONS

The neuron is the basic functional unit of the nervous system. If it is destroyed by trauma or disease it is not replaced. It is incapable of undergoing cell division. Millions of neurons are present within the nervous system, and they are linked together to form functional conducting pathways. They are supported by a framework of nonconducting cells referred to as the neuroglia.

Neurons may be classified according to the number of their processes as unipolar, bipolar, or multipolar; they also may be classified according to their size, the large Golgi type I neurons with long axons and the smaller Golgi type II neurons with short axons. All neurons have the common function of conducting impulses and serving the general function of control and integration. By this means, the activities of separate structures are integrated for the good of the entire body.

It has been seen that the neuron consists of the cell body and its processes, the axons, and the dendrites. All three parts are concerned with the process of conduction. It should be remembered, however, that the cell body is necessary for the normal metabolism of all its processes. Should these processes become separated from the cell body, as the result of disease or simple trauma, they will quickly degenerate. The complex physical and chemical processes involved in the response of a neuron to a stimulus and the mechanisms of nerve conduction will be discussed in a later chapter (see p. 105).

An examination of the structure of a neuron allows one to postulate the possible functions of its constituent parts. For example, the large numbers of unattached ribosomes are present presumably for the synthesis of enzymes and structural macromolecules. The presence of rough and smooth endoplasmic reticulum within the cell body indicates that the cell is producing large amounts of material that could be used for transcellular secretion. These synthetic functions are limited to the cell body and dendrites and are absent from the axon. This would explain the necessity for the transport of macromolecules down the axon from the cell body and also emphasizes the dependence of the axon on the cell body. The rate of axoplasmic transport is, however, insufficient to satisfy the release of transmitter substances at the nerve terminals. This problem is overcome in two ways. First, enzymes are present within the nerve terminals in order to synthesize the transmitters from amino acids derived from the extracellular fluid, and, second, at some terminals the transmitter is reabsorbed back into the terminal following its release. Clinically, it is possible, by the use of drugs, to influence this reuptake mechanism.

REACTION OF A NEURON TO INJURY

The first reaction of a nerve cell to injury is loss of function. Whether the cell recovers or dies will depend on the severity and duration of the damaging agent. If death occurs quickly, say in a few minutes from lack of oxygen, no morphological changes will be immediately apparent. Morphological evidence of cell injury requires a minimum of 6 to 12 hours of survival (Robbins and Angell, 1971). The nerve cell becomes swollen and rounded off, the nucleus swells and is displaced toward the periphery of the cell, and the Nissl granules become dispersed toward the periphery of the cytoplasm. At this stage the neuron could recover. If the kind of neuronal injury were not so severe as to cause death, the reparative changes would start to appear. The cell would resume its former size and shape, the nucleus would return to the center of the cell body, and the Nissl granules would take up their normal position.

When cell death is imminent or has just occurred, the cell cytoplasm stains dark with basic dyes (hyperchromatism) and the nuclear structure becomes unclear. The final stage occurs after cell death. The cytoplasm becomes vacuolated and the nucleus and cytoplasmic organelles disintegrate. The neuron now is dissolved and removed by the activity of the phagocytes. In the central nervous system this function is performed by the microglial cells and in the peripheral nervous system by local members of the reticuloendothelial system.

In chronic forms of injury, the size of the cell body is reduced, the nucleus and cytoplasm show hyperchromatism, and the nuclear membranes and those of the cytoplasmic organelles show irregularity.

Axonal Reaction or Axonal Degeneration

Axonal reaction or axonal degeneration are the changes that take place in a nerve cell when its axon is cut or injured. The changes start to appear within 24 to 48 hours after injury; the degree of change will depend on the severity of the injury to the axon, and will be greater if the injury occurred close to the cell body. The nerve cell becomes rounded off and swollen, the nucleus swells and becomes eccentrically placed, and the Nissl granules become dispersed toward the periphery of the cytoplasm. These changes reach their maximum in about 12 days.

In the peripheral nervous system, section of an axon is followed by attempts at regeneration and reparative changes take place in the cell body.

In the central nervous system there is degeneration that is not followed by regeneration. If the corticospinal tracts, for example, are destroyed by disease, the nerve cells that give rise to these axons degenerate and disappear completely.

There is an important exception to the axonal reaction of nerve cells described above. This occurs in the nerve cells of posterior root ganglia of spinal nerves. If the peripheral axons are sectioned, the nerve cells show degenerative changes; if, however, the central axons are sectioned or destroyed by disease, such as tabes dorsalis, the nerve cells show no degenerative changes.

TUMORS OF NEURONS

When considering tumors of the nervous system one must not forget that the nervous system is made up of many different types of tissues. In the central nervous system there are neurons, neuroglia, blood vessels, and meninges and in the peripheral nervous system there are neurons, Schwann cells, connective tissue, and blood vessels. Tumors of neurons in the central nervous system are rare but tumors of peripheral neurons are not uncommon (Florey, 1970).

The **neuroblastoma** occurs in association with the suprarenal gland; it is highly malignant and occurs in infants and children. The **ganglioneuroma** occurs in the suprarenal medulla or sympathetic ganglia; it is benign and occurs in children and adults. The **phaeochromocytoma** occurs in the suprarenal medulla; it is usually benign and gives rise to hypertension, since it secretes norepinephrine and epinephrine.

SYNAPTIC BLOCKING AGENTS

Transmission of a nervous impulse across a synapse is accomplished by the release of neurotransmitters into the synaptic gutter. Transmission occurs in one direction and subthreshold stimulation of many synapses leads to summation. The released transmitter then exerts its effect on the postsynaptic membrane, by increasing the permeability of the postsynaptic membrane to sodium and causing excitation or by increasing the permeability of the postsynaptic membrane to chloride and causing inhibition.

The synapse is a region in which transmission is easily blocked. As a general rule, long chains of neurons with multiple synapses are more easily blocked than shorter, simpler chains of neurons. General anesthetic agents are effective because they have the ability to block synaptic transmission.

At autonomic ganglia, preganglionic fibers enter the ganglia and synapse with the postganglionic sympathetic or parasympathetic neurons. The nerve impulse, on reaching the termination of the preganglionic nerve, brings about the release of **acetylcholine**, which excites a nervous impulse in the postganglionic neuron.

Ganglionic blocking agents may be divided into three groups, depending on their mechanism of action. The first group, which include the **hexamethonium** and **tetraethylammonium salts**, resemble acetylcholine at the postsynaptic membrane; they thus inhibit transmission across a synapse. The second group, which include **nicotine**, have the same action as acetylcholine on the postsynaptic membrane but they are not destroyed by the cholinesterase. This results in a prolonged depolarization of the postsynaptic membrane, so that it is insensitive to further stimulation by acetylcholine. Unfortunately, this depolarization block is associated with initial stimulation and therefore these drugs are not suitable for clinical use. The third group, which include **procaine**, inhibit the release of acetylcholine from the preganglionic fibers.

In the central nervous system, it is much more difficult to demonstrate the release of a particular transmitter substance at specific synapses due to inaccessibility. For example, with present techniques it is impossible to perfuse specific localized brain areas through their vascular system and it is very difficult to stimulate an isolated neuronal pathway within the brain or spinal cord. The motor neuron collaterals to the Renshaw cells have been shown to liberate acetylcholine at their endings. There is increasing evidence that many synapses in the central nervous system are also cholinergic.

The nonuniform concentrations of norepinephrine in the central nervous system have led many investigators to believe that it might function as a central neurotransmitter. The concentrations are greater in gray matter than in white matter and the highest concentrations are found in the hypothalamus. Dopamine is found in high concentrations in the central nervous system and is secreted by neurons that originate in the substantia nigra.

Many of the cholinergic blocking agents used in the peripheral nervous system have little or no effect on the cholinergic synapses of the central nervous system because they are unable to cross the blood-brain barrier in significant concentrations. **Atropine**, **scopolamine**, and **diisopropylphos-** phorofluoridate (DPF) can effectively cross the barrier and their effects on human behavior have been extensively studied. Similarly, it is believed that many psychotropic drugs bring about changes in the activities of the central nervous system by influencing the release of catecholamines at synaptic sites. The **phenothiazines**, for example, are thought to block dopamine receptors on postsynaptic neurons.

TREATMENT OF CERTAIN NEUROLOGICAL DISEASES BY THE MANIPULATION OF NEUROTRANSMITTERS

The increasing numbers of neurotransmitters being discovered in the central nervous system and the location of their site of action are raising the possibility that certain diseases can be modified by the administration of specific drugs. In Huntington's chorea, for example, there is a loss of neurons that use GABA and acetylcholine as transmitters. GABA is unable to cross the blood-brain barrier, but physostigmine, a cholinesterase inhibitor that can cross the barrier, has brought about some improvement. The use of L-dopa in the treatment of parkinsonism has been most successful; in this disease it replaces the deficiency of dopamine, which is normally released to the basal ganglia by the neurons of the substantia nigra.

CLINICAL PROBLEMS

Answers on Page 586

1. From 1 to 2 percent of the population of the United States suffer from mental deficiency of such severity to prevent them from becoming self-sufficient. Realizing that mental deficiency is a symptom that is initiated by a number of disease mechanisms, can you make a list of common diseases that have an effect on the normal development and function of neurons?

2. During an operation for repair of the radial nerve, which had been sectioned where it passes around the lateral aspect of the humerus and through the lateral intermuscular septum, the surgeon asked a medical student if the nerve fibers contained within the radial nerve were axons or dendrites, or was the nerve made up of a mixture of axons and dendrites. How would you have answered that question?

3. In a histological section of nervous tissue, one of the characteristic features noted is the large size of the nucleoli. What is the function of a nucleolus and why do you think it is large in nerve cells?

4. A well-known textbook of neurosurgery makes these statements regarding the prognosis following peripheral nerve repair: (a) The younger the patient, the better the return of function. (b) The more distal the injury to a nerve, the more effective regeneration will be. (c) The closer a lesion is to the nerve cell body, the more profound will be the effect on this trophic cen-

ter. (d) Sensory nerve cells are affected more by this retrograde phenomenon than are motor nerve cells. Comment on these statements.

5. An 18-year-old male patient was examined by a neurosurgeon 12 months after injury to the right forearm in which the median nerve was severed. At the initial operation, shortly after the injury had occurred, debridement was performed and the separated nerve ends were tagged with radiopaque sutures. Unfortunately, the wound was infected and surgical repair of the nerve was deferred. Is it practical to consider repairing a peripheral nerve after a delay of 12 months?

6. While examining a patient, a neurologist turned to a medical student and said, "The pyramidal cells in the cerebral cortex are type I Golgi neurons. What is the structural difference between type I and type II Golgi neurons?" How would you have answered this question?

7. During the examination of a cell body of a neuron in an electron micrograph, a student was puzzled by the number and varied appearance of membrane-bound vesicles seen within the cytoplasm. How would you classify the different types of vesicles found in the cytoplasm?

8. While examining a pathology specimen of nervous tissue under a microscope, the pathologist was able to determine the sex of the individual from whom the tissue had been removed. How would you be able to do this?

9. Axoplasmic flow is believed to be involved in the buildup of materials at the axon terminals for the production of transmitter substances. This is sometimes referred to as anterograde flow. Retrograde axoplasmic flow is also thought to occur. What structures present in the cytoplasm of the neuron are possibly involved in these processes?

10. According to Walton (1977), about 1 percent of all deaths are due to intracranial tumors. One must remember, however, that many different types of tissues are present within the skull in addition to the nervous system. Moreover, the nervous system itself is composed of many different types of tissues. In fact, tumors that arise as neoplasms of nerve cells and fibers are rare. Name the different types of tissues that are found in the central nervous system and in the peripheral nervous system.

11. When a nerve cell is stimulated the permeability of the plasma membrane changes, permitting certain ionic movements to take place across the membrane. (1) What is the structure of the plasma membrane? (2) Is the permeability of the plasma membrane increased or decreased when the nerve cell is stimulated? (3) What is the action of local analgesics on the cell membrane?

12. Define the following terms: (a) *synapse*, (b) *synaptic spine*, (c) *synaptic cleft*, and (d) *presynaptic vesicles*. (e) Give some examples of neurotransmitter substances found at synapses.

13. The synapse is a region where nervous transmission is easily blocked. Clinically, the ganglion-blocking drugs used act by competing with acetylcholine released from the nerve endings in the ganglia. Name two groups of drugs that have been used for this purpose and indicate the site at which they act.

14. With our present methods of investigation it is very difficult to determine the different types of neurotransmitters that act at specific synapses within the central nervous system. Name three possible chemicals that have been identified within the central nervous system and that may serve as neurotransmitters.

15. A 2-year-old boy was taken to a pediatrician because his mother had noticed that his right eye was protruding (proptosis). When questioned, the mother stated that she had first noticed this protrusion one month previously and that it had progressively worsened since that time. The child was otherwise perfectly fit. On physical examination, the child was observed to be healthy in every respect except for the marked proptosis of the right eye. A careful palpation of the abdomen, however, revealed a large, soft mass in the upper part of the abdomen that extended across the midline. X-ray examination, including a CT body scan, revealed a large, soft tissue mass that displaced the right kidney downward. A diagnosis of malignant tumor of the suprarenal or neighboring sympathetic nervous tissue was made with metastases in the right orbital cavity, the latter being responsible for the right-side proptosis. Name a tumor of the suprarenal gland or sympathetic nervous tissue that occurs commonly in children and may metastasize in the bones of the orbit.

NATIONAL BOARD TYPE QUESTIONS

Answers on Page 619

IN EACH OF THE FOLLOWING QUESTIONS, ANSWER:
- (a) IF (1) ONLY IS CORRECT
- (b) IF (2) ONLY IS CORRECT
- (c) IF BOTH (1) AND (2) ARE CORRECT, OR
- (d) IF NEITHER (1) NOR (2) IS CORRECT

1. Which of the following statements is (are) cor rect?
   - (1) A unipolar neuron is one that gives rise to a single neurite that remains unbranched until it reaches its destination and synapses with a second neuron. It is found in the anterior gray horn of the spinal cord.
   - (2) A bipolar neuron is one that gives rise to a neurite that emerges from each end of the cell body. The sensory ganglia of the vestibulocochlear nerve (eighth cranial nerve) possess bipolar neurons.

2. (1) Nissl substance is not found in the axon of a neuron.
   - (2) The Golgi apparatus is important in the synthesis of cell membranes.

3. (1) Melanin granules are found in the neurons of the substantia nigra, and it is these neurons that are responsible for the neurotransmitter dopamine.
   - (2) The protein molecules projecting from the surface of the microfilaments take part in a ratchetlike action in rapid transport in axoplasm.

4. (1) The protein molecules that extend through the full thickness of the plasma membrane of a neuron possibly serve as sodium and potassium channels.
   - (2) There is strong experimental evidence to suggest that the gates of the sodium and potassium channels are formed by actin molecules.

Select the best response:

5. The following statements concerning the axon are true **except**:
   - (a) The initial segment of the axon is the first 50 to 100 μm after it leaves the axon hillock.
   - (b) The nerve impulse generated by a neuron does not originate at the initial segment of an axon but on the dendrite.
   - (c) The action potential is produced by the sudden influx of Na^+ ions into the cytoplasm.
   - (d) Following the influx of Na^+ ions in the production of the action potential, the permeability for Na^+ ions ceases and that for K^+ ions increases, so that K^+ ions start to flow from the cell cytoplasm.
   - (e) The spread of the action potential along the plasma membrane of the axon constitutes the nerve impulse.

6. The following statements concerning a nerve impulse are true **except**:
   - (a) The refractory period is the duration of the nonexcitable state of the plasma membrane following the passage of a wave of depolarization.
   - (b) Subthreshold stimuli when applied to the surface of a neuron can be summated.
   - (c) Inhibitory stimuli are believed to produce their effect by causing an influx of K^+ ions through the plasma membrane of the neuron.
   - (d) Hyperpolarization can be produced by causing an influx of Cl^- ions through the plasma membrane.
   - (e) The axolemma is the site of nerve conduction.

7. The following statements concerning the structure of a synapse are true **except**:
   - (a) Synapses may be axodendritic, axosomatic, or axoaxonic.
   - (b) The synaptic cleft is the space between the presynaptic and postsynaptic membranes and measures about 20 nm.
   - (c) The subsynaptic web lies beneath the postsynaptic membrane.
   - (d) Presynaptic vesicles may contain the neurotransmitter substance.
   - (e) Most neurons produce and release many different types of transmitter substances at their nerve endings.

In the following questions, answer:
- (a) IF (1), (2), AND (3) ONLY ARE CORRECT
- (b) IF (1) AND (3) ONLY ARE CORRECT
- (c) IF (2) AND (4) ONLY ARE CORRECT
- (d) IF (4) ONLY IS CORRECT, OR
- (e) IF ALL ARE CORRECT

8. Which of the following statements is (are) correct concerning the neuron?
   (1) Nerve fibers are the dendrites and axons of a neuron.
   (2) Golgi type II neurons have very long axons.
   (3) Golgi type I neurons form the Purkinje cells of the cerebellar cortex.
   (4) The volume of cytoplasm within the nerve cell body always far exceeds that found in the neurites.
9. Which of the following statements is (are) correct concerning the neuron organelles and inclusions?
   (1) The Nissl substance fills the axon hillock but is absent from other areas of the cytoplasm.
   (2) Centrioles are found in dividing nerve cells but are not seen in mature cells.
   (3) Lipofuscin granules are found in immature nerve cells and later disappear.
   (4) Microfilaments contain actin and myosin and probably assist in cell transport.
10. Which of the following statements is (are) correct concerning a dendrite?
    (1) A dendrite conveys a nerve impulse toward the nerve cell body.

    (2) Dendritic spines are small projections of the plasma membrane to increase the receptor surface area of the dendrite.
    (3) The cytoplasm of dendrites contains Nissl granules, mitochondria, microtubules, microfilaments, ribosomes, and agranular endoplasmic reticulum.
    (4) Most dendrites expand in width as they extend from the nerve cell body.

Match the structures associated with a neuron listed below on the left with appropriate structures listed below on the right. Answers may be used more than once.

11. Lysosome
12. Terminal bouton
13. Receptor
14. Microtubule
15. Nissl substance

(a) Rough endoplasmic reticulum
(b) Membrane-bound vesicle
(c) Presynaptic part of axon
(d) Protein molecule on postsynaptic membrane
(e) None of the above

ADDITIONAL READING

Aguayo, A. J., Benfey, M., and David, S. A. Potential for axonal regeneration in neurons of the adult mammalian nervous system. *Birth Defects* 19(4):327, 1983.

Barr, M. L. The significance of the sex chromatin. *Int. Rev. Cytol.* 19:35, 1966.

Bernstein, J. J., and Bernstein, E. M. Axonal regeneration and formation of synapses proximal to the site of lesion following hemisection of the rat spinal cord. *Exp. Neurol.* 30:336, 1971.

Berry, M. Regeneration of axons in the central nervous system. In V. Navaratnam and R. J. Harrison (eds.) *Progress in Anatomy*. New York: Cambridge University Press, 1983. Vol. 3, p. 213.

Bodian, D. Synaptic types on spinal motorneurons: An electron microscopic study. *Johns Hopkins Med. J.* 119:16, 1966.

Catterall, W. A. The molecular basis of neural excitability. *Science* 223:653, 1984.

Cooper, J. R., Bloom, F. E., and Roth, R. H. *The Biochem-*

ical Basis of Neuropharmacology (4th ed.). New York: Oxford University Press, 1983.

Grafstein, B., and Forman, D. S. Intracellular transport in neurons. *Physiol. Rev.* 60:1167, 1980.

Heuser, J. E., and Reese, T. S. Evidence for recycling of synaptic vesicle membrane during transmitter release of the frog neuromuscular junction. *J. Cell. Biol.* 57:315, 1973.

Hille, B. *Ionic Channels in Excitable Membranes*. Sunderland, Massachusetts: Sinauer Associates, 1984.

Kelly, R. B., et al. Biochemistry of neurotransmitter release. *Annu. Rev. Neurosci.* 2:399, 1979.

Krogsgaard-Larsen, P., et al. (eds.). *GABA-Neuro-transmitters*. New York: Academic, 1979.

Kupfermann, I. Modulatory actions of neurotransmitters. *Annu. Rev. Neurosci.* 2:447, 1979.

Langer, S. Z. Presynaptic regulation of the release of catecholamines. *Pharmacol. Rev.* 32:337, 1980.

McEwen, B. S., and Grafstein, B. Fast and slow components in axonal transport of protein. *J. Cell. Biol.* 38:494, 1968.

Moore, R. Y., and Bloom, F. E. Central catecholamine neuron systems: Anatomy and physiology of the dopamine systems. *Annu. Rev. Neurosci.* 1:129, 1978.

Mugnaini, E. The relation between cytogenesis and the formation of different types of synaptic contact. *Brain Res.* 17:169, 1970.

Nicoll, R. A., et al. Substance P as a transmitter candidate. *Annu. Rev. Neurosci.* 3:227, 1980.

Robbins, S. L., Cotran, R. S., and Kumar, V. *Pathologic Basis of Disease* (3rd ed.). Philadelphia: Saunders, 1984.

Siegel, G. J., Albers, R. W., Katzman, R., and Agranoff, B. W. *Basic Neurochemistry* (2nd ed.). Boston: Little, Brown, 1976.

Simon, P. (Ed.). *Neurotransmitters*. New York: Pergamon, 1979.

Stevens, C. F. The neuron. *Sci. Am.* 241:54, 1979.

Veraa, R. P., and Grafstein, B. Cellular mechanisms for recovery from nervous system injury. *Exp. Neurol.* 71:6, 1981.

Walton, J. N. *Brain's Diseases of the Nervous System* (9th ed.). New York: Oxford University Press, 1984.

Chapter 3
Neuroglia

The neurons of the central nervous system are supported by several varieties of nonexcitable cells, which together are called **neuroglia** (Fig. 3-1). Neuroglial cells are generally smaller than neurons and outnumber them 5 to 10 times; they comprise about half the total volume of the brain and spinal cord.

There are four types of neuroglial cells: (1) astrocytes, (2) oligodendrocytes, (3) microglia, and (4) ependyma (Fig. 3-1).

ASTROCYTES

Astrocytes have small cell bodies with branching processes that extend in all directions. There are two types of astrocytes: fibrous and protoplasmic.

Fibrous astrocytes are found mainly in the white matter, where their processes pass between the nerve fibers (Fig. 3-2). Each process is long, slender, smooth, and not much branched. The cell bodies and processes contain many filaments in their cytoplasm.

Protoplasmic astrocytes are found mainly in the gray matter, where their processes pass between the nerve cell bodies (Figs. 3-3 and 3-4). The processes are shorter, thicker, and more branched than those of the fibrous astrocyte. The cytoplasm of these cells contains fewer filaments than that of the fibrous astrocyte.

Many of the processes of astrocytes end in expansions on blood vessels (perivascular feet), where they form an almost complete covering on the external surface of capillaries. Large numbers of astrocytic processes are interwoven at the outer and inner surfaces of the central nervous system, where they form the **outer** and **inner glial limiting membranes**. Thus the outer glial limiting membrane is found beneath the pia mater and the inner glial limiting membrane is situated beneath the ependyma lining the ventricles of the brain and the central canal of the spinal cord.

Astrocytic processes are also found in large numbers around the initial segment of most axons and in the bare segments of axons at the nodes of Ranvier. Axon terminals at many sites are separated from other nerve cells and their processes by an envelope of astrocytic processes.

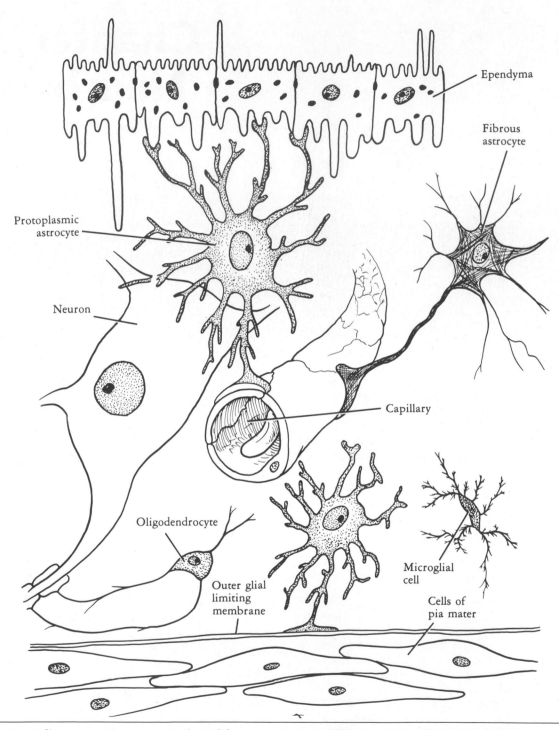

Ependyma

Fibrous
astrocyte

Protoplasmic
astrocyte

Neuron

Capillary

Oligodendrocyte

Outer glial
limiting
membrane

Microglial
cell

Cells of
pia mater

Fig. 3-1. A diagrammatic representation of the arrangement of different types of neuroglial cells.

Capillary with astrocytic foot processes   Microglial cell   Oligodendrocyte

A Fibrous astrocytes   **B**   Astrocyte   Microglial cell

Fig. 3-2. A. Photomicrograph of section of gray matter of spinal cord showing fibrous astrocytes.
B. Electron micrograph showing an astrocyte.
(Courtesy Dr. J. M. Kerns.)

Functions of Astrocytes

Astrocytes with their branching processes form a supporting framework for the nerve cells and nerve fibers. In the embryo they serve as a scaffolding for the migration of immature neurons. By covering the synaptic contacts between neurons they may serve as electrical insulators preventing axon terminals from influencing neighboring and unrelated neurons. They may even form barriers for the spread of neurotransmitter substances released at synapses. Astrocytes have been shown to absorb gamma-aminobutyric acid (GABA) and glutamic acid secreted by the nerve terminals, thereby limiting the influence of these neurotransmitters. Astrocytes appear to be able to take up excess K^+ ions from the extracellular space. They store glycogen within their cytoplasm. The glycogen can be broken down into glucose and released to surrounding neurons in response to norepinephrine.

Astrocytes may serve as phagocytes by taking up degenerating synaptic axon terminals. Following the death of neurons due to disease, they proliferate and fill in the spaces previously occupied by the

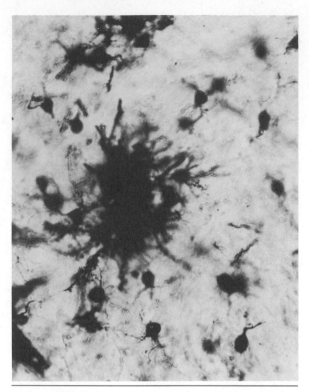

Fig. 3-3. Photomicrograph of a protoplasmic astrocyte in the cerebral cortex.

neurons, a process called **replacement gliosis**. It is possible that astrocytes can serve as a conduit for the passage of metabolites or raw materials from blood capillaries to the neurons through their perivascular feet. The fact that astrocytes are linked together by gap junctions would enable ions to pass from one cell to another without entering the extracellular space. Astrocytes may produce substances that have a trophic influence on neighboring neurons.

OLIGODENDROCYTES

Oligodendrocytes have small cell bodies and a few delicate processes; there are no filaments in their cytoplasm. Oligodendrocytes are frequently found in rows along myelinated nerve fibers and surround nerve cell bodies (Fig. 3-5). Electron micrographs show the processes of a single oligodendrocyte join the myelin sheaths of several nerve fibers

(Fig. 3-6). However, only one process joins the myelin between two adjacent nodes of Ranvier.

Functions of Oligodendrocytes

Oligodendrocytes are responsible for the formation of the myelin sheath of nerve fibers in the central nervous system, much as the myelin of peripheral nerves is formed from Schwann cells (see p. 91). Because oligodendrocytes have several processes, unlike Schwann cells, they can each form several internodal segments of myelin on the same or different axons. A single oligodendrocyte can form as many as sixty internodal segments. Myelination begins at about the sixteenth week of intrauterine life and continues postnatally until practically all the major nerve fibers are myelinated by the time the child is walking.

Oligodendrocytes also surround nerve cell bodies (satellite oligodendrocytes) and probably have a similar function to the satellite or capsular cells of peripheral sensory ganglia. They are thought to influence the biochemical environment of neurons.

MICROGLIA

The microglial cells are the smallest of the neuroglial cells and are found scattered throughout the central nervous system (Fig. 3-7). From their small cell bodies arise wavy branching processes that give off numerous spinelike projections. They closely resemble connective tissue macrophages. They migrate into the nervous system during fetal life. Microglial cells increase in number in the presence of damaged nervous tissue and many of these new cells are monocytes that have migrated from the blood.

Function of Microglial Cells

Microglial cells in the normal brain and spinal cord appear to be inactive and are sometimes called **resting microglial cells**. In inflammatory and degenerative lesions of the central nervous system, they retract their processes and migrate to the site of the lesion. Here they proliferate and are actively phagocytic; their cytoplasm becomes filled with lipids and cell remnants. The microglial cells are joined by monocytes from neighboring blood vessels.

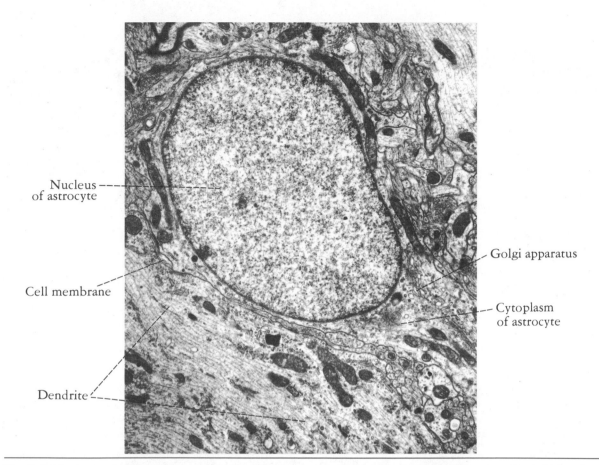

Nucleus of astrocyte

Cell membrane

Dendrite

Golgi apparatus

Cytoplasm of astrocyte

Fig. 3-4. Electron micrograph of a protoplasmic astrocyte in the cerebral cortex. (Courtesy Dr. A. Peters.)

EPENDYMA

Ependymal cells line the cavities of the brain and the central canal of the spinal cord. They form a single layer of cells that are cuboidal or columnar in shape and possess microvilli and cilia (Fig. 3-8). The cilia are often motile and their movements contribute to the flow of the cerebrospinal fluid. The bases of the ependymal cells lie on the internal glial limiting membrane.

Ependymal cells may be divided into three groups:

1. **Ependymocytes**, which line the ventricles of the brain and the central canal of the spinal cord and are in contact with the cerebrospinal fluid. Their adjacent surfaces have gap junctions, but the cerebrospinal fluid is in free communication with the intercellular spaces of the central nervous system.

2. **Tanycytes**, which line the floor of the third ventricle overlying the median eminence of the hypothalamus. These cells have long basal processes that pass between the cells of the median eminence and place end feet on blood capillaries.

3. **Choroidal epithelial cells**, which cover the surfaces of the choroid plexuses. The sides and bases of these cells are thrown into folds and near their luminal surfaces the cells are held together by tight junctions that encircle the cells. The presence of tight junctions prevents the leakage of cerebrospinal fluid into the underlying tissues.

Oligodendrocytes

A

B

Fig. 3-5. A. Photomicrograph of a group of oligodendrocytes.
B. Electron micrograph of two oligodendrocytes.
(Courtesy Dr. J. M. Kerns.)

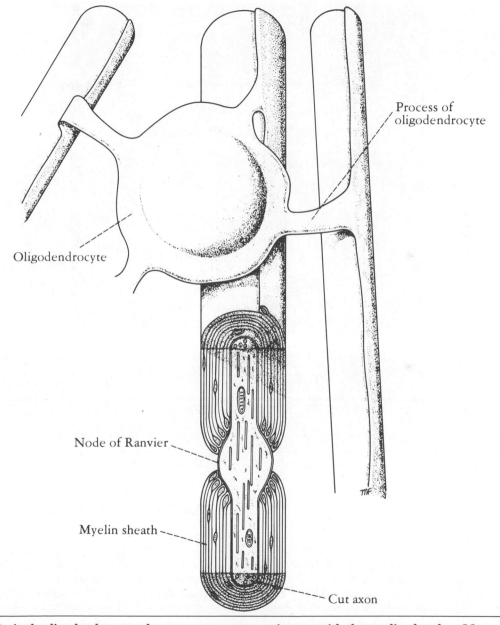

Process of
oligodendrocyte

Oligodendrocyte

Node of Ranvier

Myelin sheath

Cut axon

Fig. 3-6. A single oligodendrocyte whose processes are continuous with the myelin sheaths of four nerve fibers within the central nervous system.

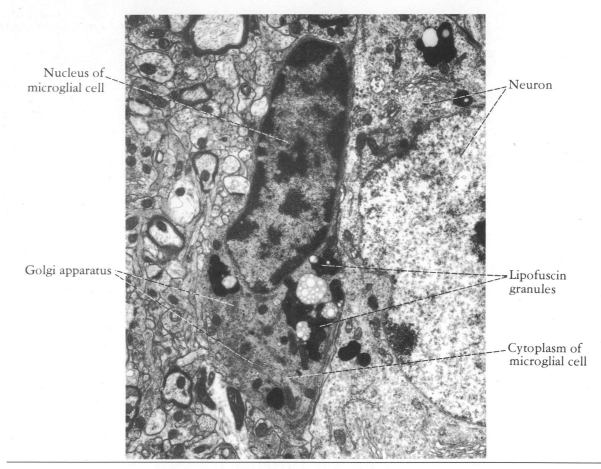

Nucleus of microglial cell

Neuron

Golgi apparatus

Lipofuscin granules

Cytoplasm of microglial cell

Fig. 3-7. Electron micrograph of a microglial cell in the cerebral cortex. (Courtesy Dr. A. Peters.)

Functions of Ependymal Cells

Ependymocytes assist in the circulation of the cerebrospinal fluid within the cavities of the brain and the central canal of the spinal cord by the movements of the cilia. The microvilli on the free surfaces of the ependymocytes would indicate that they also have an absorptive function. Tanycytes are thought to transport chemical substances from the cerebrospinal fluid to the hypophyseal portal system. In this manner they may play a part in the control of the hormone production by the anterior lobe of the pituitary. Choroidal epithelial cells are involved in the production and secretion of cerebrospinal fluid from the choroid plexuses.

EXTRACELLULAR SPACE

When nervous tissue is examined under an electron microscope, a very narrow gap separates the neurons and the neuroglial cells. These gaps are linked together and filled with tissue fluid; they are called the **extracellular space**. The extracellular space is in almost direct continuity with the cerebrospinal

Fig. 3-8. A. Photomicrograph of ependymal cells lining central canal of spinal cord.
B. Electron micrograph of ependymal cells lining cavity of third ventricle.
(Courtesy Dr. J. M. Kerns.)

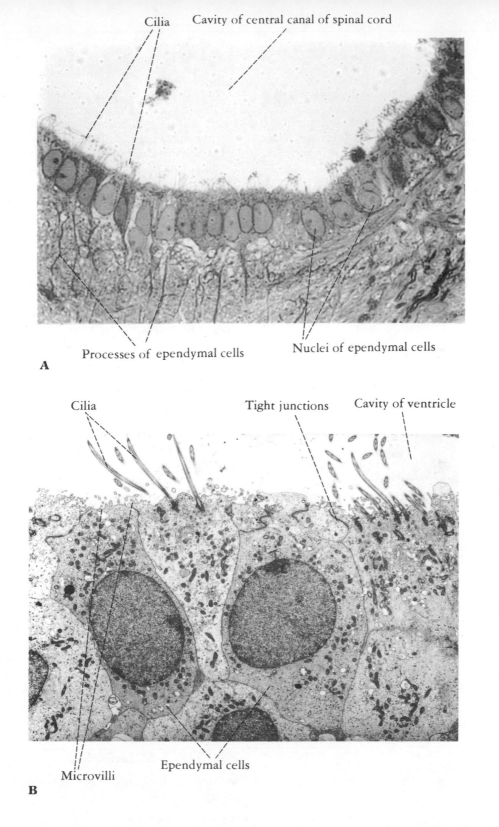

Cilia

Cavity of central canal of spinal cord

Processes of ependymal cells

Nuclei of ependymal cells

A

Cilia

Tight junctions

Cavity of ventricle

Microvilli

Ependymal cells

B

fluid in the subarachnoid space externally and with the cerebrospinal fluid in the ventricles of the brain and the central canal of the spinal cord internally. The extracellular space also surrounds the blood capillaries in the brain and spinal cord. (There are no lymphatic capillaries in the central nervous system.)

The extracellular space thus provides a pathway for the exchange of ions and molecules between the blood and the neurons and glial cells. The plasma membrane of the endothelial cells of most capillaries is impermeable to many chemicals, and this forms the blood-brain barrier (see p. 355).

CLINICAL NOTES

Neuroglial cells, in contrast to neurons, are nonexcitable and do not have axons, nor do axon terminals synapse upon them. They are smaller than neurons and yet outnumber them 5 to 10 times. They comprise about one-half the total volume of the central nervous system.

Four types have been described: (1) astrocytes, (2) oligodendrocytes, (3) microglial cells, and (4) ependymal cells. Clinicians often refer to astrocytes and oligodendrocytes as **macroglial cells** to distinguish them from the microglial cells, which are very much smaller.

REACTIONS OF NEUROGLIA TO INJURY

The reaction of neuroglial cells to injury, whether caused by physical trauma or by vascular occlusion, is characterized by the hyperplasia and hypertrophy of the astrocytes, which become fibrous irrespective of their antecedent morphology. The proliferation of the astrocytes is referred to as **astrocytosis** or **gliosis**. The loss of neuronal tissue is not compensated for in volume by the glial hypertrophy. The cytoplasm of the enlarged astrocytes contains large numbers of fibrils and glycogen granules. The dense feltwork of astrocytic processes that occurs in the areas of neuronal degeneration produces the so-called **gliotic scar**. The degree of gliosis is much greater in the presence of residual damaged neuronal tissue as compared with a clean surgical excision in which no traumatized brain remains. This is why, in patients with focal epilepsy due to a large gliotic scar, the scar is excised surgically, leaving a minimal glial reaction.

Oligodendrocytes respond to injury by expanding and showing vacuolation of their cytoplasm; the nuclei also tend to become pyknotic. Severe damage to oligodendrocytes would result in demyelination.

Microglial cells in inflammatory and degenerative lesions of the central nervous system retract their processes and migrate to the site of the lesion. Here they proliferate and are actively phagocytic and their cytoplasm becomes filled with lipids and cell remnants. They are joined in their scavenger activity by monocytes that migrate from the neighboring blood vessels.

NEOPLASMS OF NEUROGLIA

According to Walton (1977) tumors of neuroglia account for 40 to 45 percent of intracranial tumors. Such tumors are referred to as *gliomas*. Tumors of astrocytes are those most commonly encountered and include *astrocytomas*, *glioblastomas*, and *medulloblastomas*. Apart from the ependymomas, tumors of the neuroglia are highly invasive. This explains the difficulty in achieving complete surgical removal and the great possibility of recurrence after surgery. Another feature is that as these tumors infiltrate they often do so without interfering with the function of neighboring neurons. As a result, the tumor is often very much larger than the symptoms and physical signs would indicate.

MULTIPLE SCLEROSIS

Multiple sclerosis (MS) is one of the most common central nervous system diseases and affects about

250,000 Americans. It is characterized by the appearance of patches of demyelination in the white matter of the central nervous system, generally starting in the optic nerve, spinal cord, or cerebellum. The myelin sheaths degenerate and the myelin is removed, leading to the proliferation of astrocytes and the formation of a gliotic scar. As demyelination occurs, the conduction of the nerve impulses in the axons is impeded. Because raising the temperature shortens the duration of the action potential, one of the early signs of multiple sclerosis is that the symptoms and signs can be improved by cooling and made worse by heating by a hot bath. Most cases occur between the ages of 20 and 40. The cause of the disease is unknown, although an interplay between a viral infection and a host immune response may be responsible.

CLINICAL PROBLEMS

Answers on Page 588

1. At an autopsy a third-year medical student was handed a slice of the cerebrum and was asked what proportion of central nervous tissue is made up by neuroglia. How would you have answered that question? Which cells are present in the largest numbers, neurons or neuroglial cells?

2. A neurologist, while discussing the different types of intracranial tumors, repeatedly used the term *macroglia*. What is macroglia? How does macroglia differ from microglia? What is neuroglia?

3. At the end of a seminar entitled "The Neuroglia," a physiologist, a pathologist, and an anatomist took part in an intense discussion on the possible functions of neuroglia in the central nervous system. What do you know about the functions of neuroglial cells?

4. A 23-year-old man, while in the army in Vietnam, received a penetrating gunshot wound to the left side of his head. At the operation the neurosurgeon was able to remove the bullet from the left frontal lobe of his brain. Apart from a slight weakness of his right leg, the patient made an uneventful recovery. Eighteen months later the patient started to have severe generalized attacks of convulsions, during which he lost consciousness. Since this time the attacks have occurred irregularly at about monthly intervals. Each attack is preceded by a feeling of mental irritability, and twitching of the right leg occurs. A diagnosis of epilepsy was made by the examining neurologist. Is it possible that this patient's attacks of epilepsy are related to his gunshot wound in Vietnam? Is traumatic epilepsy a common condition? What treatment would you recommend?

5. A 42-year-old woman visited her physician because she was suffering from very severe headaches. Until six months ago she experienced only an occasional mild headache. Since that time her headaches gradually have become more severe and their duration has increased. They now last three or four hours and are so intense that she has to lie down. She has felt sick on two occasions but she has vomited on only one occasion. The headaches are generalized in nature and are made worse by coughing or straining. A physical examination revealed swelling of both optic discs with congestion of the retinal veins and the presence of multiple retinal hemorrhages. Weakness of the lateral rectus muscle of the right eye also was detected. Anteroposterior radiographs of the skull showed displacement of the calcified pineal gland to the left side. Anteroposterior and lateral radiographs of the skull showed some degree of calcification in a localized area in the right cerebral hemisphere. These findings, together with those obtained from CT scans of the brain and MRIs, made the diagnosis of a right-sided cerebral tumor certain. Surgical exploration confirmed the presence of a large infiltrating tumor of the right parietal lobe. What is the commonest type of tumor found in such a site in a middle-aged patient? How would you treat such a patient?

NATIONAL BOARD TYPE QUESTIONS

Answers on Page 619.

In each of the following questions, answer:
- (a) If (1) only is correct
- (b) If (2) only is correct
- (c) If both (1) and (2) are correct, or
- (d) If neither (1) nor (2) is correct

1. Which of the following statements is (are) correct?
   (1) Fibrous astrocytes are located mainly in the white matter of the central nervous system.
   (2) Replacement gliosis follows the death of neurons in the central nervous system and is due to the proliferation of oligodendrocytes.

2. Which of the following statements is (are) correct?
   (1) The inner glial limiting membrane is formed by the processes of astrocytes situated beneath the pia mater.
   (2) Astrocytes are involved in the absorption of gamma-aminobutyric acid (GABA) secreted by the nerve terminals.

3. Which of the following statements is (are) correct?
   (1) Oligodendrocytes are responsible for the formation of the myelin of nerve fibers in the central nervous system.
   (2) Unlike Schwann cells in the peripheral nervous system, a single oligodendrocyte can form by means of its many processes several internodal segments of myelin on the same or different axons.

Select the best response:

4. The following statements concerning the microglial cells is (are) correct **except**:
   (a) Microglial cells resemble connective tissue macrophages.
   (b) Microglial cells are smaller than astrocytes or oligodendrocytes.
   (c) Microglial cells migrate into the central nervous system during fetal life.
   (d) In the presence of damaged neurons microglial cells increase in number.
   (e) In degenerative lesions of the central nervous system, the circulating blood contributes no cells to the population of microglial cells.

5. The following statements concerning the ependymal cells is (are) correct **except**:
   (a) The ependymal cells form a single layer and many possess microvilli and cilia.
   (b) The ependymocytes line the ventricular system but permit the cerebrospinal fluid to enter the extracellular spaces of the nervous tissue.
   (c) Tanycytes have long, branching basal processes, many of which have end feet placed on the capillaries of the median eminence.
   (d) Choroidal epithelial cells secrete cerebrospinal fluid.
   (e) Ependymal cells are incapable of absorbing substances from the cerebrospinal fluid.

6. The following statements concerning the extracellular space is (are) true **except**:
   (a) The space is formed by the gaps between the neurons and the neuroglial cells.
   (b) The space surrounds the lymphatic capillaries present in the brain and spinal cord.
   (c) The space is in almost direct continuity with the subarachnoid space.
   (d) The space is filled with tissue fluid.
   (e) The space is continuous with the synaptic cleft between two neurons.

In the following questions, answer:
- (a) If (1), (2), and (3) only are correct
- (b) If (1) and (3) only are correct
- (c) If (2) and (4) only are correct
- (d) If (4) only is correct, or
- (e) If all are correct

7. Which of the following statements is (are) correct concerning tumors of neuroglia?
   (1) They form about 40 to 45 percent of all intracranial tumors.
   (2) Apart from the ependymomas, tumors of neuroglia are highly invasive.
   (3) They commonly infiltrate between neurons causing initially the minimum disturbance of function.
   (4) They are nonmalignant and easily removed surgically.

8. Which of the following statements is (are) correct concerning the neuroglial cells?
    (1) They tend to be larger than nerve cell bodies.
    (2) Multiple sclerosis is a disease involving the oligodendrocyte.
    (3) Oligodendrocytes are confined to the neurites of a neuron and are not found close to nerve cell bodies.
    (4) Heat reduces the action potential in an axon and accentuates the signs and symptoms in multiple sclerosis.

Match the features listed below on the left with the appropriate neuroglial cells listed below on the right. Answers may be used more than once.

9. Wavy processes with spinelike projections
10. Forms scaffold for developing neurons
11. Processes are continuous with myelin sheath
12. Cilia

(a) Ependyma
(b) Microglia
(c) Astrocytes
(d) Oligodendrocytes
(e) None of the above

ADDITIONAL READING

Bannister, R. *Brain's Clinical Neurology* (6th ed.). London and New York: Oxford University Press, 1985.

Berry, M. Neurogenesis and gliogenesis in the human brain. *Food Chem. Toxicol.* 24:79, 1986.

Hayes, G. M., Woodroofe, M. N., and Cuzner, M. L. Characterization of microglia isolated from adult human brain. *J. Neuroimmunol.* 19:177, 1988.

Henn, F. A., and Henn, S. W. The psychopharmacology of astroglial cells. *Prog. Neurobiol.* 15:1, 1983.

Hertz, L. Functional Interactions between Astrocytes and Neurons. In *Glial and Neuronal Cell Biology.* New York: Liss, 1981, p. 45.

Imamoto, V. Origin of Microglia: Cell Transformation from Blood Monocytes into Macrophagic Ameboid Cells and Microglia. In *Glial and Neuronal Cell Biology.* New York: Liss, 1981, p. 125.

Kuffler, S. W., and Nicholls, J. G. *From Neuron to Brain.* Sunderland, Massachusetts: Sinauer Associates, 1976.

Peters, A., Palay, S. L., and Webster, H. *The Fine Structure of the Nervous System: The Neurons and Supporting Cells.* Philadelphia: Saunders, 1976.

Robbins, S. L., Cortran, R. S., and Kumar, V. *Pathologic Basis of Disease* (3rd ed.). Philadelphia: Saunders, 1984.

Robertson, M. Nerves, myelin and multiple sclerosis. *Nature (Lond.)* 290:357, 1981.

Sudarsky, L. *Pathophysiology of the Nervous System.* Boston: Little, Brown, 1990.

Varon, S. S., and Somjen, G. G. (eds.). Neuron-glia interactions. *Neurosci. Res. Progr. Bull.* 17:1, 1979.

Watson, W. E. Physiology of neuroglia. *Physiol. Rev.* 54:245, 1974.

Chapter 4
Nerve Fibers and Peripheral Nerves

NERVE FIBERS

A nerve fiber is the name given to an axon (or a dendrite) of a nerve cell. The structure of axons and dendrites is described on page 62. Bundles of nerve fibers found in the central nervous system are often referred to as **nerve tracts** (Fig. 4-1); bundles of nerve fibers found in the peripheral nervous system are called **peripheral nerves** (Fig. 4-2).

Two types of nerve fibers are present in the central and peripheral parts of the nervous system, namely, myelinated and nonmyelinated fibers.

MYELINATED NERVE FIBERS

A myelinated nerve fiber is one that is surrounded by a myelin sheath. The myelin sheath is not part of the neuron but is formed by a supporting cell (Figs. 4-2 and 4-3). In the central nervous system the supporting cell is called the oligodendrocyte; in the peripheral nervous system it is called the Schwann cell.

The myelin sheath is a segmented, discontinuous layer interrupted at regular intervals by the **nodes of Ranvier** (Figs. 4-4 and 4-6). Each segment of the myelin sheath measures approximately 0.5 to 1 mm in length. In the central nervous system each oligodendrocyte may form and maintain myelin sheaths for as many as 60 nerve fibers (axons). In the peripheral nervous system there is only one Schwann cell for each segment of one nerve fiber.

Formation of Myelin

Myelin sheaths begin to form before birth and during the first year postnatally. The process has been studied with the electron microscope.

In the **peripheral nervous system**, the nerve fiber or axon first indents the side of a Schwann cell (Fig. 4-4). Later, as the axon sinks farther into the Schwann cell, the external plasma membrane of the Schwann cell forms a **mesaxon**, which suspends the axon within the Schwann cell. Subsequently, it is thought, the Schwann cell rotates on the axon so that the plasma membrane becomes

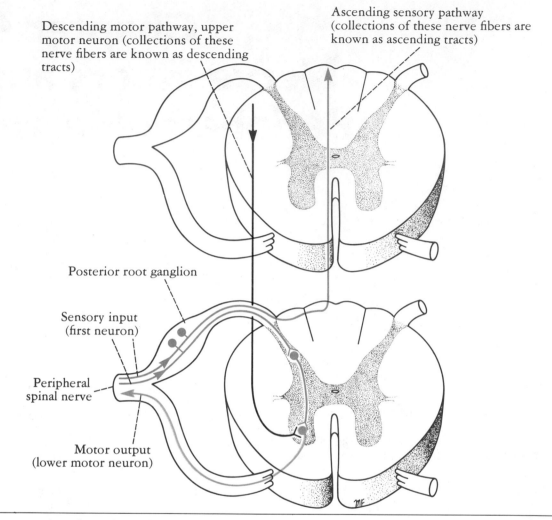

Descending motor pathway, upper motor neuron (collections of these nerve fibers are known as descending tracts)

Ascending sensory pathway (collections of these nerve fibers are known as ascending tracts)

Posterior root ganglion

Sensory input (first neuron)

Peripheral spinal nerve

Motor output (lower motor neuron)

Fig. 4-1. Sections through the thoracic region of the spinal cord showing examples of nerve fibers entering or leaving the central nervous system; ascending and descending nerve fibers (tracts or pathways) are also shown.

Fig. 4-2. Exploded view of a peripheral nerve, showing the connective tissue sheaths and the structure of myelinated and nonmyelinated nerve fibers.

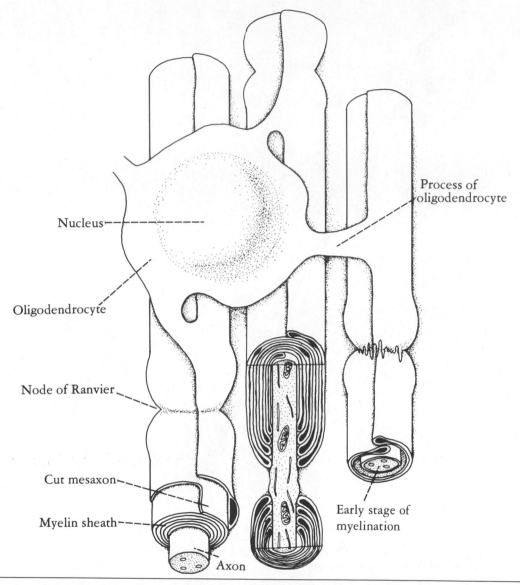

Nucleus

Process of oligodendrocyte

Oligodendrocyte

Node of Ranvier

Cut mesaxon

Myelin sheath

Axon

Early stage of myelination

Fig. 4-3. The relationship between an oligodendrocyte and myelinated nerve fibers in the central nervous system.

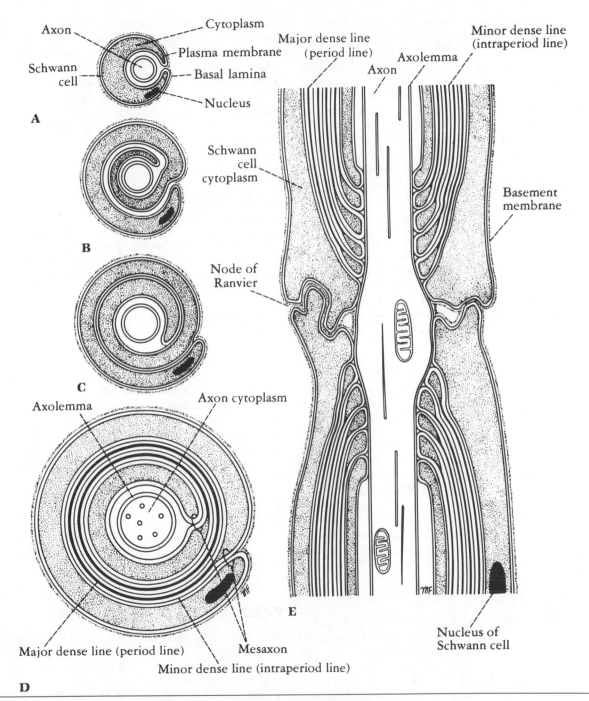

Fig. 4-4. A myelinated nerve fiber in the peripheral nervous system.
A, B, C, and D. Cross sections showing the stages in the formation of the myelin sheath.
E. A longitudinal section of a mature myelinated nerve fiber showing a node of Ranvier.

wrapped around and around the axon in a spiral. The direction of the spiral is clockwise in some segments and counterclockwise in others. To begin with, the wrappings are loose, but gradually the cytoplasm between the layers of the cell membrane disappears, leaving cytoplasm near the surface and in the region of the nucleus. The wrappings become tight with maturation of the nerve fiber. The thickness of the myelin depends on the number of spirals of Schwann cell membrane. Some nerve fibers are surrounded by only a few turns of the membrane while others have as many as 50 turns. In electron micrographs of cross sections of mature myelinated nerve fibers, the myelin is seen to be laminated (Fig. 4-5). Each lamella measures 13 to 18 nm thick. The dark **major dense line**, about 2.5 nm thick, consists of two inner protein layers of the plasma membrane that are fused together. The lighter **minor dense line**, about 10 nm thick, is formed by the approximation of the outer surfaces of adjacent plasma membranes and is made up of lipid. The fused outer protein layers of the plasma membranes are very thin and form a thin intraperiod line situated in the center of the lighter lipid layer (Figs. 4-4 and 4-5). At the node of Ranvier, two adjacent Schwann cells terminate and the myelin sheaths become thinner by the turning off of the lamellae (Fig. 4-6). At these regions the plasma membrane of the axon, the axolemma, is exposed.

The **incisures of Schmidt-Lanterman** are seen on longitudinal sections of myelinated nerve fibers. They represent areas where the dark major dense line is not formed as a result of the localized persistence of Schwann cell cytoplasm (Fig. 4-7). This persistence of cytoplasm involves all the layers of the myelin and thus there is a continuous spiral of cytoplasm from the outermost region of the Schwann cell to the region of the axon. This spiral of cytoplasm may provide a pathway for the conduction of metabolites from the surface region of the Schwann cell to the axon.

In the **central nervous system**, oligodendrocytes are responsible for the formation of the myelin sheaths. The plasma membrane of the oligodendrocyte becomes wrapped around the axon and the number of layers will determine the thickness of the myelin sheath (Fig. 4-3). The **nodes of Ranvier** are situated in the intervals between adjacent oligodendrocytes. A single oligodendrocyte may be connected to the myelin sheaths for as many as 60 nerve fibers. For this reason, the process of myelination in the central nervous system cannot take place by rotation of the oligodendrocyte on the axon, as did the Schwann cell in the peripheral nervous system. It is possible that myelination in the central nervous system occurs by the growth in length of the process of the oligodendrocyte, the process wrapping itself around the axon. There are incisures of Schmidt-Lanterman in nerve fibers of the central nervous system.

NONMYELINATED NERVE FIBERS

The smaller axons of the central nervous system, the postganglionic axons of the autonomic part of the nervous system, and some fine sensory axons associated with the reception of pain are nonmyelinated.

In the **peripheral nervous system** each axon, which is usually less than 1 μm in diameter, indents the surface of the Schwann cell so that it lies within a trough (Fig. 4-2). As many as 15 or more axons may share a single Schwann cell, each lying within its own trough or sometimes sharing a trough. In some situations the troughs are deep and the axons are embedded deep in the Schwann cells, forming a **mesaxon** from the Schwann cell plasma membrane (Figs. 4-5 and 4-8). The Schwann cells lie close to one another along the length of the axons and there are no nodes of Ranvier.

In areas where there are synapses or where motor transmission occurs, the axon emerges from the trough of the Schwann cell for a short distance, thus exposing the active region of the axon (Fig. 4-9).

In the **central nervous system** nonmyelinated nerve fibers run in small groups and are not particularly related to the oligodendrocytes.

PERIPHERAL NERVES

The peripheral nerves are the cranial and spinal nerves. Each peripheral nerve consists of parallel bundles of nerve fibers, which may be efferent or afferent axons, and may be myelinated or nonmyelinated, and are surrounded by connective tissue sheaths (Figs. 4-10 and 4-11).

The nerve trunk is surrounded by a dense con-

Fig. 4-5. Electron micrograph of a transverse section of a peripheral nerve, showing a myelinated axon with spiral myelin lamellae (center). Note the mesaxon (arrow). Parts of two other myelinated fibers are also shown. A number of nonmyelinated axons are enclosed in the peripheral cytoplasm of a Schwann cell (top). The mesaxons are indicated by arrows. (× 28,000) (Courtesy Dr. H. de F. Webster.)

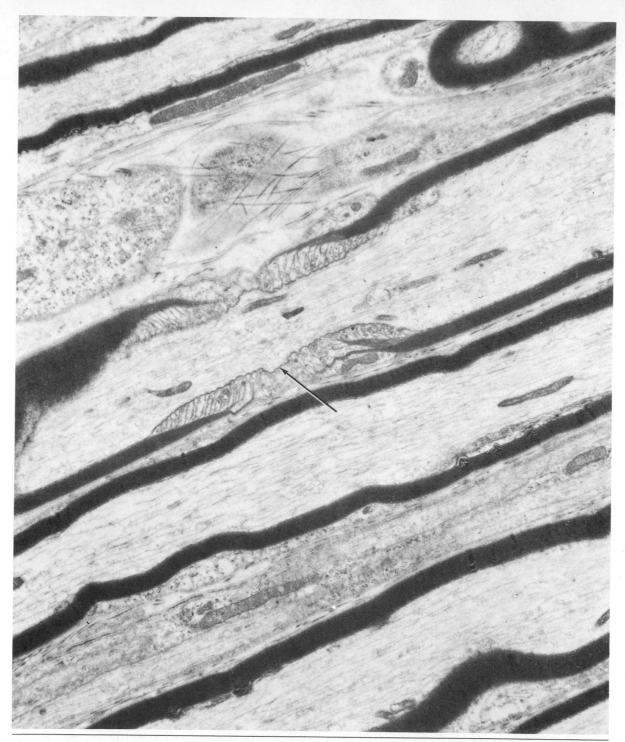

Fig. 4-6. Electron micrograph of a longitudinal section of several myelinated axons, showing the structure of a node of Ranvier (arrow). At the node, two adjacent Schwann cells terminate and the myelin sheaths become thinner by the turning off of the lamellae. Note the many microtubules and microfilaments within the axons. (× 12,220) (Courtesy Dr. H. de F. Webster.)

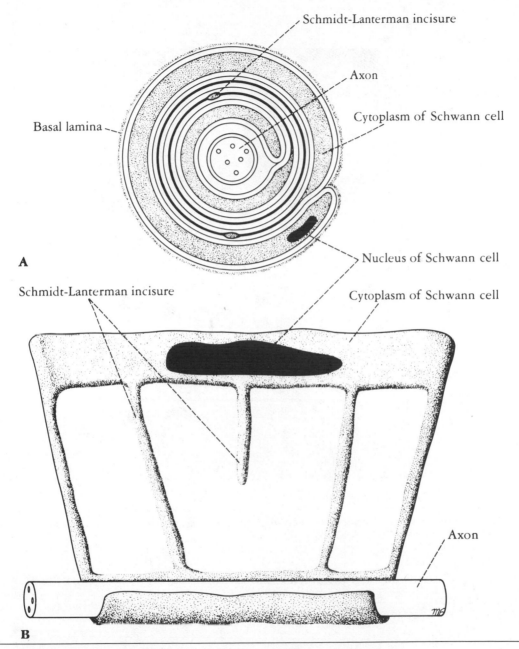

Fig. 4-7. Schmidt-Lanterman incisures in the myelin sheath of a peripheral nerve.
A. Transverse section of a myelinated nerve fiber.
B. Schematic diagram of a myelinated nerve fiber in which the myelin sheath has been unrolled.

Schwann cell nucleus

Axon

Myelin sheath

Nonmyelinated
axons

Schwann cell
cytoplasm

Processes of Schwann cells

Fig. 4-8. Electron micrograph of a transverse section of a myelinated nerve fiber and several nonmyelinated nerve fibers. (Courtesy Dr. J. M. Kerns.)

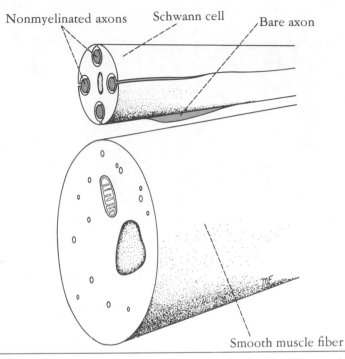

Nonmyelinated axons Schwann cell Bare axon

Smooth muscle fiber

Fig. 4-9. An autonomic neuromuscular junction between a nonmyelinated axon and a smooth muscle fiber.

Node of Ranvier Endoneurium

Axon Myelin sheath

Fig. 4-10. Photomicrograph of a longitudinal section of a peripheral nerve stained with hematoxylin and eosin. (× 400)

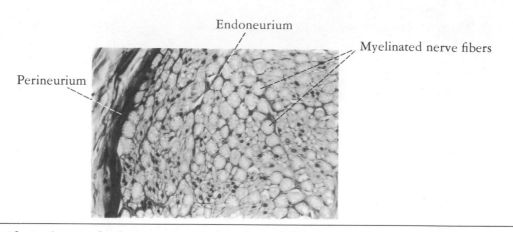

Fig. 4-11. Photomicrograph of a transverse section of a peripheral nerve stained with hematoxylin and eosin. (× 275)

nective tissue sheath called the **epineurium** (Fig. 4-12). Within the sheath are bundles of nerve fibers, each of which is surrounded by a connective tissue sheath called the **perineurium**. Between the individual nerve fibers is a loose, delicate connective tissue referred to as the **endoneurium**. The connective tissue sheaths serve to support the nerve fibers and their associated blood vessels and lymph vessels.

Peripheral nerve fibers may be classified into three groups, depending on their size and speed of conduction:

Group A fibers are 1 to 20 μm in diameter and they conduct at the rate of 5 to 120 meters per second. They are myelinated somatic efferent and afferent fibers.

Group B fibers are 1 to 3 μm in diameter and they conduct at 3 to 15 meters per second. They are myelinated efferent preganglionic autonomic fibers.

Group C fibers are 0.5 to 2 μm in diameter and they conduct at 0.5 to 2 meters per second. They are nonmyelinated efferent postganglionic autonomic fibers.

SPINAL NERVES AND SPINAL NERVE ROOTS

There are 31 pairs of spinal nerves, which leave the spinal cord and pass through intervertebral foramina in the vertebral column. (For details, see p. 25.) Each spinal nerve is connected to the spinal cord by **two roots**: the **anterior root** and the **posterior root** (Fig. 4-13). The **anterior root** consists of bundles of nerve fibers carrying nerve impulses away from the central nervous system; these nerve fibers are called **efferent fibers**. The **posterior root** consists of bundles of nerve fibers carrying nerve impulses to the central nervous system; these nerve fibers are called **afferent fibers**. Because these fibers are concerned with conveying information to the central nervous system, they are called **sensory fibers**. The cell bodies of these nerve fibers are situated in a swelling on the posterior root called the **posterior root ganglion**.

CRANIAL NERVES

There are 12 pairs of cranial nerves (Fig. 4-13), which leave the brain and pass through foramina in the skull. Some of these nerves are composed entirely of afferent nerve fibers bringing sensations to the brain (olfactory, optic, vestibulo-cochlear), others are composed entirely of efferent fibers (oculomotor, trochlear, abducent, accessory, hypoglossal), while the remainder possess both afferent and efferent fibers (trigeminal, facial, glossopharyngeal, and vagus). The cranial nerves are described in detail in Chapter 23.

SENSORY GANGLIA

The sensory ganglia of the posterior spinal nerve roots and of the trunks of the trigeminal, facial,

Nerve fibers

Endoneurium

Perineurium

Epineurium

Fig. 4-12. The structure of a peripheral nerve.

glossopharyngeal, and vagal cranial nerves have the same structure. Each ganglion is surrounded by a layer of connective tissue that is continuous with the epineurium and perineurium of the peripheral nerve. The neurons are unipolar, possessing cell bodies that are rounded or oval in shape (Fig. 4-14). The cell bodies tend to be aggregated and separated by bundles of nerve fibers. A single nonmyelinated process leaves each cell body and after a convoluted course bifurcates at a T junction into peripheral and central branches. The former axon

terminates in a series of dendrites in a peripheral sensory ending, and the latter axon enters the central nervous system. The nerve impulse, on reaching the T junction, passes directly from the peripheral axon to the central axon, thus bypassing the nerve cell body.

Each nerve cell body is closely surrounded by a layer of flattened cells called **capsular cells** or **satellite cells** (Fig. 4-14). The capsular cells are similar in structure to Schwann cells and are continuous with these cells as they envelop the peripheral and central processes of each neuron.

AUTONOMIC GANGLIA

The autonomic ganglia (sympathetic and parasympathetic ganglia) are situated at a distance from the brain and spinal cord. They are found in the sympathetic trunks, in prevertebral autonomic plexuses—for example, in the cardiac, celiac, and mesenteric plexuses—and as ganglia in or close to viscera. Each ganglion is surrounded by a layer of connective tissue that is continuous with the epineurium and perineurium of the peripheral nerve. The neurons are multipolar and possess cell bodies that are irregular in shape (Fig. 4-15). The dendrites of the neurons make synaptic connections with the myelinated axons of preganglionic neurons. The axons of the neurons are of small diameter (C fibers) and unmyelinated, and they pass to viscera, blood vessels, and sweat glands.

Each nerve cell body is closely surrounded by a layer of flattened cells called **capsular cells** or **satellite cells**. The capsular cells, like those of sensory ganglia, are similar in structure to Schwann cells and are continuous with them as they envelop the peripheral and central processes of each neuron.

PERIPHERAL NERVE PLEXUSES

Peripheral nerves are composed of bundles of nerve fibers. In their course, peripheral nerves sometimes divide into branches that join neighboring peripheral nerves. If this should occur frequently, a network of nerves is formed called a **nerve plexus**. It should be emphasized that the formation of a nerve plexus allows individual nerve fibers to pass from one peripheral nerve to another and **in most instances branching of nerve fibers does not take place**. A plexus thus permits

Posterior root ganglion

Thoracic segment of spinal cord

Spinal nerve

Anterior root

A

Motor nucleus of trigeminal nerve

Main sensory nucleus of trigeminal nerve

Pons

Fig. 4-13. A. Transverse section of the thoracic region of the spinal cord, showing the formation of a spinal nerve from the union of an anterior and a posterior nerve root.
B. Transverse section of the pons showing the sensory and motor roots of the trigeminal nerve.

Capsular cells

Cell bodies of neurons

Fig. 4-14. Photomicrograph of longitudinal section of posterior root ganglion of spinal nerve. Stained with hematoxylin and eosin. (× 400)

Fig. 4-15. Photomicrograph of longitudinal section of ganglion of the sympathetic trunk. Stained with hematoxylin and eosin. (× 300)

a redistribution of the nerve fibers within the different peripheral nerves.

At the root of the limbs the anterior rami of the spinal nerves form complicated plexuses. The cervical and brachial plexuses are at the root of the upper limbs (Fig. 4-16), and the lumbar and sacral plexuses are at the root of the lower limbs. This allows the nerve fibers derived from different segments of the spinal cord to be arranged and distributed efficiently in different nerve trunks to the various parts of the upper and lower limbs.

Cutaneous nerves, as they approach their final destination, commonly form fine plexuses that again permit a rearrangement of nerve fibers before they reach their terminal sensory endings.

The autonomic nervous system also possesses numerous nerve plexuses that consist of pre- and postganglionic nerve fibers and ganglia.

CONDUCTION IN PERIPHERAL NERVES

In the resting unstimulated state a nerve fiber is polarized so that the interior is negative to the ex-

terior; the potential difference across the axolemma is about 80 mV and is called the **resting membrane potential** (Fig. 4-17). As has been explained previously, this so-called resting potential is produced by the diffusion of sodium and potassium ions through the plasma membrane and is maintained by the sodium-potassium pump. The pump involves active transport across the membrane and requires adenosine triphosphate (ATP) to provide the energy.

A nerve impulse (action potential) starts at the initial segment of the axon and is a self-propagating wave of electrical negativity that passess along the surface of the plasma membrane (axolemma). The wave of electrical negativity is initiated by an adequate stimulus being applied to the surface of the neuron. Under normal circumstances this occurs at the initial segment of the axon, which is the most sensitive part of the neuron. The stimulus alters the permeability of the membrane to Na^+ ions at the point of stimulation. Now Na^+ ions rapidly enter the axon (Fig. 4-17). The positive ions outside the axolemma quickly decrease to zero. The membrane potential therefore is reduced to zero and is said to be depolarized. A typical resting potential is 80 mV, with the outside of the membrane positive to the inside; the action potential is about 40 mV, with the outside of the membrane negative to the inside.

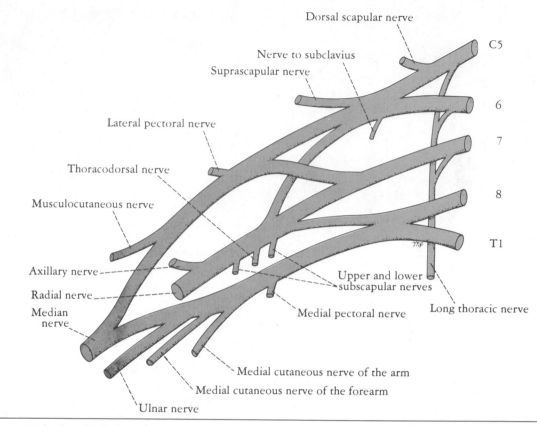

Fig. 4-16. The brachial plexus.

The negatively charged point on the outside of the axolemma now acts as a stimulus to the adjacent positively charged axolemma and in less than 1 msec the polarity of the adjacent resting potential is reversed (Fig. 4-17). The action potential now has moved along the axolemma from the point originally stimulated to the adjacent point on the membrane. It is in this manner that the action potential travels along the full length of a nerve fiber.

As the action potential moves along the nerve fiber, the entry of the Na$^+$ ions into the axon ceases and the permeability of the axolemma to K$^+$ ions increases. Now K$^+$ ions rapidly diffuse outside the axon (since the concentration is much higher within the axon than outside), so that the original resting membrane potential is restored. The permeability of the axolemma now decreases and the status quo is restored by the active transport of the Na$^+$ ions out of the axon and the K$^+$ ions into the axon. The outer surface of the axolemma is again electrically positive compared to the inner surface.

For a short time after the passage of a nerve impulse along a nerve fiber, while the axolemma is still depolarized, a second stimulus, however strong, is unable to excite the nerve. This period of time is called the **absolute refractory period**. This period is followed by a further short interval during which the excitability of the nerve gradually returns to normal. This latter period is called the **relative refractory period**. It is clear from this

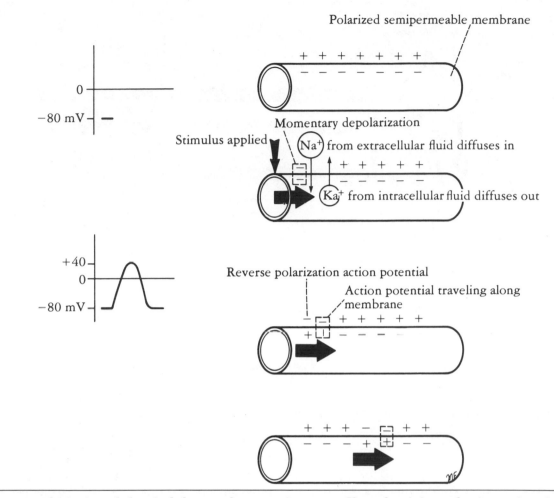

Fig. 4-17. The ionic and electrical changes that occur in a nerve fiber when it is conducting an impulse.

that the refractory period makes a continuous excitatory state of the nerve impossible and it limits the frequency of the impulses.

The **conduction velocity** of a nerve fiber is proportional to the cross-sectional area of the axon, the thicker fibers conducting more rapidly than those of smaller diameter. In the large motor fibers (alpha fibers), the rate may be as high as 80 to 120 meters per second; the smaller sensory fibers have slower conduction rates.

In nonmyelinated fibers, the action potential passes continuously along the axolemma, progressively exciting neighboring areas of membrane (Fig. 4-18). In myelinated fibers, the presence of a myelin sheath serves as an insulator. Consequently, a myelinated nerve fiber can be stimulated only at the nodes of Ranvier, where the axon is naked and the ions can pass freely through the plasma membrane between the extracellular fluid and the axoplasm. In these fibers the action potential jumps from one node to the next (Fig. 4-18). The action potential at one node sets up a current in the surrounding tissue fluid, which quickly produces depolarization at the next node. This leaping of the

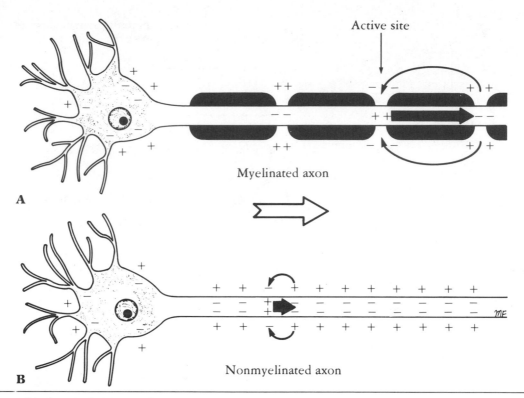

Active site

Myelinated axon

A

Nonmyelinated axon

B

Fig. 4-18. The electrical changes that occur in:
A. A stimulated myelinated axon (saltatory conduction).
B. A stimulated nonmyelinated axon.

action potential from one node to the next is re-ferred to as **saltatory conduction** (Fig. 4-18). This is a more rapid mechanism than is found in non-myelinated fibers (120 meters per second in a large myelinated fiber compared with 0.5 meter per sec-ond in a very small unmyelinated fiber).

CLINICAL NOTES

RESPONSE OF NEURONS TO INJURY

The survival of the cytoplasm of a neuron depends on its being connected, however indirectly, with the nucleus. The nucleus plays a key role in the synthe-sis of proteins, which pass into the cell processes and replace proteins that have been metabolized by the cell activity. Thus, the cytoplasm of axons and dendrites will undergo degeneration quickly if these processes are separated from the nerve cell body.

Injury of the Nerve Cell Body

Severe damage of the nerve cell body due to trauma, interference with the blood supply, or dis-ease may result in degeneration of the entire neu-ron, including its dendrites and synaptic endings. In the brain and spinal cord, the neuronal debris and the fragments of myelin (if the processes are myelinated) are engulfed and phagocytosed by the microglial cells. Later, the neighboring astrocytes proliferate and replace the neuron with scar tissue.

In the peripheral nervous system, the tissue macrophages remove the debris and the local fibroblasts replace the neuron with scar tissue.

Injury of the Nerve Cell Process

If the axon of the nerve cell is divided, degenerative changes will take place in (1) the distal segment that is separated from the cell body, (2) a portion of the axon proximal to the injury, and (3) possibly the cell body from which the axon arises.

Changes in the Distal Segment of the Axon

The changes spread distally from the site of the lesion (Fig. 4-19) and include its terminations; the process is referred to as **wallerian degeneration**. In the peripheral nervous system, on the first day the axon becomes swollen and irregular, and by the third or fourth day the axon is broken into fragments (Fig. 4-19) and the debris is digested by the surrounding Schwann cells and tissue macrophages. The entire axon is destroyed within a week.

Meanwhile, the myelin sheath slowly breaks down and lipid droplets appear within the Schwann cell cytoplasm (Fig. 4-19). Later, the droplets are extruded from the Schwann cell and subsequently are phagocytosed by tissue macrophages. The Schwann cells now begin to proliferate rapidly and become arranged in parallel cords within the persistent basement membrane. The endoneurial sheath and the contained cords of Schwann cells are sometimes referred to as a **band fiber**. If regeneration does not occur the axon and the Schwann cells are replaced by fibrous tissue produced by local fibroblasts.

In the central nervous system, degeneration of the axons and the myelin sheaths follows a similar course, and the debris is removed by the phagocytic activity of the microglial cells. Little is known about the role of oligodendrocytes in this process. The astrocytes now proliferate and replace the axons.

Changes in the Proximal Segment of the Axon

The changes in the proximal segment of the axon are similar to those that take place in the distal segment (Fig. 4-19) but extend only proximally

above the lesion as far as the first node of Ranvier. The proliferating cords of Schwann cells in the peripheral nerves bulge from the cut surfaces of the endoneurial tubes.

Changes in the Nerve Cell Body from Which the Axon Arises

The changes that may occur in the cell body following injury to its axon are referred to as **retrograde degeneration**; the changes that take place in the proximal segment of the axon commonly are included under this heading.

The most characteristic change occurs in the cell body within the first two days following injury and reaches its maximum within two weeks. The Nissl material becomes fine, granular (Figs. 4-20 and 4-21), and dispersed throughout the cytoplasm, a process known as **chromatolysis**. Chromatolysis begins near the axon hillock and spreads to all parts of the cell body. In addition, the nucleus moves from its central location toward the periphery of the cell and the cell body swells and becomes rounded (Fig. 4-21). The degree of chromatolysis and the degree of swelling of the cell are greatest when the injury to the axon is close to the cell body. In some neurons, very severe damage to the axon close to the cell body may lead to death of the neuron. On the other hand, damage to the most distal process may lead to little or no detectable change in the cell body. The dispersal of the Nissl material, that is, the cytoplasmic RNA, and the swelling of the cell are caused by cellular edema. The apparent loss of staining affinity of the Nissl material is due to the wide dispersal of the cytoplasmic RNA. The movement of the nucleus away from the center of the cell may be due to the cellular edema.

RECOVERY OF NEURONS FOLLOWING INJURY

In contrast to the rapid onset of retrograde degeneration, the recovery of the nerve cell body and regeneration of its processes may take several months.

RECOVERY OF THE NERVE CELL BODY

The nucleolus moves to the periphery of the nucleus and polysome clusters reappear in the cyto-

Fig. 4-19. A, B, C, and D. Degeneration and regeneration in a divided nerve.

A   B

Fig. 4-20. Photomicrographs of motor neurons of the anterior gray column of the spinal cord.
A. Nissl substance in normal neurons.
B. Following section of anterior roots of spinal nerve, showing chromatolysis.

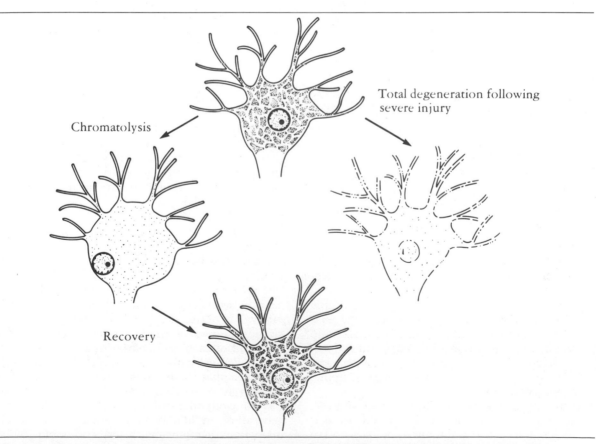

Total degeneration following
severe injury

Chromatolysis

Recovery

Fig. 4-21. The changes that may take place in a nerve cell body following division of one of its processes.

plasm. This indicates that RNA and protein synthesis is being accelerated in preparation for the reformation of the axon. Thus, there is a reconstitution of the original Nissl structure, a decrease in the swelling of the cell body, and a return of the nucleus to its characteristic central position (see Fig. 4-21).

Regeneration of the Axons

Regrowth of the axons is possible in peripheral nerves and appears to depend on the presence of endoneurial tubes and the special qualities possessed by Schwann cells. In the central nervous system there is an attempt at regeneration of the axons, as evidenced by sprouting of the axons, but the process ceases after about 2 weeks. There is no evidence that restoration of function takes place. The regeneration process is aborted by the absence of endoneurial tubes (which are necessary to guide the regenerating axons), the failure of oligodendrocytes to serve in the same manner as Schwann cells, and the laying down of scar tissue by the active astrocytes. It has also been suggested that there is an absence of nerve growth factors in the central nervous system or that the neuroglial cells may produce nerve growth–inhibiting factors.

Regeneration of Axons in Peripheral Nerves

The satisfactory regeneration of axons and the return of normal function will depend on the following factors:

1. In crush nerve injuries, where the axon is divided or its blood supply has been interfered with but the endoneurial sheaths remain intact, the regenerative process may be very satisfactory.
2. In nerves that have been completely severed there is much less chance of recovery, because the regenerating fibers from the proximal stump may be directed to an incorrect destination in the distal stump, i.e., cutaneous fibers entering incorrect nerve endings or motor nerves supplying incorrect muscles.
3. If the distance between the proximal and distal stumps of the completely severed nerve is greater than a few millimeters, or the gap becomes filled with proliferating fibrous tissue or

is simply filled by adjacent muscles that bulge into the gap, then the chances of recovery are very poor. The outgrowing axonal sprouts escape into the surrounding connective tissue and form a tangled mass or **neuroma**. In these cases, early close surgical approximation of the severed ends, if possible, greatly facilitates the chances of recovery.

4. When mixed nerves (those containing sensory, motor, and autonomic fibers) are completely severed, the chances of a good recovery are very much less than if the nerve is purely sensory or purely motor. The reason for this is that the regenerating fibers from the proximal stump may be guided to an incorrect destination in the distal stump, e.g., cutaneous fibers may enter motor endoneurial tubes and vice versa.
5. Inadequate physiotherapy to the paralyzed muscles will result in their degenerating before the regenerating motor axons have reached them.
6. The presence of infection at the site of the wound will seriously interfere with the process of regeneration.

If one assumes that the proximal and distal stumps of the severed nerve are in close apposition, the following regenerative processes take place (Fig. 4-19). The Schwann cells, having undergone mitotic division, now fill the space within the basal lamina of the endoneurial tubes of the proximal stump as far proximally as the next node of Ranvier, and in the distal stump as far distally as the end-organs. Where a small gap exists between the proximal and distal stumps, the multiplying Schwann cells form a number of cords to bridge the gap.

Each proximal axon end now gives rise to multiple fine sprouts or filaments with bulbous tips. These filaments, as they grow, advance along the clefts between the Schwann cells and thus cross the interval between the proximal and distal nerve stumps. Many such filaments now enter the proximal end of each endoneurial tube and grow distally in contact with the Schwann cells (Fig. 4-22). It is clear that the filaments from many different axons may enter a single endoneurial tube. However, only one filament persists, the remainder degenerating, and that one filament grows distally to reinnervate a motor or sensory end-organ. While crossing the gap between the severed nerve ends,

Fragmentation of axons and myelin

Axons growing along endoneurial tubes

Fig. 4-22. Photomicrograph of longitudinal section of distal stump of sciatic nerve, showing evidence of degeneration and axon regeneration following injury. (Courtesy Dr. M. J. T. Fitzgerald.)

many filaments fail to enter an endoneurial tube and grow out into the surrounding connective tissue. It is interesting to note that the formation of multiple sprouts or filaments from a single proximal axon greatly increases the chances that a neuron will become connected to a sensory or motor ending. It is not known why one filament within a single endoneurial tube should be selected to persist while the remainder degenerate.

Once the axon has reached the end-organ, the adjacent Schwann cells start to lay down a myelin sheath. This process begins at the site of the original lesion and extends in a distal direction. By this means, the nodes of Ranvier and the Schmidt-Lanterman incisures are formed.

Many months may elapse before the axon reaches its appropriate end-organ, depending on the site of the nerve injury. The rate of growth has been estimated to be of the order of 2 to 4 mm per day. If, however, one takes into consideration the almost certain delay incurred by the axons as they cross the site of the injury, an overall regeneration rate of 1.5 mm per day is a useful figure to remember for clinical use. Even if all the difficulties outlined above are overcome and a given neuron reaches the original end-organ, the enlarging axonal filament within the endoneurial tube reaches only about 80 percent of its original diameter. For this reason the conduction velocity will not be as great as the original axon. Moreover, a given motor

axon tends to innervate more muscle fibers than formerly, so that the control of muscle is less precise.

TRANSNEURONAL DEGENERATION

The responses of a single neuron to injury have been considered in the previous section. In the central nervous system it is recognized that if one group of neurons is injured then a second group farther along the pathway, serving the same function, may also show degenerative changes. This phenomenon is referred to as **anterograde transneuronal degeneration**. For example, if the axons of the ganglion cells of the retina are severed, not only do the distal ends of the axons that go to the lateral geniculate bodies undergo degeneration, but the neurons in the lateral geniculate bodies with which these axons form synapses also undergo degeneration. In fact, a further set of neurons may be involved in the degenerative process in the visual cortex.

In situations in the central nervous system where multiple neurons synapse with a single distal neuron, injury to one of the proximal neurons is not followed by degeneration of the distal neuron.

Experimentation on animals with artificial lesions of the central nervous system has shown that

retrograde transneuronal degeneration may occur in certain situations.

NEURONAL DEGENERATION ASSOCIATED WITH SENESCENCE

Many neurons degenerate and disappear during fetal development. This process is believed to be due to their failure to establish adequate functional connections. During postnatal life further gradual neuronal degeneration continues to occur. It has been estimated that in old age an individual may have lost up to 20 percent of the original number of neurons. This may account to some extent for the loss of efficiency of the nervous system that is associated with senescence.

ATROPHY OF VOLUNTARY MUSCLE AND OTHER END-ORGANS FOLLOWING PERIPHERAL NERVE DEGENERATION

Voluntary muscle undergoes degenerative changes following motor nerve section. First, there is an altered response to acetylcholine, followed by gradual wasting of the sarcoplasm, and finally loss of the fibrils and striations. Eventually the muscle completely atrophies and is replaced by fibrous tissue. Reinnervation of the muscle halts its degeneration, and if the muscle atrophy is not too advanced, normal structure and function return.

Furthermore, if the motor nerve that supplies fast white voluntary muscle fibers is exchanged for a motor nerve that supplies slow red voluntary muscle fibers, the muscle fibers change their structural and functional properties to comply with the new type of innervation. This experimental result strongly suggests that not only are voluntary muscle cells dependent on the presence of intact motor nerves, but that the nerve has some trophic influence on the muscle and even determines the type of muscle that it innervates.

Another end-organ, the taste bud, also depends on the integrity of the sensory nerve. If the nerve is sectioned, the taste bud quickly atrophies. Once the sensory nerve regenerates into the mucous membrane new taste buds develop.

TRAUMATIC LESIONS OF PERIPHERAL NERVES

Seddon (1944) describes three clinical types of nerve injury:

Neuropraxia is the term applied to a transient block. The paralysis is incomplete, recovery is rapid and complete, and there is no microscopic evidence of nerve degeneration. Pressure is the most common cause. It is essentially a temporary interference in function.

Axonotmesis is the term applied to a nerve lesion in which the axons are damaged but the surrounding connective tissue sheaths remain more or less intact. Wallerian degeneration occurs peripherally. Functional recovery is more rapid and more complete than after complete section of the nerve trunk. The explanation of the more rapid and more complete recovery is that the nerve fibers, although severely damaged, for the most part retain their normal anatomical relationships to one another, owing to the preservation of the connective tissue sheaths. Crush injuries, traction, and compression are the most common causes.

Neurotmesis is the term applied to complete section of the nerve trunk.

SYMPTOMS AND SIGNS OF NEUROTMESIS

Motor Changes

The muscles innervated show flaccid paralysis and rapidly waste. The reflexes in which the muscles participate are lost. The paralyzed muscle ceases to respond to faradic stimulation after 4 to 7 days. After 10 days the muscle responds only sluggishly to galvanic stimulation and the strength of the current must be greater than that required for normal innervated muscle. This altered response of muscle to electrical stimulation is known as the **reaction of degeneration**.

Sensory Changes

There is a total loss of cutaneous sensibility over the area exclusively supplied by the nerve. This area is surrounded by a zone of partial sensory loss where adjacent sensory nerves overlap. The skin area in which the sensation of light touch is lost is much greater than the area lost to pin prick.

Vasomotor, Sudomotor, and Trophic Changes

Section of a peripheral nerve results in the interruption of postganglionic sympathetic fibers traveling in the nerve. As a result of the loss of vascular control, the skin area at first becomes red and hot. Later, the affected area becomes blue and colder than normal, especially in cold weather. Because of the loss of sudomotor control, the sweat glands cease to produce sweat and the skin becomes dry and scaly. Nail growth becomes retarded as the direct result of poor peripheral circulation. If a large area of the body is denervated, as, for example, in cases in which the sciatic nerve is sectioned, the bones undergo decalcification as a result of disuse and loss of circulatory control.

SYMPTOMS AND SIGNS OF RECOVERY FOLLOWING NEUROTMESIS

Assuming that the divided peripheral nerve has been carefully sutured together, a physician must be aware of the symptoms and signs of recovery and their sequence.

Motor Recovery

Regenerating motor axons grow at an average rate of about 1.5 mm per day. The proximal muscles will recover first and the distal muscles later. The muscles may respond to faradic stimulation before voluntary control returns.

Sensory Recovery

Sensory recovery occurs before there is a return of voluntary movement. The part of the nerve distal to the section becomes very sensitive to mechanical stimulation once the regenerating sensory axons have entered the distal segment. Simple tapping of the distal nerve trunk gives rise to a tingling sensation in the area of cutaneous distribution of the nerve. This sign is referred to as **Tinel's sign**. Re-

covery of deep cutaneous sensibility, i.e., pain caused by deep pressure, is the first sign of recovery. This is followed by the return of poorly localized, superficial cutaneous pain. Vasomotor control also returns at about this time. Later, the sensations of heat and cold are recovered. Light touch and tactile discrimination are the last sensations to return, many months later, and they are often incomplete.

SOME BASIC CLINICAL PRINCIPLES UNDERLYING PERIPHERAL NERVE INJURIES

In open, dirty wounds, where there is a high risk of infection, the sectioned nerve should be ignored and the wound infection should be treated. Later, when the wound has healed satisfactorily, the nerve should be explored and the cut ends of the nerve sutured together.

If a patient visits a physician with a healed wound and there is no evidence of nerve recovery, the treatment should be conservative. Sufficient time should be allowed to elapse to enable the regenerating nerve fibers to reach the proximal muscles. If recovery fails to occur, the nerve should be explored surgically.

In those cases in which connective tissue, bone fragments, or muscles come to lie between the cut ends of a severed nerve, the nerve should be explored and, if possible, the cut ends of the nerve should be brought together and sutured.

The nutrition of the paralyzed muscles must be maintained with adequate physiotherapy. Warm baths, massage, and warm clothing help to maintain adequate circulation.

The paralyzed muscles must not be allowed to be stretched by antagonist muscles or by gravity. Moreover, excessive shortening of the paralyzed muscles leads to contracture of these muscles.

The joints must be kept mobile by daily passive movements of all joints. Failure to do this results in the formation of adhesions and consequent limitation of movement.

Once voluntary movement returns in the most proximal muscles, the physiotherapist can assist the patient in performing active exercises. This not only aids in the return of a normal circulation to the affected part but helps the patient to learn once again the complicated muscular performance of skilled movements.

NERVE TRANSPLANTATION

Nerve grafts have been used with some success to restore muscle tone in facial nerve palsy. In mixed nerve injuries nerve grafts have succeeded only in restoring some sensory function and slight muscle activity. The presence of two suture lines and the increased possibility of mixing the nerve fibers is probably the reason for the lack of success with nerve grafts. In most nerve injuries, even when the gap between the proximal and distal ends is as great as 10 cm, it is usually possible to mobilize the nerve or alter its position in relation to joints so that the proximal and distal ends may be brought together without undue tension; the ends are then sutured together.

TUMORS OF PERIPHERAL NERVES

A peripheral nerve consists essentially of nerve fibers (axons), each of which is associated with Schwann cells; the fibers are either myelinated or nonmyelinated. The nerve fibers are arranged in parallel bundles and are surrounded by connective tissue sheaths.

A **benign fibroma** or a **malignant sarcoma** may arise in the connective tissue of the nerve and does not differ from similar tumors elsewhere. **Neurolemmomas** are believed to arise from Schwann cells. They arise from any nerve trunk, cranial or spinal, and in any part of its course. Primary tumors of the axons are very rare.

BLOOD VESSELS, LYMPHATICS, AND ENDONEURIAL SPACES WITHIN PERIPHERAL NERVES

Peripheral nerves receive branches from arteries in the regions through which they pass. The anastomotic network that exists within a nerve is considerable and local ischemia does not occur should a single artery be obstructed.

A plexus of lymph vessels lies within the epineurial connective tissues and this drains to regional lymph nodes.

As the result of experiments in which dyes have been injected into peripheral nerves, spaces have been demonstrated between individual nerve fibers. There seems to be little doubt that these endoneurial spaces provide a potential route for the ascent of tetanus toxin to the spinal cord.

ACTION OF LOCAL ANESTHETICS ON NERVE CONDUCTION

Local anesthetics are drugs that block nerve conduction when applied locally to a nerve fiber in suitable concentrations. Their site of action is the axolemma and they interfere with the transient increase in permeability of the axolemma to Na^+, K^+, and other ions. The sensitivity of nerve fibers to local anesthetics is related to the size of the nerve fibers. Small nerve fibers are more susceptible than are large fibers; small fibers are also slower to recover.

Cocaine has been used clinically to block nerve conduction. Unfortunately, it is a strong stimulant of the cerebral cortex and readily causes addiction. **Procaine** is a synthetic compound that is widely used as a local anesthetic agent.

APPARENT RECOVERY OF FUNCTION OF THE CENTRAL NERVOUS SYSTEM FOLLOWING INJURY

Axon regeneration in the brain and spinal cord is minimal following a lesion, and yet considerable functional recovery often occurs. Several explanations exist and more than one mechanism may be involved.

1. The function of nerve fibers may be interfered with as the result of compression by edema fluid. Once the edema subsides a substantial recovery may take place.
2. The damaged nerve fiber proximal to the lesion may form new synapses with neighboring normal neurons.
3. Following a lesion of an afferent neuron, an increased number of receptor sites may develop on a postsynaptic membrane. This may result in the

second neuron responding to neurotransmitter substances from neighboring neurons.

4. Nonfunctioning neurons may take over the function of damaged neurons.

5. It is possible with intensive physiotherapy for patients to be trained to use other muscles to compensate for the loss of paralyzed muscles.

HERPES ZOSTER

Herpes zoster or shingles is a relatively common condition caused by the reactivation of the latent varicella-zoster virus in a patient who has previously had chickenpox. The infection is found in the first sensory neuron in a cranial or spinal nerve. The lesion is seen as an inflammation and degeneration of the sensory neuron with the formation of vesicles with inflammation of the skin. The first symptom is pain in the distribution of the sensory

neuron followed in a few days by a skin eruption. The condition occurs most frequently in patients over the age of 50.

POLYNEUROPATHY

Polyneuropathy is an impairment of function of many peripheral nerves simultaneously. There are many causes, including infection (endotoxin of diphtheria, Guillain-Barré syndrome), metabolic disorders (vitamin B_1 and B_{12} deficiency, poisoning by heavy metals, drugs), and endocrine disorders (diabetes). Axon degeneration and/or segmental demyelination may take place and the neuron cell body may be involved. In mild cases the condition is reversible, but in severe cases it may be permanent. Both sensory and motor symptoms and signs may be evident.

CLINICAL PROBLEMS

Answers on Page 589

1. A surgeon meticulously examined a patient, who had a stab wound in the arm, for evidence that the median nerve had been severed. The median nerve is a peripheral nerve. What is the structure of a peripheral nerve?

2. A 20-year-old man was seen in the emergency room following an automobile accident. A diagnosis of fracture dislocation of the fourth thoracic vertebra was made, with injury to the spinal cord as a complication. It was decided to perform a laminectomy because it was felt that the spinal cord should be decompressed to avoid permanent injury to the tracts of the cord. What is a nerve tract in the spinal cord? How does this differ in structure from a peripheral nerve?

3. Define the following terms: (a) *myelin sheath*, (b) *node of Ranvier*, (c) *Schmidt-Lanterman incisure*, (d) *satellite cells in sensory and autonomic ganglia*.

4. Multiple sclerosis is an example of a demyelinating disease of the nervous system. There are many other examples of diseases of the nervous system that have the common pathological feature of destruction of the myelin sheaths of nerve fibers. How does myelination normally take place in (a) peripheral nerves and (b) cen-

tral nervous system tracts? When does myelination of nerves normally take place?

5. The myelin sheath is said to be formed in the peripheral nervous system by the rotation of the Schwann cells on the axon so that the plasma membrane becomes wrapped around and around the axon in a spiral. In the central nervous system, do the oligodendrocytes rotate on the axons in a similar manner to form myelin?

6. Give three examples of nonmyelinated nerve fibers in the nervous system.

7. During a neurobiology lecture the professor repeatedly referred to such terms as *type A and B nerve fibers, resting membrane potential, absolute refractory period, conduction velocity,* and *saltatory conduction.* Can you define each of these terms?

8. A 26-year-old man was involved in a street brawl and received a knife wound of the right arm at about the midhumeral level. Physical examination revealed that the median nerve had been sectioned. Motor loss consisted of paralysis of the pronator muscles of the forearm and the long flexor muscles of the wrist and fingers, with the exception of the flexor carpi ulnaris and the medial half of flexor digitorum

profundus. As a result of this, the right forearm was kept in the supine position; wrist flexion was weak and was accompanied by adduction. The latter deviation was due to the paralysis of the flexor carpi radialis and the strength of both the flexor carpi ulnaris and the medial half of flexor digitorum profundus. No flexion was possible at the interphalangeal joints of the index and middle fingers, although weak flexion of the metacarpophalangeal joints of these fingers was attempted by the interossei. When the patient was asked to make a fist of his right hand, the index and, to a lesser extent, the middle fingers tended to remain straight, while the ring and little fingers flexed. The latter two fingers were weakened by the loss of the flexor digitorum superficialis. Flexion of the terminal phalanx of the thumb was lost due to paralysis of the flexor pollicis longus. The muscles of the thenar eminence were paralyzed and the right thumb was laterally rotated and adducted.

Sensory loss of the skin of the right hand involved the lateral half of the palm and the palmar aspect of the lateral three and one-half fingers. There was also sensory loss of the skin of the distal parts of the dorsal surfaces of the lateral three and one-half fingers.

The skin areas involved in sensory loss became warmer and drier than normal, evidencing vasomotor changes. This was due to arteriolar dilatation and absence of sweating resulting from loss of sympathetic nervous control.

(a) Describe the changes that would take place in the median nerve proximal and distal to the site of section. (b) How would you treat this case? (c) What will be the first signs and symptoms to indicate that the nerve is regenerating adequately? (d) Which function will return first, sensory or muscular? (e) About how long will it take for the nerve to regenerate and reach its end-organs?

9. What is meant by the following terms: (a) *wallerian degeneration*, (b) *band fiber*, (c) *transneuronal degeneration?*

10. A 45-year-old woman with a right-sided facial palsy was examined. When questioned, she said that 3 years previously she had experienced a weakness of the right side of the face and some degree of loss of taste sensation following a ride in an open car on a cold day. A diagnosis of Bell's palsy was made. What is Bell's palsy? How would you treat this patient?

11. A family with five small children moved into an old house. Six months later the mother noticed that her 1-year-old son was becoming somnolent and quiet. Whereas previously he was very active and crawled around the house, he now tended to lie about the floor, uninterested in his toys. He had also stopped eating well and was very constipated. The mother decided to take the child to a pediatrician when, as she put it, he suddenly "threw a fit." On examination, there was an absence of positive physical signs except for a dark line between the gums and teeth. When questioned further, the mother admitted that the child liked sucking the peeling paint on the railings outside the house. A diagnosis of chronic lead poisoning was made. This was confirmed by finding that the blood lead level was in excess of 50 μg per 100 ml. What effect does lead have on the nervous system?

12. A 54-year-old man suddenly developed severe pain down both legs in the distribution of the sciatic nerve. He also noticed numbness in the buttocks and perineum and recently noted that he could not feel the passage of urine or feces. A diagnosis was made of central protrusion posteriorly of the intervertebral disc between the third and fourth lumbar vertebrae. From the symptoms it was clear that the cauda equina was being pressed upon. Does regeneration occur in the cauda equina?

13. By what anatomical route is tetanus toxin believed to pass from a wound to the central nervous system?

14. Name two tumors that occur in peripheral nerves. In each case state the cell of origin of the tumor.

15. Following an automobile accident, a 35-year-old man was seen in the emergency room with fractures of the fifth and sixth ribs on the right side. In order to relieve the pain and discomfort experienced by the patient when breathing, the physician decided to block the right fifth and sixth intercostal nerves by injecting a local anesthetic, xylocaine, around the nerve trunks. What is the effect of the local anesthetic agent on the nerve fibers? Are the large diameter or

the small diameter nerve fibers more suscepti- ble to the action of the drug?

16. A 65-year-old man, on returning home from a party, found that he could not climb the stairs. He had consumed several large whiskeys and seemed to have lost control of his legs. He sat down on a chair in the hallway and was soon in a deep, stuporous sleep, with his right arm suspended over the back of the chair. Next morning he awoke with a severe headache and loss of the use of his right arm and hand. Dur- ing examination in the emergency room, it was found that the patient had severe paralysis in- volving branches of the medial cord of the bra- chial plexus and the radial nerve. The diagnosis was neuropraxia, which occurred as the result of the pressure of the back of the chair on the involved nerves. What is neuropraxia? How

does this differ from axonotmesis and neurot- mesis? What is the prognosis in this patient? How would you treat this case?

17. A well-known politician was attending a rally when a youth suddenly stepped forward and shot him in the back. During examination in the emergency room, it was found that the bul- let had entered the back obliquely and was lodged in the vertebral canal at the level of the eighth thoracic vertebra. The patient could not feel anything below this level and was para- lyzed from the waist downward. At the opera- tion a laminectomy was performed and the bullet was removed. Considerable damage to the spinal cord was noted. What changes take place in the spinal cord when the nerve fibers are damaged? Does regeneration take place in the central nervous system?

NATIONAL BOARD TYPE QUESTIONS

Answers on Page 619

IN EACH OF THE FOLLOWING QUESTIONS, ANSWER:
   (a) IF (1) ONLY IS CORRECT
   (b) IF (2) ONLY IS CORRECT
   (c) IF BOTH (1) AND (2) ARE CORRECT, OR
   (d) IF NEITHER (1) NOR (2) IS CORRECT

1. Which of the following statements is (are) cor- rect?
   (1) A nerve tract is the name given to a nerve fiber in the central nervous system.
   (2) The supporting cell of a myelinated nerve fiber in the central nervous system is called an oligodendrocyte.

2. Which of the following statements is (are) cor- rect?
   (1) A node of Ranvier in peripheral nerves is where two Schwann cells terminate and the plasma membrane of the axon is exposed.
   (2) Nodes of Ranvier are absent from my- elinated nerve fibers in the central nervous system.

3. Which of the following statements is (are) cor- rect?
   (1) The major dense line of myelin consists of the lipid layers of the plasma membrane.
   (2) The minor dense line of myelin consists of the two inner protein layers of the plasma membrane fused together.

4. Which of the following statements is (are) cor- rect?
   (1) The incisures of Schmidt-Lanterman are caused by the mesaxons of the Schwann cells.
   (2) As many as 15 or more unmyelinated axons may share a single Schwann cell in the pe- ripheral nervous system.

Select the best response:

5. The following statements concerning an oligo- dendrocyte are true **except**:
   (a) A single oligodendrocyte may be associated with several segments of myelin on a single axon.
   (b) A single oligodendrocyte may be associated with the myelin sheaths of as many as 60 axons.
   (c) Myelination in the central nervous system occurs by the growth in length of the oli- godendrocytic process and the wrapping of it around the axon.
   (d) A nonmyelinated axon in the central ner- vous system has a special relationship with the oligodendrocyte.

(e) The incisures of Schmidt-Lanterman are present in the myelinated fibers of the central nervous system.

6. The following statements concerning spinal nerves are true **except**:
   (a) There are 31 pairs.
   (b) They are formed by the union of anterior and posterior nerve roots.
   (c) The posterior ramus contains only sensory axons.
   (d) The anterior root contains only motor axons.
   (e) The posterior root ganglion contains unipolar neurons enveloped in capsular cells.

7. The following statements concerning peripheral nerve plexuses are true **except**:
   (a) They are formed by a network of nerve fibers.
   (b) Bundles of nerve fibers branch, but in most instances the individual nerve fibers do not branch.
   (c) The plexuses at the roots of the limbs are formed from posterior rami of spinal nerves.
   (d) The plexuses of the autonomic nervous system possess a network of nerve fibers and nerve cells.
   (e) A plexus situated at the root of a limb permits nerve fibers from different segments of the spinal cord to become rearranged so that they more easily travel to different parts of the limb.

In the following questions, answer:
   (a) If (1), (2), and (3) only are correct
   (b) If (1) and (3) only are correct
   (c) If (2) and (4) only are correct
   (d) If (4) only is correct, or
   (e) If all are correct

8. Which of the following statements is (are) correct concerning nerve conduction?
   (1) An adequate stimulus alters the permeability of the axolemma to Na^+ ions at the point of stimulation.
   (2) A typical action potential is about 40 mV.
   (3) As the action potential moves along the axon, the entry of Na^+ ions into the axon ceases and the permeability to K^+ ions increases.
   (4) During the absolute refractory period no stimulus, no matter how strong, will excite the nerve fiber.

9. Which of the following statements is (are) correct concerning the propagation of a nerve impulse?
   (1) The conduction velocity of a nerve fiber is inversely proportional to the cross-sectional area of the axon.
   (2) In nonmyelinated fibers the action potential occurs randomly along the length of the fiber.
   (3) Saltatory conduction occurs only in the central nervous system.
   (4) A myelinated nerve fiber can be stimulated only at the nodes of Ranvier, where the axon is naked.

10. Which of the following statements is (are) correct concerning wallerian degeneration?
   (1) The myelin breaks down into droplets that are phagocytosed by the Schwann cells.
   (2) The axon is broken down into fragments.
   (3) The Schwann cells multiply.
   (4) In the central nervous system the debris is removed by the microglial cells.

11. Which of the following explanations is (are) correct concerning the failure of regeneration in the central nervous system?
   (1) Absence of endoneurial tubes
   (2) Failure of oligodendrocytes to multiply and form a band fiber as do Schwann cells in the peripheral nervous system
   (3) Absence of nerve growth factors
   (4) Lack of adequate blood supply to the nervous tissue

12. The following factor(s) may explain the partial return of function following injury to the central nervous system.
   (1) The subsiding of the edema at the site of injury
   (2) The complete regeneration of axons
   (3) Nonfunctional neurons taking over the function of damaged neurons
   (4) The injection of growth hormone intravenously

Match the features of a nerve cell or nerve fiber listed below on the left with an appropriate structure or function listed below on the right. Answers may be used more than once.

13. Schmidt-Lanterman incisure
14. Epineurium
15. Node of Ranvier

16. Chromatolysis
17. Axolemma

(a) Site of nerve activity
(b) Connective tissue
(c) Persistence of cytoplasm of Schwann cells or oligodendrocytes
(d) Nerve injury
(e) None of the above

ADDITIONAL READING

Aguayo, A. J., Benfey, M., and David, S. A potential for axonal regeneration in neurons of the adult mammalian nervous system. *Birth Defects* 19(4):327, 1983.

Almers, W. Gating Currents and Charge Movements in Excitable Membranes. In R. H. Adrian et al. (eds.). *Reviews of Physiology, Biochemistry, and Pharmacology.* New York: Springer-Verlag, 1978, p. 96.

Barron, K. D. Axon Reaction and Central Nervous System Regeneration. In *Nerve, Organ, and Tissue Regeneration: Research Perspectives.* New York: Academic, 1983, p. 3.

Baxter, C. F. Some Thoughts Concerning the Study of Intrinsic and Extrinsic Factors That Promote Neuronal Injury and Recovery. In B. Haber, J. R. Perez-Polo, G. A. Hashim, and A. M. Guiffrida Stella (eds.). *Nervous System Regeneration.* New York: Raven, 1983, Vol. 19, p. 241.

Berry, M. Regeneration of Axons in the Central Nervous System. In V. Navaratnam and R. J. Harrison (eds.). *Progress in Anatomy.* Cambridge: Cambridge University Press, 1983, Vol. 3, p. 213.

Dawson, D. M., Hallett, M., and Millender, L. H. *Entrapment Neuropathies* (2nd ed.). Boston: Little, Brown, 1990.

Fozzard, H. A. Conduction of the Action Potential. In R. M. Berne et al. (eds.). *Handbook of Physiology.* Baltimore: Williams & Wilkins, 1979, Sec. 2, Vol. 1, p. 335.

Guth, L., Reier, P. J., Barrett, C. P., and Donati, E. J. Repair of the mammalian spinal cord. *Trends Neurosci.* 5:20, 1983.

Hodgkin, A. L., and Huxley, A. F. Movement of sodium and potassium ions during nervous activity. *Cold Spring Harbor Symp. Quant. Biol.* 17:43, 1952.

Landon, D. N. (ed.). *The Peripheral Nerve.* New York: Wiley, 1976.

Marx, J. Regeneration in the central nervous system. *Science* 209:378, 1980.

Peters, A., Palay, S. L., and Webster, H. *The Fine Structure of the Nervous System: The Neurons and Supporting Cells.* Philadelphia: Saunders, 1976.

Pollock, M., and Harris, A. J. Accuracy in peripheral nerve regeneration. *Trends Neurosci.* 2:18, 1981.

Risling, M., Dalsgaard, C. J., Cukierman, A., and Cuello, A. C. Electron microscopic and immunohistochemical evidence that unmyelinated ventral root axons make U-turns or enter the spinal pia mater. *J. Comp. Neurol.* 225:53, 1984.

Seddon, H. J. Three types of nerve injury. *Brain* 66:237, 1944.

Seddon, H. J. *Surgical Disorders of Peripheral Nerves.* Edinburgh and London: Longman, 1972.

Snell, R. S. Changes in the histochemical appearances of cholinesterase in a mixed peripheral nerve following nerve section and compression injury. *Br. J. Exp. Pathol.* 38:34, 1957.

Sunderland, S. *Nerves and Nerve Injuries* (2nd ed.). Edinburgh: Churchill Livingstone, 1979.

Thomas, P. K., and King, R. H. M. The degeneration of unmyelinated axons following nerve section: An ultrastructural study. *J. Neurocytol.* 3:497, 1974.

Trojaborg, W. Rate of recovery in motor and sensory fibers of the radial nerve: Clinical and electrophysiological aspects. *J. Neurol. Neurosurg. Psychiatry* 33:625, 1970.

Veraa, R. P., and Grafstein, B. Cellular mechanisms for recovery from nervous system injury. *Exp. Neurol.* 71:6, 1981.

Waxman, S. G. (ed.). *Physiology and Pathobiology of Axons.* New York: Raven, 1978.

Chapter 5
Receptor and Effector Endings

RECEPTOR ENDINGS

An individual receives impressions from the outside world and from within the body by special sensory nerve endings or receptors.

Sensory receptors can be classified into five basic functional types.

Mechanoreceptors. These respond to mechanical deformation.

Thermoreceptors. These respond to changes in temperature; some receptors respond to cold and others to heat.

Nociceptors. These respond to any stimuli that bring about damage to the tissue.

Electromagnetic receptors. The rods and cones of the eyes are sensitive to changes in light intensity and wave length.

Chemoreceptors. These respond to chemical changes associated with taste and smell and oxygen and carbon dioxide concentrations in the blood.

ANATOMICAL TYPES OF RECEPTORS

For convenience the sensory endings can be classified, on a structural basis, into nonencapsulated and encapsulated receptors.

Nonencapsulated Receptors

Free Nerve Endings

Free nerve endings are widely distributed throughout the body (Fig. 5-1). They are found between the epithelial cells of the skin, the cornea, and the alimentary tract, and in connective tissues, including the dermis, fascia, ligaments, joint capsules, tendons, periosteum, perichondrium, Haversian systems of bone, tympanic membrane, and dental pulp, and they are also present in muscle.

The afferent nerve fibers from the free nerve endings are of small diameter and are either my-

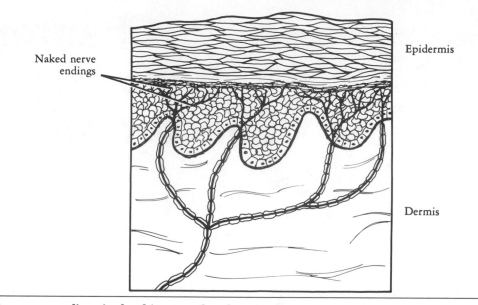

Naked nerve endings

Epidermis

Dermis

Fig. 5-1. Free nerve endings in the skin. Note that the nerve fibers in the epidermis are naked.

elinated or nonmyelinated. The terminal endings are devoid of a myelin sheath and there are no Schwann cells covering their tips.

Most of these endings detect pain, while others detect crude touch, pressure, and tickle sensations, and possibly cold and heat.

Merkel's Discs

Merkel's discs are found in hairless skin, e.g., the fingertips (Figs. 5-2 and 5-3), and in hair follicles. The nerve fiber passes into the epidermis and terminates as a disc-shaped expansion that is applied closely to a dark-staining epithelial cell in the deeper part of the epidermis, called the **Merkel cell**. In hairy skin, clusters of Merkel's discs, known as **tactile domes**, are found in the epidermis between the hair follicles.

Merkel's discs are slowly adapting touch receptors that transmit information about the degree of pressure exerted on the skin, as for example, when one is holding a pen.

Hair Follicle Receptors

Nerve fibers wind around the follicle in its outer connective tissue sheath below the sebaceous gland. Some branches surround the follicle, while others run parallel to its long axis (Figs. 5-4 and 5-5). Many naked axon filaments terminate among the cells of the outer root sheath.

Bending of the hair stimulates the follicle receptor, which belongs to the rapidly adapting group of mechanoreceptors. While the hair remains bent the receptor is silent, but when the hair is released, a further burst of nerve impulses is initiated.

Encapsulated Receptors

These receptors show wide variations in size and shape and the termination of the nerve is covered by a capsule.

Meissner's Corpuscles

Meissner's corpuscles are located in the dermal papillae of the skin (Figs. 5-6 and 5-7), especially that of the palm of the hand and the sole of the foot. Many also are present in the skin of the nipple and the external genitalia. Each corpuscle is ovoid in shape and consists of a stack of modified flattened Schwann cells arranged transversely across the long axis of the corpuscle. The corpuscle is enclosed by a capsule of connective tissue that is continuous

Epidermis

Tactile cell

Schwann cell   Naked axon

Dermis

A   B

Fig. 5-2. Merkel's discs in the skin. (A) Low magnification. (B) A Merkel's disc showing expanded ending of axon with stippled tactile cell.

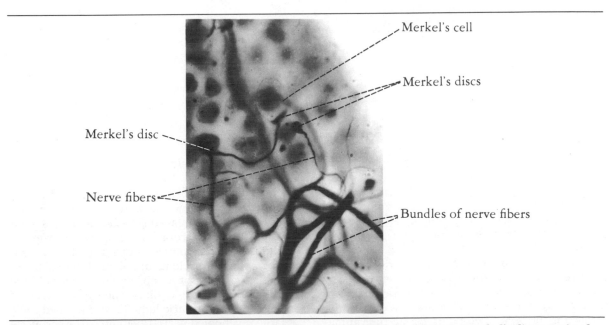

Merkel's cell

Merkel's discs

Merkel's disc

Nerve fibers

Bundles of nerve fibers

Fig. 5-3. Photomicrograph of digital skin showing fine nerve terminals ending in Merkel's discs. Stained by silver method. (Courtesy Dr. N. Cauna.)

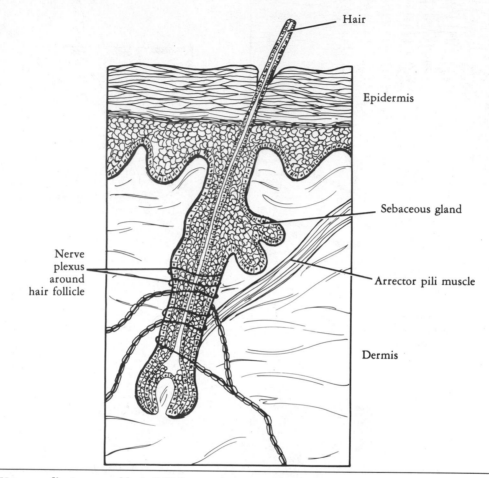

Fig. 5-4. Nerve endings around hair follicle.

with the endoneurium of the nerves that enter it. A few myelinated nerve fibers enter the deep end of the corpuscle; myelinated and unmyelinated branches decrease in size and ramify among the Schwann cells. There is a considerable reduction in the number of Meissner's corpuscles between birth and old age.

Meissner's corpuscles are very sensitive to touch and are rapidly adapting mechanoreceptors. They enable an individual to distinguish between two pointed structures when they are placed close together on the skin (two-point tactile discrimination).

Pacinian Corpuscles

Pacinian corpuscles (Figs. 5-8 and 5-9) are widely distributed throughout the body and are abundant in the dermis, subcutaneous tissue, ligaments, joint capsules, pleura, peritoneum, nipples, and external genitalia. Each corpuscle is ovoid in shape, measuring about 2 mm long and about 100 to 500 μm across. It consists of a capsule and a central core containing the nerve ending. The capsule consists of numerous concentric lamellae of flattened cells. A large myelinated nerve fiber enters the corpuscle and loses its myelin sheath and then its Schwann

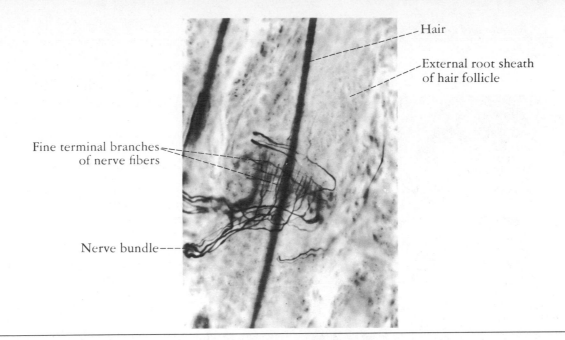

Fine terminal branches
of nerve fibers

Nerve bundle

Hair

External root sheath
of hair follicle

Fig. 5-5. Photomicrograph of nerve endings around hair follicle. Stained by silver method. (Courtesy Dr. M. J. T. Fitzgerald.)

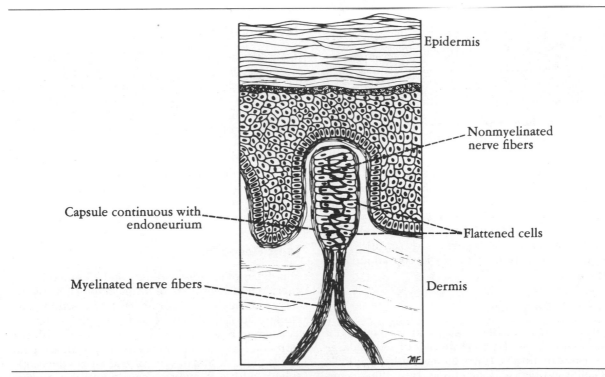

Epidermis

Nonmyelinated
nerve fibers

Capsule continuous with
endoneurium

Flattened cells

Myelinated nerve fibers

Dermis

Fig. 5-6. Detailed structure of Meissner's corpuscle in skin.

Fig. 5-7. Photomicrograph of Meissner's corpuscle of skin. (Courtesy Dr. N. Cauna.)

cell covering. The naked axon, surrounded by lamellae formed of flattened cells, passes through the center of the core and terminates in an expanded end.

The pacinian corpuscle is a rapidly adapting mechanoreceptor that is particularly sensitive to vibration. It can respond to up to 600 stimuli per second.

Ruffini's Corpuscles

Ruffini's corpuscles are located in the dermis of hairy skin. Each corpuscle consists of several large unmyelinated nerve fibers ending within a bundle of collagen fibers and surrounded by a cellular capsule. These slowly adapting mechanoreceptors are

stretch receptors, which respond when the skin is stretched.

Function of Cutaneous Receptors

In the past it was believed that the different histological types of receptors corresponded to specific types of sensation. It was soon pointed out that there are areas of the body that have only one or two histological types of receptors and yet they are sensitive to a variety of different stimuli. Moreover, although the body has these different receptors, all nerves only transmit nerve impulses. It is now generally agreed that the type of sensation felt is determined by the specific area of the central nervous system to which the afferent nerve fiber passes. For example, if a pain nerve fiber is stimulated by heat, cold, touch, or pressure, the individual will experience only pain.

Transduction of Sensory Stimuli into Nerve Impulses

Transduction is the process by which one form of energy (the stimulus) is changed into another form of energy (electrochemical energy of the nerve impulse). The stimulus when applied to the receptor brings about a change in potential of the plasma membrane of the nerve ending. Since this process takes place in the receptor, it is referred to as the **receptor potential**. If large enough, the receptor potential will generate an action potential that will travel along the afferent nerve fiber to the central nervous system.

Joint Receptors

Four types of sensory endings can be located in the capsule and ligaments of synovial joints. Three of these endings are encapsulated and resemble pacinian, Ruffini's, and tendon stretch receptors. They provide the central nervous system with information regarding the position and movements of the joint. A fourth type of ending is nonencapsulated and is thought to be sensitive to excessive movements and to transmit pain sensations.

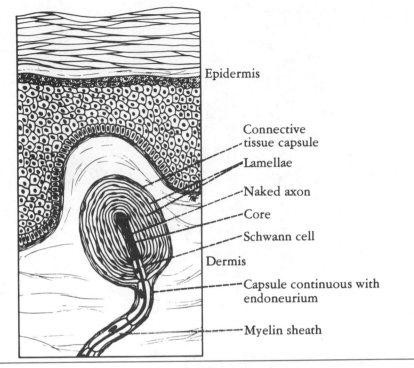

Fig. 5-8. Detailed structure of pacinian corpuscle in skin.

Epidermis

Connective tissue capsule

Lamellae

Naked axon

Core

Schwann cell

Dermis

Capsule continuous with endoneurium

Myelin sheath

Neuromuscular Spindles

Neuromuscular spindles, or muscular spindles (Figs. 5-10 and 5-11), are found in skeletal muscle and are most numerous toward the tendinous attachment of the muscle. They provide sensory information that is used by the central nervous system in the control of muscle activity. Each spindle measures about 1 to 4 mm in length and is surrounded by a fusiform capsule of connective tissue. Within the capsule are 6 to 14 slender **intrafusal muscle fibers**; the ordinary muscle fibers situated outside the spindles are referred to as **extrafusal fibers**. The intrafusal fibers of the spindles are of two types: the **nuclear bag** and **nuclear chain** fibers. The nuclear bag fibers are recognized by the presence of numerous nuclei in the equatorial region, which consequently is expanded; also, cross-striations are absent in this region. In the nuclear chain fibers, the nuclei form a single longitudinal row or chain in the center of each fiber at the equatorial region. The nuclear bag fibers are larger in

Fig. 5-9. Photomicrograph of part of pacinian corpuscle of skin seen in transverse section, showing concentric lamellae of flattened cells. (Courtesy Dr. N. Cauna.)

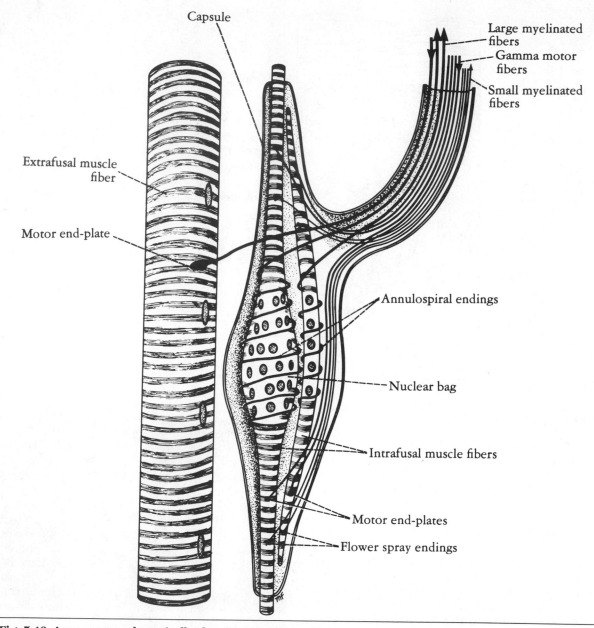

Fig. 5-10. A neuromuscular spindle showing two types of intrafusal fibers: the nuclear bag and nuclear chain fibers.

Bundle of nerve fibers

Annulospiral ending around intrafusal muscle fiber

Muscle fibers

Fig. 5-11. Photomicrograph of a neuromuscular spindle.

diameter than the nuclear chain fibers, and they extend beyond the capsule at each end to be attached to the endomysium of the extrafusal fibers.

There are two types of sensory innervation of muscle spindles: the annulospiral and the flower spray. The **annulospiral endings** are situated at the equator of the intrafusal fibers. As the large myelinated nerve fiber pierces the capsule, it loses its myelin sheath and the naked axon winds spirally around the nuclear bag or chain portions of the intrafusal fibers.

The **flower spray endings** are situated mainly on the nuclear chain fibers some distance away from the equatorial region. A slightly smaller myelinated nerve fiber than that for the annulospiral ending pierces the capsule and loses its myelin sheath and the naked axon branches terminally and ends as varicosities; it resembles a spray of flowers.

Stretching (elongation) of the intrafusal fibers results in stimulation of the annulospiral and flower spray endings, and nerve impulses pass to the spinal cord in the afferent neurons.

Motor innervation of the intrafusal fibers is provided by fine gamma motor fibers. The nerves terminate in small motor end-plates situated at both ends of the intrafusal fibers. Stimulation of the motor nerves causes both ends of the intrafusal fibers to contract and activate the sensory endings. The

equatorial region, which is without cross-striations, is noncontractile. The extrafusal fibers of the remainder of the muscle receive their innervation in the usual way from large alpha-size axons.

Function of the Neuromuscular Spindle

Under resting conditions, the muscle spindles give rise to afferent nerve impulses all the time, and most of this information is not consciously perceived. When muscle activity occurs, either actively or passively, the intrafusal fibers are stretched and there is an increase in the rate of passage of nerve impulses to the spinal cord or brain in the afferent neurons. Similarly, if the intrafusal fibers are now relaxed due to the cessation of muscle activity, the result is a decrease in the rate of passage of nerve impulses to the spinal cord or brain. The neuromuscular spindle thus plays a very important role in keeping the central nervous system informed about muscle activity, thereby indirectly influencing the control of voluntary muscle.

Stretch Reflex

The neurons of the spinal cord involved in the simple stretch reflex are as follows. Stretching a muscle results in the elongation of the intrafusal fibers of the muscle spindle and stimulation of the annulospiral and flower spray endings. The nerve impulses reach the spinal cord in the afferent neurons and synapse with the large alpha motor neurons situated in the anterior gray horns of the spinal cord. Nerve impulses now pass via the efferent motor nerves and stimulate the extrafusal muscle fibers and the muscle contracts. This simple stretch reflex depends on a two-neuron arc consisting of an afferent neuron and an efferent neuron. It is interesting to note that the muscle spindle afferent impulses inhibit the alpha motor neurons supplying the antagonist muscles. This effect is called **reciprocal inhibition**.

Control of the Intrafusal Fibers of the Neuromuscular Spindle

In the brain and spinal cord there are centers that give rise to tracts that synapse with gamma motor neurons in the spinal cord. The reticular formation, the basal ganglia, and the cerebellum are examples of such centers. It is by these means that these centers can greatly influence voluntary muscle activity. The gamma efferent motor fibers cause shortening of the intrafusal fibers, stretching the equatorial regions and stimulating the annulospiral and flower spray endings. This in turn initiates the reflex contraction of the extrafusal fibers described previously.

It is estimated that about one-third of all the motor fibers passing to a muscle are gamma efferents; the remaining two-thirds are the large alpha motor fibers. It is believed that the nuclear bag fibers are concerned with dynamic responses and are associated more with position and velocity of contraction, whereas the nuclear chain fibers are associated with slow static contractions of voluntary muscle.

NEUROTENDINOUS SPINDLES (GOLGI TENDON ORGANS)

Neurotendinous spindles are present in tendons and are located near the junctions of tendons with muscles (Fig. 5-12). Each spindle consists of a fibrous capsule that surrounds a small bundle of loosely arranged tendon (collagen) fibers (intrafusal fibers). The tendon cells are larger and more numerous than those found elsewhere in the tendon. One or more myelinated sensory nerve fibers pierce the capsule, lose their myelin sheath, branch, and terminate in club-shaped endings.

The nerve endings are activated by being squeezed by the adjacent tendon fibers within the spindle when tension develops in the tendon. Unlike the neuromuscular spindle, which is sensitive to changes in muscle length, the neurotendinous organ detects changes in muscle tension.

Function of the Neurotendinous Spindle

Increased muscle tension stimulates the neurotendinous spindles and an increased number of nerve impulses reach the spinal cord through the afferent nerve fibers. These fibers synapse with the large alpha motor neurons situated in the anterior gray horns of the spinal cord. Unlike the muscle spindle reflex, this reflex is inhibitory and inhibits muscle contraction. In this manner the tendon reflex prevents the development of too much tension in the muscle. Although this function is probably important as a protective mechanism, its main function is to provide the central nervous system with information that can influence voluntary muscle activity.

EFFECTOR ENDINGS

Innervation of Skeletal Muscle

Skeletal muscle is innervated by one or more nerves. In the limbs and head and neck the innervation is usually single, but in the large muscles of the abdominal wall the innervation is multiple, the latter muscles having retained their embryonic segmental nerve supply.

The nerve supply and blood supply to a muscle enter it at a more or less constant position called the **neurovascular hilus**. The nerve to a muscle contains motor and sensory fibers. The motor fibers are of three types: (1) large alpha myelinated fibers,[*] (2) small gamma myelinated fibers, and

---

*Class A fibers (see p. 102) are subdivided into alpha, beta, and gamma fibers. The alpha fibers are large and fast-conducting, and average about 17 μm in diameter. The gamma fibers are the smallest fibers, measure about 2 to 10 μm in diameter, and are slow-conducting.

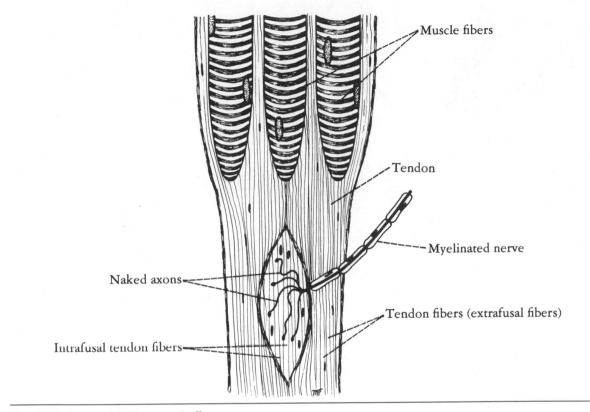

Fig. 5-12. A neurotendinous spindle.

(3) fine unmyelinated fibers. The large myelinated axons of the alpha anterior horn cells supply the extrafusal fibers that form the main mass of the muscle. The small gamma myelinated fibers supply the intrafusal fibers of the neuromuscular spindles. The fine unmyelinated fibers are postganglionic autonomic efferents that supply the smooth muscle in the walls of blood vessels.

The sensory fibers are of three main types: (1) the myelinated fibers, which originate in the annulospiral and flower spray endings of the neuromuscular spindles, (2) the myelinated fibers, which originate in the neurotendinous spindles, and (3) the myelinated and nonmyelinated fibers, which originate from a variety of sensory endings in the connective tissue of the muscle.

Motor Unit

The motor unit may be defined as the single alpha motor neuron and the muscle fibers that it inner-

vates (Fig. 5-13). The muscle fibers of a single motor unit are widely scattered throughout the muscle. Where fine, precise muscle control is required, such as in the extraocular muscles or the small muscles of the hand, the motor units possess only a few muscle fibers. However, in a large limb muscle, such as the gluteus maximus, where precise control is not necessary, a single motor nerve may innervate many hundreds of muscle fibers.

Neuromuscular Junctions in Skeletal Muscle

As each large alpha myelinated fiber enters a skeletal muscle it branches many times. The number of branches depends on the size of the motor unit. A single branch then terminates on a muscle fiber at a site referred to as a **neuromuscular junction** or **motor end-plate** (Figs. 5-14 and 5-15). The great majority of muscle fibers are innervated by just one motor end-plate. On reaching the muscle

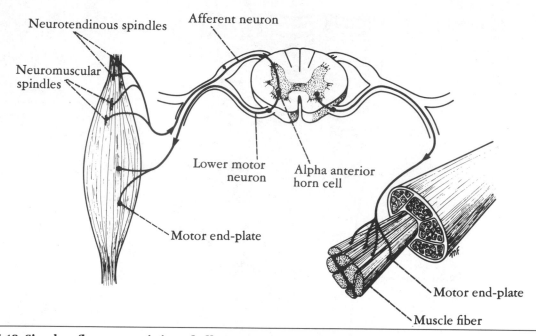

Fig. 5-13. Simple reflex arc consisting of afferent neuron arising from neuromuscular spindles and neuro-tendinous spindles and efferent lower motor neuron whose cell body is an alpha anterior horn cell within the spinal cord. Note that the efferent neuron terminates on muscle fibers at motor end-plates.

fiber, the nerve loses its myelin sheath and breaks up into a number of subsidiary branches. Each branch ends as a naked axon and constitutes the **neural element** of the motor end-plate (Fig. 5-16). The axon is expanded slightly and contains numerous mitochondria and vesicles (approximately 45 nm in diameter). At the site of the motor end-plate the surface of the muscle fiber is elevated slightly to form the **muscular element** of the plate, often referred to as the **sole plate** (see Fig. 5-14). The elevation is due to the local accumulation of granular sarcoplasm beneath the sarcolemma and the presence of numerous nuclei and mitochondria.

The expanded naked axon lies in a groove on the surface of the muscle fiber. Each groove is formed by the infolding of the sarcolemma. The groove may branch many times, each branch containing a division of the axon. It is important to realize that the axons are truly naked; the Schwann cells merely serve as a cap or roof to the groove and never project into it. The floor of the groove is formed of sarcolemma, which is thrown into numerous folds,

called **junctional folds**; these serve to increase the surface area of the sarcolemma that lie close to the naked axon (Fig. 5-17). The plasma membrane of the axon (the axolemma or presynaptic membrane) is separated, by a space about 20 to 50 nm wide, from the plasma membrane of the muscle fiber (the sarcolemma or postsynaptic membrane). This space constitutes the **synaptic cleft**. The synaptic cleft is filled with the basement membranes of the axon and the muscle fiber (Fig. 5-14). The motor end-plate is strengthened by the connective tissue sheath of the nerve fiber, the endoneurium, which becomes continuous with the connective tissue sheath of the muscle fiber, the endomysium.

A nerve impulse, on reaching a motor end-plate, causes the release of acetylcholine from some of the axonal vesicles. The acetylcholine is discharged into the synaptic cleft by a process of **exocytosis** and diffuses through the basement membranes to reach the receptors on the postsynaptic membrane. This makes the postsynaptic membrane more permeable to Na^+ ions and a local potential is cre-

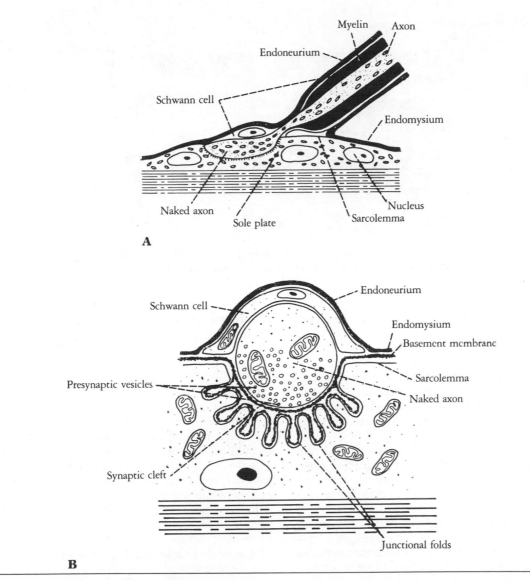

**Fig. 5-14. A. A skeletal neuromuscular junction.
B. Enlarged view of muscle fiber showing terminal naked axon lying in surface groove of muscle fiber.**

Nerve fibers and bundles
of nerve fibers

Acetylcholinesterase
at motor end-plates

Fig. 5-15. Photomicrograph showing nerve fibers terminating on skeletal muscle fibers at motor end-plates. Stained histochemically for acetylcholinesterase and counterstained with silver. (Courtesy Dr. M. J. T. Fitzgerald.)

ated called the **end-plate potential**. If the end-plate potential is large enough, an action potential will be initiated that will spread along the surface of the sarcolemma. The wave of depolarization is carried into the muscle fiber to the contractile myofibrils through the system of T tubules. This leads to the release of Ca^+ ions from the sarcoplasmic reticulum that in turn causes the muscle to contract.

The amount of acetylcholine released at the motor end-plate will depend on the number of nerve impulses arriving at the nerve terminal. Once the acetylcholine crosses the synaptic cleft it immediately undergoes hydrolysis due to the presence of **acetylcholinesterase (AChE)** (Fig. 5-15) in the basement membranes and the postsynaptic membrane or sarcolemma. The acetylcholine remains for about 1 millisecond in contact with the postsynaptic membrane, and it is rapidly destroyed to prevent reexcitation of the muscle fiber.

Skeletal muscle fiber contraction is thus controlled by the frequency of the nerve impulses that arrive at the motor nerve terminal. A resting muscle fiber shows small occasional depolarizations (end-plate potentials) at the motor end-plate, which are insufficient to cause an action potential and make the fiber contract. These are believed to be due to the sporadic release of acetylcholine into the synaptic cleft from a single presynaptic vesicle.

Neuromuscular Junctions in Smooth Muscle

In smooth muscle, where the action is slow and widespread, such as within the wall of the intestine, the autonomic nerve fibers branch extensively, so that a single neuron exerts control over a large number of muscle fibers. In some areas, for example, the longitudinal layer of smooth muscle in the intestine, only a few muscle fibers are associated with autonomic endings, the wave of contraction passing from one muscle cell to another by means of gap junctions (Fig. 5-18).

In smooth muscle, in which the action is fast and precision is required, such as in the iris, the branching of the nerve fibers is less extensive, so that a single neuron exerts control over only a few muscle fibers.

The autonomic nerve fibers, which are postganglionic (see p. 485), are nonmyelinated and terminate as a series of varicosed branches. An interval of from 10 to 100 nm may exist between the axon and the muscle fiber. At the site where transmission is to occur, the Schwann cell is retracted so that the axon lies within a shallow groove on its surface (Fig. 5-18). Part of the axon thus is naked, permitting free diffusion of the transmitter substance from the axon to the muscle cell (Fig. 5-18). Here the axoplasm contains numerous vesicles sim-

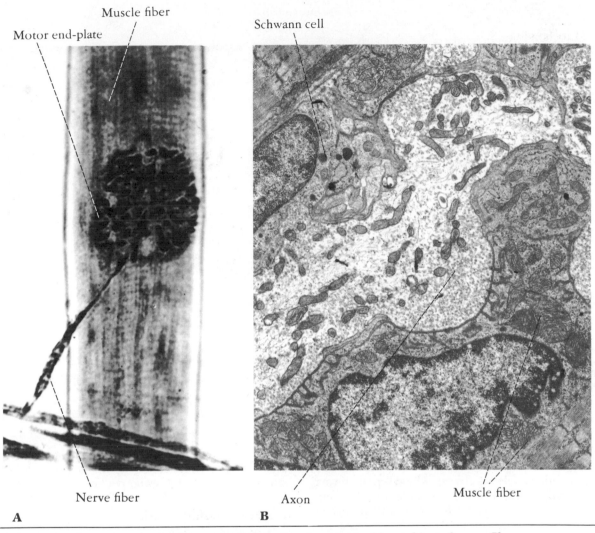

A

B

Fig. 5-16. A. Photomicrograph of motor end-plate showing terminal branching of nerve fiber. B. Electron micrograph of terminal axon at motor end-plate. Shows axon lying in a groove on the surface of the muscle fiber. (Courtesy Dr. J. M. Kerns.)

Fig. 5-17. Electron micrograph of cross section of axon at motor end-plate. Shows axon lying in a groove of folded sarcolemma. (Courtesy Dr. J. M. Kerns.)

ilar to those seen at the motor end-plate of skeletal muscle.

Smooth muscle is innervated by sympathetic and parasympathetic parts of the autonomic system. Those nerves that are cholinergic liberate acetylcholine at their endings by a process of exocytosis, the acetylcholine being present in the vesicles at the nerve ending. Those nerves that are noradrenergic liberate **norepinephrine** at their endings by a process of exocytosis, the norepinephrine being present in dark-cored vesicles at the nerve endings. Both the acetylcholine and norepinephrine bring about depolarization of the muscle fibers innervated, which thereupon contract. The fate of these neurotransmitter substances differs. The acetylcholine is hydrolyzed in the presence of acetylcholinesterase in the sarcolemma of the muscle fiber and the norepinephrine is taken up by the nerve endings. It is important to note that in some areas of the body

(e.g., bronchial muscle) the norepinephrine liberated from postganglionic sympathetic fibers causes smooth muscle to relax and not contract.

Neuromuscular Junctions in Cardiac Muscle

Nonmyelinated postganglionic autonomic nerves extend into the connective tissue between the muscle fibers and terminate in close proximity to the individual cardiac muscle fibers. At the site where transmission takes place, the axon becomes naked because of the retraction of the Schwann cell. This permits free diffusion of the neurotransmitter substance from the axon to the muscle fiber. Because of the presence of intermittent desmosomes and gap junctions between abutting muscle fibers, excitation and contraction of one muscle fiber rapidly spreads from fiber to fiber.

Naked axons

Schwann cell

Smooth muscle fibers

Gap junctions

Fig. 5-18. An autonomic neuromuscular junction. Shows the exposed axons close to the smooth muscle fibers.

Acinus

Naked axons

Duct

Fig. 5-19. Nerve fibers ending around glandular acini.

Nerve Endings on Secretory Cells of Glands

Nonmyelinated postganglionic autonomic nerves extend into the connective tissue of glands and branch close to the secretory cells (Fig. 5-19). In many glands the nerve fibers have been found to innervate only the blood vessels.

CLINICAL NOTES

RECEPTORS

Sensory endings are found throughout the body in both somatic and visceral areas. It is fortunate that they are so widely distributed, because they enable the human subject to react to changes in the external and internal environment.

A physician, in order to make a diagnosis or study the effect of treatment on a disease process, relies almost entirely on the patient's ability to describe changes in subjective sensations, or to respond to specific stimuli during a physical examination. Such statements as "knifelike pain," "dull aching pain," "colicky pain," "pins and needles," "cannot feel anything, doctor," are symptoms that are very familiar to the practicing physician. Each main type of sensation that can be experienced, such as pain, temperature, and touch and pressure, is called a **modality** of sensation. The type of modality felt by a patient from a particular part of the body is determined by the specific area of the central nervous system to which the afferent nerve fiber passes. However, it is clinically useful to remember that axons that carry specific modalities are associated with one or more anatomically distinct receptors.

Receptor	Associated Function
Free nerve endings	Pain, touch, pressure, tickle
	Sensations, ? cold and heat
Merkel's discs	Touch and pressure
Hair follicle receptor	Touch
Meissner's corpuscles	Touch (two-point tactile discrimination)
Pacinian corpuscles	Pressure and vibration
Ruffini's corpuscles	Stretch
Neuromuscular spindles	Elongation of muscle (stretch)
Neurotendinous spindles	Tension

EXAMINATION OF INDIVIDUAL SENSORY MODALITIES

An accurate physical examination may enable the neurologist to make a precise diagnosis. He may be able to determine whether a particular sensation can or cannot be appreciated, or whether it is less than normal. He will be able to determine the precise area over the surface of the body where impairment of sensation is found. The following sensations are usually tested:

1. **Light touch**. This is tested by gently touching the skin with a wisp of cotton; the patient has his eyes closed and responds "yes" whenever he feels the stimulus. It is important to realize that different areas of the skin normally exhibit different thresholds for touch. The back and buttocks are less sensitive than the face or fingertips. On hairy surfaces, the slightest movement of a hair usually can be felt.
2. **Localization of touch**. After the patient has detected the light touch with his eyes closed, he is asked to place a finger on the exact site touched. Failure to accomplish this may be due to damage to the cerebral cortex.
3. **Two-point tactile discrimination**. Two blunt points are applied to the skin surface with the patient's eyes closed. Gradually the points are brought closer together until the patient is unable to distinguish two definite points. A normal person is able to distinguish two separate points on the tip of the index finger when they are separated by a distance greater than about 3 mm. On the back, however, they have to be separated by as much as 3 to 4 cm.
4. **Pain**. The skin may be touched with the sharp end of a pin. First the pain threshold is established, and the areas of diminished or lost pain sensation are mapped out. It is advisable to apply the stimulus in an irregular manner, first

using the sharp end of the pin, and then the dull head, the patient responding "sharp" or "dull." In certain diseases, such as tabes dorsalis or polyneuropathy (polyneuritis), there is a delay of up to 3 seconds before the patient recognizes the sharp pain.

5. **Pressure pain**. This is a poorly localized pain, which is perceived by deep pressure on a muscle or by squeezing a tendon.

6. **Temperature testing**. Test tubes filled with hot or cold water may be used. When they are applied to the skin the patient responds with either "warm" or "cold." First the temperature threshold is established and then the areas of diminished or lost temperature sensation are mapped out.

7. **Vibration**. When the handle of a vibrating tuning fork is applied to the skin over bone (e.g., the medial malleolus of the tibia or the olecranon process of the ulna), a tingling sensation is felt. This is due to the stimulation of superficial and deep pressure receptors. The patient is asked to respond when he first feels the vibration and when he no longer can detect the vibration. The perception of vibration in the legs is usually diminished after the age of 60.

8. **Appreciation of form (stereognosis)**. Have the patient close his eyes and place common objects such as coins or keys in his hands. The patient normally should be able to identify objects by moving them around in his hand and feeling them with his fingers.

9. **Passive movements of joints**. This test may be carried out on the fingers or toes. With the patient completely relaxed and in the supine position with his eyes closed, the digit is flexed or extended irregularly. After each movement, the patient is asked, "Is the digit 'up' or 'down'?" A normal individual not only can determine that passive movement is taking place but also is aware of the direction of the movement.

10. **Postural sensibility**. This is the ability to describe the position of a limb when it is placed in that position while the patient's eyes are closed. Another way to perform the test is to ask the patient, with his eyes closed, to place the limb on the opposite side in the same position as the other limb. The application and interpretation of the results of these tests will be understood more fully when the afferent or sensory pathways have been discussed (See p. 363.)

PHANTOM LIMB

It has been established that wherever a particular sensory pathway is stimulated along its course from the receptor to the sensory cortex of the brain, the sensation experienced by the individual is referred to the site of the receptor. For example, if the pain fibers from the receptors in the little finger are stimulated in the ulnar nerve at the elbow, the individual will experience pain in the little finger and not at the elbow.

Following the amputation of a limb, the patient may experience severe pain in the absent limb due to pressure on the nerve fibers at the end of the stump. This phenomenon is referred to clinically as **phantom limb**.

ACTION OF DRUGS AND OTHER AGENTS ON SKELETAL NEUROMUSCULAR JUNCTIONS

Neuromuscular Blocking Agents

D-Tubocurarine produces flaccid paralysis of skeletal muscle first affecting the extrinsic muscles of the eyes and then those of the face, the extremities, and finally the diaphragm. **Dimethyl tubocurarine**, **gallamine**, and **benzoquinonium** have similar effects.

These drugs combine with the receptor sites at the postsynaptic membrane normally used by acetylcholine, and thus block the neurotransmitter action of acetylcholine. They are therefore referred to as competitive blocking agents, since they are competing for the same receptor site as does acetylcholine. As these drugs are slowly metabolized, the paralysis passes off.

Decamethonium and **succinylcholine** also paralyze skeletal muscle, but their action differs from that of competitive blocking agents because they produce their effect by causing depolarization of the motor end-plate. Acting like acetylcholine, they produce depolarization of the postsynaptic membrane and the muscle contracts once. This is followed by a flaccid paralysis and a blockage of neuromuscular activity. Although the blocking action endures for some time, the drugs are metabolized and the paralysis passes off. The actual paralysis is produced by the continued depolarization of the postsynaptic membrane. It must be remembered that continuous depolarization does not produce continuous skeletal muscle contraction. Repolarization has to take place before further depolarization can occur.

Neuromuscular blocking agents are commonly used with general anesthetics to produce the desired degree of muscle relaxation without using larger doses of general anesthetics. Because the respiratory muscles are paralyzed, facilities for artificial respiration are essential.

Anticholinesterases

Physostigmine and **neostigmine** have the capacity to combine with acetylcholinesterase and prevent the esterase from inactivating acetylcholine. In addition, neostigmine has a direct stimulating action on skeletal muscle. The actions of both drugs are reversible and they have been used with success in the treatment of myasthenia gravis.

Bacterial Toxins

Clostridium botulinum, the causative organism in certain cases of food poisoning, produces a toxin that inhibits the release of acetylcholine at the neuromuscular junction. Death results from paralysis of the respiratory muscles.

Motor Nerve and Skeletal Muscle

Not only does the motor nerve control the activity of the muscle it supplies, but its integrity is essential for the muscle's normal maintenance. Following section of a motor nerve, the muscle fibers rapidly atrophy and are replaced by connective tissue. The total bulk of the muscle may be reduced by three-quarters in as little as three months. This degree of atrophy does not occur if the muscle simply is immobilized, i.e., it is not just disuse atrophy. It is apparent that the maintenance of normal muscle is dependent on the continued reception of

acetylcholine at the postsynaptic membrane at the neuromuscular junction.

Denervation Supersensitivity of Skeletal Muscle

After approximately two weeks of denervation, skeletal muscle fibers respond to externally applied acetylcholine at sites other than the neuromuscular junctions. This supersensitivity could be explained on the basis that many new acetylcholine receptors have developed along the length of the muscle fibers following denervation.

Myasthenia Gravis

Myasthenia gravis is a disease characterized by drooping of the upper eyelids (ptosis), double vision (diplopia), difficulty in swallowing (dysphagia), difficulty in talking (dysarthria), and general muscular weakness and fatigue. Initially, the disease most commonly involves the muscles of the eye and pharynx and the symptoms may be relieved with rest. In the progressive form of the disease, the weakness becomes steadily worse and ultimately death occurs.

The condition is an autoimmune disorder, in which there is a reduced responsiveness of the postsynaptic membrane to acetylcholine. The T-lymphocytes produced by the thymus in some way affect the receptor sites. The condition can be temporarily relieved by anticholinesterase drugs such as **neostigmine**, which potentiate the action of acetylcholine. Thymectomy is recommended in severe progressive cases.

Hypokalemic Periodic Paralysis and Hyperkalemic Paralysis

These are diseases due to lowered or raised blood potassium levels. It is known that the ability of acetylcholine to initiate electrical changes in the postsynaptic membrane of the neuromuscular junction can be greatly influenced by the level of blood potassium, and it is this blood change that is responsible for the paralysis in these patients.

ACTION OF DRUGS ON NEUROMUSCULAR JUNCTIONS IN SMOOTH MUSCLE, CARDIAC MUSCLE, AND NERVE ENDINGS ON SECRETORY CELLS

It has been stated that, in normal body physiology, acetylcholine released from postganglionic parasympathetic fibers can bring about depolarization and resulting contraction of smooth muscle fibers. Acetylcholine, however, is a useless drug to be administered by the physician, because it is rapidly destroyed by the **cholinesterases**, and because its actions are so widespread it cannot be used selectively. By slightly changing the structure, as in the case of **methacholine chloride** or **carbechol chloride**, the drugs are less susceptible to destruction by the cholinesterases but still possess the ability to react with the receptors.

Atropine and **scopolamine** are drugs that compete with acetylcholine for the same receptors. These drugs are competitive antagonists of acetylcholine at receptor sites of smooth muscle, cardiac muscle, and various secretory cells.

Norepinephrine is released from postganglionic sympathetic fibers and can bring about depolarization of smooth muscle in the walls of arteries, for example, resulting in their contraction. At other sites, such as the bronchi, it causes smooth muscle relaxation. In 1948 Ahlquist classified sympathetic receptors as alpha and beta. The functions associated with alpha receptors are vasoconstriction, mydriasis (dilatation of pupil), and relaxation of the smooth muscle of the intestine. Beta receptors are associated with vasodilatation, cardioacceleration, bronchial relaxation, and intestinal relaxation.

Phenoxybenzamine has been found to block alpha receptors while **propranolol** blocks beta receptors. The structure of these receptors is not known.

CLINICAL PROBLEMS   *Answers on Page 591*

1. An 18-year-old woman visited her physician because she had burns, which she had not felt, on the tips of the fingers of the right hand. She also mentioned that she had weakness of her right hand. On physical examination severe scarring of the fingers of the right hand was noted. Obvious atrophy of the small muscles of the right hand was also found. Testing the sensory modalities of the skin of the entire patient showed total loss of pain and temperature sensation of the distal part of the right upper limb. There was diminished sensibility to pain and temperature of the left hand. Definite muscular weakness was demonstrated in the small muscles of the right hand and a small amount of weakness also was found in the muscles of the left hand. A diagnosis of syringomyelia was made. (a) Using your neuroanatomical knowledge, can you describe the type of sensory nerve endings that are sensitive to pain and temperature? (b) How would you examine a patient to determine if there is cutaneous pain and temperature sensory loss?

2. A 35-year-old man, while walking past some workmen who were digging a hole in the road, suddenly became aware of a foreign body in his left eye. Since the cornea is extremely sensitive, he suffered considerable discomfort. What sensory endings are present in the cornea? Is the cornea sensitive to stimuli other than pain?

3. If you wished to carry out some physiological research involving the implantation of electrodes into sensory receptors, you would probably do the work on the larger receptors. What is the name of the largest sensory receptor (excluding the eye and the ear) and what are its approximate dimensions?

4. While performing a complete neurological examination on a patient, a fourth-year medical student was asked by a physician if there is any anatomical basis for cutaneous sensations. How would you have answered that question?

5. A 60-year-old man visited his physician because for the past three months he had been experiencing an agonizing stabbing pain over the middle part of the right side of his face. The stabs would last a few seconds but might be repeated several times. "The pain is the worst I have ever experienced," he told his physician. He had noticed particularly that a draft of cold

air on his face or the touching of a few scalp hairs in the temporal region could trigger the pain. Physical examination revealed no sensory or motor loss of the trigeminal nerve. A diagnosis of trigeminal neuralgia was made. Using your knowledge of neuroanatomy, can you explain why hairs are so sensitive to touch?

6. A 50-year-old man was diagnosed as suffering from tabes dorsalis. On physical examination, many signs of the syphilitic disease were present, including a total lack of deep sensation to pain. Intense squeezing of the tendo calcaneus or the testicles produced no response. Using your knowledge of neuroanatomy, explain how deep pain sensation is normally experienced.

7. What is the function of intrafusal fibers in a neuromuscular spindle? Is there more than one type of intrafusal muscle fiber? What is the significance of a gamma efferent motor fiber entering a muscle spindle?

8. While carrying out a physical examination of a patient, the physician asked the patient to cross his knees and relax his leg muscles. The left ligamentum patellae was then struck smartly with a reflex hammer, and this immediately produced an involuntary partial extension of the left knee joint (the knee-jerk test was positive). How does the central nervous system receive nervous information from the quadriceps femoris muscle in order that it may respond reflexly by extending the knee?

9. Name four types of sensory nerve endings found in muscle; indicate the probable function of each of these endings.

10. Define the terms (a) *motor unit*, (b) *neurovascular hilus*, (c) *sole plate*, (d) *junctional folds of motor end-plate*, and (e) *synaptic cleft of motor end-plate*.

11. A 55-year-old man suffering from syphilis of the spinal cord presented characteristic symptoms and signs of tabes dorsalis. He had experienced severe stabbing pains in the abdomen and legs for the last 6 months. When asked to walk, the patient was seen to do so with a broad base, slapping the feet on the ground. How would you test the patient's ability to perceive the position of his lower extremities and his vibratory sense? Using your knowledge of neuroanatomy, explain how a normal individual is able to perceive the position of his extremities and detect vibrations.

12. Using your knowledge of pharmacology, name two drugs that act as competitive blocking agents on skeletal neuromuscular junctions. Name the chemical substance against which these agents are competing. Name the sites at which the blocking agents are believed to act.

13. Name a drug that will bring about flaccid paralysis of skeletal muscle by causing depolarization of the postsynaptic membrane.

14. In cases of severe food poisoning the organism *Clostridium botulinum* may be found to be responsible. How does this organism cause paralysis of the respiratory muscles?

15. An orthopedic surgeon stated, during a ward round, that the degree of muscular atrophy that occurs in a limb immobilized in a cast is totally different from the degree of muscular atrophy that follows section of the motor nerve supply to muscles. The surgeon asked a medical student to explain this difference. How would you account for this difference in the degree of muscular atrophy?

16. A 35-year-old woman visited her physician because she had noticed that her upper eyelid drooped, especially when she was tired or emotionally upset. She had first noticed this 6 months before. Two months before, she had started to have double vision, which was very slight to begin with and lasted for only a few hours. During the last week the double vision had returned, was more severe, and lasted for several hours. Her friends have remarked that she doesn't seem to smile as much as she used to. On questioning she admitted that talking tires her and her throat feels particularly tired after eating a large meal. On physical examination the patient had slight ptosis (drooping of the upper lid) of the right eye. The eye movements appeared to be normal but the face seemed to be unnaturally immobile. In her attempts to smile the expression was more of a snarl than a happy expression. It was also noted that the patient responded to questions in a rather feeble voice with a nasal quality. When asked to hold her arms outstretched in front of her, the patient became quickly fatigued. What is the diagnosis? What is the cause of this condition?

17. Following an abdominal operation for peptic ulcer, the surgeon was concerned that the patient had not voluntarily urinated for 14 hours. Before catheterizing the patient, the resident decided to use a cholinergic drug in order to stimulate the detrusor muscle of the bladder. How does an autonomic nerve terminate in the region of a smooth muscle fiber? Name a cholinergic drug that could be used to bring about contraction of the detrusor muscle.

NATIONAL BOARD TYPE QUESTIONS

Answers on Page 619

IN EACH OF THE FOLLOWING QUESTIONS, ANSWER:
   (a) IF (1) ONLY IS CORRECT
   (b) IF (2) ONLY IS CORRECT
   (c) IF BOTH (1) AND (2) ARE CORRECT, AND
   (d) IF NEITHER (1) NOR (2) IS CORRECT

1. Which of the following statements is (are) correct?
   (1) The rods and cones of the eyes are examples of electromagnetic receptors.
   (2) The taste and smell endings are chemoreceptors.
2. Which of the following statements is (are) correct?
   (1) Free nerve endings have no Schwann cells covering their tips.
   (2) Merkel's discs are fast-adapting touch receptors.
3. Which of the following statements is (are) correct?
   (1) Meissner's corpuscles are absent from the skin of the palm of the hand and the sole of the foot.
   (2) There is a considerable reduction in the number of Meissner's corpuscles between birth and old age.
4. Which of the following statements concerning a pacinian corpuscle is (are) correct?
   (1) It is a rapidly adapting mechanoreceptor.
   (2) Each corpuscle consists of a lamellated capsule and a central core containing the nerve ending.

Select the best response:

5. The following statements concerning Ruffini's corpuscles are true **except**:
   (a) They are located in the dermis of hairy skin.
   (b) Each consists of several unmyelinated nerve fibers surrounded by a cellular capsule.
   (c) They are fast-adapting mechanoreceptors.
   (d) They are stretch receptors.
   (e) The nerve fibers end among collagen fibers.
6. The following statements concerning cutaneous receptors are true **except**:
   (a) Although there are a variety of histological types of receptors, nerves only transmit nerve impulses.
   (b) The type of sensation felt is determined by the specific area of the central nervous system to which the sensory nerve fiber passes.
   (c) Transduction at the receptor is the process by which the energy of the stimulus is changed into electrochemical energy of the nerve impulse.
   (d) When applied to the receptor, the stimulus brings about a change in the potential of the plasma membranes of the capsule cells and not the nerve ending.
   (e) If large enough, the receptor potential will generate an action potential in the afferent sensory nerve fiber.
7. The following statements concerning the function of a neuromuscular spindle are true **except**:
   (a) It gives rise to afferent nerve impulses all the time.
   (b) When active or passive muscle movement occurs, there is an increase in the rate of passage of nerve impulses in the afferent nerve fiber.
   (c) The neuromuscular spindle keeps the central nervous system informed about muscle activity.
   (d) The neuromuscular spindle indirectly influences the control of voluntary movement.
   (e) The flower spray endings are situated mainly on the nuclear bag fibers close to the equatorial region.

In the following questions, answer:
  (a) IF (1), (2), AND (3) ONLY ARE CORRECT
  (b) IF (1) AND (3) ONLY ARE CORRECT
  (c) IF (2) AND (4) ONLY ARE CORRECT
  (d) IF (4) ONLY IS CORRECT, OR
  (e) IF ALL ARE CORRECT

8. Which of the following statements is (are) correct concerning the neurotendinous spindles?
  (1) They are situated in tendons close to the musculotendinous junction.
  (2) Each has a fibrous capsule, loosely arranged collagen fibers, and tendon cells.
  (3) The nerve ends by branching and terminating in club-shaped endings.
  (4) The neurotendinous spindle is activated by changes in muscle tension and inhibits muscle contraction.

9. Which of the following statements is (are) correct concerning the neuromuscular junctions in skeletal muscle?
  (1) Each terminal branch of the motor nerve ends as a naked axon.
  (2) Each axon lies in a groove on the surface of the muscle fiber formed by the infolding of the sarcolemma.
  (3) Acetylcholine is released from the axon terminal when the nerve impulse reaches the neuromuscular junction.
  (4) Having caused depolarization of the postsynaptic membrane, acetylcholine is reabsorbed into the axon terminal.

10. Which of the following statements is (are) correct concerning the neuromuscular junctions on smooth and cardiac muscle?
  (1) In smooth muscle the autonomic nerve fiber exerts control over a single muscle fiber.
  (2) In smooth muscle the wave of contraction does not pass from one muscle fiber to another by means of gap junctions.
  (3) The autonomic nerve fibers terminate on smooth muscle as myelinated fibers.
  (4) In cardiac muscle the wave of contraction spreads rapidly from one muscle fiber to another by way of desmosomes and gap junctions.

Match the features of sensory and effector endings listed below on the left with appropriate structures listed below on the right. Answers may be used more than once.

11. Lamellated capsule of flattened cells
12. Annulospiral endings
13. Sole plate
14. T tubules
15. Junctional folds

  (a) Muscular element of myoneural junction
  (b) Derived from sarcolemma
  (c) Pacinian corpuscle
  (d) Intrafusal muscle fibers
  (e) None of the above

ADDITIONAL READING

Bannister, L. H. Sensory Terminals of Peripheral Nerves. In D. N. Landon (ed.), *The Peripheral Nerve.* London: Chapman and Hall, 1976, p. 396.

Barker, D. The morphology of muscle receptors. In C. D. Hunt (ed.), *Handbook of Physiology,* Vol. 111/2: *Muscle Receptors.* Berlin: Springer-Verlag, 1974, p. 1.

Binder, M. D., and Stuart, D. G. Motor unit–muscle receptor interactions: Design features of the neuromuscular control system. *Prog. Clin. Neurophysiol.* 8:72, 1980.

Burke, D., McKeon, B., and Skuse, N. F. The muscle spindle, muscle tone and proprioceptive reflexes in normal man. In D. Ganick (ed.), *Proprioception, Posture and Emotion.* New South Wales: Committee on Postgraduate Education, 1982, p. 121.

Cargo, P. E., Houk, J. C., and Rymer, W. Z. Sampling of total muscle force by tendon organs. *J. Neurophysiol.* 47:1069, 1982.

Cauna, N. The free penicillate nerve endings of the human hairy skin. *J. Anat.* 115:277, 1973.

Cauna, N., and Mannan, G. The structure of human digital pacinian corpuscles (corpusculae lamellosae) and its functional significance. *J. Anat.* 92:1, 1958.

Cauna, N., and Ross, L. L. The fine structure of Meissner's touch corpuscle of human fingers. *J. Biophys. Biochem. Cytol.* 8:467, 1960.

Couteaux, R. Localization of cholinesterase at neuromuscular junctions. *Int. Rev. Cytol.* 4:335, 1955.

Cunningham, F. O., and Fitzgerald, M. J. T. Encapsulated nerve endings in hairy skin. *J. Anat.* 112:93, 1972.

Desaki, J., and Vehara, Y. The overall morphology of neuromuscular junctions as revealed by scanning electron microscopy. *J. Neurocytol.* 10:101, 1981.

Drachman, D. B. Myasthenia gravis: Immunobiology of a receptor disorder. *Trends Neurosci.* 6:446, 1983.

Duchen, L. W., and Gale, A. N. The Motor End Plate. In M. Swash and C. Kennard (eds.), *Scientific Basis of Clinical Neurology.* Edinburgh: Churchill Livingstone, 1985, p. 400.

Ganong, W. F. *Review of Medical Physiology* (12th ed.). Los Altos, California: Lange, 1985.

Guyton, A. C. *Textbook of Medical Physiology* (6th ed.). Philadelphia: Saunders, 1981.

Halata, Z., and Munger, B. L. Identification of the Ruffini corpuscle in human hairy skin. *Cell Tissue Res.* 219:437, 1981.

Horsch, K. W., Tuckett, R. P., and Burgess, P. R. A key to the classification of cutaneous mechanoreceptors. *J. Invest. Dermatol.* 69:75, 1977.

Houk, J. C., Crago, P. E., and Rymer, P. Z. Functional properties of the golgi tendon organs. *Prog. Clin. Neurophysiol.* 8:33, 1980.

Iggo, A., and Andres, K. H. Morphology of cutaneous receptors. *Annu. Rev. Neurosci.* 5:1, 1982.

Kennedy, W. R. Innervation of normal human muscle spindles. *Neurology (N.Y.)* 20:463, 1970.

LaMotte, R. H. Cutaneous nociceptors and pain sensation in normal and hyperalgesic skin. In L. Kruger and J. C. Liebeskind (eds.). *Advances in Pain Research and Therapy.* New York: Raven, 1984, Vol. 6, p. 69.

McCloskey, D. L. Kinesthetic sensibility. *Physiol. Rev.* 58:763, 1978.

Perl, E. R. Afferent basis of nociception and pain: Evidence from the characteristics of sensory receptors and their projections to the spinal dorsal horn. In J. J. Bonica (ed.). *Pain.* New York: Raven, 1980, Vol. 58, p. 19.

Snell, R. S., and McIntyre, N. Changes in the histochemical appearances of cholinesterase at the motor endplate following denervation. *Br. J. Exp. Pathol.* 37:44, 1956.

Swash, M., and Fox, K. P. Muscle spindle innervation in man. *J. Anat.* 112:61, 1972.

Tracey, D. J. Joint receptors and the control of movement. *Trends Neurosci.* 2:253, 1980.

Chapter 6
Dermatomes and Muscular Activity

SEGMENTAL INNERVATION OF SKIN

The area of skin supplied by a single spinal nerve, and, therefore, a single segment of the spinal cord, is called a **dermatome**. On the trunk the dermatomes extend round the body from the posterior to the anterior median plane. Adjacent dermatomes overlap considerably, so that to produce a region of complete anesthesia at least three contiguous spinal nerves have to be sectioned. It should be noted that the area of tactile loss is always greater than the area of loss of painful and thermal sensations. The reason for this difference is that the degree of overlap of fibers carrying pain and thermal sensations is much more extensive than the overlap of fibers carrying tactile sensations. Dermatomal charts for the anterior and posterior surfaces of the body are shown in Figures 6-1 and 6-2.

In the limbs the arrangement of the dermatomes is more complicated, and the reason for this is the embryological changes that take place as the limbs grow out from the trunk. (For details, see Figs. 6-1 and 6-2.)

SEGMENTAL INNERVATION OF MUSCLES

Skeletal muscle also receives a segmental innervation. Most of these muscles are innervated by more than one spinal nerve and, therefore, by the same number of segments of the spinal cord. Thus, to paralyze a muscle completely it would be necessary to section several spinal nerves or destroy several segments of the spinal cord.

To learn the segmental innervation of all the muscles of the body is an impossible task. Nevertheless, the segmental innervation of the following muscles should be known, because it is possible to test them by eliciting simple muscle reflexes in the patient (Fig. 6-3):

Biceps Brachii Tendon Reflex C5-**6** (flexion of the elbow joint by tapping the biceps tendon).
Triceps Tendon Reflex C6-**7**, and **8** (extension of the elbow joint by tapping the triceps tendon).
Brachioradialis Tendon Reflex C5-**6**, and 7 (supination of the radioulnar joints by tapping the insertion of the brachioradialis tendon).

C2
C3
C4
C5
T2
C6
T1
C8
C7
L1
S3
S4
L2
L3
L4
L5
S1

T3
T4
T5
T6
T7
T8
T9
T10
T11
T12

Transverse cutaneous nerve of neck

Supraclavicular nerves

Anterior cutaneous branch of second
intercostal nerve

Upper lateral cutaneous nerve of arm

Medial cutaneous nerve of arm

Lower lateral cutaneous nerve of arm

Medial cutaneous nerve of forearm

Lateral cutaneous nerve of forearm

Lateral cutaneous branch of
subcostal nerve

Femoral branch of genitofemoral
nerve

Median nerve

Ulnar nerve

Ilioinguinal nerve

Lateral cutaneous nerve of thigh

Obturator nerve

Medial cutaneous nerve of thigh

Intermediate cutaneous nerve of thigh

Infrapatellar branch of saphenous nerve

Lateral sural cutaneous nerve

Saphenous nerve

Superficial peroneal nerve

Deep peroneal nerve

Fig. 6-1. Anterior aspect of body, showing distribution of cutaneous nerves on left side and dermatomes on the right side.

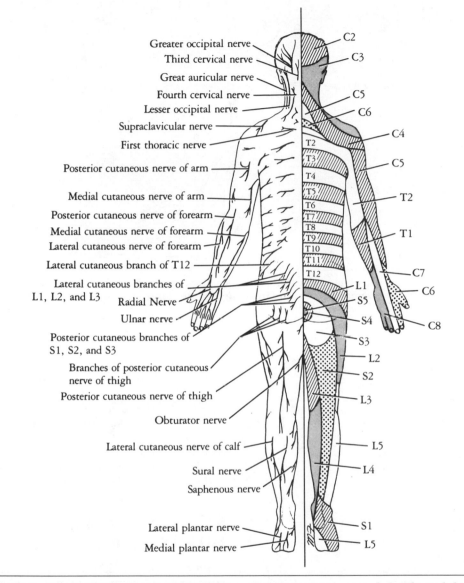

Greater occipital nerve — C2
Third cervical nerve — C3
Great auricular nerve
Fourth cervical nerve — C5
Lesser occipital nerve — C6
Supraclavicular nerve — C4
First thoracic nerve — T2
Posterior cutaneous nerve of arm — C5
T3
T4
Medial cutaneous nerve of arm — T5 — T2
T6
Posterior cutaneous nerve of forearm — T7
Medial cutaneous nerve of forearm — T8 — T1
Lateral cutaneous nerve of forearm — T9
T10
Lateral cutaneous branch of T12 — T11
T12 — C7
Lateral cutaneous branches of — L1 — C6
L1, L2, and L3 Radial Nerve — S5
Ulnar nerve — S4 — C8
Posterior cutaneous branches of — S3
S1, S2, and S3 — L2
Branches of posterior cutaneous — S2
nerve of thigh
Posterior cutaneous nerve of thigh — L3
Obturator nerve
Lateral cutaneous nerve of calf — L5
Sural nerve — L4
Saphenous nerve
Lateral plantar nerve — S1
Medial plantar nerve — L5

Fig. 6-2. Posterior aspect of body, showing distribution of cutaneous nerves on left side and dermatomes on right side.

C5 to 6

Fig. 6-3. Biceps brachii tendon reflex. Note that reflex arc passes through fifth and sixth cervical segments of spinal cord and is monosynaptic, that is, the internuncial neuron (black) is usually absent.

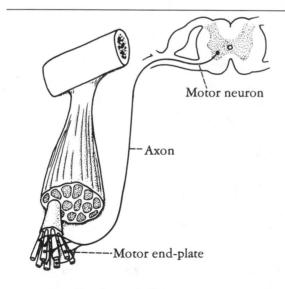

Motor neuron

Axon

Motor end-plate

Bundle of muscle fibers

Fig. 6-4. Components of a motor unit.

Abdominal Superficial Reflexes (contraction of underlying abdominal muscles by stroking the skin). Upper abdominal skin T6–7; middle abdominal skin T8–9; lower abdominal skin T10–12.

Patellar Tendon Reflex (knee jerk) L2, **3** and **4** (extension of knee joint on tapping the patellar tendon).

Achilles Tendon Reflex (ankle jerk) S**1** and 2 (plan(plantar flexion of ankle joint on tapping the Achilles tendon—tendo calcaneus).

MUSCLE TONE AND MUSCLE ACTION

A **motor unit** consists of a motor neuron in the anterior gray column (horn) of the spinal cord and all the muscle fibers it supplies (Fig. 6-4). In a large buttock muscle, such as the gluteus maximus, where fine control is unnecessary, a given motor neuron may supply as many as 200 muscle fibers. In contrast, in the small muscles of the hand or the extrinsic muscles of the eyeball, where fine control is required, one nerve fiber supplies only a few muscle fibers.

Every skeletal muscle, while resting, is in a partial state of contraction. This condition is referred to as **muscle tone**. Since there is no intermediate stage, muscle fibers are either fully contracted or relaxed; it follows that a few muscle fibers within a muscle are fully contracted all the time. To bring about this state, and to avoid fatigue, different groups of motor units, and thus different groups of muscle fibers, are brought into action at different times. This is accomplished by the asynchronous discharge of nervous impulses in the motor neurons in the anterior gray horn of the spinal cord.

Basically, muscle tone is dependent on the integrity of a simple monosynaptic reflex arc composed of two neurons in the nervous system (Fig. 6-5). The lengthening and shortening in a muscle are detected by sensitive sensory endings called **muscle spindles** (see p. 129) and the tension is detected by **tendon spindles** (see p. 132). The nervous impulses travel in the large afferent fibers to the spinal cord. There, they synapse with the motor neurons situated in the anterior gray column, which, in turn, send impulses down their axons to the muscle fibers (Fig. 6-5). The muscle spindles themselves are innervated by small gamma efferent fibers that regulate the response of the muscle spindles, acting synergically with external stretch. In this manner, muscle tone is maintained reflexly

and adjusted to the needs of posture and movement.

Should the afferent or efferent pathways of the reflex arc be cut, the muscle would lose its tone immediately and become flaccid. A flaccid muscle, on palpation, feels like a mass of dough and has completely lost its resilience. It quickly atrophies and becomes reduced in volume. It is important to realize that the degree of activity of the motor anterior column cells, and therefore the degree of muscle tone, depends on the summation of the nerve impulses received by these cells from other neurons of the nervous system.

Muscle movement is accomplished by bringing into action increasing numbers of motor units and, at the same time, reducing the activity of the motor units of muscles that will oppose or antagonize the movement. When the maximum effort is required, all the motor units of a muscle are thrown into action.

SUMMATION OF MOTOR UNITS

When a muscle begins to contract, the smaller motor units are stimulated first. The reason for this is that the smaller motor units are innervated by

Fig. 6-5. Simple reflex arc consisting of afferent neuron arising from neuromuscular spindles, neurotendinous spindles, and efferent neuron whose cell body lies in anterior gray column (horn) of spinal cord. Note that for simplicity the afferent fibers from the neurotendinous spindle and the neuromuscular spindle are shown as one pathway; in fact, the neurotendinous receptor is inhibitory and reduces tone whereas the neuromuscular spindle is excitatory and increases tone.

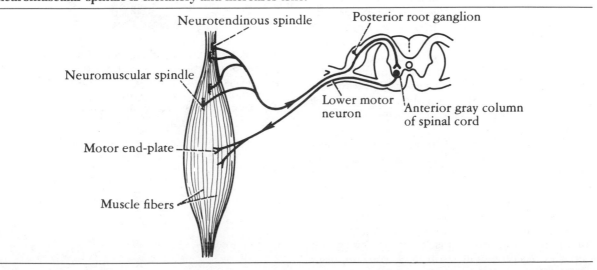

Neurotendinous spindle

Posterior root ganglion

Neuromuscular spindle

Lower motor neuron

Anterior gray column of spinal cord

Motor end-plate

Muscle fibers

smaller neurons in the spinal cord and brainstem and they have a lower threshold of excitability. As the contraction increases, progressively larger motor units are brought into action. This phenomenon causes a gradual increase in muscle strength as the muscle contracts.

MUSCLE FATIGUE

The progressive loss of strength of a muscle with prolonged strong contraction is due to the reduction in the amounts of adenosine triphosphate (ATP) within the muscle fibers. Nerve impulses continue to arrive at the neuromuscular junction and normal depolarization of the plasma membrane of the muscle fiber occurs.

POSTURE

Posture may be defined as the position adopted by the individual within his environment. In the standing position the line of gravity passes through the odontoid process of the axis, behind the centers of the hip joints, and in front of the knee and ankle joints (Fig. 6-6). In order to stabilize the body and prevent it from collapsing, it is not surprising to find that in humans the antigravity muscles are well developed and exhibit the greatest degree of tone. One can therefore say that posture depends on the degree and distribution of muscle tone, which in turn depends on the normal integrity of simple reflex arcs centered in the spinal cord.

An individual may assume a particular posture (sitting or standing) over long periods of time with little evidence of fatigue. The reason for this is that muscle tone is maintained through different groups of muscle fibers contracting in relays, only a small number of muscle fibers within a muscle being in a state of contraction at any one time. The active muscle fiber groups are scattered throughout the muscle.

In order to maintain posture, the simple myotatic reflex, upon which muscle tone is dependent, must receive adequate nervous input from higher levels of the nervous system (Fig. 6-7). For example, impulses arising from the labyrinths and neck muscles, information arising from the cerebellum, midbrain, and cerebral centers, general information arising from other muscle groups, joints, and even skin receptors will result in nervous impulses

Fig. 6-6. Lateral view of skeleton, showing line of gravity. Since greater part of body weight lies anterior to vertebral column, deep muscles of back are important in maintaining normal postural curves of vertebral column in standing position.

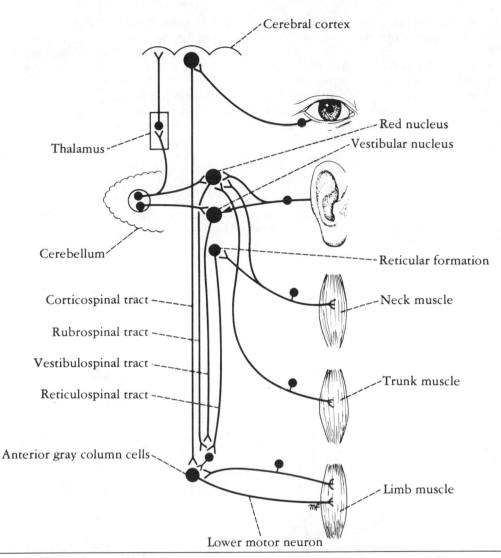

Fig. 6-7. Nervous input from higher levels of the central nervous system, which can influence the activity of the anterior gray column (horn) cells of the spinal cord.

impinging on the large anterior gray column cells (i.e., the final common pathway) controlling the muscle fibers.

When an individual assumes a given posture, the tone of the muscles controlling that posture is constantly undergoing fine adjustments so that the posture is maintained. Normal posture thus depends not only on the integrity of the reflex arc but also on the summation of the nervous impulses received by the motor anterior gray column cells from other neurons of the nervous system (Fig. 6-8). The detail of the different nervous pathways involved in bringing the information to the anterior gray column cells will be dealt with in Chapters 20 and 21, which are concerned with the ascending and descending tracts of the spinal cord.

Fig. 6-8. Normal postural tone of skeletal muscle is dependent not only on the integrity of the reflex arc, but also on the summation of the nervous impulses received by the motor anterior gray column (horn) cells from other neurons of the nervous system.

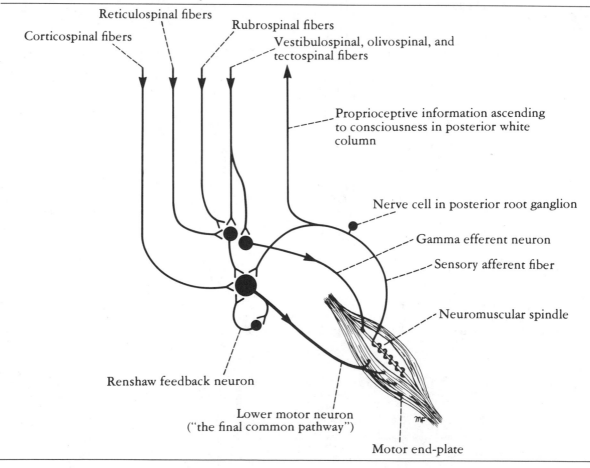

CLINICAL NOTES

SEGMENTAL INNERVATION OF THE SKIN

Because large nerve plexuses are present at the roots of the upper and lower limbs, it follows that a single spinal nerve may send both motor and sensory fibers to several peripheral nerves, and, conversely, a single peripheral nerve may receive nerve fibers from many spinal nerves. Moreover, it follows that a lesion of a segment of the spinal cord, or posterior root, or spinal nerve will result in a sensory loss that is different from that occurring after a lesion of a peripheral nerve.

The area of skin supplied by a single spinal nerve, and, therefore, a single segment of the spinal cord, is called a **dermatome**. A physician should remember that dermatomes overlap and that in the trunk at least three contiguous spinal nerves have to be sectioned to produce a region of complete anesthesia. A physician should remember also that the degree of overlap for painful and thermal sensations is much greater than for tactile sensation. A physician should have a working knowledge of the segmental (dermatomal) innervation of skin, since with the help of a pin or a piece of cotton he can determine whether or not the sensory function of a particular spinal nerve or segment of the spinal cord is normal. When examining the dermatomal charts, one should note that because of the development of the upper limbs the anterior rami of the lower cervical and first thoracic spinal nerves have lost their cutaneous innervation of the trunk anteriorly, and at the level of the second costal cartilage the fourth cervical dermatome is contiguous with the second thoracic dermatome. In the sensory innervation of the head, the trigeminal (fifth cranial) nerve supplies a large area of the face and scalp, and its cutaneous area is contiguous with that of the second cervical segment.

Since the dermatomes run longitudinally along the long axis of the upper limbs, sensation should be tested by dragging a wisp of cotton or a pin along the long axis of the medial and lateral borders of the limbs. On the trunk the dermatomes run almost horizontally, so the stimulus should be applied by moving in a vertical direction.

SEGMENTAL INNERVATION OF THE MUSCLES

It is important to remember that most skeletal muscles are innervated by more than one spinal nerve and, therefore, by the same number of segments of the spinal cord. Complete destruction of one segment of the spinal cord as the result of trauma or pressure from a tumor will cause weakness of all the muscles that are innervated from that segment. To paralyze a muscle completely, several adjacent segments of the spinal cord have to be destroyed.

Because of the presence of the cervical, brachial, and lumbosacral plexuses the axons of motor anterior gray column cells are redistributed into a number of peripheral nerves. A physician, knowing this, is able to distinguish between a lesion of a segment of the spinal cord, an anterior root, or a spinal nerve, on the one hand, and a lesion of a peripheral nerve on the other. For example, the musculocutaneous nerve of the arm, which receives nerve fibers from the fifth, sixth, and seventh cervical segments of the spinal cord, supplies a finite number of muscles, namely, the biceps brachii, the brachialis, and the coracobrachialis muscles, and section of that nerve would result in total paralysis of these muscles; a lesion of the fifth, sixth, and seventh cervical spinal segments, or their anterior roots, or their spinal nerves, would result in paralysis of these muscles and also partial paralysis of many other muscles, including the deltoid, supraspinatus, teres minor, and infraspinatus.

The segmental innervation of the biceps brachii, triceps, brachioradialis, muscles of the anterior abdominal wall, quadriceps femoris, gastrocnemius, and soleus should be memorized, because it is possible to test them easily by eliciting their reflex contraction (for details, see pp. 149 and 152).

MUSCLE TONE

Skeletal muscle tone is due to the presence of a few muscle fibers within a muscle being in a state of full contraction all the time. Muscle tone is controlled reflexly from afferent nerve endings situated in the muscle itself. It follows, therefore, that any disease process that interferes with any part of the reflex arc will abolish the muscle tone. Some examples are: syphilitic infection of the posterior root (tabes dorsalis); destruction of the motor anterior gray column cells, as in poliomyelitis or syringomyelia; destruction of a segment of the spinal cord by trauma or pressure from a tumor; section of an anterior root; pressure on a spinal nerve by a prolapsed intervertebral disc; and section of a peripheral nerve, as in a stab wound. All these clinical conditions will result in loss of muscle tone.

While it has been emphasized that the basic mechanism underlying muscle tone is the integrity of the spinal segmental reflex, it must not be forgotten that this reflex activity is influenced by nervous impulses received by the anterior horn cells from all levels of the brain and spinal cord. Spinal shock, which follows injury to the spinal cord and is caused by loss of functional activity of neurons, will result in diminished muscle tone. Cerebellar disease also results in diminished muscle tone, because the cerebellum facilitates the stretch reflex. The reticular formation normally tends to increase muscle tone, but its activity is inhibited by higher cerebral centers. Therefore, it follows that if the higher cerebral control is interfered with by trauma or disease, the inhibition is lost and the muscle tone is exaggerated (decerebrate rigidity). It must not be forgotten that primary degeneration of the muscles themselves (myopathies) can cause loss of muscle tone.

POSTURE

The posture of an individual depends on the degree and distribution of muscle tone and, therefore, on the activity of the motor neurons that supply the muscles. The motor neurons in the anterior gray columns of the spinal cord are the points upon which converge the nervous impulses from many posterior nerve roots, and the descending fibers from many different levels of the brain and spinal cord. The successful coordination of all these nervous influences results in a normal posture.

When one is in the standing posture there is remarkably little muscular activity taking place in the muscles of the limbs and trunk. The reason for this is that the center of gravity of any part of the body is mainly above the joints upon which its weight is directed. Moreover, in many joints, for example, the hip and the knee, the ligaments are very strong and support the body in the erect posture. However, it must be stressed that a person cannot remain standing if all muscles are paralyzed. Once a person starts to fall, either forward, backward, or laterally, the muscle spindles and other stretch receptors immediately increase their activity and the reflex arcs come into play, so that reflex compensatory muscle contractions take place to restore the state of balance. The eyes and the receptors in the membranous labyrinth also play a vital part in the maintenance of balance. The importance of the eyes in maintaining the erect position can easily be tested in a normal person. Once the eyes are closed, the person shows a tendency to sway slightly, because he now must rely exclusively on his muscle and labyrinthine receptors to preserve his balance.

It follows that a pathological alteration in muscle tone will affect posture. For example, in hemiplegia or in Parkinson's disease, in which there is hypertonicity, posture will be changed. As with cerebellar disease, hypotonicity will cause drooping of the shoulder on the affected side. Lesions involving peripheral nerves that innervate antigravity muscles will produce wrist drop (radial nerve) and foot drop (common peroneal nerve).

CLINICAL OBSERVATION OF MUSCULAR ACTIVITY

Muscular Power

Ask the patient to perform movements for which the muscle under examination is primarily responsible. Next, ask the patient to perform each movement against resistance and compare the strengths of the muscles on the two sides of the body. Section of the peripheral nerve that supplies the muscle or disease affecting the anterior gray column cells, e.g., poliomyelitis, will clearly reduce the power of or paralyze the muscles involved.

Muscle Wasting

This occurs within two to three weeks after section of the motor nerve. In the limbs it is easily tested by measuring the diameter of the limbs at a given point over the involved muscle and comparing the measurement obtained with that at the same site on the opposite limb.

Muscular Fasciculation

Twitching of groups of muscle fibers is seen most often in patients with chronic disease that affects the anterior horn cells—for example, progressive muscular atrophy.

Muscular Contracture

Muscular contracture occurs most commonly in the muscles that normally oppose paralyzed muscles. The muscles contract and undergo permanent shortening.

Muscle Tone

A muscle without tone, i.e., one in which the simple spinal reflex arcs are not functioning, is noncontractile and is doughlike on palpation. Degrees of loss of tone may be tested by passively moving the joints and comparing the resistance to the movements by the muscles on the two sides of the body. Increase in muscle tone can occur following the removal of the cerebral inhibition on the reticular formation (see p. 396).

Muscular Coordination

Ask the patient to touch, with his eyes open, the tip of his nose with the tip of his forefinger, then ask him to repeat the process with his eyes closed. A similar test of the lower limbs may be carried out with the patient lying down. Ask him to place one heel on the opposite knee, with his eyes open, then ask him to repeat the process with his eyes closed.

Another test is to ask the patient to quickly supinate and pronate both forearms simultaneously. Disease of the cerebellum, for example, which coordinates muscular activity, would result in impaired ability to perform these rapid repetitive movements.

INVOLUNTARY MOVEMENT OF MUSCLES

Tic. This is a coordinated, repetitive movement involving one or more muscles.

Choreiform movements. These are quick, jerky, irregular movements that are nonrepetitive. Swift grimaces and sudden movements of the head or limbs are examples of this condition.

Athetosis. This consists of slow, sinuous, writhing movements that most commonly involve the distal segments of the limbs.

Tremor. This is the alternating contraction of the agonists and antagonists of a joint.

Myoclonus. This consists of shocklike muscular contractions of a portion of a muscle, or an entire muscle, or a group of muscles.

Tonic spasm. This term refers to a sustained contraction of a muscle or group of muscles, as in the tonic phase of an epileptic seizure.

CLINICAL PROBLEMS

Answers on Page 594

1. A 55-year-old man visited his physician because of pain in the right buttock that extended down the right leg, the back of the thigh, the outer side and back of the calf, and the outer border of the foot. The patient gave no history of previous injury, but stated that the pain started about three months ago as a dull, low backache. Since that time the pain has increased in intensity and has spread down the right leg. When asked if the pain had ever disappeared, he replied that on two separate occasions the pain had diminished in intensity, but his back remained "stiff" all the time. He said the pain was aggravated by stooping or by coughing and sneezing. Sometimes he experienced pins and needles along the outer border of his right foot. After a complete physical examination, a diagnosis was made of herniation of a lumbar intervertebral disc. Using your knowledge of anatomy, state which intervertebral disc is most likely to have been herniated.

2. A 60-year-old woman was seen by her physician because she was experiencing a shooting, burning pain in the left side of her chest. Three days later a group of localized papules appeared on the skin covering the left fifth inter-

costal space. One day later the papules became vesicular; a few days later the vesicles dried up into crusts, and these later separated, leaving small permanent scars. The patient also noticed that there was some loss of sensibility over the left side of the chest. A diagnosis of herpes zoster was made. Using your knowledge of anatomy, state the segment of the spinal cord involved with the disease.

3. While examining the sensory innervation of the skin of the head and neck in a patient, a medical student had difficulty remembering the dermatomal pattern at the junction of the head with the neck and at the junction of the neck with the thorax. Are the dermatomes arranged in a special manner in these areas? If so, what is the underlying reason for this?

4. A 30-year-old man was found, on physical examination, to have weakness and diminished tone of the rhomboid muscles, deltoids, and biceps brachii on both sides of the body. The degree of weakness was greater on the right side. The biceps tendon jerk was absent on the right side and diminished on the left side. The triceps jerks were normal on both sides of the body. The muscles of the trunk and lower limb showed increased tone and exhibited spastic paralysis. Radiology of the vertebral column revealed the presence of vertebral destruction due to a tumor arising within the vertebral canal. Using your knowledge of anatomy, answer the following questions: (a) Which vertebra is likely to have the tumor within the vertebral canal? (b) Name the segments of the spinal cord that are being pressed upon by the tumor. (c) Which segments of the spinal cord participate in the reflex arcs responsible for the biceps brachii tendon jerk? (d) Why do the rhomboid and deltoid muscles exhibit diminished muscle tone, whereas the muscles of the lower limb exhibit increased tone?

5. Name three clinical conditions that could result in a loss of tone of skeletal muscle.

6. A 60-year-old man with advanced tabes dorsalis was asked to stand with his toes and heels together and his eyes closed. He immediately started to sway violently and if the nurse had not held on to his arm he would have fallen to the ground (positive Romberg test). Why was it vital for this patient to keep his eyes open in order to remain upright?

7. A 60-year-old man with moderately advanced Parkinson's syndrome was disrobed and asked to walk in a straight line in the examining room. The physician observed that the patient had his head and shoulders stooped forward, the arms slightly abducted, the elbow joints partly flexed, and the wrists slightly extended with the fingers flexed at the metacarpophalangeal joints and extended at the interphalangeal joints. It was noted that on starting to walk, the patient leaned forward and slowly shuffled his feet. The farther he leaned forward the more quickly he moved his legs, so that by the time he had crossed the room he was almost running. The patient's face was masklike and exhibited few emotional movements. The hands showed a coarse tremor and the muscles of the upper and lower limbs showed increased tone in the opposing muscle groups when the joints were passively moved. Parkinson's disease, or the parkinsonian syndrome, can be caused by a number of pathological conditions but they usually interfere in the normal function of the corpus striatum or the substantia nigra or both. Using your knowledge of the anatomy and physiology of muscle action, attempt to explain the different signs seen in this important syndrome.

8. A 10-year-old girl was taken to a neurologist because of a six-month history of epileptic attacks. The parents described the attacks as starting with sudden involuntary movements of the trunk, arms, or legs. Sometimes the muscle movements were slight, but at other times they were so violent that she had been known to throw an object in her hand across the room. At other times the patient just fell to the ground, as the result of a sudden loss of muscle tone. Having hit the ground, the patient would immediately rise to her feet. On one occasion she severely bruised her head and shoulder by striking a chair and a table. One month ago the parents noticed that their daughter appeared to lose consciousness briefly. At the time, she was carrying on a normal conversation, when she suddenly stopped and her gaze became fixed. After a few seconds she became alert and con-

tinued her conversation. This patient is suffering from a form of epilepsy known as petit mal. What is the correct term for the sudden involuntary contraction of the muscles of the trunk or extremities? Do you know the name for the condition of a patient who suddenly loses all muscle tone and falls to the ground?

9. A 45-year-old man suffering from amyotrophic lateral sclerosis was examined by a third-year medical student. The student found that the flexor and extensor muscles of the knee and ankle joints of the right leg were weaker than those of the left leg. However, he was of the opinion that the muscles of the left leg also were somewhat weaker than normal. On palpation of the extensor muscles of the right thigh it was possible to detect a twitching of the muscle fibers in the quadriceps muscle. Marked atrophy of the muscles of both legs also was noted. There was no evidence of cutaneous sensation on either limb. Amyotrophic lateral scle-

rosis is a condition in which there is degeneration of the motor anterior horn cells of the spinal cord and brainstem with secondary degeneration of the nervous tracts in the lateral and anterior portions of the spinal cord. Why do you think this patient had weakness and atrophy of the muscles of the lower limbs? What is the correct clinical term for the twitching of the muscle fibers in the extensor muscles of the right knee?

10. A 12-year-old girl was diagnosed as suffering from a medulloblastoma of the cerebellum. Clinical and radiological examinations revealed that the tumor was predominantly invading the right cerebellar hemisphere. Knowing that the cerebellum is concerned with the coordination of motor activity so that complex voluntary movements involving antagonistic muscle groups can take place in a precise manner, what tests would you perform on this patient to demonstrate loss of cerebellar function?

NATIONAL BOARD TYPE QUESTIONS

Answers on Page 619

IN EACH OF THE FOLLOWING QUESTIONS, ANSWER:
  (a) IF (1) ONLY IS CORRECT
  (b) IF (2) ONLY IS CORRECT
  (c) IF BOTH (1) AND (2) ARE CORRECT, AND
  (d) IF NEITHER (1) NOR (2) IS CORRECT

1. Which of the following statements is (are) correct?
   (1) To produce on the trunk a region of complete anesthesia, only two segments of the spinal cord have to be damaged.
   (2) When contiguous spinal nerves are sectioned, it is noted that the area of tactile loss is always smaller than the area of loss of painful and thermal sensations.

2. Which of the following statements is (are) correct?
   (1) The dermatome present on the medial side of the wrist is T2.
   (2) The dermatome present on the point of the shoulder is C5 and C6.

3. Which of the following statements is (are) correct?
   (1) The biceps brachii tendon reflex involves C5 and C6 segments of the spinal cord.

   (2) The triceps tendon reflex involves the T1 segment of the spinal cord.

4. Which of the following statements is (are) correct?
   (1) The patellar tendon reflex (knee jerk) involves L2, 3, and 4 segments of the spinal cord.
   (2) A tumor pressing on the third and fourth sacral segments of the spinal cord is likely to interfere with the ankle jerk.

5. Which of the following statements is (are) correct?
   (1) The Achilles tendon reflex (ankle jerk) involves S1 and 2 segments of the spinal cord.
   (2) The abdominal superficial reflexes involve T6–12 segments of the spinal cord.

6. Which of the following statements is (are) correct?
   (1) The dermatomes for the limbs run almost horizontally.
   (2) The degree of overlap of dermatomes for painful and thermal sensations is much greater than for tactile sensations.

Select the best response:

7. The following statements concerning the dermatomes of the trunk and lower limbs are true **except**:
   (a) T10 dermatome includes the skin of the umbilicus.
   (b) L1 dermatome lies over the inguinal ligament.
   (c) L2 dermatome lies over the medial side of the knee joint.
   (d) S1 dermatome runs along the lateral side of the foot.
   (e) L3 and L5 dermatomes lie over the lateral side of the knee joint.

8. The following statements concerning muscle innervation are correct **except**:
   (a) A motor unit consists of the posterior root ganglion and all the neuromuscular spindles it is connected to.
   (b) In the small muscles of the hand one nerve fiber supplies only a few muscle fibers.
   (c) Neurotendinous spindles are innervated by myelinated nerve fibers.
   (d) Muscle tone is dependent on the integrity of a simple monosynaptic reflex arc.
   (e) The gamma motor efferent fibers innervate the intrafusal fibers of a muscle spindle.

In the following questions, answer:
   (a) If (1), (2) AND (3) ONLY ARE CORRECT
   (b) If (1) AND (3) ONLY ARE CORRECT
   (c) If (2) AND (4) ONLY ARE CORRECT
   (d) If (4) ONLY IS CORRECT, OR
   (e) If ALL ARE CORRECT

9. Which of the following statements is (are) correct concerning muscle action?
   (1) When a muscle begins to contract, the smaller motor units are stimulated first.
   (2) Muscle fatigue is caused by an exhaustion of the presynaptic vesicles at the neuromuscular junction.
   (3) When a prime mover contracts, the antagonistic muscles are inhibited.
   (4) When a muscle is paralyzed, it retains its normal tone for three weeks.

10. Which of the following statements is (are) correct concerning posture?
    (1) In the standing position, the line of gravity passes through the odontoid process of the axis, behind the centers of the hip joints, and in front of the knee and ankle joints.
    (2) Posture depends on the degree and distribution of muscle tone.
    (3) A particular posture can often be maintained for long periods by different groups of muscle fibers in a muscle contracting in relays.
    (4) Nerve impulses arising in the eyes and ears can influence posture.

11. The following conditions can bring about a pathological change in posture.
    (1) Disease of the cerebellum
    (2) Disease of muscles (myopathies)
    (3) Tabes dorsalis
    (4) Prolapsed intervertebral disc

12. The following clinical observations can be made on muscle activity.
    (1) Muscle contracture is a condition in which the muscle contracts for a long period of time.
    (2) Muscular fasciculation is seen with chronic disease that affects anterior horn cells or motor nuclei of cranial nerves.
    (3) Muscle wasting does not occur if only the efferent motor nerve fibers to a muscle are sectioned.
    (4) Muscle atrophy takes place when a limb is immobilized in a cast.

ADDITIONAL READING

Critchley, M., O'Leary, J. L., and Jennett, B. *Scientific Foundations of Neurology.* Philadelphia: Davis, 1972.

Guyton, A. C. *Textbook of Medical Physiology* (7th ed.). Philadelphia: Saunders, 1986.

Judge, R. D., and Zuidema, G. D. *Physical Diagnosis: A Physiologic Approach to the Clinical Examination* (3rd ed.). Boston: Little, Brown, 1974.

Lance, J. W., and McLeod, J. G. *A Physiological Approach to Clinical Neurology* (3rd ed.). London: Butterworth, 1981.

Lavine, R. A. *Neurophysiology: The Fundamentals.* Lexington, Mass., and Toronto: Collamore–Heath, 1983.

Ottoson, D. *Physiology of the Nervous System.* Oxford: Oxford University Press, 1983.

Walton, J. N. *Brain's Diseases of the Nervous System.* New York and London: Oxford University Press, 1977.

Williams, P. L., and Warwick, R. *Gray's Anatomy* (37th ed.). Philadelphia: Saunders, 1989.

Chapter 7
The Spinal Cord

The spinal cord, as noted in Chapter 1, is roughly cylindrical in shape. It begins superiorly at the foramen magnum in the skull, where it is continuous with the **medulla oblongata** of the brain, and it terminates inferiorly in the adult at the level of the **lower border of the first lumbar vertebra.** In the young child, it is relatively longer and usually ends at the upper border of the third lumbar vertebra. Thus it occupies the upper two-thirds of the **vertebral canal** of the vertebral column and is surrounded by the three meninges, the **dura mater,** the **arachnoid mater,** and the **pia mater.** Further protection is provided by the **cerebrospinal fluid,** which surrounds the spinal cord in the **subarachnoid space.**

In the cervical region, where it gives origin to the brachial plexus, and in the lower thoracic and lumbar regions, where it gives origin to the lumbosacral plexus, the spinal cord is fusiformly enlarged; the enlargements are referred to as the **cervical** and **lumbar enlargements** (Fig. 7-1). Inferiorly, the spinal cord tapers off into the **conus medullaris,** from the apex of which a prolongation of the pia mater, the **filum terminale,** descends to be attached to the posterior surface of the coccyx. The cord possesses, in the midline anteriorly, a deep longitudinal fissure, the **anterior median fissure,** and on the posterior surface, a shallow furrow, the **posterior median sulcus** (Fig. 7-1).

Along the entire length of the spinal cord are attached 31 pairs of spinal nerves by the **anterior**[*] or **motor roots** and the **posterior** or **sensory roots** (Fig. 7-1). Each root is attached to the cord by a series of rootlets, which extend the whole length of the corresponding segment of the cord. Each posterior nerve root possesses a **posterior root ganglion,** the cells of which give rise to peripheral and central nerve fibers.

---

[*]Since much of the early neurobiological research was performed on animals, many investigators refer to the posterior roots and anterior roots as dorsal roots and ventral roots, respectively. This designation results in confusion, especially because, regarding the gray and white matter of the spinal cord in man, reference is generally made to anterior gray columns, posterior white columns, and so on. For this reason the terminology used for spinal nerve roots in this section will be followed throughout this text.

Fig. 7-1. Spinal cord.
A. Posterior view, showing cervical and lumbar enlargements.
B. Three segments of the spinal cord, showing the coverings of dura mater, arachnoid mater, and pia mater.

STRUCTURE OF SPINAL CORD

The spinal cord is composed of an inner core of **gray matter,** which is surrounded by an outer covering of **white matter** (Figs. 7-2 through 7-6); there is no indication that the cord is segmented.

Gray Matter

On cross section, the gray matter is seen as an H-shaped pillar with **anterior and posterior gray columns, or horns,** united by a thin **gray commissure** containing the small **central canal** (Fig. 7-2). A small **lateral gray column or horn** is present in the thoracic and upper lumbar segments of the cord. The amount of gray matter present at any given level of the spinal cord is related to the amount of muscle innervated at that level. Thus, its size is greatest within the cervical and lumbosacral enlargements of the cord, which innervate the muscles of the upper and lower limbs, respectively (Figs. 7-2 through 7-6).

Structure of Gray Matter

As in other regions of the central nervous system, the gray matter of the spinal cord consists of a mixture of nerve cells and their processes, neuroglia, and blood vessels. The nerve cells are multipolar and the neuroglia forms an intricate network around the nerve cell bodies and their neurites.

Nerve Cell Groups in the Anterior Gray Columns

Most nerve cells are large and multipolar, and their axons pass out in the anterior roots of the spinal nerves as **alpha efferents,** which innervate skeletal muscles. The smaller nerve cells are also multipolar and the axons of many of these pass out in the anterior roots of the spinal nerves as **gamma efferents,** which innervate the intrafusal muscle fibers of neuromuscular spindles.

For practical purposes,* the nerve cells of the an-

*In thick sections of the spinal cord, the gray matter appears to have a laminar (layered) appearance. Rexed (1952) described 10 layers of neurons in the cat spinal cord. This detailed cytoarchitectural lamination is useful for researchers but of little value to the practicing neurologist.

terior gray column may be divided into three basic groups or columns—medial, central, and lateral (Fig. 7-2).

The medial group is present in most segments of the spinal cord and is responsible for innervating the skeletal muscles of the neck and trunk, including the intercostal and abdominal musculature.

The central group is the smallest and is present in some cervical and lumbosacral segments (Figs. 7-2 and 7-3). In the cervical part of the cord some of these nerve cells (segments C3, 4, and 5) specifically innervate the diaphragm and are collectively referred to as the **phrenic nucleus** (Fig. 7-2). In the upper five or six cervical segments, some of the nerve cells innervate the sternocleidomastoid and trapezius muscles and are referred to as the **accessory nucleus** (Figs. 7-2 and 7-3). The axons of these cells form the spinal part of the accessory nerve. The **lumbosacral nucleus** present in the second lumbar down to the first sacral segments of the cord is made up of nerve cells whose axons have an unknown distribution.

The lateral group is present in the cervical and lumbosacral segments of the cord and is responsible for innervating the skeletal muscles of the limbs (Figs. 7-2, 7-3, 7-5, and 7-6).

Nerve Cell Groups in the Posterior Gray Columns

There are four nerve cell groups of the posterior gray column, two that extend throughout the length of the cord and two that are restricted to the thoracic and lumbar segments.

The **substantia gelatinosa group** is situated at the apex of the posterior gray column throughout the length of the spinal cord (Figs. 7-2 through 7-6). It is largely composed of Golgi type II neurons and receives afferent fibers concerned with pain, temperature, and touch from the posterior root. Furthermore, it receives input from descending fibers from supraspinal levels. It is believed that the input of the sensations of pain and temperature are modified by excitatory or inhibitory information from other sensory inputs and by information from the cerebral cortex.

The **nucleus proprius** is a group of large nerve cells situated anterior to the substantia gelatinosa throughout the spinal cord (Figs. 7-2 through 7-6).

Fig. 7-2. Transverse sections of the spinal cord at different levels, showing the arrangement of the gray matter and white matter.

Fig. 7-3. Transverse section of the spinal cord at the level of the fifth cervical segment. (Weigert stain.)

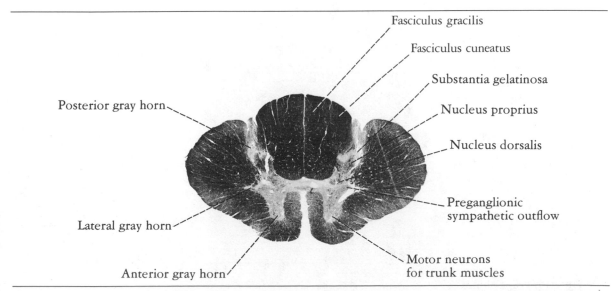

Fig. 7-4. Transverse section of the spinal cord at the level of the second thoracic segment. (Weigert stain.)

Central canal

Posterior median sulcus

Fasciculus gracilis

Posterior gray column

Substantia gelatinosa

Nucleus proprius

Nucleus dorsalis

Motor neurons for lower limb muscles

Anterior gray column

Anterior white commissure

Anterior median fissure

Motor neurons for trunk muscles

Fig. 7-5. Transverse section of the spinal cord at the level of the fourth lumbar segment. (Weigert stain.)

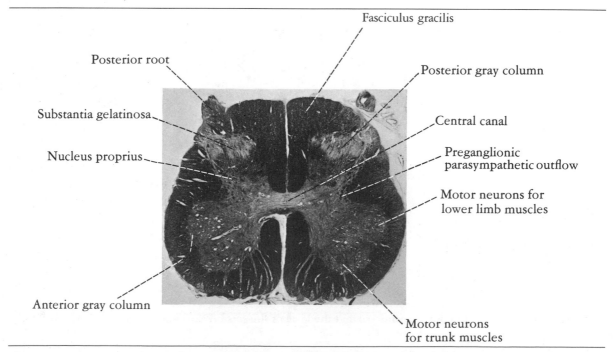

Fasciculus gracilis

Posterior root

Posterior gray column

Substantia gelatinosa

Central canal

Nucleus proprius

Preganglionic parasympathetic outflow

Motor neurons for lower limb muscles

Anterior gray column

Motor neurons for trunk muscles

Fig. 7-6. Transverse section of the spinal cord at the level of the second sacral segment. (Weigert stain.)

This nucleus constitutes the main bulk of cells present in the posterior gray column and receives fibers from the posterior white column that are associated with the senses of position and movement (proprioception), two-point discrimination, and vibration.

The **nucleus dorsalis (Clark's column)** is a group of nerve cells situated at the base of the posterior gray column and extending from the eighth cervical segment caudally to the third or fourth lumbar segments (Figs. 7-2, 7-4, and 7-5). Most of the cells are comparatively large and are associated with proprioceptive endings (neuromuscular spindles and tendon spindles).

The **visceral afferent nucleus** is a group of nerve cells of medium size situated lateral to the nucleus dorsalis; it extends from the first thoracic to the third lumbar segment of the spinal cord. It is believed to be associated with receiving visceral afferent information.

Nerve Cell Groups in the Lateral Gray Columns

The intermediolateral group of cells form the small lateral gray column, which extends from the first thoracic to the second or third lumbar segments of the spinal cord (Figs. 7-2 and 7-4). The cells are relatively small and give rise to preganglionic sympathetic fibers.

A similar group of cells found in the second, third, and fourth sacral segments of the spinal cord give rise to preganglionic parasympathetic fibers (Figs. 7-2 and 7-6).

The Gray Commissure and Central Canal

In transverse sections of the spinal cord, the anterior and posterior gray columns on each side are seen to be connected by a transverse **gray commissure,** so that the gray matter resembles the letter H (Figs. 7-2 through 7-6). In the center of the gray commissure is situated the **central canal.** The part of the gray commissure that is situated posterior to the central canal is often referred to as the **posterior gray commissure;** similarly, the part that lies anterior to the canal is called the **anterior gray commissure.**

The central canal is present throughout the spinal cord (Figs. 7-2 through 7-6). Superiorly, it is continuous with the central canal of the caudal half of the medulla oblongata and above this it opens into the cavity of the fourth ventricle. Inferiorly in the conus medullaris, it expands into the fusiform **terminal ventricle** and terminates below within the root of the filum terminale. It is filled with cerebrospinal fluid and is lined with ciliated columnar epithelium, the **ependyma.** Thus it is seen that the central canal is closed inferiorly and opens superiorly into the fourth ventricle.

White Matter

The white matter, for purposes of description, may be divided into **anterior, lateral,** and **posterior white columns** or **funiculi** (Figs. 7-1 through 7-6). The anterior column on each side lies between the midline and the point of emergence of the anterior nerve roots; the lateral column lies between the emergence of the anterior nerve roots and the entry of the posterior nerve roots; the posterior column lies between the entry of the posterior nerve roots and the midline.

Structure of White Matter

As in other regions of the central nervous system, the white matter of the spinal cord consists of a mixture of nerve fibers, neuroglia, and blood vessels. It surrounds the gray matter and its white color is due to the high proportion of myelinated nerve fibers.

Arrangement of Nerve Fiber Tracts

The arrangement of the nerve fiber tracts within the spinal cord has been deduced as the result of animal experimentation and study of the human spinal cord for degenerative nerve fibers resulting from injury or disease. Although some nerve tracts are concentrated in certain areas of the white matter, it is now generally accepted that considerable overlap is present. For purposes of description, the spinal tracts are divided into ascending, descending, and intersegmental tracts and their relative positions in the white matter are described below. A detailed description of the connections and function of the various tracts is given in Chapters 20 and 21. A simplified diagram, showing the general arrangement of the major tracts, is shown in Figure 7-7.

Ascending Tracts

Tracts in the Posterior White Column

The **fasciculus gracilis and cuneatus** are two large ascending tracts, which are separated from each other by a septum (Fig. 7-7). These tracts convey information of proprioceptive sensibility, vibration sense, and tactile discrimination.

Tracts in the Lateral White Column

1. The **posterior spinocerebellar tract** is a flat band of fibers situated at the periphery of the lateral white column (Fig. 7-7). It conveys proprioceptive information and additional contributions from touch and pressure receptors. This information enables the cerebellum to participate in the control of voluntary movements.

2. The **anterior spinocerebellar tract** is a flat band of fibers situated at the periphery of the lateral white column (Fig. 7-7). Like the posterior cerebellar tract, it conveys proprioceptive information and contributions from touch and pressure receptors. This information enables the cerebellum to participate in the control of voluntary movements.

3. The **lateral spinothalamic tract** is situated medial to the anterior spinocerebellar tract in the lateral white column (Fig. 7-7). It conveys information concerned with pain and temperature sensibility.

4. The **spinotectal tract** is situated medial to the anterior spinocerebellar tract and anterior to the lateral spinothalamic tract (Fig. 7-7). It is concerned with providing an ascending pathway for spinovisual reflexes.

5. The **posterolateral tract (Lissauer's tract)** is situated between the tip of the posterior gray column and the surface of the spinal cord close to the posterior roots (Fig. 7-7). It is made up of fibers of the lateral part of the posterior roots,

Fig. 7-7. Transverse section of spinal cord at midcervical level, showing the general arrangement of the ascending tracts on the right and the descending tracts on the left.

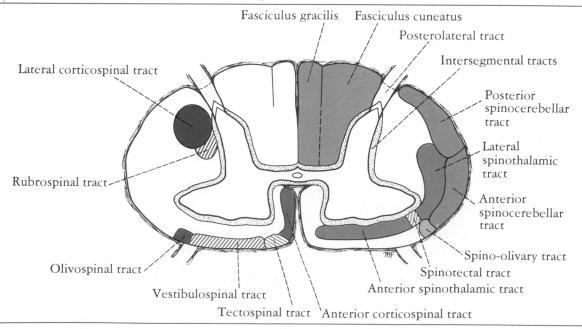

which divide into ascending and descending branches. (For details concerning function, see pp. 365, 366, and 368.)

6. The **spinoreticular tract** is mixed with the lateral spinothalamic tract (Fig. 7-7). (For details concerning function, see pp. 308, 315, and 373.)
7. The **spino-olivary tract** is situated at the junction of the anterior and lateral white columns (Fig. 7-7). It conveys information from cutaneous and proprioceptive organs.

Tracts in the Anterior White Column

The **anterior spinothalamic tract** lies medial to the anterior nerve roots and is concerned with conveying tactile and pressure sensibilities (Fig. 7-7).

Descending Tracts

Tracts in the Posterior White Column

A number of small tracts have been described by workers whose observations have been based on studies of clinical material. Until more information is available, no further details will be given here.

Tracts in the Lateral White Column

1. The **lateral corticospinal tract** is situated anterior to the posterior gray column and medial to the posterior spinocerebellar tract (Fig. 7-7). In the lumbar and sacral regions, where the posterior spinocerebellar tract is not present, the lateral corticospinal tract extends laterally to the surface of the spinal cord. The lateral corticospinal tract is an important motor pathway concerned with voluntary movement.
2. The **rubrospinal tract** forms a small band situated anterior to the lateral corticospinal tract (Fig. 7-7). It conveys impulses concerned with muscular activity.
3. The **lateral reticulospinal tract** almost certainly exists in the human subject but its position has not been established. In animals, it is situated medial to the rubrospinal and corticospinal tracts. This tract is thought to play an important role in muscular activity.
4. The **descending autonomic fibers** are thought to be situated mainly in the lateral white column. Some authorities believe they are located

close to the lateral corticospinal tract; others believe they are diffusely dispersed throughout the white columns of the cord. The autonomic fibers are concerned with controlling visceral functions.

5. The **olivospinal tract** is situated lateral to the anterior nerve roots and is present only in the upper cervical segments (Fig. 7-7). Its precise function is unknown, although it may be associated with muscular activity.

Tracts in the Anterior White Column

1. The **anterior corticospinal tract** is small and is situated alongside the anterior median fissure (Fig. 7-7). It is confined to the cervical and superior half of the thoracic region of the spinal cord. Although its precise function is unknown, it forms an important pathway concerned with voluntary movement.
2. The **vestibulospinal tract** is a flat band of fibers situated at the periphery of the anterior white column (Fig. 7-7). It conveys information concerned with equilibratory control to the anterior gray horn cells and therefore is associated with the control of muscle tone.
3. The **tectospinal tract** is small and is situated lateral to the margin on the anterior median fissure (Fig. 7-7). It forms part of a reflex nervous pathway associated with rotation of the head and moving of the arms in response to visual stimuli.
4. The **reticulospinal fibers** are scattered throughout the anterior white column and are concerned with motor function.

Intersegmental Tracts

Tracts in the Posterior White Column

The **posterior intersegmental tract** is a thin band of fibers situated posterior to the gray commissure (Fig. 7-7). As its name implies, its fibers run from one segment of the cord to another, thus establishing important intersegmental spinal reflexes.

Tracts in the Lateral White Column

The **lateral intersegmental tract** is a thin band of fibers situated immediately lateral to the gray matter of the spinal cord (Fig. 7-7). Its function is similar to that of the posterior intersegmental tract, but it is also believed to contain within it some reticulospinal and descending autonomic fibers.

Tracts in the Anterior White Column

The **anterior intersegmental tract** is a thin band of fibers situated immediately anterior to the gray matter of the spinal cord (Fig. 7-7). Its functions are believed to be identical to those of the posterior and lateral intersegmental tracts.

It must be emphasized that the above description of the arrangement of the different tracts within the spinal cord is the barest outline. Nevertheless, the information provided is sufficient for the physician. Those wishing to obtain further details should consult the original publications listed at the end of this chapter.

MENINGES OF THE SPINAL CORD

The spinal cord, like the brain, is surrounded by three meninges: the dura mater, the arachnoid mater, and the pia mater.

Dura Mater of the Spinal Cord

The dura mater is a dense, strong, fibrous membrane that encloses the spinal cord and cauda equina (Figs. 7-1 and 1-6). It is continuous above through the foramen magnum with the meningeal layer of dura covering the brain. Inferiorly, it ends on the filum terminale at the level of the lower border of the second sacral vertebra. The dural sheath lies loosely in the vertebral canal and is separated from the walls of the canal by the **extradural space.** This contains loose aerolar tissue and the **internal vertebral venous plexus.** The dura mater extends along each nerve root and becomes continuous with the connective tissue surrounding each spinal nerve (epineurium). The inner surface of the dura mater is in contact with the arachnoid mater (Fig. 7-1).

Arachnoid Mater of the Spina Cord

The arachnoid mater is a delicate impermeable membrane that covers the spinal cord and lies between the pia mater internally and the dura mater externally (Fig. 7-1). It is separated from the pia mater by a wide space, the **subarachnoid space,** which is filled with **cerebrospinal fluid** (Fig. 7-1). The subarachnoid space is crossed by a number of fine strands of connective tissue. The arachnoid mater is continuous above through the foramen magnum with the arachnoid covering the brain. Inferiorly, it ends on the filum terminale at the level of the lower border of the second sacral vertebra (see Fig. 1-6). The arachnoid mater continues along the spinal nerve roots, forming small lateral extensions of the subarachnoid space.

Pia Mater of the Spinal Cord

The pia mater, a vascular membrane that closely invests the spinal cord (Fig. 7-1), is thickened on either side between the nerve roots to form the **ligamentum denticulatum,** which passes laterally to adhere to the arachnoid and dura. It is by this means that the spinal cord is suspended in the middle of the dural sheath. The pia mater extends along each nerve root and becomes continuous with the connective tissue surrounding each spinal nerve (Fig. 7-1).

CEREBROSPINAL FLUID

The cerebrospinal fluid is produced mainly by the **choroid plexuses** within the lateral, third, and fourth ventricles of the brain; small amounts are produced by the ependymal cells lining the ventricles and from the brain through the perivascular spaces. The cerebrospinal fluid escapes from the ventricular system of the brain through the three foramina in the roof of the fourth ventricle and so enters the subarachnoid space (see p. 11). The fluid now circulates both superiorly over the surface of the cerebral hemispheres and inferiorly around the spinal cord. The spinal part of the subarachnoid space extends down as far as the lower border of the second sacral vertebra (see Fig. 1-6). Eventually, the fluid enters the bloodstream by passing into the **arachnoid villi** and diffusing through their walls.

In addition to removing waste products associated with neuronal activity, the cerebrospinal fluid provides a medium that surrounds the spinal cord. This fluid, together with the bony and ligamentous walls of the vertebral canal, effectively protects the spinal cord from trauma.

BLOOD SUPPLY OF THE SPINAL CORD

The spinal cord receives its arterial supply from three small arteries, the two posterior spinal arteries and the anterior spinal artery. These longitudinally running arteries are reinforced by small segmentally arranged arteries that enter the vertebral canal through the intervertebral foramina. These vessels anastomose on the surface of the cord and send branches into the substance of the white and gray matter. Considerable variation exists as to the size and segmental levels at which the reinforcing arteries occur.

Posterior Spinal Arteries

The posterior spinal arteries arise either directly from the vertebral arteries inside the skull or indirectly from the posterior inferior cerebellar arteries. Each artery descends on the posterior surface of the spinal cord close to the posterior nerve roots and gives off branches that enter the substance of the cord (Fig. 7-8). The posterior spinal arteries supply the posterior one-third of the spinal cord.

It should be noted that the posterior spinal arteries are small in the upper thoracic region and that the first three thoracic segments of the spinal cord are particularly vulnerable to ischemia should the segmental or radicular arteries in this region be occluded.

Anterior Spinal Artery

The anterior spinal artery is formed by the union of two arteries, each of which arises from the vertebral artery inside the skull. The anterior spinal

Fig. 7-8. Transverse section of spinal cord, showing arterial supply and venous drainage.

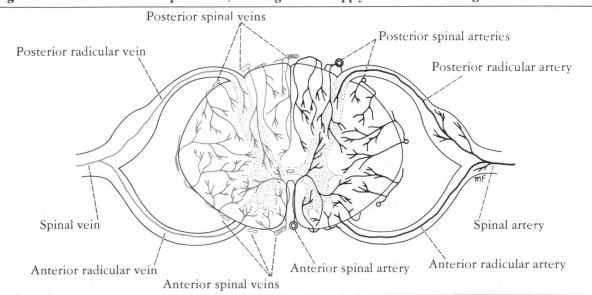

artery then descends on the anterior surface of the spinal cord within the anterior median fissure (Fig. 7-8). Branches from the anterior spinal artery enter the substance of the cord and supply the anterior two-thirds of the spinal cord.

In the upper and lower thoracic segments of the spinal cord the anterior spinal artery may be extremely small. Should the segmental or radicular arteries be occluded in these regions, the fourth thoracic and the first lumbar segments of the spinal cord would be particularly liable to ischemic necrosis.

Segmental Spinal Arteries

At each intervertebral foramen the longitudinally running posterior and anterior spinal arteries are reinforced by small segmental arteries on both sides (Fig. 7-8). The arteries are branches of arteries outside the vertebral column (deep cervical, intercostal, and lumbar arteries). Having entered the vertebral canal, each segmental spinal artery gives rise to **anterior and posterior radicular arteries**

that accompany the anterior and posterior nerve roots to the spinal cord.

Additional **feeder arteries** enter the vertebral canal and anastomose with the anterior and posterior spinal arteries; however, the number and size of these arteries vary considerably from one individual to another. One large and important feeder artery, the **great anterior medullary artery of Adamkiewicz,** arises from the aorta in the lower thoracic or upper lumbar vertebral levels; it is unilateral and in the majority of persons enters the spinal cord from the left side. The importance of this artery lies in the fact that it may be the major source of blood to the lower two-thirds of the spinal cord.

Veins of the Spinal Cord

The veins of the spinal cord drain into six tortuous longitudinal channels that communicate superiorly within the skull with the veins of the brain and the venous sinuses. They drain mainly into the internal vertebral venous plexus.

CLINICAL NOTES

GENERAL ANATOMICAL FEATURES OF CLINICAL IMPORTANCE

The spinal cord may be described, for practical purposes, as consisting of columns of motor and sensory nerve cells, the gray matter, surrounded by ascending and descending tracts, the white matter. It lies within the vertebral canal and is protected by three surrounding fibrous membranes, the meninges. It is cushioned against trauma by the cerebrospinal fluid and is held in position by the denticulate ligaments on each side and the filum terminale inferiorly. The spinal cord is segmented, and paired posterior (sensory) and anterior (motor) roots corresponding to each segment of the cord leave the vertebral canal through the intervertebral foramina.

The spinal cord is shorter than the vertebral column and terminates inferiorly in the adult at the level of the lower border of the first lumbar vertebra. The subarachnoid space extends inferiorly be-

yond the end of the cord and ends at the level of the lower border of the second sacral vertebra.

Because of the shortness of the spinal cord relative to the length of the vertebral column, the nerve roots of the lumbar and sacral segments have to take an oblique course downward to reach their respective intervertebral foramina; the resulting leach of nerve roots forms the cauda equina.

A lumbar puncture needle may be inserted into the subarachnoid space below the level of the second lumbar vertebra without damaging the spinal cord. (For details, see p. 32.)

Ischemia of the Spinal Cord

The blood supply to the spinal cord is surprisingly meager considering the importance of this nervous tissue. The posterior and anterior spinal arteries are of small and variable diameter and the reinforcing segmental arteries vary in number and size. Ischemia of the spinal cord can easily follow minor damage to the arterial supply, as the result of nerve block procedures, aortic surgery, or any operation in which severe hypotension occurs. The fourth thoracic and first lumbar segments of the cord are particularly prone to ischemia.

Anterior and Posterior Nerve Roots

Each nerve root has a covering of pia, arachnoid, and dura mater. The anterior and posterior roots unite in the intervertebral foramina to form the spinal nerves. Here the meninges fuse with the epineurium of the spinal nerves. Either or both spinal nerve roots may be involved in syphilitic spinal meningitis or pyogenic meningitis. The posterior roots may be involved in tabes dorsalis and herpes zoster. Their anatomical location, both in the vertebral canal and in the intervertebral foramina, exposes them to compression from tumors of the vertebral column and to irritation from abnormal constituents of the cerebrospinal fluid, such as blood following a subarachnoid hemorrhage. A herniated intervertebral disc, a primary or secondary vertebral tumor, vertebral destruction by tumor or infection, or a fracture dislocation can press upon the spinal nerve roots in the intervertebral foramina. Even severe scoliosis may result in compression of the nerve roots.

A lesion of one posterior spinal nerve root will produce pain in the area of skin innervated by that root, and also in the muscles that receive their sensory nerve supply from that root. Movements of the vertebral column in the region of the lesion will heighten the pain, and coughing and sneezing will also make it worse by raising the pressure within the vertebral canal. Before there is actual loss of sensation in the dermatome there may be evidence of hyperalgesia and hyperesthesia.

A lesion of an anterior root will result in paralysis of any muscle that is supplied exclusively by that root and a partial paralysis of any muscle that is supplied partially by that root. In both cases, fasciculation and muscle atrophy occur.

ACUTE SPINAL CORD INJURIES

The incidence of acute spinal cord injuries in the United States is about 10,000 per year. The injury is catastrophic, since little or no regeneration of the severed nerve tracts takes place (see p. 112) and the individual is permanently disabled. Treatment has been restricted to anatomical realignment and stabilization of the vertebral column or decompression of the spinal cord. During the recovery process the patient goes through intensive rehabilitation to optimize the remaining neurological function. Apart from improved management of medical complications, very little new therapy has been successful in spite of an enormous amount of research into the problem of neuronal regeneration in the spinal cord. Recently, the use of certain drugs (GM_1 ganglioside and methylprednisolone) administered to the patient soon after injury has resulted in some improvement in the neurological deficit. Animal experiments appear to indicate that these drugs enhance the functional recovery of damaged neurons.

COMPRESSION OF THE SPINAL CORD

If injuries to the spinal cord are excluded (see p. 29), the causes of compression may be divided into extradural and intradural. The intradural causes may be divided into those that arise outside the spinal cord (extramedullary) and those that arise within the cord (intramedullary).

The extradural causes include herniation of an intervertebral disc, infection of the vertebrae with tuberculosis, and primary and secondary tumors of the vertebra; leukemic deposits and extradural abscesses may also compress the spinal cord. The two common extramedullary tumors are meningiomas and nerve fibromas. Intramedullary causes include primary tumors of the spinal cord, such as gliomas.

The clinical signs and symptoms are produced by an interference with the normal anatomical and physiological functions of the spinal cord. Pressure on the spinal arteries causes ischemia of the spinal cord with degeneration of nerve cells and their fibers. Pressure on the spinal veins causes edema of the spinal cord with interference in the function of the neurons. Finally, direct pressure on the white and gray matter of the spinal cord and the spinal nerve roots interferes with nerve conduction. At the same time, the circulation of the cerebrospinal fluid is obstructed, and the composition of the fluid changes below the level of obstruction.

Clinical Signs

One of the earliest signs is pain. This may be local pain in the vertebra involved or pain radiating along the distribution of one or more spinal nerve roots. The pain is made worse by coughing or sneezing and is usually worse at night, when the patient is recumbent.

Interference with motor function occurs early. Involvement of the anterior gray column motor cells at the level of the lesion results in partial or complete paralysis of muscles, with loss of tone and muscle wasting. The early involvement of the corticospinal and other descending tracts produces muscular weakness, increased muscle tone (spasticity), increased tendon reflexes below the level of the lesion, and an extensor plantar response. The degree of sensory loss will depend on the nerve tracts involved. A lesion of the posterior white columns of the spinal cord will cause loss of muscle joint sense (proprioception), vibration sense, and tactile discrimination below the level of the lesion on the same side. Involvement of the lateral spinal thalamic tracts will cause loss of pain and heat and cold sensations on the opposite side of the body below the level of the lesion. A more detailed discussion of the clinical signs and symptoms associated with lesions of the spinal cord appears following the description of the ascending and descending tracts of the spinal cord. (See pp. 376, 395, and 398.)

Since many spinal tumors are benign and can be successfully removed (provided that irreversible damage to the spinal cord has not occurred as a result of compression of the blood supply), an early accurate diagnosis is essential. The following investigations should be performed: (1) radiography of the vertebral column, including CT scanning and MRI, (2) lumbar puncture, and (3) myelography.

Examination of Cerebrospinal Fluid

Performing a lumbar puncture (spinal tap) is of great value in making a diagnosis of compression of the spinal cord. (For details, see p. 32.) Normal cerebrospinal fluid is clear and colorless and it has the following constituents:

Protein: 15–45 mg per 100 ml
Glucose: 50–85 mg per 100 ml
Chloride: 720–750 mg per 100 ml
Cells: 0–3 lymphocytes per cu mm

The normal pressure of cerebrospinal fluid with the patient lying quietly on his side and breathing through his mouth is between 60 mm and 150 mm of water.

If the cause of the compression is obstructing the flow of cerebrospinal fluid in the subarachnoid space, the normal variations in pressure corresponding to the pulse and respiration are reduced or absent. Compression of the internal jugular veins in the neck raises the cerebral venous pressure and inhibits the absorption of cerebrospinal fluid in the arachnoid granulations, thus producing a rise in the manometric reading of the cerebrospinal fluid pressure. If this fails to occur, the subarachnoid space is blocked and the patient is exhibiting a positive **Queckenstedt's sign.**

Should the tumor completely occupy the vertebral canal in the region of the cauda equina, no cerebrospinal fluid may flow out of the lumbar puncture needle.

Normally the cerebrospinal fluid is clear. In the presence of a tumor the cerebrospinal fluid may become yellow and clot spontaneously owing to the rise in protein content.

Radiographic Appearances of the Vertebral Column

The views commonly used in radiography are anteroposterior, lateral, and oblique. Vertebral destruction owing to tuberculosis or to primary or secondary tumors of the vertebrae, or fractures owing to trauma usually can be revealed by radiographic examination. Erosion of the pedicles by a tumor within the intervertebral foramina may be seen. Narrowing of the space between the vertebral bodies with bony spurs because of osteoarthritic changes in adjacent vertebral bodies can also be seen.

CT Scans and MRI of the Vertebral Column and Spinal Cord

CT scans can be obtained of the vertebrae and their joints (Fig. 7-9). A protrusion of an intervertebral

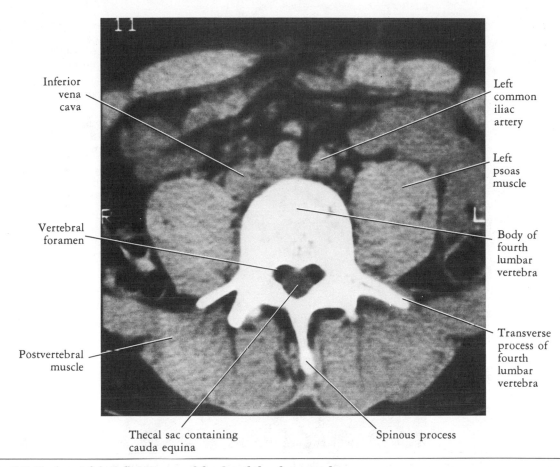

Inferior vena cava

Left common iliac artery

Left psoas muscle

Vertebral foramen

Body of fourth lumbar vertebra

Transverse process of fourth lumbar vertebra

Postvertebral muscle

Thecal sac containing cauda equina

Spinous process

Fig. 7-9. Horizontal (axial) CT scan of the fourth lumbar vertebra.

disc can be identified and the presence of narrowing of the vertebral canal (**spinal stenosis**) can be diagnosed.

Sagittal MR images are increasingly being used to replace CT scans and myelography. The parts of a vertebra, the intervertebral disc, the posterior longitudinal ligament, and the meningeal sac (**thecal sac**) can easily be identified (Fig. 7-10).

Myelography

The subarachnoid space may be studied radiographically by the injection of a contrast medium into the subarachnoid space by lumbar puncture. Iodized oil has been used with success. This tech-

nique is referred to as **myelography** (Figs. 7-11 and 7-12).

If the patient is sitting in the upright position, the oil sinks to the lower limit of the subarachnoid space at the level of the lower border of the second sacral vertebra. By placing the patient on a tilting table, the oil can be made to gravitate gradually to higher levels of the vertebral column.

A normal myelogram will show pointed lateral projections at regular intervals at the intervertebral space levels. The reason for this is that the opaque medium fills the lateral extensions of the subarachnoid space around each spinal nerve. The presence of a tumor or a prolapsed intervertebral disc may obstruct the movement of the oil from one region to another when the patient is tilted.

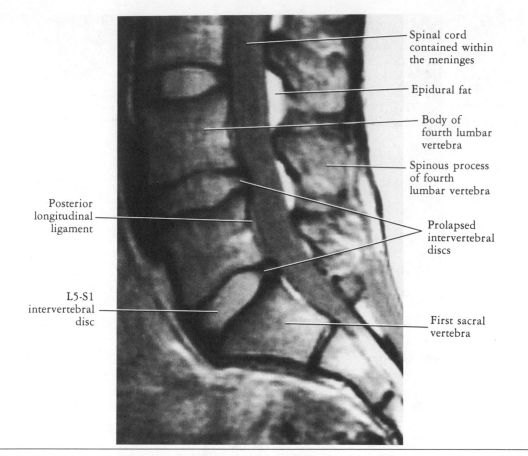

Spinal cord
contained within
the meninges

Epidural fat

Body of
fourth lumbar
vertebra

Spinous process
of fourth
lumbar vertebra

Prolapsed
intervertebral
discs

First sacral
vertebra

Posterior
longitudinal
ligament

L5-S1
intervertebral
disc

Fig. 7-10. Sagittal MR scan of the lumbosacral part of the vertebral column. Shows several prolapsed intervertebral discs. (Courtesy of Dr. Pait.)

Fig. 7-11. Posteroanterior myelogram of the cervical region of a 22-year-old woman.

Fig. 7-12. Diagrammatic explanation of myelogram shown in Figure 7-11.

CLINICAL PROBLEMS

Answers on Page 595

1. A 53-year-old widower was admitted to the hospital complaining of a burning pain over his right shoulder region and the upper part of his right arm. The pain had started three weeks previously and since that time had progressively worsened. The pain was accentuated by moving his neck and by coughing. Two years previously he had been treated for osteoarthritis of his vertebral column. The patient stated that he had been a football player at college and since that time he continued to take an active part in the game until his forty-second year. Physical examination revealed weakness, wasting, and fasciculation of the right deltoid and biceps brachii muscles. The right biceps tendon reflex was absent. Radiological examination revealed extensive spur formation on the bodies of the fourth, fifth, and sixth cervical vertebrae. The patient demonstrated hyperesthesia and partial analgesia in the skin over the lower part of the right deltoid and down the lateral side of the arm. Using your knowledge of neuroanatomy, make the diagnosis. How is the pain produced? Why is the pain made worse by coughing?

2. A 66-year-old woman was admitted to the hospital because of her increasing difficulty in walking. Two weeks before admission she had been able to walk with the help of a stick. Since that time walking had become increasingly difficult and for the past two days she could not walk at all. She had complete control of micturition and defecation. On examination, the handgrip was weak on both sides but power was normal in the proximal segments of the upper extremities. The tendon reflexes of the upper limbs and the sensory function were normal. Both lower limbs showed muscular weakness with increased muscle tone, especially on the left side. The knee jerks and ankle jerks (tendon reflexes) in both lower limbs were grossly exaggerated and there were bilateral extensor plantar responses. The patient had a loss of sensation of pain below the fifth thoracic dermatome on both sides of the body. Postural sense was impaired in both great toes and vibration sense was absent below the fifth thoracic segmental level. Radiological examination of the vertebral column showed nothing abnormal. A myelogram in the lumbar region revealed a complete block at the lower border of the fourth thoracic vertebra. Using your knowledge of neuroanatomy, make the diagnosis. How would you treat this patient? Name the tracts in the spinal cord that are responsible for conduction of the sensation of pain. What is the position of these tracts in the spinal cord? Name the tracts responsible for the conduction of postural sense and vibration sense from the spinal cord to the brain. Why did the patient have increasing difficulty in walking? Why were the tendon reflexes in the lower limbs exaggerated, and why did the patient exhibit bilateral extensor plantar responses?

3. How would you perform a lumbar puncture? What important information can be obtained by carrying out this form of examination? What is the normal pressure of cerebrospinal fluid with the patient lying on his side? What is the normal concentration of protein, chloride, and glucose in the cerebrospinal fluid? What color is the normal cerebrospinal fluid? Can one inject foreign substances into the subarachnoid space?

4. A patient's notes state that he has a positive Queckenstedt's sign. What does this mean?

5. What is the blood supply to the spinal cord? Which areas of the spinal cord are supplied by the anterior spinal artery? Which regions of the spinal cord are most suceptible to ischemia?

6. Draw a cross-sectional diagram of the spinal cord at the level of the fourth thoracic segment. Label the gray and white matter. Indicate the position of the major groups of nerve cells in the gray matter.

7. Draw a cross-sectional diagram of the spinal cord in the lower cervical region. Indicate the positions of the major ascending and descending tracts in the white matter. Now imagine that this patient has syringomyelia*; place in position the lesion and identify the nerve tracts and nerve cells that will be pressed upon by the

---

*Developmental abnormality of the central canal of the spinal cord resulting in the presence of expanding cavities close to the central canal.

expanding lesion. What symptoms and signs would you expect from such a patient?

8. A myelogram was performed on a 35-year-old man who visited a neurologist with a history of pain in the fourth left thoracic dermatome that he had had for three months. The radiopaque iodized oil was introduced into the subarachnoid space with the patient in the vertical position on a tilting table. Altering the tilt of the table caused the oil to gravitate to higher levels, but there was no evidence of blockage in the subarachnoid space. However, it was noted that the lateral extension of the space around the fourth left thoracic spinal nerve did not show up on the myelogram. Using your knowledge of neuroanatomy, give the diagnosis. What is the lateral extension of the subarachnoid space around the spinal nerve? In anatomical terms, how far does this extension pass laterally?

9. A neurologist made the statement in a lecture that the nerve cell groups found in the gray matter of the spinal cord are not small, isolated groups of cells but, rather, should be considered as columns of cells extending along the spinal cord. Do you agree with this statement?

10. Define each of the following terms: (a) *ligamentum denticulatum*, (b) *filum terminale*, (c) *substantia gelatinosa*, (d) *nucleus proprius*, and (e) *anterior gray commissure*.

NATIONAL BOARD TYPE QUESTIONS

Answers on Page 620

IN EACH OF THE FOLLOWING QUESTIONS, ANSWER:
   (a) IF (1) ONLY IS CORRECT
   (b) IF (2) ONLY IS CORRECT
   (c) IF BOTH (1) AND (2) ARE CORRECT, AND
   (d) IF NEITHER (1) NOR (2) IS CORRECT

1. Which of the following statements concerning the spinal cord is (are) correct?
   (1) The anterior and posterior gray columns on the two sides are united by a gray commissure.
   (2) The central canal expands superiorly into the terminal ventricle.

2. Which of the following statements concerning the anterior gray columns of the spinal cord is (are) correct?
   (1) The larger nerve cell bodies give rise to the alpha efferent fibers that leave the cord in the anterior roots.
   (2) For practical purposes the nerve cells may be divided into medial, central, and lateral groups.

3. Which of the following statements concerning the posterior gray columns of the spinal cord is (are) correct?
   (1) The substantia gelatinosa groups of cells are located at the base of each column.
   (2) The nucleus dorsalis (Clark's column) is a group of nerve cells found only in the cervical segments of the cord.

Match the tracts listed on the left with the appropriate white column listed on the right:

4. Posterior spinocerebellar tract   (a) Posterior white column
5. Lateral spinothalamic tract   (b) Anterior white column
6. Anterior corticospinal tract   (c) Lateral white column
7. Fasciculus gracilis   (d) None of the above
8. Rubrospinal tract

Select the best response:

9. The following statements concerning the spinal cord are correct **except**:
   (a) The spinal cord has a cervical enlargement for the brachial plexus.
   (b) It possesses 34 pairs of spinal nerves.
   (c) In the adult, the spinal cord usually ends inferiorly at the lower border of the first lumbar vertebra.
   (d) The ligamentum denticulatum anchors the spinal cord to the dura mater along each side.
   (e) The central canal communicates with the fourth ventricle of the brain.

10. The following statements concerning the blood supply of the spinal cord are true **except**:
    (a) The posterior spinal arteries supply the posterior third of the spinal cord.
    (b) The veins communicate with the veins of the brain and the venous sinuses.
    (c) The arteria radicularis magna (artery of Adamkiewicz) arises in the upper thoracic region from the arch of the aorta.
    (d) The anterior spinal artery is single but usually arises from both vertebral arteries.
    (e) The spinal arteries are reinforced by radicular arteries, which are branches of local arteries.

11. The following statements concerning the cerebrospinal fluid are correct **except**:
    (a) With the patient lying on his side, the normal pressure is between 60 and 150 mm of water.
    (b) The normal glucose content is 50 to 85 mg per 100 ml.
    (c) It is a clear, colorless fluid.
    (d) The cells are polymorphonuclear leucocytes.
    (e) Compression of the internal jugular veins raises the cerebrospinal fluid pressure.

12. The following statements concerning the meninges of the spinal cord are correct **except**:
    (a) The dura mater is a delicate impermeable membrane.
    (b) The pia mater is a vascular membrane that closely invests the cord.
    (c) The arachnoid mater continues along the spinal nerve roots forming small lateral extensions of the subarachnoid space.
    (d) The dura mater is continuous above through the foramen magnum with the meningeal layer of dura covering the brain.
    (e) The extradural space contains the internal vertebral venous plexus.

In Figure 7-13, match the numbers listed on the left with the appropriate structure listed on the right.

13. Number 1
14. Number 2
15. Number 3
16. Number 4
17. Number 5
18. Number 6

(a) Nucleus proprius
(b) Preganglionic sympathetic outflow
(c) Nucleus dorsalis
(d) Substantia gelatinosa
(e) None of the above

Fig. 7-13.

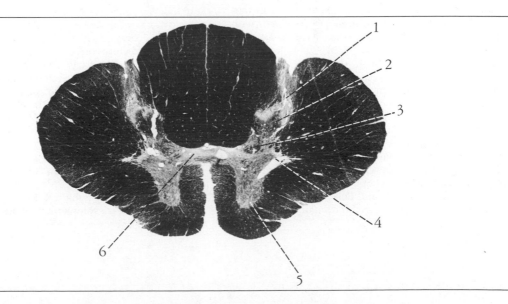

Match the structures listed below on the left with the appropriate answers listed below on the right. The answers may be used more than once.

19. Location of conus medullaris
20. Filum terminale is formed by
21. Lateral gray column is located in
22. Gamma efferent nerve cells are located in
23. Lining of central canal is formed of

(a) Pia mater
(b) Thoracic and upper lumbar segments of spinal cord
(c) Lower end of spinal cord
(d) Anterior gray column
(e) None of the above

ADDITIONAL READING

Austin, G. *The Spinal Cord.* New York: Igaku Shoin, 1981.

Barson, A. J. The vertebral level of termination of the spinal cord during normal and abnormal development. *J. Anat.* 106:489, 1970.

Basbaum, A. I., and Fields, H. L. Endogenous pain control systems: Brainstem spinal pathways and endorphin circuitry. *Annu. Rev. Neurosci.* 7:309, 1984.

Bennett, G. J., Abdelmoumine, M., Hayashi, H., and Dubner, R. Physiology and morphology of substantia gelatinosa neurons intracellularly stained with horseradish peroxidase. *J. Comp. Neurol.* 194:809, 1980.

Bracken, M. B., Shepard, M. J., Collins, W. F., et al. A randomized, controlled trial of methylprednisolone or naloxone in the treatment of acute spinal-cord injury: Results of the second national acute spinal cord injury study. *N. Engl. J. Med.* 322:1405, 1990.

Carpenter, M. B., and Sutin, J. *Human Neuroanatomy* (8th ed.). Baltimore: Williams & Wilkins, 1983.

Ekerot, C. F., Larson, B., and Oscarsson, O. Information carried by the spinocerebellar tracts. *Prog. Brain Res.* 50:79, 1979.

Geisler, F. H., Dorsey, F. C., and Coleman, W. P. Recovery of motor function after spinal cord injury: A randomized, placebo-controlled trial with G. M.-1 ganglioside. *N. Engl. J. Med.* 344 (26): 1829, 1991.

Kerr, F. W. L., and Fukushima, T. New observations on the anatomy of the spinothalamic tract. *Pain* 58:47, 1980.

Lazorthes, G., Gouaze, A., Zadeh, J. O., et al. Arterial vascularization of the spinal cord. *J. Neurosurg.* 35: 253, 1971.

Rexed, B. A. Cytoarchitectonic atlas of the spinal cord in the cat. *J. Comp. Neurol.* 100:297, 1954.

Ross, E. D., Kirkpatrick, J. B., and Lastimoso, A. C. B. Position and vibration sensations: Function of the dorsal spinocerebellar tracts? *Ann. Neurol.* 5:171, 1979.

Smith, M. C., and Deacon, P. Topographical anatomy of the posterior columns of the spinal cord in man: The long ascending fibers. *Brain* 107:671, 1984.

Walton, J. N. *Brain's Diseases of the Nervous System* (8th ed.). New York and London: Oxford University Press, 1977.

Williams, P. L., Warwick, R., Dyson, M., and Bannister, L. H. *Gray's Anatomy* (37th Brit. ed.). Philadelphia: Saunders, 1989.

Willis, W. D., and Coggeshall, R. E. *Sensory Mechanisms of the Spinal Cord.* New York: Plenum, 1978.

Chapter 8
The Medulla Oblongata

GROSS APPEARANCE

The medulla oblongata connects the pons superiorly with the spinal cord inferiorly (Fig. 8-1). The junction of the medulla and spinal cord is at the origin of the anterior and posterior roots of the first cervical spinal nerve, which corresponds approximately to the level of the foramen magnum. The medulla oblongata is conical in shape, its broad extremity being directed superiorly. The **central canal** of the spinal cord continues upward into the lower half of the medulla; in the upper half of the medulla it expands as the **cavity of the fourth ventricle** (Fig. 8-1).

On the anterior surface of the medulla is the anterior median fissure, which is continuous inferiorly with the **anterior median fissure** of the spinal cord (Fig. 8-1). On each side of the median fissure there is a swelling called the **pyramid.** The pyramids are composed of bundles of nerve fibers, corticospinal fibers, which originate in large nerve cells in the precentral gyrus of the cerebral cortex. The pyramids taper inferiorly and it is here that the majority of the descending fibers cross over to the

opposite side, forming the **decussation of the pyramids** (Fig. 8-1). The **anterior external arcuate fibers** are a few nerve fibers that emerge from the anterior median fissure above the decussation and pass laterally over the surface of the medulla oblongata. Posterolateral to the pyramids are the **olives,** which are oval elevations produced by the underlying **inferior olivary nuclei.** In the groove between the pyramid and the olive emerge the rootlets of the hypoglossal nerve. Posterior to the olives are the **inferior cerebellar peduncles** (Fig. 8-1), which connect the medulla to the cerebellum. In the groove between the olive and the inferior cerebellar peduncle emerge the roots of the glossopharyngeal and vagus nerves and the cranial roots of the accessory nerve (Fig. 8-1).

The posterior surface of the superior half of the medulla oblongata forms the lower part of the **floor of the fourth ventricle** (Fig. 8-1). The posterior surface of the inferior half of the medulla is continuous with the posterior aspect of the spinal cord and possesses a **posterior median sulcus.** On each side of the median sulcus there is an elongated swelling, the **gracile tubercle,** produced by

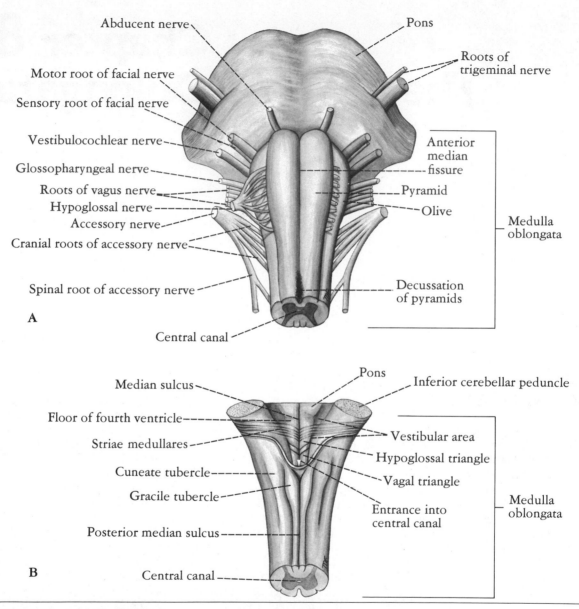

Fig. 8-1. The medulla oblongata.
A. Anterior view.
B. Posterior view. Note that the roof of the fourth ventricle and the cerebellum have been removed.

the underlying **gracile nucleus** (Fig. 8-1). Lateral to the gracile tubercle is a similar swelling, the **cuneate tubercle,** produced by the underlying **cuneate nucleus.**

INTERNAL STRUCTURE OF THE MEDULLA OBLONGATA

As in the spinal cord, the medulla oblongata consists of white matter and gray matter, but a study of transverse sections of this region shows that they have been extensively rearranged. This rearrangement can be explained embryologically by the expansion of the **neural tube** to form the **hindbrain vesicle,** which becomes the **fourth ventricle** (Fig. 8-2). The extensive lateral spread of the fourth ventricle results in an alteration in the position of the derivatives of the **alar** and **basal plates** of the embryo. To assist in understanding this concept, remember that in the spinal cord the derivatives of the alar and basal plates are situated posterior and anterior to the **sulcus limitans,** respectively, and in the case of the medulla oblongata they are situated lateral and medial to the sulcus limitans, respectively (Fig. 8-2).

The internal structure of the medulla oblongata will be considered at four levels: (1) level of decussation of pyramids, (2) level of decussation of lemnisci, (3) level of the olives, and (4) level just inferior to the pons.

Level of Decussation of Pyramids

A transverse section through the inferior half of the medulla oblongata (Figs. 8-3A and 8-4) passes through the **decussation of the pyramids,** the great motor decussation. In the superior part of the medulla the corticospinal fibers occupy and form the pyramid, but inferiorly about three-quarters of the fibers cross the median plane and continue down the spinal cord in the lateral white column as the **lateral corticospinal tract.** As these fibers cross the midline, they sever the continuity between the anterior column of the gray matter of the spinal cord and the gray matter that surrounds the central canal.

The **fasciculus gracilis** and the **fasciculus cuneatus** continue to ascend superiorly posterior to the central gray matter (Figs. 8-3A and 8-4). The **nucleus gracilis** and the **nucleus cuneatus** appear as posterior extensions of the central gray matter.

The **substantia gelatinosa** in the posterior gray column of the spinal cord becomes continuous with the inferior end of the **nucleus of the spinal tract of the trigeminal nerve.** The fibers of the tract of the nucleus are situated between the nucleus and the surface of the medulla oblongata.

The lateral and anterior white columns of the spinal cord are easily identified in these sections and their fiber arrangement is unchanged (Figs. 8-3A and 8-4).

Level of Decussation of Lemnisci

A transverse section through the inferior half of the medulla oblongata, a short distance above the level of the decussation of the pyramids, passes through the **decussation of lemnisci,** the great sensory decussation (Figs. 8-3B and 8-5). The decussation of the lemnisci takes place anterior to the central gray matter and posterior to the pyramids. It should be understood that the lemnisci have been formed from the **internal arcuate fibers,** which have emerged from the anterior aspects of the **nucleus gracilis** and **nucleus cuneatus.** The internal arcuate fibers first travel anteriorly and laterally round the central gray matter. They then curve medially toward the midline, where they decussate with the corresponding fibers of the opposite side (Figs. 8-3B and 8-5).

The **nucleus of the spinal tract of the trigeminal nerve** lies lateral to the internal arcuate fibers. The **spinal tract of the trigeminal nerve** lies lateral to the nucleus (Figs. 8-3B and 8-5).

The **lateral and anterior spinothalamic tracts and the spinotectal tracts** occupy an area lateral to the decussation of the lemnisci (Fig. 8-3B). They are very close to one another and collectively are known as the **spinal lemniscus.** The **spinocerebellar, vestibulospinal,** and the **rubrospinal tracts** are situated in the anterolateral region of the medulla oblongata.

Level of the Olives

A transverse section through the olives passes across the inferior part of the fourth ventricle (Figs. 8-6 and 8-7). The amount of gray matter has increased at this level owing to the presence of the

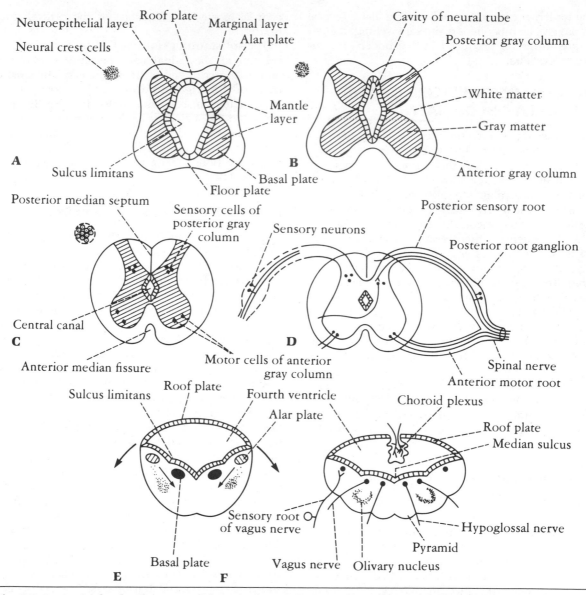

Fig. 8-2. Stages in the development of the spinal cord (A, B, C, D) and the medulla oblongata (E, F). The neural crest cells will form the first afferent sensory neurons in the posterior root ganglia of the spinal nerves and the sensory ganglia of the cranial nerves.

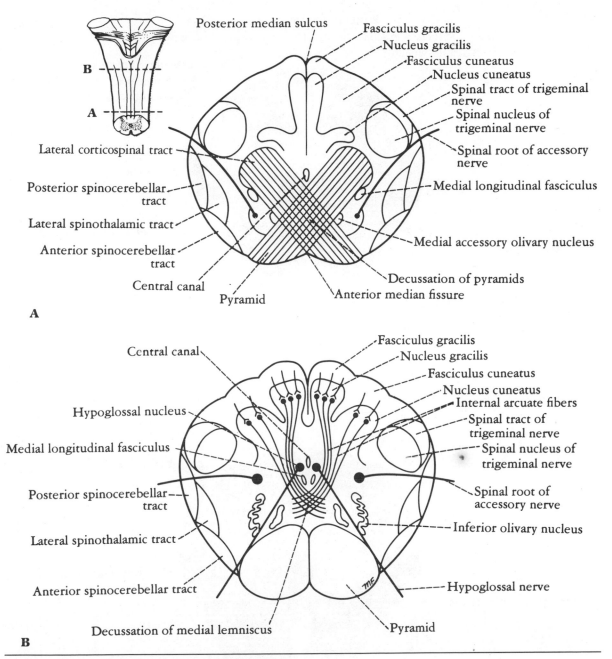

Fig. 8-3. Transverse sections of the medulla oblongata.
A. Level of decussation of the pyramids.
B. Level of decussation of the medial lemnisci.

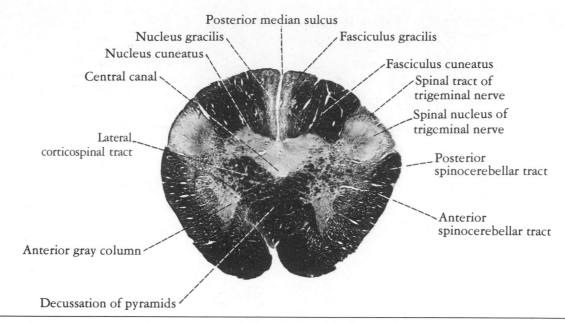

Posterior median sulcus
Nucleus gracilis
Nucleus cuneatus
Central canal
Lateral corticospinal tract
Anterior gray column
Decussation of pyramids

Fasciculus gracilis
Fasciculus cuneatus
Spinal tract of trigeminal nerve
Spinal nucleus of trigeminal nerve
Posterior spinocerebellar tract
Anterior spinocerebellar tract

Fig. 8-4. Transverse section of the medulla oblongata at the level of the decussation of the pyramids. (Weigert stain.)

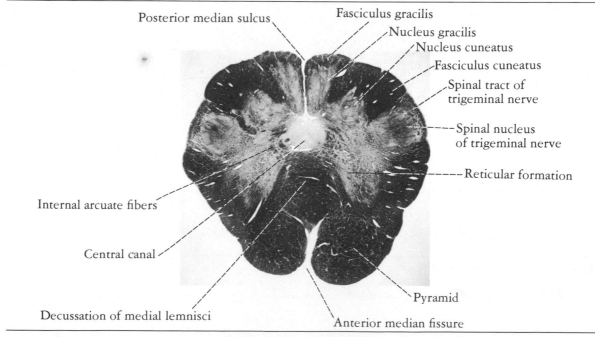

Posterior median sulcus
Internal arcuate fibers
Central canal
Decussation of medial lemnisci

Fasciculus gracilis
Nucleus gracilis
Nucleus cuneatus
Fasciculus cuneatus
Spinal tract of trigeminal nerve
Spinal nucleus of trigeminal nerve
Reticular formation
Pyramid
Anterior median fissure

Fig. 8-5. Transverse section of the medulla oblongata at the level of decussation of the medial lemnisci. (Weigert stain.)

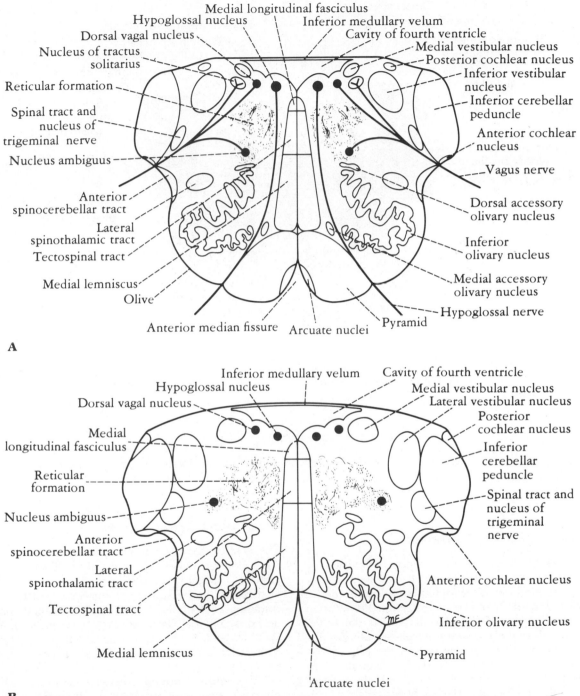

Fig. 8-6. Transverse sections of the medulla oblongata at the level of:
A. Middle of the olivary nuclei.
B. Superior part of the olivary nuclei just inferior to the pons.

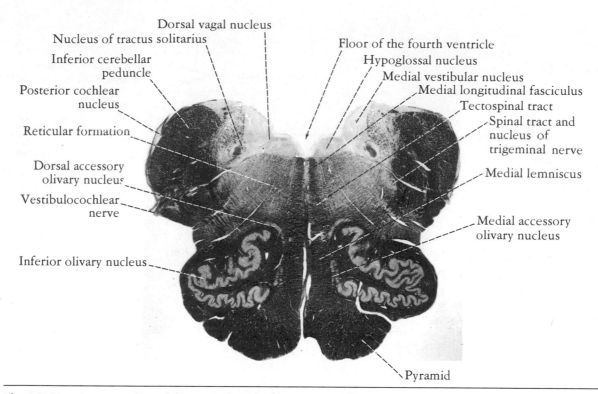

Dorsal vagal nucleus

Nucleus of tractus solitarius

Inferior cerebellar peduncle

Posterior cochlear nucleus

Reticular formation

Dorsal accessory olivary nucleus

Vestibulocochlear nerve

Inferior olivary nucleus

Floor of the fourth ventricle

Hypoglossal nucleus

Medial vestibular nucleus

Medial longitudinal fasciculus

Tectospinal tract

Spinal tract and nucleus of trigeminal nerve

Medial lemniscus

Medial accessory olivary nucleus

Pyramid

Fig. 8-7. Transverse section of the medulla oblongata at the level of the middle of the olivary nuclei. (Weigert stain.)

olivary nuclear complex, the nuclei of the vestibulocochlear, glossopharyngeal, vagus, accessory, and hypoglossal nerves, and the arcuate nuclei.

Olivary Nuclear Complex

The largest nucleus of this complex is the **inferior olivary nucleus** (Figs. 8-6 and 8-7). The gray matter is shaped like a crumpled bag with its mouth directed medially; it is responsible for the elevation on the surface of the medulla called the **olive.** Smaller **dorsal and medial accessory olivary nuclei** also are present. The cells of the inferior olivary nucleus send fibers medially across the midline to enter the cerebellum through the inferior cerebellar peduncle. Afferent fibers reach the inferior olivary nuclei from the spinal cord (the **spino-olivary tracts**) and from the cerebellum

and cerebral cortex. The function of the olivary nuclei is associated with voluntary muscle movement.

Vestibulocochlear Nuclei

The **vestibular nuclear complex** is made up of the following nuclei: (1) **medial vestibular nucleus,** (2) **inferior vestibular nucleus,** (3) **lateral vestibular nucleus,** and (4) **superior vestibular nucleus.** The details of these nuclei and their connections will be discussed later (see p. 436). It should be noted that the medial and inferior vestibular nuclei can be seen on section at this level (Figs. 8-6 and 8-7).

The **cochlear nuclei** are two in number. The **anterior cochlear nucleus** is situated on the anterolateral aspect of the inferior cerebellar peduncle and the **posterior cochlear nucleus** is situated on the posterior aspect of the peduncle lateral to the floor of the fourth ventricle (Figs. 8-6 and 8-7). The connections of these nuclei will be described later (see p. 436).

The Nucleus Ambiguus

The nucleus ambiguus consists of large motor neurons and is situated deep within the reticular formation (Figs. 8-6 and 8-8). The emerging nerve fibers join the glossopharyngeal, vagus, and cranial part of the accessory nerve and are distributed to voluntary skeletal muscle.

Central Gray Matter

The central gray matter lies beneath the floor of the fourth ventricle at this level (Figs. 8-6 and 8-7). Passing from medial to lateral (Fig. 8-8), the following important structures may be recognized: (1) the **hypoglossal nucleus,** (2) the **dorsal nucleus of the vagus,** (3) the **nucleus of the tractus solitarius,** and (4) the **medial and inferior vestibular nuclei** (see above). The nucleus ambiguus, referred to above, has become deeply placed within the reticular formation (Fig. 8-6). The connections and functional significance of these nuclei will be described in Chapter 23.

Fig. 8-8. Position of the cranial nerve nuclei within the brainstem. The hatched area indicates the position of the vestibular nuclei.

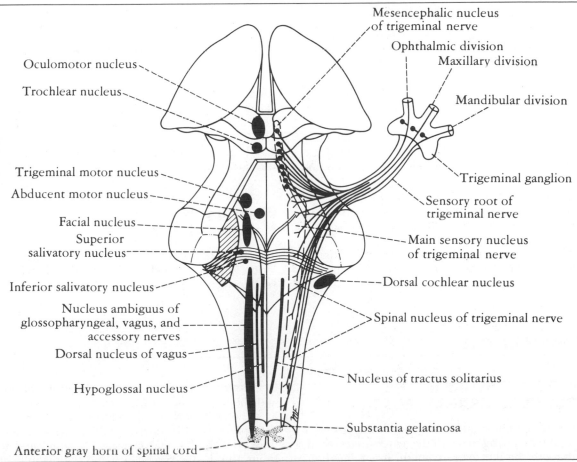

The arcuate nuclei are thought to be inferiorly displaced **pontine nuclei** (see p. 203) and are situated on the anterior surface of the pyramids (see Fig. 8-6). They receive nerve fibers from the cerebral cortex and send efferent fibers to the cerebellum through the **anterior external arcuate fibers.**

The **pyramids** containing the corticospinal and some corticonuclear fibers are situated in the anterior part of the medulla separated by the anterior median fissure (see Figs. 8-6 and 8-7); the corticospinal fibers descend to the spinal cord and the corticonuclear fibers are distributed to the motor nuclei of the cranial nerves situated within the medulla.

The **medial lemniscus** forms a flattened tract on each side of the midline posterior to the pyramid (Figs. 8-6 and 8-7). These fibers emerge from the decussation of the lemnisci and convey sensory information to the thalamus.

The **medial longitudinal fasciculus** forms a small tract of nerve fibers situated on each side of the midline posterior to the medial lemniscus and anterior to the hypoglossal nucleus (Figs. 8-6 and 8-7). It consists of ascending and descending fibers, the connections of which will be described on page 202.

The **inferior cerebellar peduncle** is situated in the posterolateral corner of the section on the lateral side of the fourth ventricle (see Figs. 8-6 and 8-7).

The **spinal tract of the trigeminal nerve and its nucleus** are situated on the anteromedial aspect of the inferior cerebellar peduncle (Figs. 8-6 and 8-7).

The **anterior spinocerebellar tract** is situated near the surface in the interval between the inferior olivary nucleus and the nucleus of the spinal tract of the trigeminal nerve (Figs. 8-6 and 8-7). The **spinal lemniscus,** consisting of the **anterior spinothalamic,** the **lateral spinothalamic and spinotectal tracts** is deeply placed.

The **reticular formation,** consisting of a diffuse mixture of nerve fibers and small groups of nerve cells, is deeply placed posterior to the olivary nucleus (Figs. 8-6 and 8-7). The reticular formation represents, at this level, only a small part of this system, which is also present in the pons and midbrain.

The **glossopharyngeal, vagus,** and **cranial part of the accessory nerves** can be seen running forward and laterally through the reticular formation (Fig. 8-6). The nerve fibers emerge between the olives and the inferior cerebellar peduncles. The **hypoglossal nerves** also run anteriorly and laterally through the reticular formation and emerge between the pyramids and the olives (see Fig. 8-6).

Level of the Medulla Oblongata Just Inferior to the Pons

There are no major changes in the distribution of the gray and white matter (Figs. 8-6 and 8-8). The lateral vestibular nucleus has replaced the inferior vestibular nucleus, and the cochlear nuclei now are visible on the anterior and posterior surfaces of the inferior cerebellar peduncle.

Blood Supply of the Medulla Oblongata

The vertebral, anterior and posterior spinal, posterior inferior cerebellar, and basilar arteries all send branches to the medulla oblongata.

CLINICAL NOTES

RAISED PRESSURE IN THE POSTERIOR CRANIAL FOSSA

The medulla oblongata is situated in the posterior cranial fossa, lying beneath the tentorium cerebelli and above the foramen magnum. It is related anteriorly to the basal portion of the occipital bone and the upper part of the odontoid process of the axis and posteriorly to the cerebellum.

In patients with tumors of the posterior cranial fossa, the intracranial pressure is raised and the brain, that is, the cerebellum and the medulla oblongata, tends to be pushed toward the area of least resistance, and there is a downward herniation of the medulla and cerebellar tonsils through the foramen magnum. This will produce the symptoms of headache, neck stiffness, and paralysis of the glossopharyngeal, vagus, accessory, and hypoglossal nerves owing to traction. In these circumstances it is extremely dangerous to perform a lumbar puncture, because the sudden withdrawal of cerebrospinal fluid may precipitate further herniation of the brain through the foramen magnum and a sudden failure of vital functions resulting from pressure and ischemia of the cranial nerve nuclei present in the medulla oblongata.

ARNOLD-CHIARI PHENOMENON

The **Arnold-Chiari malformation** is a congenital anomaly in which there is a herniation of the tonsils of the cerebellum and the medulla oblongata through the foramen magnum into the vertebral canal. This results in the blockage of the exits in

the roof of the fourth ventricle to the cerebrospinal fluid, causing internal hydrocephalus. It is commonly associated with craniovertebral anomalies or various forms of spina bifida. Signs and symptoms related to pressure on the cerebellum and medulla oblongata and involvement of the last four cranial nerves are associated with this condition.

VASCULAR DISORDERS OF THE MEDULLA OBLONGATA

Lateral Medullary Syndrome of Wallenberg

The lateral part of the medulla oblongata is supplied by the posterior inferior cerebellar artery, which is usually a branch of the vertebral artery. Thrombosis of either of these arteries (Fig. 8-9) produces the following signs and symptoms: dysphagia and dysarthria due to paralysis of the ipsilateral palatal and laryngeal muscles (innervated by the nucleus ambiguus); analgesia and thermo-

Fig. 8-9. Transverse section of the medulla oblongata at the level of the inferior olivary nuclei, showing the extent of the lesion producing the lateral medullary syndrome.

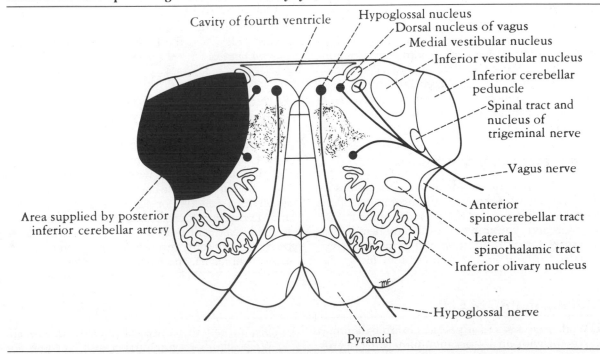

Cavity of fourth ventricle
Hypoglossal nucleus
Dorsal nucleus of vagus
Medial vestibular nucleus
Inferior vestibular nucleus
Inferior cerebellar peduncle
Spinal tract and nucleus of trigeminal nerve
Vagus nerve
Anterior spinocerebellar tract
Lateral spinothalamic tract
Inferior olivary nucleus
Area supplied by posterior inferior cerebellar artery
Hypoglossal nerve
Pyramid

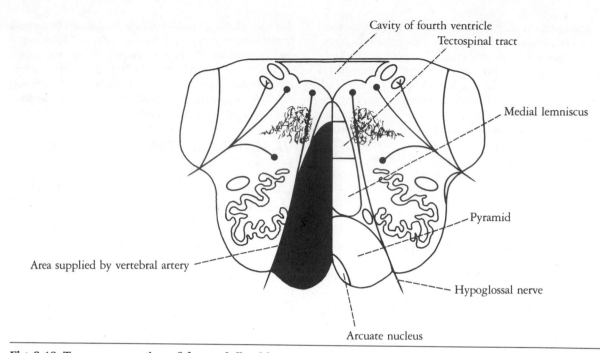

Fig. 8-10. Transverse section of the medulla oblongata at the level of the inferior olivary nuclei, showing the extent of the lesion producing the medial medullary syndrome.

anesthesia on the ipsilateral side of the face (nucleus and spinal tract of the trigeminal nerve); vertigo, nausea, vomiting, and nystagmus (vestibular nuclei); ipsilateral Horner's syndrome (descending sympathetic fibers); ipsilateral cerebellar signs—gait and limb ataxia (cerebellum or inferior cerebellar peduncle); and contralateral loss of sensations of pain and temperature (spinal lemniscus—spinothalamic tract).

Medial Medullary Syndrome

The medial part of the medulla oblongata is supplied by the vertebral artery. Thrombosis of the medullary branch (Fig. 8-10) produces the following signs and symptoms: contralateral hemiparesis (pyramidal tract); contralateral impaired sensations of position and movement and tactile dis-

crimination (medial lemniscus); and ipsilateral paralysis of tongue muscles with deviation to paralyzed side when the tongue is protruded (hypoglossal nerve).

FUNCTIONAL SIGNIFICANCE OF THE MEDULLA OBLONGATA

It is important to remember that the medulla oblongata not only contains many cranial nerve nuclei that are concerned with vital functions (e.g., regulation of heart rate and respiration), but it also serves as a conduit for the passage of ascending and descending tracts connecting the spinal cord to the higher centers of the nervous system. These tracts may become involved in demyelinating diseases, neoplasms, and vascular disorders.

CLINICAL PROBLEMS

Answers on Page 597

1. While carrying out a physical examination of a patient with an intracranial tumor, the neurol-

ogist turned to a medical student and asked, "What signs or symptoms would you look for that would enable you to localize the tumor to the region of the medulla oblongata?" How would you have answered that question?

2. A 6-month-old boy died with hydrocephalus and a myelocele in the lower thoracic region. At autopsy the hindbrain was found to be deformed. The lower part of the medulla oblongata extended inferiorly through the foramen magnum into the vertebral canal as far as the third cervical vertebra. The lower four cranial nerves were longer than normal and the upper cervical nerve roots ascended to reach their exit from the vertebral canal. The cerebellum on the left side extended inferiorly through the foramen magnum to the third cervical vertebra, where it was adherent to the spinal cord. The roof of the fourth ventricle was abnormally low. (a) What is the name of this malformation? (b) Is hydrocephalus common in this condition? (c) Is there a possible association between the thoracic myelocele and the presence of part of the hindbrain in the vertebral canal?

3. A 68-year-old man was admitted to the hospital with the sudden onset of severe dizziness (vertigo), hiccups, and vomiting. He also complained of a hot, painful sensation in the skin of the right side of the face. On physical examination the soft palate was drawn up to the left side when the patient was asked to say "ah," and there was lack of mobility of the right vocal cord as seen on laryngoscopic examination. The patient also showed drooping of the right upper eyelid (ptosis), sunken right eye (enophthalmos), and a constricted right pupil (myosis). When asked to protrude his tongue straight out of his mouth, the patient tried to do so but the tip of the tongue pointed to the right side. There was evidence of impairment of pain and temperature sensation in the trunk and extremities on the left side. Using your knowledge of anatomy, make the diagnosis.

4. The pathologist, while exploring the posterior cranial fossa during an autopsy, was endeavoring to determine where the ninth, tenth, and cranial part of the eleventh cranial nerves emerged from the hindbrain. Can you answer that question?

NATIONAL BOARD TYPE QUESTIONS

Answers on Page 620

IN EACH OF THE FOLLOWING QUESTIONS, ANSWER:
   (a) IF (1) ONLY IS CORRECT
   (b) IF (2) ONLY IS CORRECT
   (c) IF BOTH (1) AND (2) ARE CORRECT, AND
   (d) IF NEITHER (1) NOR (2) IS CORRECT

1. Concerning the anterior surface of the medulla oblongata, which of the following statements is (are) correct?
   (1) On each side of the midline there is an ovoid swelling called the olive, which contains the corticospinal fibers.
   (2) The pyramids taper inferiorly and give rise to the decussation of the pyramids.

2. Concerning the emergence of the cranial nerves from the medulla oblongata, which of the following statements is (are) correct?
   (1) The hypoglossal nerve emerges between the pyramid and the olive.
   (2) The vagus nerve emerges between the olive and the inferior cerebellar peduncle.

3. Concerning the posterior surface of the medulla oblongata, which of the following statements is (are) correct?
   (1) On each side of the median sulcus there is an elongated swelling, the gracile tubercle, produced by the underlying gracile nucleus.
   (2) The superior half forms the entire floor of the fourth ventricle.

Select the best response:

4. The following statements concerning the interior of the lower part of the medulla are true **except**:
   (a) The decussation of the pyramids represents the crossing over from one side of the medulla to the other of three-quarters of the corticospinal fibers.
   (b) The central canal of the spinal cord continues upward into the medulla.

(c) The substantia gelatinosa becomes continuous with the nucleus of the spinal tract of the trigeminal nerve.

(d) The medial lemniscus is formed by the anterior spinothalamic tract and the spinotectal tract.

(e) The internal arcuate fibers emerge from the nucleus gracilis and nucleus cuneatus.

5. The following statements concerning the interior of the upper part of the medulla are true **except**:

(a) The reticular formation consists of a mixture of nerve fibers and small groups of nerve cells.

(b) The nucleus ambiguus constitutes the motor nucleus of the vagus, cranial part of the accessory, and hypoglossal nerves.

(c) Beneath the floor of the fourth ventricle are located the dorsal nucleus of the vagus and the vestibular nuclei.

(d) The medial longitudinal fasciculus is a bundle of ascending and descending fibers that lie posterior to the medial lemniscus on each side of the midline.

(e) The inferior cerebellar peduncle connects the medulla to the cerebellum.

In the following questions, answer:

(a) IF (1), (2), AND (3) ONLY ARE CORRECT

(b) IF (1) AND (3) ONLY ARE CORRECT

(c) IF (2) AND (4) ONLY ARE CORRECT

(d) IF (4) ONLY IS CORRECT, OR

(e) IF ALL ARE CORRECT

6. Which of the following statements is (are) correct concerning the Arnold-Chiari phenomenon?

(1) It is a congenital anomaly.

(2) The exits in the roof of the fourth ventricle are blocked.

(3) It is commonly associated with various forms of spina bifida.

(4) The cerebellum never herniates through the foramen magnum.

7. Which of the following statements is (are) correct concerning the medial medullary syndrome?

(1) The tongue is paralyzed on the contralateral side.

Fig. 8-11.

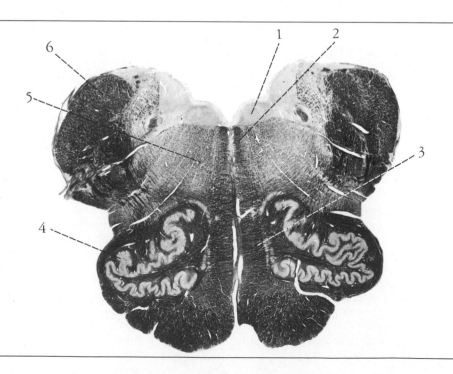

(2) There is contralateral hemiparesis.

(3) There are ipsilateral impaired sensations of position and movement.

(4) It is commonly caused by thrombosis of a branch of the vertebral artery to the medulla oblongata.

8. Which of the following statements is (are) correct concerning the lateral medullary syndrome?

(1) The condition may be caused by a thrombosis of the posterior inferior cerebellar artery.

(2) The nucleus ambiguus of the same side may be damaged.

(3) There may be analgesia and thermoanesthesia on the ipsilateral side of the face.

(4) There may be nausea and vomiting.

In Figure 8-11, match the numbers listed on the left with the appropriate structure listed on the right.

9. Number 1   (a) Inferior cerebellar
10. Number 2   peduncle
11. Number 3   (b) Medial lemniscus
12. Number 4   (c) Hypoglossal
13. Number 5   nucleus
14. Number 6   (d) Reticular formation
                 (e) None of the above

Match the structures listed below on the left that are located within the brainstem with the appropriate levels listed below on the right. Each answer may be used more than once.

15. Decussation of pyramids

16. Lower part of fourth ventricle

17. Decussation of medial lemnisci

18. Nucleus gracilis

19. Central canal

20. Facial colliculus

(a) Rostral half of medulla oblongata

(b) Caudal half of medulla oblongata

(c) None of the above

ADDITIONAL READING

Crosby, E. C., Humphrey, T., and Lauer, E. W. *Correlative Anatomy of the Nervous System.* New York: Macmillan, 1962.

Patten, J. P. *Neurological Differential Diagnosis.* London: Harold Stark, 1980.

Rowland, L. P. (Ed.). *Merritt's Textbook of Neurology* (7th ed.). Philadelphia: Lea & Febiger, 1984.

Walton, J. N. *Brain's Diseases of the Nervous System* (8th ed.). New York and London: Oxford University Press, 1977.

Chapter 9
The Pons

GROSS APPEARANCE

The pons is anterior to the cerebellum (Fig. 9-1) and connects the medulla oblongata to the midbrain. It is about 1 inch (2.5 cm) long and owes its name to the appearance presented on the anterior surface, which is that of a bridge connecting the right and left cerebellar hemispheres.

The anterior surface is convex from side to side and shows many transverse fibers that converge on each side to form the **middle cerebellar peduncle** (Fig. 9-1). There is a shallow groove in the midline, the **basilar groove,** which lodges the basilar artery. On the anterolateral surface of the pons the **trigeminal nerve** emerges on each side. Each nerve consists of a smaller, medial part—the **motor root**—and a larger, lateral part—the **sensory root.** In the groove between the pons and the medulla oblongata there emerge, from medial to lateral, the **abducent, facial,** and **vestibulocochlear nerves** (Fig. 9-1).

The posterior surface of the pons is hidden from view by the cerebellum (Fig. 9-2). It forms the upper half of the floor of the fourth ventricle and is triangular in shape. The posterior surface is limited laterally by the **superior cerebellar peduncles** and is divided into symmetrical halves by a **median sulcus.** Lateral to this sulcus is an elongated elevation, the **medial eminence,** which is bounded laterally by a sulcus, the **sulcus limitans** (Fig. 9-2). The inferior end of the medial eminence is slightly expanded to form the **facial colliculus,** which is produced by the root of the facial nerve winding around the nucleus of the abducent nerve (Fig. 9-3). The floor of the superior part of the **sulcus limitans** is bluish-gray in color and is called the **substantia ferruginea;** it owes its color to a group of deeply pigmented nerve cells. Lateral to the sulcus limitans is the **area vestibuli** produced by the underlying vestibular nuclei (Fig. 9-2).

INTERNAL STRUCTURE OF THE PONS

For purposes of description, the pons is commonly divided into a posterior part, the **tegmentum,** and

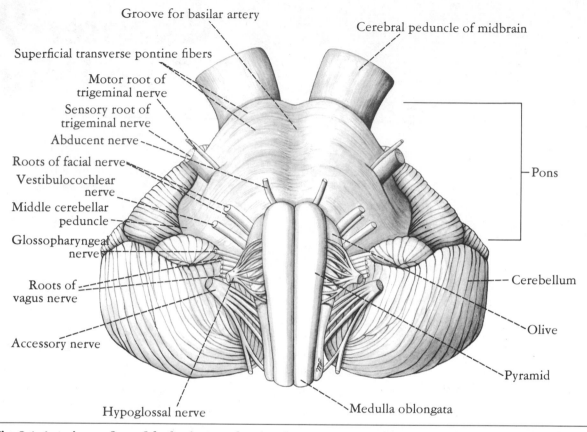

Fig. 9-1. Anterior surface of the brainstem showing the pons.

an anterior **basal part** by the transversely running fibers of the **trapezoid body** (Fig. 9-3).

The structure of the pons may be studied at two levels: (1) transverse section through the caudal part, passing through the facial colliculus, and (2) transverse section through the cranial part, passing through the trigeminal nuclei.

Transverse Section through the Caudal Part of the Pons

The **medial lemniscus** rotates as it passes from the medulla into the pons. It is situated in the most anterior part of the tegmentum with its long axis running transversely (Fig. 9-3).

The **facial nucleus** lies posterior to the lateral part of the medial lemniscus. The fibers of the facial nerve wind round the **nucleus of the abdu-**

cent nerve, producing the **facial colliculus** (Fig. 9-3). The fibers of the facial nerve then pass anteriorly between the facial nucleus and the superior end of the nucleus of the spinal tract of the trigeminal nerve.

The **medial longitudinal fasciculus** is situated beneath the floor of the fourth ventricle on either side of the midline (Fig. 9-3). The medial longitudinal fasciculus is the main pathway that connects the vestibular and cochlear nuclei with the nuclei controlling the extraocular muscles (oculomotor, trochlear, and abducent nuclei).

The **medial vestibular nucleus** is situated lateral to the abducent nucleus (Fig. 9-3) and is in close relationship to the inferior cerebellar peduncle. The superior part of the lateral and the inferior part of the superior vestibular nucleus are found at this level. The **posterior and anterior cochlear nuclei** are also found at this level (p. 440).

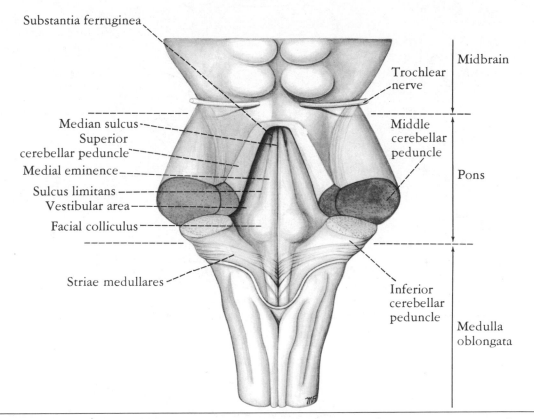

Substantia ferruginea

Trochlear nerve

Midbrain

Median sulcus
Superior cerebellar peduncle
Medial eminence
Sulcus limitans
Vestibular area
Facial colliculus

Middle cerebellar peduncle

Pons

Striae medullares

Inferior cerebellar peduncle

Medulla oblongata

Fig. 9-2. Posterior surface of the brainstem showing the pons. The cerebellum has been removed.

The **spinal nucleus of the trigeminal nerve and its tract** lie on the anteromedial aspect of the inferior cerebellar peduncle (Fig. 9-3).

The **trapezoid body** is made up of fibers derived from the cochlear nuclei and the nuclei of the trapezoid body. They run transversely (Fig. 9-3) in the anterior part of the tegmentum (p. 440).

The basilar part of the pons, at this level, contains small masses of nerve cells called **pontine nuclei** (Fig. 9-3). The **corticopontine fibers** of the crus cerebri of the midbrain terminate in the pontine nuclei. The axons of these cells give origin to the **transverse fibers** of the pons, which cross the midline and intersect the corticospinal and corticonuclear tracts, breaking them up into small bundles. The transverse fibers of the pons enter the middle cerebellar peduncle and are distributed to the cerebellar hemisphere. This connection forms the main pathway linking the cerebral cortex to the cerebellum.

Transverse Section through the Cranial Part of the Pons

The internal structure of the pons is similar to that seen at the caudal level (Figs. 9-4 through 9-6), but it now contains the motor and principal sensory nuclei of the trigeminal nerve.

The **motor nucleus of the trigeminal nerve** is situated beneath the lateral part of the fourth ventricle within the reticular formation (Figs. 9-4 and 9-5). The emerging motor fibers travel anteriorly through the substance of the pons and exit on its anterior surface.

The **principal sensory nucleus of the trigeminal nerve** is situated on the lateral side of the motor nucleus (Figs. 9-4 and 9-5); it is continuous inferiorly with the nucleus of the spinal tract. The entering sensory fibers travel through the substance of the pons and lie lateral to the motor fibers (Fig. 9-4).

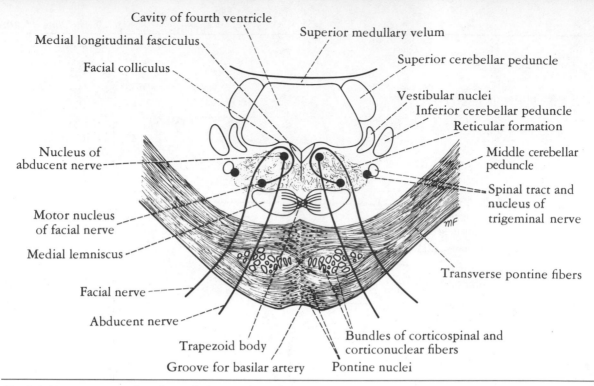

Fig. 9-3. Transverse section through the caudal part of the pons at the level of the facial colliculus.

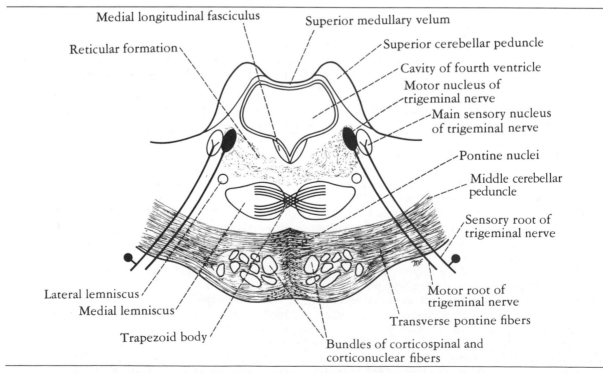

Fig. 9-4. Transverse section through the pons at the level of the trigeminal nuclei.

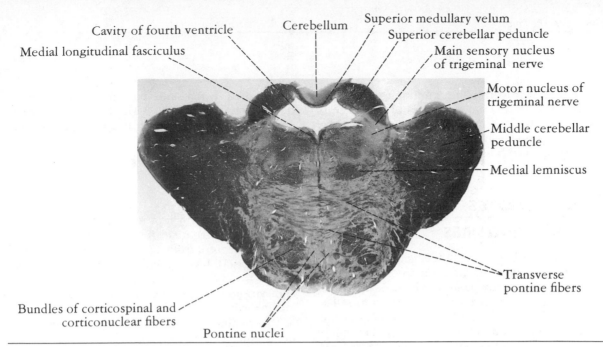

Fig. 9-5. Photomicrograph of transverse section of the pons at the level of the trigeminal nuclei.

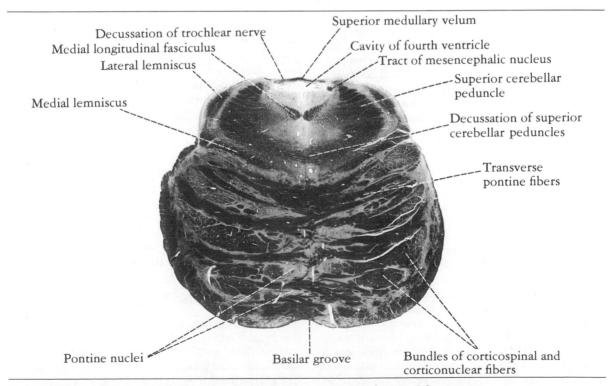

Fig. 9-6. Photomicrograph of transverse section of the most rostral part of the pons.

The **superior cerebellar peduncle** is situated posterolateral to the motor nucleus of the trigeminal nerve (Figs. 9-4 and 9-5). It is joined by the **anterior spinocerebellar tract.**

The **trapezoid body** and the **medial lemniscus** are situated in the same position as they were in the previous section (Fig. 9-4). The **lateral lemniscus** lies at the lateral extremity of the medial lemniscus (Figs. 9-4 and 9-6).

CLINICAL NOTES

GENERAL FEATURES

The pons, like the medulla oblongata and the cerebellum, is situated in the posterior cranial fossa lying beneath the tentorium cerebelli. It is related anteriorly to the basilar artery, the dorsum sellae of the sphenoid bone, and the basilar part of the occipital bone. In addition to forming the upper half of the floor of the fourth ventricle, it possesses several important cranial nerve nuclei (trigeminal, abducent, facial, and vestibulocochlear) and serves as a conduit for important ascending and descending tracts (corticonuclear, corticopontine, corticospinal, medial longitudinal fasciculus, and medial and lateral lemnisci). It is not surprising, therefore, that tumors, hemorrhage, or infarcts in this area of the brain produce a variety of symptoms and signs. For example, involvement of the corticopontocerebellar tracts will produce marked cerebellar ataxia, and voluntary movements are accompanied by a rhythmic tremor that develops and becomes further accentuated as the movements proceed (intention tumor).

Tumors of the Pons

Astrocytoma of the pons occurring in childhood (Walton, 1977) is the most common tumor of the brainstem. The symptoms and signs are those of ipsilateral cranial nerve paralysis and contralateral hemiparesis: weakness of the facial muscles on the same side (facial nerve nucleus); weakness of the lateral rectus muscle on one or both sides (abducent nerve nucleus); nystagmus (vestibular nucleus); weakness of the jaw muscles (trigeminal nerve nucleus); impairment of hearing (cochlear nuclei); contralateral hemiparesis; quadriparesis (corticospinal fibers); anesthesia to light touch with the preservation of appreciation of pain over the skin of the face (principal sensory nucleus of trigeminal nerve involved, leaving spinal nucleus and tract of trigeminal intact); and contralateral sensory defects of trunk and limbs (medial and lateral lemnisci). Involvement of the corticopontocerebellar tracts may cause ipsilateral cerebellar signs and symptoms. There may be impairment of conjugate deviation of the eyeballs due to involvement of the medial longitudinal fasciculus, which connects the oculomotor, trochlear, and abducent nerve nuclei.

Pontine Hemorrhage

The pons is supplied by the basilar artery and the anterior, inferior, and superior cerebellar arteries. If the hemorrhage occurs from one of those arteries and is unilateral, there will be facial paralysis on the side of the lesion (involvement of the facial nerve nucleus and, therefore, a lower motor neuron palsy) and paralysis of the limbs on the opposite side (involvement of the corticospinal fibers as they pass through the pons). There is often paralysis of conjugate ocular deviation (involvement of the abducent nerve nucleus and the medial longitudinal fasciculus).

When the hemorrhage is extensive and bilateral the pupils may be "pinpoint" (involvement of the ocular sympathetic fibers); there is commonly bilateral paralysis of the face and the limbs. The patient may become poikilothermic because severe damage to the pons has cut off the body from the heat-regulating centers in the hypothalamus.

Infarctions of the Pons

Usually this is due to thrombosis or embolism of the basilar artery or its branches. If it involves the paramedian area of the pons the corticospinal tracts, the pontine nuclei, and the fibers passing to the cerebellum through the middle cerebellar peduncle may be damaged. A laterally situated infarct will involve the trigeminal nerve, the medial lemniscus, and the middle cerebellar peduncle; the corticospinal fibers to the lower limbs also may be affected.

The clinical conditions mentioned above will be understood more clearly after you have studied the ascending and descending tracts of the brain and spinal cord (see Chapters 20 and 21).

CLINICAL PROBLEMS

Answers on Page 598

1. A 10-year-old girl was taken to a physician because her mother had noticed that the right half of her face was weak and did not appear to react to emotional changes. It was noted also that her mouth was pulled over slightly to the left, especially when she was tired. On questioning, the patient admitted that food tended to stick inside her right cheek and that the right side of her face "felt funny." The mother had first noticed the facial changes three months previously and the condition had progressively worsened. On examination, there was definite weakness of the facial muscles on the right side; the facial muscles on the left side were normal. Skin sensation on stimulation of the face was normal. On testing of the ocular movements there was evidence of slight weakness of the lateral rectus muscle on the right side. Examination of the movements of the arm and leg showed slight weakness on the left side. Using your knowledge of neuroanatomy, relate these symptoms and signs to a lesion in the pons.
2. A 65-year-old man was admitted to the emergency room with a diagnosis of a severe pontine hemorrhage. On examination, he was found to have bilateral "pinpoint" pupils and quadriplegia. How can you explain the presence of the "pinpoint" pupils?
3. A 46-year-old man visited his physician with symptoms of deafness, vertigo, and double vision (diploplia). On questioning, he said that he also suffered from severe headaches, which were increasing in frequency and severity. The week before he vomited several times during one of the headache attacks. On examination, he was found to have a slight right internal strabismus and there were a flattening of the skin furrows on the right side of his forehead and a slight drooping of the right corner of his mouth. There was definite evidence of impairment of hearing on the right side. On testing for sensory loss, there was definite sensory impairment on the right side of the face in the areas supplied by the maxillary and mandibular divisions of the trigeminal nerve. Using your knowledge of anatomy, explain the symptoms and signs.

NATIONAL BOARD TYPE QUESTIONS

Answers on Page 620

In each of the following questions, answer:
   (a) If (1) only is correct.
   (b) If (2) only is correct.
   (c) If both (1) and (2) are correct, and
   (d) If neither (1) nor (2) is correct.

1. Which of the following statements is (are) correct concerning the anterior surface of the pons?
   (1) The trigeminal nerve emerges on each side as two parts, the larger medial motor part and the smaller lateral sensory part.
   (2) In the groove between the pons and the medulla oblongata there emerge, from medial to lateral, the abducent, the vestibulocochlear, and the facial nerves.

2. Which of the following statements is (are) correct concerning the posterior surface of the pons?
   (1) It forms the upper half of the floor of the fourth ventricle.
   (2) It is limited laterally by the superior cerebellar peduncles.

Select the best response:
3. The following statements concerning the posterior surface of the pons are correct **except**:
   (a) Lateral to the median sulcus is an elongated swelling called the medial eminence.
   (b) The facial colliculus is produced by the root

of the abducent nerve winding around the nucleus of the facial nerve.

(c) The floor of the superior part of the sulcus limitans is pigmented and is called the substantia ferruginea.

(d) The vestibular area lies lateral to the sulcus limitans.

(e) The cerebellum lies posterior to the pons.

4. The following statements concerning a transverse section through the caudal part of the pons are correct **except**:

(a) The medial longitudinal fasciculus lies beneath the floor of the fourth ventricle on either side of the midline.

(b) The vestibular nuclei lie lateral to the abducent nucleus.

(c) The trapezoid body is made up of fibers derived from the facial nerve nuclei.

(d) The tegmentum is the part of the pons lying posterior to the trapezoid body.

(e) In the midline anteriorly there is a groove for the basilar artery.

In the following questions, answer:

(a) IF (1), (2), AND (3) ONLY ARE CORRECT

(b) IF (1) AND (3) ONLY ARE CORRECT

(c) IF (2) AND (4) ONLY ARE CORRECT

(d) IF (4) ONLY IS CORRECT, OR

(e) IF ALL ARE CORRECT

5. Which of the following statements concerning a transverse section through the rostral part of the pons is (are) correct?

(1) The motor nucleus of the trigeminal nerve lies medial to the main sensory nucleus in the tegmentum.

(2) The medial lemniscus has rotated so that it lies lateral to the lateral lemniscus.

(3) Bundles of corticospinal fibers lie in among the transverse pontine fibers.

(4) The medial longitudinal fasciculus joins the

Fig. 9-7.

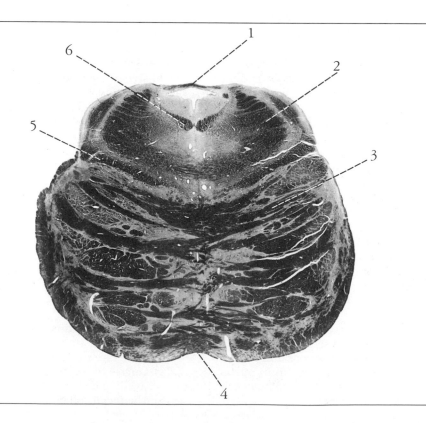

thalamus to the spinal nucleus of the trigeminal nerve.

6. Which of the following statements concerning the pons is (are) correct?
   (1) It is related anteriorly to the dorsum sellae of the sphenoid bone.
   (2) It lies in the posterior cranial fossa.
   (3) The corticopontine fibers terminate in the pontine nuclei.
   (4) Glial tumors of the pons are rare.

In Figure 9-7, match the numbers listed on the left with the appropriate structures listed on the right.

7. Number 1   (a) Basilar groove
8. Number 2   (b) Medial longitudinal
9. Number 3   fasciculus
10. Number 4   (c) Superior cerebellar
11. Number 5   peduncle
12. Number 6   (d) Superior medullary
                               velum
                           (e) None of the above

Match the structures listed below on the left that are located within the brainstem with the appropriate level listed below on the right. Answers may be used more than once.

13. Red nucleus   (a) Rostral part of
                               pons
14. Facial colliculus   (b) Caudal part of
                               pons
15. Abducent nucleus   (c) None of the above
16. Spinal tract of the
    trigeminal nerve
17. Motor nucleus of
    trigeminal nerve

ADDITIONAL READING

Crosby, E. C., Humphrey, T., and Lauer, E. W. *Correlative Anatomy of the Nervous System.* New York: Macmillan, 1962.

Rowland, L. P. (ed.). *Merritt's Textbook of Neurology* (7th ed.). Philadelphia: Lea & Febiger, 1984.

Walton, J. N. *Brain's Diseases of the Nervous System* (8th ed.). New York and London: Oxford University Press, 1977.

Williams, P. L., Warwick, R., Dyson M., and Bannister, L. H. *Gray's Anatomy* (37th Brit. ed.). Philadelphia: Saunders, 1989.

Chapter 10
The Structure
of the Cerebellum

This chapter considers the structure of the cerebellum. This important part of the central nervous system unconsciously controls the smooth contraction of voluntary muscles and carefully coordinates their actions, together with the relaxation of their antagonists. Each cerebellar hemisphere controls the muscles on the same side of the body. In Chapter 22 the precise neuronal connections of the cerebellum will be described; it will become apparent how the cerebellum exerts its influence over skeletal muscle, in both postural and voluntary movements.

GROSS APPEARANCE

The cerebellum, the largest part of the hindbrain, lies posterior to the pons and the medulla oblongata (Fig. 10-1). It is somewhat ovoid in shape and constricted in its median part. It is situated in the posteral cranial fossa and is covered superiorly by the tentorium cerebelli. The cerebellum consists of two **cerebellar hemispheres** joined by a narrow median **vermis.**

In this description, the cerebellum is divided into three main lobes: the **anterior lobe,** the **middle lobe,** and the **flocculonodular lobe.** The **anterior lobe** may be seen on the superior surface of the cerebellum and is separated from the middle lobe by a wide V-shaped fissure called the **primary fissure** (Figs. 10-2 and 10-3). The **middle lobe** (sometimes called the posterior lobe), which is the largest part of the cerebellum, is situated between the primary and **uvulonodular fissures.** The **flocculonodular lobe** is situated posterior to the uvulonodular fissure (Fig. 10-3). A deep **horizontal fissure** that is found along the margin of the cerebellum separates the superior from the inferior surfaces; it is of no morphological or functional significance (Figs. 10-2 and 10-3).

The anterior lobe, uvula, and pyramid of the vermis (Fig. 10-3) constitute the **paleocerebellum,** which is functionally related to the gross movements of the head and body. The middle lobe (except for the uvula and pyramid) constitutes the **neocerebellum** and is associated with fine voluntary movements (Fig. 10-3). The flocculonodular

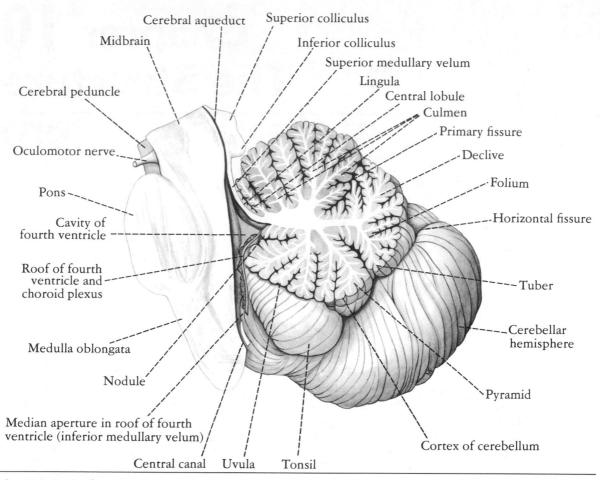

Fig. 10-1. Sagittal section through the brainstem and the cerebellum.

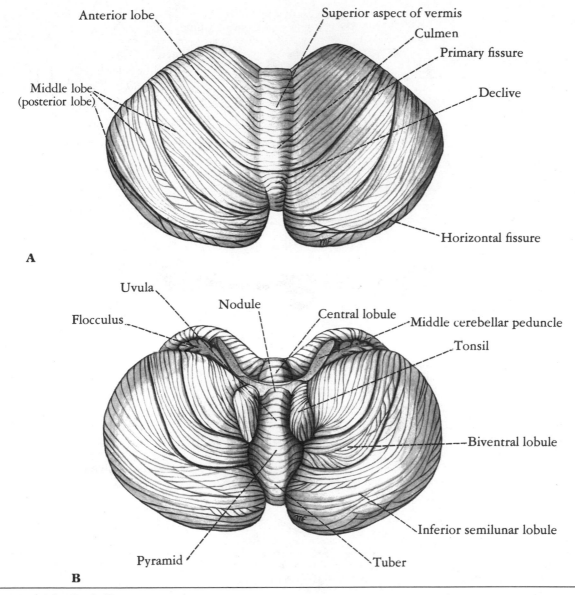

Fig. 10-2. The cerebellum.
A. Superior view.
B. Inferior view.

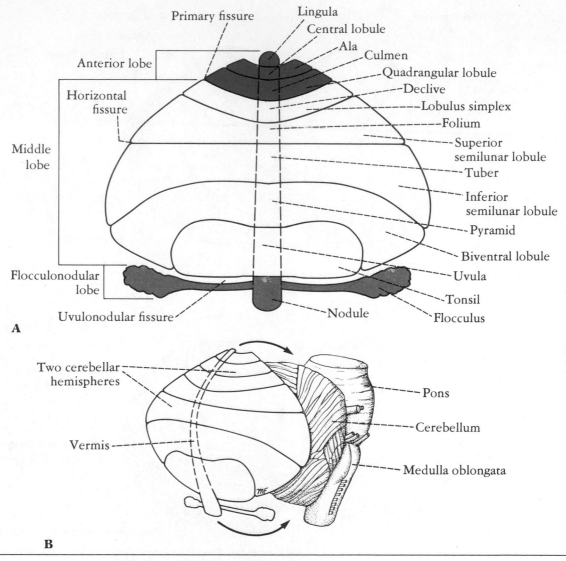

**Fig. 10-3. A. Main cerebellar lobes, lobules, and fissures.
B. Relationship between the diagram in A and the cerebellum.**

lobe is phylogenetically the oldest portion of the cerebellum and constitutes the **archicerebellum,** which is associated with the vestibular system (Fig. 10-3).

The superior surface of the cerebellum shows the superior aspect of the vermis as a ridge that is not separated from the hemispheres by grooves or fissures (Fig. 10-2). The primary fissure, noted above, is visible on this surface.

The inferior surface of the cerebellum shows a deep groove, the **vallecula,** the floor of which is formed by the inferior aspect of the vermis (Fig. 10-2).

The **cortex** of the cerebellum is much folded, the folds or **folia** being separated by numerous transverse fissures. Each folium has a core of white matter and an outer covering of gray matter (Fig. 10-1). A section made through the cerebellum parallel with the median plane divides the folia at right angles, and the cut surface has a branched appearance, called the **arbor vitae** (Fig. 10-1).

INTERNAL STRUCTURE OF THE CEREBELLUM

The internal structure of the cerebellum is made up of gray matter and white matter. The gray matter is found mainly covering the surface of the cerebellum as **cortex;** small aggregations of gray matter are also found in the interior of the cerebellum.

GRAY MATTER OF THE CEREBELLUM

Cerebellar Cortex

The cortex of the cerebellum is folded by many parallel transverse fissures into the cerebellar folia (see Fig. 10-1). Each folium contains a core of white matter covered superficially by gray matter (Fig. 10-4). The cerebellar cortex throughout its extent has a uniform structure. The cortex may be divided into three layers: (1) an external layer, the **molecular layer;** (2) a middle layer, the **Purkinje cell layer;** and (3) an internal layer, the **granular layer** (Figs. 10-4 and 10-5).

The Molecular Layer

The molecular layer contains two types of neurons: the outer **stellate cell** and the inner **basket cell** (Fig. 10-4). These neurons are scattered among dendritic arborizations and numerous thin axons that run parallel to the long axis of the folia. Neuroglial cells are found between these structures.

Purkinje Cell Layer

The Purkinje cells are large Golgi type I neurons. They are flask-shaped and are arranged in a single layer (Figs. 10-4 and 10-5). In a plane transverse to the folium, the dendrites of these cells are seen to pass into the molecular layer, where they undergo profuse branching (Figs. 10-4 and 10-5). The primary and secondary branches are smooth and subsequent branches are covered by short, thick **dendritic spines.** It has been shown that the spines form synaptic contacts with the parallel fibers derived from the granule cell axons.

At the base of the Purkinje cell, the axon arises and passes through the granular layer to enter the white matter. On entering the white matter, the axon acquires a myelin sheath and it terminates by synapsing with cells of one of the intracerebellar nuclei. Collateral branches of the Purkinje axon make synaptic contacts with the dendrites of basket and stellate cells of the granular layer in the same area or in distant folia. A few of the Purkinje cell axons pass directly to end in the vestibular nuclei of the brainstem.

Granular Layer

The granular layer is packed with small cells with densely staining nuclei and scanty cytoplasm (Figs. 10-4 and 10-5). Each cell gives rise to four or five dendrites, which make clawlike endings and have synaptic contact with mossy fiber input (see p. 406). The axon of each granule cell passes into the molecular layer, where it bifurcates at a T junction, the branches running parallel to the long axis of the cerebellar folium (Fig. 10-4). These fibers, known as **parallel fibers,** run at right angles to the dendritic processes of the Purkinje cells. Most of the parallel fibers make synaptic contacts with the spinous processes of the dendrites of the Purkinje

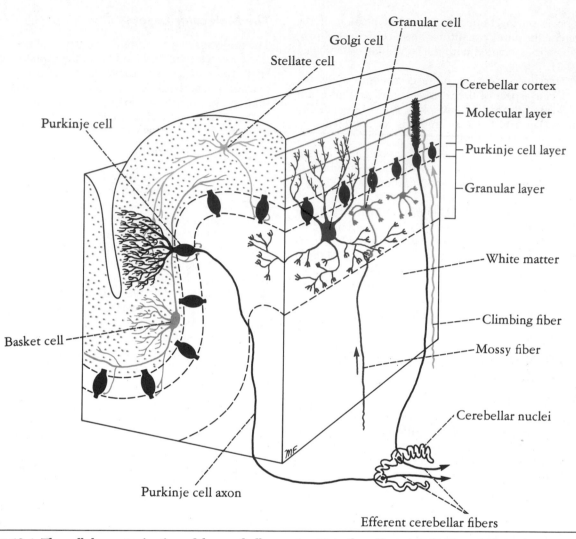

Fig. 10-4. The cellular organization of the cerebellar cortex. Note the afferent and efferent fibers.

cells. Neuroglial cells are found throughout this layer. Scattered throughout the granular layer are Golgi cells (Fig. 10-4). Their dendrites ramify in the molecular layer and their axons terminate by splitting up into branches that synapse with the dendrites of the granular cells (Fig. 10-5).

INTRACEREBELLAR NUCLEI

Four masses of gray matter are embedded in the white matter of the cerebellum on each side of the midline (Fig. 10-6). From lateral to medial these nuclei are the **dentate,** the **emboliform,** the **globose,** and the **fastigial.**

The **dentate nucleus,** the largest of the cerebellar nuclei, is situated in the white matter of each cerebellar hemisphere (Fig. 10-6). It has the shape of a crumpled bag with the opening facing medially (Fig. 10-6). The interior of the bag is filled with white matter made up of efferent fibers that leave the nucleus through the opening to form a large part of the superior cerebellar peduncle.

Molecular layer

Purkinje cell

Granular layer

Fig. 10-5. Photomicrograph of a cross section of a cerebellar folium, showing the three layers of the cerebellar cortex.

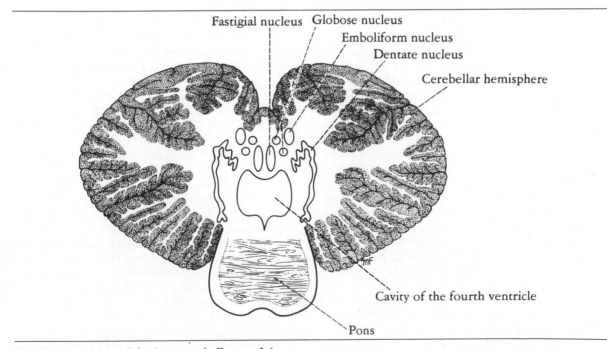

Fastigial nucleus Globose nucleus

Emboliform nucleus

Dentate nucleus

Cerebellar hemisphere

Cavity of the fourth ventricle

Pons

Fig. 10-6. Position of the intracerebellar nuclei.

The **emboliform nucleus** is ovoid and is situated medial to the dentate nucleus, partially covering its hilus (Fig. 10-6).

The **globose nucleus** consists of one or more rounded cell groups that lie medial to the emboliform nucleus (Fig. 10-6).

The **fastigial nucleus** lies near the midline in the vermis and close to the roof of the fourth ventricle; it is larger than the globose nucleus (Fig. 10-6).

The intracerebellar nuclei are composed of large, multipolar neurons with simple branching dendrites. The axons form the cerebellar outflow in the superior and inferior cerebellar peduncles.

WHITE MATTER OF THE CEREBELLUM

There is a small amount of white matter in the vermis and it closely resembles the trunk and branches of a tree—the **arbor vitae** (Fig. 10-1). There is a large amount of white matter in each cerebellar hemisphere.

The white matter is made up of three groups of fibers: (1) intrinsic, (2) afferent, and (3) efferent.

The **intrinsic fibers** do not leave the cerebellum but connect up different regions of the organ. Some interconnect folia of the cerebellar cortex and vermis on the same side; others connect the two cerebellar hemispheres together.

The **afferent fibers** form the greater part of the white matter and proceed to the cerebellar cortex. They enter the cerebellum mainly through the inferior and middle cerebellar peduncles.

The **efferent fibers** constitute the output of the cerebellum and commence as the axons of the Purkinje cells of the cerebellar cortex. The great majority of the Purkinje cell axons pass to and synapse with the neurons of the cerebellar nuclei (fastigial, globose, emboliform, and dentate). The axons of the neurons then leave the cerebellum. A few Purkinje cell axons in the flocculonodular lobe and in parts of the vermis bypass the cerebellar nuclei and leave the cerebellum without synapsing.

Fibers from the dentate, emboliform, and globose nuclei leave the cerebellum through the superior cerebellar peduncle. Fibers from the fastigial nucleus leave through the inferior cerebellar peduncle.

CEREBELLAR PEDUNCLES

The cerebellum is linked to other parts of the central nervous system by numerous efferent and afferent fibers that are grouped together on each side into three large bundles, or peduncles (Fig. 10-7). The superior cerebellar peduncles connect the cerebellum to the midbrain, the middle cerebellar peduncles connect the cerebellum to the pons, and the inferior cerebellar peduncles connect the cerebellum to the medulla oblongata (Fig. 10-7).

The **inferior cerebellar peduncle** is formed on the posterolateral aspect of the superior half of the medulla oblongata (Fig. 10-7). The two peduncles diverge as they ascend and pass into their respective cerebellar hemispheres. The inferior cerebellar peduncle is made up largely of afferent fibers, which pass to the cerebellum (Fig. 10-8) and include the following: (1) the posterior spinocerebellar tract, which passes from the spinal cord and is distributed to the paleocerebellum; (2) the cuneocerebellar tract (posterior external arcuate fibers), which passes from the cells of the cuneate nucleus to the vermis; (3) the olivocerebellar tract, which passes from the inferior olivary nuclei to the cortex of the neocerebellum; (4) the reticulocerebellar tract, which passes from the reticular formation in the medulla to the vermis; and (5) the vestibulocerebellar tract, which passes from the vestibular nuclei and the vestibulocochlear nerve to the archicerebellum.

The tracts leaving the cerebellum in the inferior cerebellar peduncle include the following: (1) cerebellovestibular fibers, which pass to the vestibular nuclei, and (2) cerebelloreticular fibers, which pass to the reticular formation in the pons and medulla oblongata.

The **middle cerebellar peduncle** is the largest of the three peduncles (Fig. 10-7). It arises from the posterolateral region of the pons and becomes continuous with the white matter within the cerebellar hemisphere. It is formed by the **transverse fibers of the pons** (Fig. 10-8). The fibers arise from the neurons of the pontine nuclei in one half of the pons and cross the midline, traversing the opposite middle cerebellar peduncle to reach the cortex of the neocerebellum of the contralateral hemisphere. The middle cerebellar peduncle, therefore, is made up of the extensive corticopontocerebellar pathway.

The **superior cerebellar peduncle** emerges

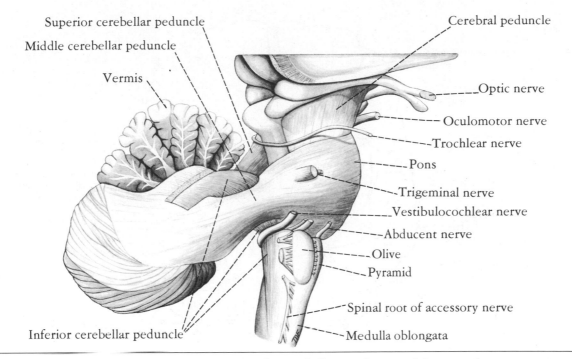

Superior cerebellar peduncle

Middle cerebellar peduncle

Vermis

Inferior cerebellar peduncle

Cerebral peduncle

Optic nerve

Oculomotor nerve

Trochlear nerve

Pons

Trigeminal nerve

Vestibulocochlear nerve

Abducent nerve

Olive

Pyramid

Spinal root of accessory nerve

Medulla oblongata

Fig. 10-7. Three cerebellar peduncles connecting the cerebellum to the rest of the central nervous system.

from the superior part of the vallecula (anterior cerebellar notch) and runs superiorly, lateral to the upper half of the fourth ventricle, to enter the lower part of the midbrain (Fig. 10-7). The great majority of the fibers within the peduncle are efferent and arise from the intracerebellar nuclei (Fig. 10-8). In addition, the superior peduncle contains afferent fibers, which include (1) the anterior spinocerebellar tract (2) rubrocerebellar fibers, and (3) the tectocerebellar fibers.

CEREBELLAR CORTICAL MECHANISMS

As the result of extensive cytological and physiological research, certain basic mechanisms have been attributed to the cerebellar cortex. The climbing and the mossy fibers constitute the two main lines of input to the cortex and are excitatory to the Purkinje cells (Fig. 10-9). The climbing fibers pass through the granular layer of the cortex and terminate by dividing repeatedly. Each climbing fiber

makes a large number of synaptic contacts with the dendrites of a single Purkinje cell. A few side branches leave each climbing fiber and synapse with the stellate cells and basket cells. The mossy fibers, on the other hand, exert a much more diffuse excitatory effect, so that a single mossy fiber may stimulate thousands of Purkinje cells through the granule cells (Fig. 10-9). The Purkinje cells, by means of their axons, exert an inhibitory effect on the intracerebellar and vestibular nuclei. What then is the function of the remaining cells of the cerebellar cortex, namely, the stellate, basket, and Golgi cells? Neurophysiological research, using microelectrodes, would indicate that they serve as inhibitory interneurons. It is believed that they not only limit the area of cortex excited but influence the degree of Purkinje cell excitation produced by the climbing and mossy fiber input. By this means, fluctuating inhibitory impulses are transmitted by the Purkinje cells to the intracerebellar nuclei, which in turn modify muscular activity through the motor control areas of the brainstem and cerebral cortex.

Fig. 10-8. Some of the main connections of the cerebellum. The cerebellar peduncles are shown as ovoid dashed lines.

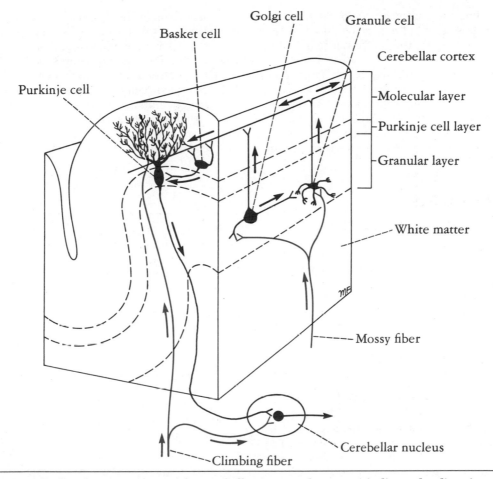

Purkinje cell

Basket cell

Golgi cell

Granule cell

Cerebellar cortex

Molecular layer

Purkinje cell layer

Granular layer

White matter

Mossy fiber

Cerebellar nucleus

Climbing fiber

Fig. 10-9. The functional organization of the cerebellar cortex. The arrows indicate the direction taken by the nervous impulses.

FUNCTIONAL ANATOMY OF THE CEREBELLUM

Brief reference has already been made to the phylogenetic development of the cerebellum (p. 211). The **archicerebellum,** phylogenetically the oldest part of the cerebellum, receives input from the vestibular nerve and the vestibular nuclei. The output to the lower motor neurons is transmitted through the vestibulospinal tract, the medial longitudinal fasciculus, and the reticulospinal fibers. This part of the cerebellum responds to vestibular stimuli from the inner ear and assists in maintaining equilibrium by bringing about modification in muscle tone.

The **paleocerebellum** receives input from the proprioceptive endings in muscles and tendons, and from touch and pressure receptors (spinocerebellar tracts, cuneocerebellar fibers, and spinoreticular and reticulocerebellar tracts). The output to the lower motor neurons, especially the gamma efferents, is transmitted through vestibulospinal, rubrospinal, and reticulospinal tracts. This part of the cerebellum is sensitive to changes in muscle and tendon tension and information on touch and deep pressure, and responds by modifying muscle tone and aiding the synergistic action of groups of muscles. It thus plays an active role in the maintenance of posture and the performance of voluntary movements.

The **neocerebellum** receives a very large input through the corticopontocerebellar tracts from the cerebral cortex of the opposite side; it also receives information through the olivocerebellar fibers. The output to the lower motor neurons travels through the thalamus to the motor area of the cerebral cor-tex, then through the corticospinal and corticonuclear fibers to the lower motor neurons. The neocerebellum thus facilitates a smooth, coordinated voluntary movement and ensures that the force, direction, and extent of the movement are accurate.

Later, when detailed studies of the connections of the cerebellum are discussed, it will become apparent that a cerebellar hemisphere influences the muscular activity of the same side of the body; this fact is of great clinical significance.

CLINICAL NOTES

GENERAL CONSIDERATIONS

The cerebellum lies in the posterior cranial fossa of the skull and forms the roof of the fourth ventricle. It is joined to the brainstem by three pairs of peduncles: the superior, middle, and inferior peduncles. The cerebellum consists of two cerebellar hemispheres joined by a narrow median vermis. The cerebellum has three main lobes: the anterior, middle, and flocculonodular lobes.

Afferent nerve fibers enter the cerebellum through all three pairs of cerebellar peduncles and terminate in the cerebellar cortex as climbing or mossy fibers. The large Purkinje cells link the cortex to the intracerebellar nuclei, namely, the dentate, emboliform, globose, and fastigial nuclei. The neurons of the nuclei form the main efferent fibers of the cerebellum, which leave through the superior and inferior cerebellar peduncles.

It is believed that within the cerebellar cortex the afferent fibers are excitatory to the Purkinje cells. The Purkinje cells exert an inhibitory influence on the intracerebellar nuclei. The axons of the cells of the nuclei exert their influence on the motor activity indirectly through the vestibular nuclei, reticular formation, red nucleus, tectum, and corpus striatum and the motor areas of the cerebral cortex. The stellate, basket, and Golgi cells of the cerebellar cortex limit the area of cortex excited by the afferent fibers and probably modify the Purkinje cell excitability.

The essential function of the cerebellum is to coordinate, by synergistic action, all reflex and voluntary muscular activity. It thus graduates and harmonizes muscle tone and maintains normal body posture. It permits voluntary movements to take place with precision and economy of effort.

There are two neuroanatomical features concerning the cerebellum that are of great clinical significance. First, the cortex of the cerebellum, unlike that of the cerebrum, has a uniform microscopic structure and physiological investigations show that the activities occurring are identical in all regions; functional localization, therefore, does not exist in the cerebellar cortex. Second, each cerebellar hemisphere is connected by nervous pathways principally with the same side of the body, so that a lesion in one cerebellar hemisphere gives rise to signs and symptoms that are limited to the same side of the body.

SIGNS AND SYMPTOMS OF CEREBELLAR DISEASE

While the importance of the cerebellum in the maintenance of muscle tone and the coordination of muscle movement has been emphasized, it should be remembered that the symptoms and signs of acute lesions differ from those produced by chronic lesions. Acute lesions produce sudden, severe symptoms and signs, but there is considerable clinical evidence to show that patients can recover completely from large cerebellar injuries. This suggests that other areas of the central nervous system can compensate for loss of cerebellar function. Chronic lesions, such as slowly enlarging tumors, produce symptoms and signs that are much less severe than those of acute lesions. The reason for this may be that other areas of the central nervous system have time to compensate for loss of cerebellar function.

The following symptoms and signs are characteristic of cerebellar dysfunction.

Hypotonia

The muscles lose resilience to palpation. There is diminished resistance to passive movements of joints. Shaking the limb produces excessive movements at the terminal joints. The condition is attributable to loss of cerebellar influence on the simple stretch reflex.

Postural Changes and Alteration of Gait

The head is often rotated and flexed and the shoulder on the side of the lesion is lower than on the normal side. The patient assumes a wide base when he stands and is often stiff-legged to compensate for loss of muscle tone. When the individual walks, he lurches and staggers toward the affected side.

Disturbances of Voluntary Movement (Ataxia)

The muscles contract irregularly and weakly. **Tremor** occurs when fine movements, such as buttoning clothes, writing, and shaving, are attempted. Muscle groups fail to work harmoniously and there is **decomposition of movement.** When the patient is asked to touch the tip of his nose with his index finger the movements are not properly coordinated and the finger either passes the nose (past-pointing) or hits the nose. A similar test can be performed on the lower limbs by asking the patient to place the heel of one foot on the shin of the opposite leg.

Dysdiadochokinesis

Dysdiadochokinesis is the inability to perform alternating movements regularly and rapidly. Ask the patient to pronate and supinate the forearms rapidly. On the side of the cerebellar lesion the movements are slow, jerky, and incomplete.

Disturbances of Reflexes

Movement produced by tendon reflexes tends to continue for a longer period of time than normal. The pendular knee jerk, for example, occurs following tapping the patellar tendon. Normally the movement occurs and is self-limited by the stretch reflexes of the agonists and antagonists. In cerebellar disease, because of loss of influence on the stretch reflexes, the movement continues as a series of flexion and extension movements at the knee joint; that is, the leg moves like a pendulum.

Disturbances of Ocular Movement

Nystagmus, which is essentially an ataxia of the ocular muscles, is a rhythmical oscillation of the eyes. It is more easily demonstrated when the eyes are deviated in a horizontal direction.

Disorders of Speech

Dysarthria occurs in cerebellar disease owing to ataxia of the muscles of the larynx. Articulation is jerky and the syllables often are separated from one another. Speech tends to be explosive and the syllables often are slurred.

It is important to remember that in cerebellar lesions there is no paralysis and there are no sensory changes. Although muscle hypotonia and incoordination may be present, the disorder is not limited to specific muscles or muscle groups; rather, an entire extremity or the entire half of the body is involved, and if both cerebellar hemispheres are involved, then the entire body may show disturbances of muscle action. Even though the muscular contractions may be weak and the patient easily fatigued, there is no atrophy.

Vermis Syndrome

The most common cause of this syndrome is a **medulloblastoma** of the vermis in children. Involvement of the flocculonodular lobe results in signs and symptoms related to the vestibular system. Since the vermis is unpaired and influences midline structures, muscle incoordination involves the head and trunk and not the limbs. There is a tendency to fall forward or backward. There is difficulty in holding the head steady and in an upright position. There also may be difficulty in holding the trunk erect.

Cerebellar Hemisphere Syndrome

Tumors of one cerebellar hemisphere may be the cause of this syndrome. The symptoms and signs are usually unilateral and involve muscles on the side of the diseased cerebellar hemisphere. Movements of the limbs, especially the arms, are disturbed. Swaying and falling to the side of the lesion often occur. Dysarthria and nystagmus are also common findings.

Common Diseases Involving the Cerebellum

The following diseases frequently involve the cerebellum: congenital agenesis or hypoplasia, neoplasms, trauma, infections, thrombosis of the cerebellar arteries, and degenerative diseases.

CLINICAL PROBLEMS

Answers on Page 598

1. A 37-year-old man visited his physician because he had noticed clumsiness of his right arm. The symptoms had started six months previously and were getting worse. He also noticed that his right hand had a tremor when he attempted fine movements or tried to insert a key in a lock. When he walks he has noticed that now and again he tends to reel over to the right, "as if he had too much alcohol to drink." On physical examination, the face was tilted slightly to the left and the right shoulder was held lower than the left. Passive movements of the arms and legs revealed hypotonia and looseness on the right side. When asked to walk heel–toe along a straight line on the floor the patient swayed over to the right side. When he was asked to touch his nose with his right index finger, the right hand displayed tremor and the finger tended to overshoot the target. Speech was normal and nystagmus was not present. Using your knowledge of neuroanatomy, explain each sign and symptom. Is the lesion of the cerebellum likely to be in the midline or to one side?

2. A 4½-year-old boy was taken to a neurologist because his mother was concerned about his attacks of vomiting on waking in the morning and his tendency to be unsteady on standing up. The mother also noticed that the child walked with an unsteady gait and often fell backward. On physical examination, the child tended to stand with the legs well apart, that is, broad-based. The head was larger than normal for his age and the suture lines of the skull could be easily felt. A retinal examination with an ophthalmoscope showed severe papilledema in both eyes. The muscles of the upper and lower limbs showed some degree of hypotonia. Nystagmus was not present and the child showed no tendency to fall to one side or the other when asked to walk. Using your knowledge of neuroanatomy, explain the symptoms and signs. Is the lesion in the cerebellum likely to be in the midline or to one side?

3. During a ward round, a third-year student was asked to explain the phenomenon of nystagmus. How would you have answered that question? Why do patients exhibit nystagmus in cerebellar disease?

4. On looking at a histological slide of the cerebellar cortex, one is struck by the uniformity of the cellular arrangement. What different types of neurons are found in the cerebellar cortex, and what may their function be?

5. What is the essential difference between the symptoms and signs of acute and chronic lesions of the cerebellum? How can you explain these differences?

6. What is meant by the terms *climbing* and *mossy fibers of the cerebellum?* Are they afferent or efferent fibers?

7. What are the cerebellar peduncles? The middle peduncle is the main connecting link between the cerebrum and the cerebellum; explain this.

8. Name the intracerebellar nuclei. Why do you think that cerebellar signs and symptoms are more permanent when these nuclei are destroyed in addition to the cerebellar cortex?

9. Two physicians were talking in the street when one turned to the other and said, "Look at that

man over there—look at the way he is walking— he is not swinging his right arm at all—it is just hanging down by his side. I wonder if he has a cerebellar lesion." Does a person with a unilateral cerebellar hemisphere tumor tend to hold his arm limply at his side when he walks?

NATIONAL BOARD TYPE QUESTIONS

Answers on Page 620

IN EACH OF THE FOLLOWING QUESTIONS, ANSWER:
- (a) IF (1) ONLY IS CORRECT
- (b) IF (2) ONLY IS CORRECT
- (c) IF BOTH (1) AND (2) ARE CORRECT, AND
- (d) IF NEITHER (1) NOR (2) IS CORRECT

1. Which of the following statements is (are) correct concerning the gross anatomy of the cerebellum?
   (1) It is separated from the occipital lobes of the cerebral hemispheres by the tentorium cerebelli.
   (2) It lies posterior to the medulla oblongata and the pons.
2. Which of the following statements is (are) correct concerning the lobes of the cerebellum?
   (1) The anterior lobe is separated from the middle (posterior) lobe by the horizontal fissure.
   (2) The flocculonodular lobe is separated from the middle (posterior) lobe by the uvulonodular fissure.
3. Which of the following statements is (are) correct concerning the phylogeny of the cerebellum?
   (1) The paleocerebellum, which is well developed in reptiles, is functionally related to the gross movements of the head and body.
   (2) The neocerebellum, which constitutes the largest part of the cerebellum in man is associated with the control of fine voluntary movements.
4. Which of the following statements is (are) correct concerning the Purkinje cells?
   (1) They are small Golgi type 2 neurons.
   (2) They exert an inhibitory influence on the intracerebellar nuclei.
5. Which of the following statements is (are) correct concerning the signs and symptoms of cerebellar disease?
   (1) Diminished resistance to passive movements.
   (2) The inability to perform alternating movements regularly and rapidly.

6. Which of the following statements is (are) correct concerning the structure and functions of the cerebellum?
   (1) Each cerebellar hemisphere controls the skeletal muscle tone on the same side of the body.
   (2) The transverse pontine fibers connect up one pontine nucleus to another and do not leave the pons.

Select the best response:

7. The following statements concerning the structure of the cerebellum are correct **except**:
   (a) The cerebellum consists of two cerebellar hemispheres joined by a narrow median vermis.
   (b) The inferior surface of the cerebellum shows a deep groove, the vallecula.
   (c) The inferior cerebellar peduncles join the cerebellum to the medulla oblongata.
   (d) The gray matter is confined to the cerebellar cortex.
   (e) The white matter and folia of the cortex have a branched appearance on the cut surface, called the arbor vitae.
8. The following statements concerning the structure of the cerebellar cortex are correct **except**:
   (a) The cortex is folded by many transverse fissures into folia.
   (b) The structure of the cortex is identical in different parts of the cerebellum.
   (c) The Purkinje cells are found in the most superficial layer of the cortex.
   (d) The Golgi cells are found in the deepest layer of the cerebellar cortex.
   (e) The axons of the Purkinje cells form the efferent fibers from the cerebellar cortex.
9. The following statements concerning the intracerebellar nuclei are correct **except**:
   (a) The nuclei are found within the substance of the white matter.
   (b) They are located in the roof of the fourth ventricle.

(c) They are composed of large multipolar neurons.

(d) Their axons form the main cerebellar outflow.

(e) The nuclei are named from medial to lateral, dentate, emboliform, globose, and fastigial.

In the following questions, answer:

(a) If (1), (2), and (3) only are correct

(b) If (1) and (3) only are correct

(c) If (2) and (4) only are correct

(d) If (4) only is correct, or

(e) If all are correct

10. Which of the following statements concerning the cerebellar peduncles is (are) correct?

(1) In the superior cerebellar peduncle most of the fibers are efferent and arise from the neurons of the intracerebellar nuclei.

(2) The middle cerebellar peduncle is formed of fibers that arise from the pontine nuclei.

(3) The anterior spinocerebellar tract enters the cerebellum through the superior cerebellar peduncle.

(4) The inferior cerebellar peduncle is made up exclusively of fibers that pass from the inferior olivary nuclei to the cortex of the neocerebellum.

11. Which of the following statements concerning the afferent fibers entering the cerebellum is (are) correct?

(1) They enter the cerebellum mainly through the inferior and middle cerebellar peduncles.

(2) The climbing and the mossy fibers constitute the two main lines of input to the cerebellar cortex.

(3) The afferent fibers are excitatory to the Purkinje cells.

(4) The mossy fibers end by making synaptic contacts with the dendrites of the Purkinje cells.

12. Which of the following statements concerning the functions of the cerebellum is (are) correct?

(1) The cerebellum influences the actions of skeletal muscle.

(2) The cerebellum controls voluntary movement by coordinating the force and extent of contraction of different muscles.

(3) It inhibits the contraction of antagonistic muscles.

(4) It has no effect on the control of smooth muscle.

ADDITIONAL READING

Angevine, J. B., Mancall, E. L., and Yakovlev, P. I. *The Human Cerebellum*. Boston: Little, Brown, 1961.

Bloomfield, S., and Marr, D. How the cerebellum may be used. *Nature (Lond.)* 227:1224, 1970.

Braitenberg, V., and Atwood, R. P. Morphological observations on the cerebellar cortex. *J. Comp. Neurol.* 109:1, 1958.

Carpenter, M. B., and Stevens, G. H. Structural and functional relationships between the deep cerebellar nuclei and the brachium conjunctivum in the rhesus monkey. *J. Comp. Neurol.* 107:109, 1957.

Chan-Palay, V. Recent advances in the morphological localization of gamma-aminobutyric acid receptors in the cerebellum by means of ^{3}H-muscimol. *Prog. Brain Res.* 51:303, 1979.

Colin, F., Manil, J., Desclin, J. C. The olivocerebellar system. 1. Delayed and slow inhibitory effects: An overlooked salient feature of cerebellar climbing fibers. *Brain Res.* 187:3, 1980.

Eccles, J. C., Ito, M., and Szentágothai, J. *The Cerebellum As a Neuronal Machine*. Berlin and Vienna: Springer-Verlag, 1967.

Fields, W. D., and Willis, W. D., Jr. *The Cerebellum in Health and Disease*. St. Louis: Green, 1970.

Fox, C. A., and Barnard, J. W. A quantitative study of the Purkinje cell dendritic branches and their relations to afferent fibers. *J. Anat.* 91:299, 1957.

Gilman, S. The mechanisms of cerebellar hypotonia. *Brain* 92:621, 1969.

Gilman, S. The Cerebellum: Its Role in Posture and Movement. In M. Swash and C. Kennedy (eds.), *Scientific Basis of Clinical Neurology*. Edinburgh: Churchill Livingstone, 1985.

Gilman, S., Bloedel, J. R., and Lechtenberg, R. *Disorders of the Cerebellum*. Philadelphia: Davis, 1981.

Ito, M. *The Cerebellum and Neural Control*. New York: Raven Press, 1984.

Jansen, J., and Brodal, A. *Aspects of Cerebellar Anatomy*. Oslo: Johan Grundt Tanum Forlag, 1954.

Kennedy, P. R., Ross, H. G., and Brooks, V. B. Participation of the principal olivary nucleus in neocerebellar motor control. *Exp. Brain Res.* 47:95, 1982.

Llinas, R. R. The cortex of the cerebellum. *Sci. Am.* 232(1):56, 1975.

Napper, R. M. A., and Harvey, R. J. Number of parallel fiber synapses on an individual Purkinje cell in the cerebellum of the rat. *J. Comp. Neurol.* 274:168, 1988.

Nieuwenhuys, R. *Chemoarchitecture of the Brain.* Berlin: Springer-Verlag, 1985.

Palay, S. L., and Chan-Palay, V. *Cerebellar Cortex: Cytol-ogy and Organization.* Berlin and Vienna: Springer-Verlag, 1974.

Schulman, J. A. Chemical neuroanatomy of the cerebellar cortex. In P. C. Emson (Ed.), *Chemical Neuroanatomy.* New York: Raven, 1983. P. 209.

Stanton, G. B. Topographical organization of ascending cerebellar projections from the dentate and interposed nuclei in Macaca mulatta: An anterograde degeneration study. *J. Comp. Neurol.* 190:699, 1980.

Chapter 11
The Fourth Ventricle

GROSS APPEARANCE

The fourth ventricle is a tent-shaped cavity filled with cerebrospinal fluid. It is situated anterior to the cerebellum and posterior to the pons and the cranial half of the medulla oblongata (Fig. 11-1). It is lined with ependyma and is continuous superiorly with the cerebral aqueduct of the midbrain and inferiorly with the central canal of the medulla oblongata.

The fourth ventricle possesses lateral boundaries, a roof and the **tela choroidea,** and a diamond-shaped anterior floor called the **rhomboid fossa.**

Lateral Boundaries

The caudal part of each lateral boundary is formed by the inferior cerebellar peduncle (Fig. 11-2). The cranial part of each lateral boundary is formed by the superior cerebellar peduncle.

Roof or Posterior Wall

The roof of the fourth ventricle extends posteriorly toward the cerebellum (Fig. 11-1). The superior part is formed by the medial borders of the two superior cerebellar peduncles and a connecting sheet of white matter called the **superior medullary velum** (Fig. 11-3). The inferior part of the roof is formed by the **inferior medullary velum,** which consists of a thin sheet devoid of nervous tissue and formed by the ventricular ependyma and its posterior covering of pia mater (Fig. 11-4). This part of the roof is pierced in the midline by a large aperture, the **median aperture** (foramen of Magendie), which connects the interior of the ventricle with the subarachnoid space (Figs. 11-1 and 11-4).

Tela Choroidea

The tela choroidea of the fourth ventricle is a double layer of pia mater that lies in the interval

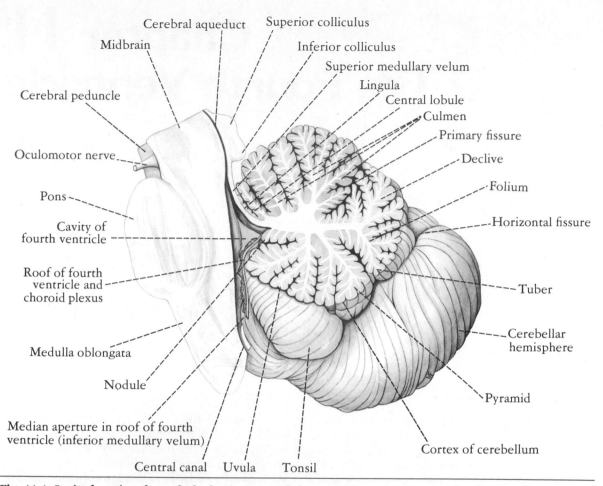

Fig. 11-1. Sagittal section through the brainstem and the cerebellum showing the fourth ventricle.

between the cerebellum and the lower part of the roof of the ventricle. In this region, the blood vessels of the tela choroidea form a rich vascular fringe that projects through the lower part of the roof of the fourth ventricle to form the **choroid plexus** (Figs. 11-1 and 11-4). In this region the cavity of the ventricle extends laterally over the surface of the inferior cerebellar peduncle to form the **lateral recess** of the ventricle (see Fig. 1-14). The lateral recess on each side opens into the subarachnoid space by a **lateral aperture** (foramen of Luschka). Thus, the cavity of the fourth ventricle communicates with the subarachnoid space through a single median opening and two lateral

apertures. These important openings permit the cerebrospinal fluid to flow from the ventricular system into the subarachnoid space.

Floor or Rhomboid Fossa

The floor is formed by the posterior surface of the pons and the cranial half of the medulla oblongata (Fig. 11-2). The floor is divided into symmetrical halves by the **median sulcus.** On each side of this sulcus there is an elevation, the **medial eminence,** which is bounded laterally by another sulcus, the **sulcus limitans.** Lateral to the sulcus

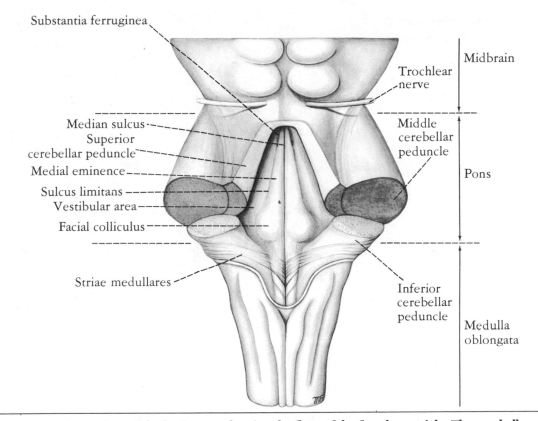

Substantia ferruginea

Median sulcus

Superior cerebellar peduncle

Medial eminence

Sulcus limitans

Vestibular area

Facial colliculus

Striae medullares

Trochlear nerve

Midbrain

Middle cerebellar peduncle

Pons

Inferior cerebellar peduncle

Medulla oblongata

Fig. 11-2. Posterior surface of the brainstem showing the floor of the fourth ventricle. The cerebellum has been removed.

limitans there is an area known as the **vestibular area** (Fig. 11-2 and 11-3). The vestibular nuclei lie beneath the vestibular area.

The **facial colliculus** is a slight swelling at the inferior end of the medial eminence that is produced by the fibers from the motor nucleus of the facial nerve looping over the abducens nucleus (Fig. 11-5). At the superior end of the sulcus limitans there is a bluish-gray area produced by a cluster of nerve cells containing melanin pigment; the cluster of cells is called the **substantia ferruginea.** Strands of nerve fibers, the **stria medullaris,** emerge from the median sulcus and pass laterally over the medial eminence and the vestibular area and enter the inferior cerebellar peduncle (Fig. 11-2).

Inferior to the stria medullaris the following features should be recognized in the floor of the ven-

tricle. The most medial is the **hypoglossal triangle,** which indicates the position of the underlying **hypoglossal nucleus** (Fig. 11-3). Lateral to this is the **vagal triangle,** beneath which lies the dorsal motor nucleus of the vagus. The **area postrema** is a narrow area between the vagal triangle and the lateral margin of the ventricle, just rostral to the opening into the central canal. The inferior part of the vestibular area also lies lateral to the vagal triangle.

The **choroid plexus** of the fourth ventricle, whose function is to produce cerebrospinal fluid, is suspended from the inferior medullary velum (Figs. 11-1 and 11-3). Here the highly vascular, fringelike processes of the tela choroidea invaginate the ependymal lining of the ventricular roof. It is the cells of the ependyma that are secretory and produce the cerebrospinal fluid.

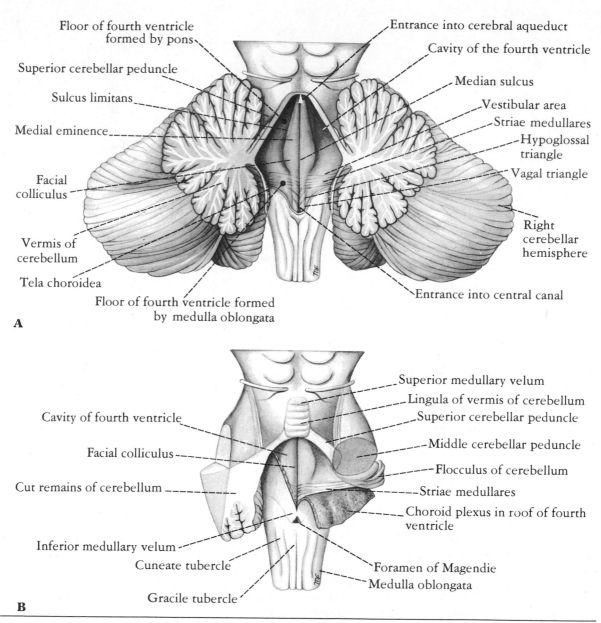

Fig. 11-3. Posterior view of the cavity of the fourth ventricle.
A. The vermis of the cerebellum has been divided in the midline and the cerebellar hemispheres have been displaced laterally.
B. The greater part of the cerebellum has been removed, leaving the superior and inferior medullary vela. Note that the right half of the inferior medullary velum has been reflected inferiorly to reveal the choroid plexus.

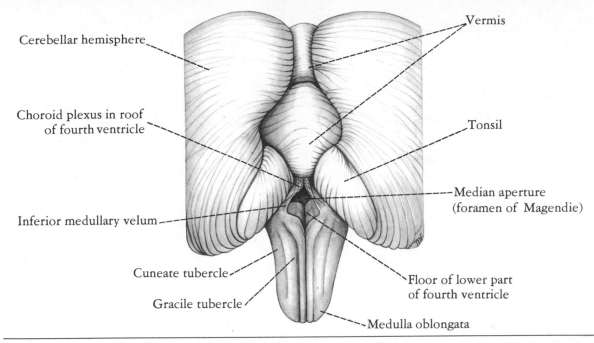

Fig. 11-4. Posterior view of the roof of the fourth ventricle. The cerebellum has been displaced superiorly to show the large median aperture (foramen of Magendie).

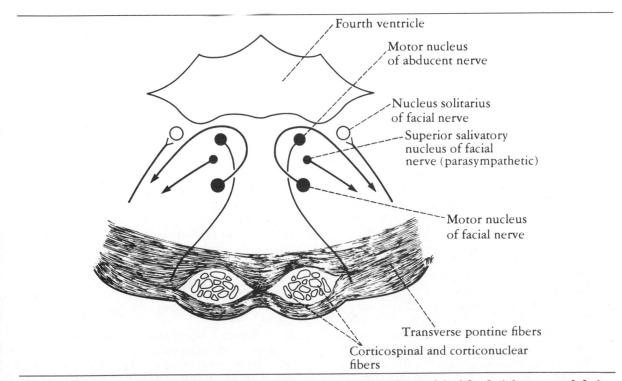

Fig. 11-5. Transverse section through the developing pons showing the nuclei of the facial nerve and their relationship to the nucleus of the abducent nerve.

CLINICAL NOTES

GENERAL CONSIDERATIONS

The fourth ventricle is the cavity of the hindbrain and is situated in the posterior cranial fossa. It is related posteriorly to the vermis of the cerebellum and anteriorly to the pons and the cranial part of the medulla oblongata. The ventricle is lined with ependyma and is continuous superiorly with the third ventricle through the cerebral aqueduct of the midbrain. Inferiorly it is continuous with the central canal of the medulla and the spinal cord. The fourth ventricle is full of cerebrospinal fluid, which leaves the ventricular system through the three apertures in the roof of the ventricle. The large median aperture, the foramen of Magendie, and the two small lateral apertures, the foramina of Luschka, are the only openings by which the cerebrospinal fluid within the ventricular system of the brain can enter the subarachnoid space.

Suspended from the roof of the fourth ventricle is the choroid plexus, which, together with similar plexuses in the third ventricle and the lateral ventricles, is the site for the secretion of cerebrospinal fluid.

Beneath the floor of the fourth ventricle are located several important nuclei that control vital functions; the hypoglossal and vagal nuclei, for example, control movements of the tongue, swallowing, respiration, heart rate, and blood pressure.

Hydrocephalus

Hydrocephalus, which may be defined as an abnormal increase in volume of the cerebrospinal fluid within the skull, may occur as the result of blockage of the foramina in the roof of the fourth ventricle. A congenital septum may be present, or adhesions occurring during meningitis, or displacement of the medulla oblongata by the pressure of an intracranial tumor; all these conditions can cause hydrocephalus.

Tumors of the Fourth Ventricle

Tumors may arise in the vermis of the cerebellum or in the pons and invade the fourth ventricle. **Ependymomas** arising from the ependymal cells lining the ventricle also occur. Tumors in this region may invade the cerebellum and produce the symptoms and signs of cerebellar deficiency, or they may press upon the vital nuclear centers situated beneath the floor of the ventricle and produce cardiac irregularities, tachycardia, irregular respiration, and vasomotor disturbances.

CLINICAL PROBLEMS

Answers on Page 599

1. A 38-year-old man was admitted to the neurosurgery ward with symptoms of persistent headache and vomiting and some unsteadiness in walking. The headache started 6 weeks previously and has become progressively worse. On examination it was found that he could not sit up in bed unsupported. The limbs on the right side of the body showed some loss of tone. Examination of the patient when he stood up showed a marked loss of equilibrium. Examination of the cranial nerves showed central deafness of the right ear. Ophthalmoscopic examination showed severe bilateral papilledema. Using your knowledge of neuroanatomy, explain the symptoms and signs experienced by this patient and try to make a diagnosis.

2. A 4-year-old girl was found to have tuberculous meningitis. She was immediately admitted to the hospital and administration of streptomycin and isoniazid was commenced. As soon as this therapy was started she was also administered steroid hormones to reduce the incidence of adhesions. She recovered fully, with no complications. Using your knowledge of neuroanatomy, explain why it is important to prevent the formation of adhesions in the subarachnoid space.

3. A freshman medical student was asked by his professor of neuroanatomy to name the five ways by which cerebrospinal fluid may leave the cavity of the fourth ventricle. The student responded by giving the three apertures in the roof

of the fourth ventricle, but he could not remember the other two. Do you remember?

4. On three occasions during a lecture a professor referred to the superior and inferior medullary vela. What are these vela, and do they perform any particular function?

5. Name the important structures that lie beneath the floor of the fourth ventricle.

NATIONAL BOARD TYPE QUESTIONS

Answers on Page 620

IN THE FOLLOWING QUESTIONS, ANSWER:

(a) IF (1), (2), AND (3) ONLY ARE CORRECT
(b) IF (1) AND (3) ONLY ARE CORRECT
(c) IF (2) AND (4) ONLY ARE CORRECT
(d) IF (4) ONLY IS CORRECT, OR
(e) IF ALL ARE CORRECT

1. Which of the following structure(s) form the roof of the fourth ventricle?
   (1) The inferior medullary velum
   (2) The occipital lobes of the cerebral hemispheres
   (3) The superior medullary velum
   (4) The floculus of the cerebellum

2. The apertures in the roof of the fourth ventricle are:
   (1) The foramina of Luschka
   (2) The interventricular foramen
   (3) The foramen of Magendie
   (4) The foramen of Monroe

3. The cerebrospinal fluid in the fourth ventricle has the following characteristics:
   (1) It is produced mainly by the choroid plexuses of the lateral, third, and fourth ventricles.
   (2) It enters the midbrain within the cerebral aqueduct.
   (3) It enters the spinal cord through the central canal.
   (4) It escapes into the subarachnoid space through the apertures in the roof of the fourth ventricle.

4. The fourth ventricle has the following lateral boundaries:
   (1) Inferior cerebellar peduncles
   (2) Middle cerebellar peduncles
   (3) Superior cerebellar peduncles
   (4) The sulcus limitans

5. The following important nuclei lie beneath the floor of the fourth ventricle:
   (1) Vestibular nuclei
   (2) Vagal nucleus
   (3) Hypoglossal nucleus
   (4) Trochlear nucleus

In each of the following questions, answer:

(a) IF (1) ONLY IS CORRECT
(b) IF (2) ONLY IS CORRECT
(c) IF BOTH (1) AND (2) ARE CORRECT, AND
(d) IF NEITHER (1) NOR (2) IS CORRECT

6. Which of the following statements concerning the fourth ventricle is (are) correct?
   (1) It is lined with ependyma.
   (2) It has a diamond-shaped floor called the rhomboid fossa.

7. Which of the following statements concerning the fourth ventricle is (are) correct?
   (1) The choroid plexus is suspended from the roof.
   (2) Nerve centers controlling the heart rate and blood pressure lie beneath the floor.

ADDITIONAL READING

Crosby, E. C., Humphrey, T., and Lauer, E. W. *Correlative Anatomy of the Nervous System*. New York: Macmillan, 1962.

Rowland, L. P. (ed.). *Merritt's Textbook of Neurology* (7th ed.). Philadelphia: Lea & Febiger, 1984.

Walton, J. N. *Brain's Diseases of the Nervous System* (8th ed.). New York and London: Oxford University Press, 1977.

Williams, P. L., Warwick, R., Dyson, M., and Bannister, L. H. (eds.). *Gray's Anatomy* (37th Brit. ed.). Philadelphia: Saunders, 1989.

Chapter 12
The Midbrain
(Mesencephalon)

GROSS APPEARANCE

The midbrain measures about 0.8 inch (2 cm) in length and connects the pons and cerebellum with the forebrain (Fig. 12-1). Its long axis inclines anteriorly as it ascends through the hiatus in the tentorium cerebelli. The midbrain is traversed by a narrow channel, the **cerebral aqueduct,** which is filled with cerebrospinal fluid (Figs. 12-2 through 12-4).

On the posterior surface are four **colliculi** (corpora quadrigemina). These are rounded eminences that are divided into superior and inferior pairs by a vertical and a transverse groove (see Fig. 1-16). The superior colliculi are centers for visual reflexes (p. 425), and the inferior are lower auditory centers. In the midline below the inferior colliculi the **trochlear** nerves emerge. These are small-diameter nerves that wind round the lateral aspect of the midbrain to enter the lateral wall of the cavernous sinus.

On the lateral aspect of the midbrain, the superior and inferior brachia ascend in an anterolateral direction (Fig. 12-1). The **superior brachium** passes from the superior colliculus to the lateral geniculate body and the optic tract. The **inferior brachium** connects the inferior colliculus to the **medial geniculate body.**

On the anterior aspect of the midbrain (Fig. 12-1) there is a deep depression in the midline, the **interpeduncular fossa,** which is bounded on either side by the **crus cerebri.** Many small blood vessels perforate the floor of the interpeduncular fossa and this region is termed the **posterior perforated substance** (Fig. 12-1). The **oculomotor** nerve emerges from a groove on the medial side of the crus cerebri and passes forward in the lateral wall of the cavernous sinus.

INTERNAL STRUCTURE OF THE MIDBRAIN

The midbrain comprises two lateral halves, called the **cerebral peduncles;** each of these is divided into an anterior part, the **crus cerebri,** and a posterior part, the **tegmentum,** by a pigmented band of gray matter, the **substantia nigra** (Fig. 12-2).

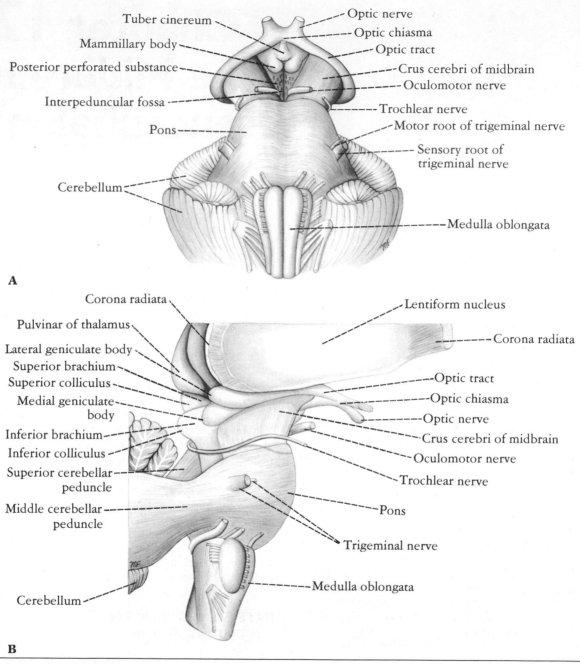

Fig. 12-1. The midbrain.
A. Anterior view.
B. Lateral view.

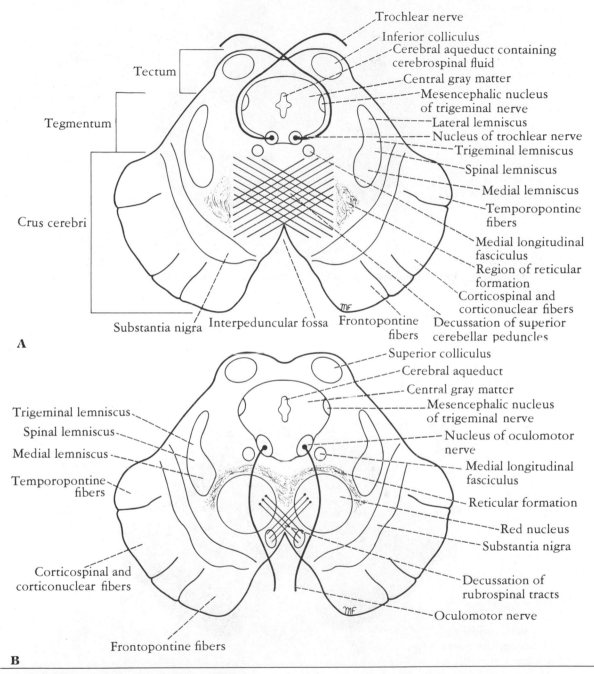

Trochlear nerve

Inferior colliculus

Cerebral aqueduct containing cerebrospinal fluid

Central gray matter

Mesencephalic nucleus of trigeminal nerve

Lateral lemniscus

Nucleus of trochlear nerve

Trigeminal lemniscus

Spinal lemniscus

Medial lemniscus

Temporopontine fibers

Medial longitudinal fasciculus

Region of reticular formation

Corticospinal and corticonuclear fibers

Decussation of superior cerebellar peduncles

Tectum

Tegmentum

Crus cerebri

Substantia nigra   Interpeduncular fossa   Frontopontine fibers

A

Superior colliculus

Cerebral aqueduct

Central gray matter

Mesencephalic nucleus of trigeminal nerve

Nucleus of oculomotor nerve

Medial longitudinal fasciculus

Reticular formation

Red nucleus

Substantia nigra

Decussation of rubrospinal tracts

Oculomotor nerve

Trigeminal lemniscus

Spinal lemniscus

Medial lemniscus

Temporopontine fibers

Corticospinal and corticonuclear fibers

Frontopontine fibers

B

Fig. 12-2. Transverse sections of the midbrain.
A. At the level of the inferior colliculus.
B. At the level of the superior colliculus.
Note that trochlear nerves completely decussate within the superior medullary velum.

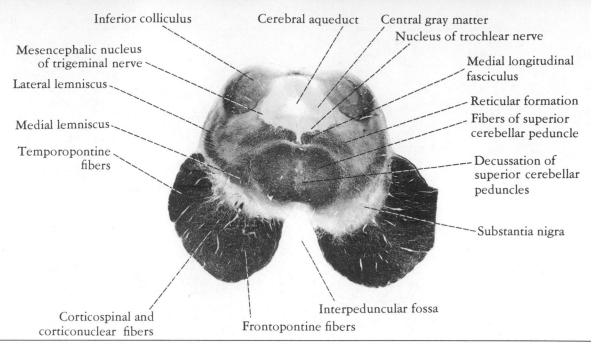

Inferior colliculus   Cerebral aqueduct   Central gray matter

Nucleus of trochlear nerve

Mesencephalic nucleus of trigeminal nerve

Medial longitudinal fasciculus

Lateral lemniscus

Reticular formation

Medial lemniscus

Fibers of superior cerebellar peduncle

Temporopontine fibers

Decussation of superior cerebellar peduncles

Substantia nigra

Corticospinal and corticonuclear fibers

Frontopontine fibers

Interpeduncular fossa

Fig. 12-3. Photomicrograph of transverse section of midbrain at the level of the inferior colliculus. (Weigert stain.)

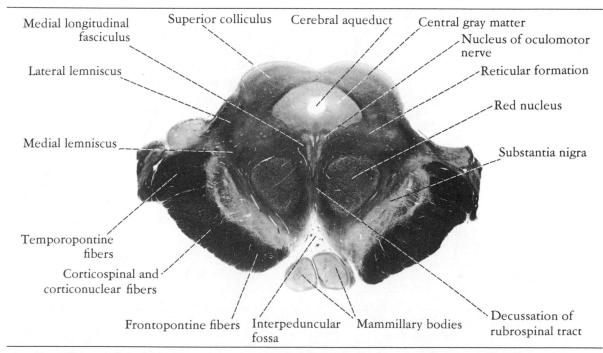

Medial longitudinal fasciculus   Superior colliculus   Cerebral aqueduct   Central gray matter

Nucleus of oculomotor nerve

Lateral lemniscus

Reticular formation

Red nucleus

Medial lemniscus

Substantia nigra

Temporopontine fibers

Corticospinal and corticonuclear fibers

Frontopontine fibers   Interpeduncular fossa   Mammillary bodies

Decussation of rubrospinal tract

Fig. 12-4. Photomicrograph of transverse section of midbrain at the level of the superior colliculus. (Weigert stain.)

The narrow cavity of the midbrain is the **cerebral aqueduct,** which connects the third and fourth ventricles. The **tectum** is the part of the midbrain posterior to the cerebral aqueduct; it has four small surface swellings referred to previously: the **two superior** and **two inferior colliculi** (Fig. 12-2). The cerebral aqueduct is lined by ependyma and is surrounded by the **central gray matter.** On transverse sections of the midbrain the interpeduncular fossa can be seen to separate the crura cerebri, whereas the tegmentum is continuous across the median plane (Fig. 12-2).

Transverse Section of the Midbrain at the Level of the Inferior Colliculi

The **inferior colliculus,** consisting of a large nucleus of gray matter, lies beneath the corresponding surface elevation and forms part of the auditory pathway (Figs. 12-2A and 12-3). It receives many of the terminal fibers of the lateral lemniscus. The pathway then continues (p. 440) through the inferior brachium to the medial geniculate body.

The **trochlear nucleus** is situated in the central gray matter close to the median plane just posterior to the **medial longitudinal fasciculus.** The emerging fibers of the trochlear nucleus pass laterally and posteriorly round the central gray matter and leave the midbrain just below the inferior colliculi. The fibers of the trochlear nerve now decussate completely in the superior medullary velum. The **mesencephalic nuclei of the trigeminal nerve** are lateral to the cerebral aqueduct (Figs. 12-2A and 12-3). The **decussation of the superior cerebellar peduncles** occupies the central part of the tegmentum anterior to the cerebral aqueduct. The **reticular formation** is smaller than that of the pons and is situated lateral to the decussation.

The **medial lemniscus** ascends posterior to the substantia nigra; the **spinal** and **trigeminal lemnisci** are situated lateral to the medial lemniscus (Figs. 12-2 and 12-3). The **lateral lemniscus** is located posterior to the trigeminal lemniscus.

The **substantia nigra** (Figs. 12-2 and 12-3) is a large motor nucleus situated between the tegmentum and the crus cerebri and is found throughout the midbrain. The nucleus is composed of medium-size multipolar neurons that possess inclusion granules of melanin pigment within their cytoplasm. The substantia nigra is concerned with muscle tone and is connected to the cerebral cortex, spinal cord, hypothalamus, and basal nuclei.

The **crus cerebri** contains important descending tracts and is separated from the tegmentum by the substantia nigra (Figs. 12-2 and 12-3). The corticospinal and corticonuclear fibers occupy the middle two-thirds of the crus. The frontopontine fibers occupy the medial part of the crus and the temporopontine fibers occupy the lateral part of the crus (Figs. 12-2 and 12-3). These descending tracts connect the cerebral cortex to the anterior gray column cells of the spinal cord, the cranial nerve nuclei, the pons, and the cerebellum.

Transverse Section of the Midbrain at the Level of the Superior Colliculi

The **superior colliculus** (Figs. 12-2B and 12-4), a large nucleus of gray matter that lies beneath the corresponding surface elevation, forms part of the visual reflexes (see p. 425). It is connected to the lateral geniculate body by the superior brachium. It receives afferent fibers from the optic nerve, the visual cortex, and the spinotectal tract. The efferent fibers form the tectospinal and tectobulbar tracts, which are probably responsible for the reflex movements of the eyes, head, and neck in response to visual stimuli. The afferent pathway for the **light reflex** ends in the **pretectal nucleus.** This is a small group of neurons situated close to the lateral part of the superior colliculus. After relaying in the pretectal nucleus, the fibers pass to the parasympathetic nucleus of the oculomotor nerve (Edinger-Westphal nucleus). The emerging fibers then pass to the oculomotor nerve. The **oculomotor nucleus** is situated in the central gray matter close to the median plane, just posterior to the **medial longitudinal fasciculus** (Figs. 12-2B and 12-4). The fibers of the oculomotor nucleus pass anteriorly through the red nucleus to emerge on the medial side of the crus cerebri in the interpeduncular fossa. The nucleus of the oculomotor nerve is divisible into a number of cell groups, the details of which are described on page 427.

The **medial, spinal,** and **trigeminal lemnisci** form a curved band posterior to the substantia nigra but the **lateral lemniscus** does not extend superiorly to this level (Figs. 12-2B and 12-4).

The **red nucleus** (Figs. 12-2B and 12-4) is a rounded mass of gray matter situated between the cerebral aqueduct and the substantia nigra. Its reddish hue, seen in fresh specimens, is due to its vascularity and the presence of an iron-containing pigment in the cytoplasm of many of its neurons. Afferent fibers reach the red nucleus from (1) the cerebral cortex through the corticospinal fibers, (2) the cerebellum through the superior cerebellar peduncle, and (3) the lentiform nucleus, subthalamic and hypothalamic nuclei, substantia nigra, and spinal cord. Efferent fibers leave the red nucleus and pass to (1) the spinal cord through the rubrospinal tract (as this tract descends it decussates), (2) the reticular formation through the rubroreticular tract, (3) the thalamus, and (4) the substantia nigra.

The **reticular formation** is situated in the tegmentum lateral and posterior to the red nucleus (Figs. 12-2B and 12-4).

The **crus cerebri** contains the identical important descending tracts, the **corticospinal, corticonuclear,** and **corticopontine fibers,** that are present at the level of the inferior colliculus.

CLINICAL NOTES

GENERAL CONSIDERATIONS

Trauma

The midbrain connects the pons and cerebellum to the forebrain and ascends through the opening in the tentorium cerebelli. Among the mechanisms of injuries to the brain, a sudden lateral movement of the head could result in the cerebral peduncles impinging against the sharp free edge of the tentorium cerebelli. Sudden movements of the head resulting from trauma cause different regions of the brain to move at different velocities relative to one another. For example, the large anatomical unit, the forebrain, may move at a different velocity from the remainder of the brain, such as the cerebellum. This will result in the midbrain being bent, stretched, or torn.

Blockage of the Cerebral Aqueduct

The cavity of the midbrain, the cerebral aqueduct, is one of the narrower parts of the ventricular system. Normally, cerebrospinal fluid that has been produced in the lateral and third ventricles passes through this channel to enter the fourth ventricle, and so escapes through the foramina in its roof to enter the subarachnoid space. In congenital hydrocephalus, the cerebral aqueduct may be blocked or replaced by numerous small tubular passages that are insufficient for the normal flow of cerebrospinal fluid. A tumor of the midbrain (Fig. 12-5A) or pressure on the midbrain from a tumor arising outside the midbrain may compress the aqueduct and produce hydrocephalus. When the cerebral aqueduct is blocked, the accumulating cerebrospinal fluid within the third and lateral ventricles produces lesions in the midbrain. The presence of the oculomotor and trochlear nerve nuclei, together with the important descending corticospinal and corticonuclear tracts, will provide symptoms and signs that are helpful in accurately localizing a lesion in the brainstem.

Involvement of the oculomotor nucleus will produce ipsilateral paralysis of the levator palpebrae superioris, the superior, inferior, and medial rectus muscles, and the inferior oblique muscle (see p. 452). Malfunction of the parasympathetic nucleus of the oculomotor nerve produces a dilated pupil that is insensitive to light and does not constrict on accommodation.

Involvement of the trochlear nucleus will produce contralateral paralysis of the superior oblique muscle of the eyeball (see p. 453). Thus it is seen that involvement of one or both of these nuclei, or the corticonuclear fibers that converge upon them, will cause impairment of ocular movements.

Weber's syndrome (Fig. 12-5B), which is commonly produced by occlusion of a branch of the posterior cerebral artery that supplies the midbrain, results in the necrosis of brain tissue involving the oculomotor nerve and the crus cerebri. There is ipsilateral ophthalmoplegia and contralateral paralysis of the lower part of the face, the tongue, and the arm and leg. The eyeball is deviated laterally because of the paralysis of the me-

A

B

C

Fig. 12-5. Pathology of the midbrain.
A. Tumor of the midbrain blocking the cerebral aqueduct.
B. Weber's syndrome, involving the oculomotor nerve and the crus cerebri following occlusion of the blood supply to the midbrain.
C. Benedikt's syndrome, involving the red nucleus and the medial lemniscus following occlusion of the blood supply to the midbrain.

dial rectus muscle; there is drooping (ptosis) of the upper lid and the pupil is dilated and fixed to light and accommodation.

Benedikt's syndrome (Fig. 12-5C), is similar to Weber's syndrome, but the necrosis involves the medial lemniscus and red nucleus, producing contralateral hemianesthesia and involuntary movements of the limbs of the opposite side.

CLINICAL PROBLEMS

Answers on Page 600

1. After a severe automobile accident that resulted in the death of the driver of one of the vehicles, an autopsy was performed and the skull was opened. A massive subdural hematoma was found in the middle cranial fossa. The rapid accumulation of blood within the skull had exerted pressure on the brain above the tentorium cerebelli. The uncus of the temporal lobe had been forced inferiorly through the hiatus in the tentorium cerebelli. What effect do you think these intracranial changes had on the midbrain of this patient?

2. A 3-month-old girl was taken to a pediatrician because her mother was concerned about the large size of her head. The child was perfectly normal in every other respect. Examination of the child showed that the diameter of the head was larger than normal for the age; the fontanelles were larger than normal and were moderately tense. The scalp was shiny and the scalp veins were dilated. The eyes were normal and the mental and physical development of the child were within normal limits. CT scans and MR images of the head revealed gross dilation of the third and lateral ventricles of the brain. What is your diagnosis? What possible treatment would have been suggested to the mother of this child?

3. A 20-year-old man was seen by a neurologist because he had a three-month history of double vision. On examination of the patient, both eyes at rest were turned downward and laterally. The patient was unable to move the eyes upward or medially. Both upper lids were drooping (ptosis). Examination of both pupils showed them to be dilated, and they did not constrict when a light was shone into either eye. Facial movements and sensation were normal. Movements of the upper and lower limbs were normal. There was no evidence of loss of or altered skin sensations in the upper or the lower limbs. Using your knowledge of neuroanatomy, make a diagnosis and accurately locate the site of the lesion. Is the lesion unilateral or bilateral?

4. A 56-year-old man with hypertension was admitted to the hospital with a diagnosis of hemorrhage into the midbrain, possibly from a branch of the posterior cerebral artery. He was found, on physical examination, to have paralysis on the right side of the levator palpebrae superioris, the superior rectus, medial rectus, inferior rectus, and inferior oblique muscle. Furthermore, his right pupil was dilated and failed to constrict on exposure to light or on accommodation. The left eye was normal in every respect. He displayed hypersensitivity to touch on the skin of the left side of his face, and loss of skin sensation on the greater part of his left arm and left leg. The left leg also displayed some spontaneous slow writhing movements (athetosis). Using your knowledge of neuroanatomy, can you explain the signs and symptoms exhibited by this patient?

5. A 42-year-old woman was diagnosed as having a lesion in the midbrain. Physical examination revealed an oculomotor nerve palsy on the left side (paralysis of the left extraocular muscles except the lateral rectus and the superior oblique muscles) and an absence of the light and accommodation reflexes on the left side. There was some weakness but no atrophy of the muscles of the lower part of the face and the tongue on the right side. There was evidence of spastic paralysis of the right arm and leg. There was no evidence of any sensory loss on either side of the head, trunk, or limbs. Using your knowledge of neuroanatomy, precisely place the lesion in the midbrain of this patient.

NATIONAL BOARD TYPE QUESTIONS

Answers on Page 620

IN EACH OF THE FOLLOWING QUESTIONS, ANSWER:
- (a) IF (1) ONLY IS CORRECT
- (b) IF (2) ONLY IS CORRECT
- (c) IF BOTH (1) AND (2) ARE CORRECT, AND
- (d) IF NEITHER (1) NOR (2) IS CORRECT

1. Which of the following statements is (are) correct concerning the midbrain?
   (1) It passes superiorly through the hiatus in the tentorium cerebelli.
   (2) The cavity of the midbrain is called the cerebral aqueduct.

2. Which of the following statements is (are) correct concerning the outer surface of the midbrain?

   (1) The oculomotor nerve emerges from the posterior surface below the inferior colliculi.
   (2) The superior brachium passes from the inferior colliculus to the lateral geniculate body.

3. Which of the following statements is (are) correct concerning the interpeduncular fossa?
   (1) It is bounded laterally by the superior cerebellar peduncles.
   (2) The oculomotor nerves are found in it.

4. Which of the following statements is (are) correct concerning the trochlear nerve?
   (1) It emerges on the posterior surface of the

midbrain and decussates completely in the superior medullary velum.

(2) The trochlear nucleus is situated in the central gray matter at the level of the inferior colliculi.

5. Which of the following statements is (are) correct concerning the lemnisci in the midbrain?
   (1) The lemnisci are situated lateral to the central gray matter.
   (2) The trigeminal lemniscus lies anterior to the medial lemniscus.

In the following questions, answer:
  (a) IF (1), (2), AND (3) ONLY ARE CORRECT
  (b) IF (1) AND (3) ONLY ARE CORRECT
  (c) IF (2) AND (4) ONLY ARE CORRECT
  (d) IF (4) ONLY IS CORRECT, OR
  (e) IF ALL ARE CORRECT

6. Which of the following statements is (are) correct concerning the internal structure of the midbrain?
   (1) The tectum is the part posterior to the cerebral aqueduct.
   (2) The crus cerebri on each side lies anterior to the substantia nigra.
   (3) The tegmentum lies posterior to the substantia nigra.
   (4) The central gray matter encircles the red nuclei.

7. Which of the following statements is (are) correct concerning the colliculi of the midbrain?
   (1) They are located within the tegmentum.
   (2) The superior colliculi are concerned with sight reflexes.
   (3) The superior colliculi lie at the level of the trochlear nerve nuclei.
   (4) The inferior colliculi are concerned with auditory reflexes.

8. Which of the following statements is (are) correct concerning the third cranial nerve nuclei?
   (1) The oculomotor nucleus is situated in the central gray matter.
   (2) The parasympathetic part of the oculomotor nucleus is called the Edinger-Westphal nucleus.
   (3) The fibers from the oculomotor nucleus pass through the red nucleus.
   (4) The oculomotor nucleus lies just posterior to the medial longitudinal fasciculus.

In Figure 12-6, match the numbers listed on the left with the appropriate structure listed on the right. The structures may be used more than once.

9. Number 1	(a) Medial longitudinal fasciculus
10. Number 2	
11. Number 3	(b) Inferior colliculus
12. Number 4	(c) Medial lemniscus
13. Number 5	(d) Trochlear nucleus
14. Number 6	(e) None of the above

Fig. 12-6.

ADDITIONAL READING

Brazis, P. W., Masdeu, J. C., and Biller, J. *Localization in Clinical Neurology* (2nd ed.). Boston: Little, Brown, 1990.

Heimer, L. *The Human Brain and Spinal Cord.* New York: Springer-Verlag, 1983.

Patten, J. P. *Neurological Differential Diagnosis.* London: Harold Stark, 1980.

Rowland, L. P. *Merritt's Textbook of Neurology* (7th ed.). Philadelphia: Lea & Febiger, 1984.

Williams, P. L., Warwick, R., Dyson, M., and Bannister, L. H. (Eds.). *Gray's Anatomy* (37th Brit. ed.). Philadelphia: Saunders, 1989.

Chapter 13
The Cerebrum

The cerebrum is the largest part of the brain and is situated in the anterior and middle cranial fossae of the skull occupying the whole concavity of the vault of the skull. It may be divided into two parts: the **diencephalon,** which forms the central core, and the **telencephalon,** which forms the **cerebral hemispheres.** The different parts of the diencephalon will be described in this chapter.

DIENCEPHALON

The diencephalon consists of the third ventricle and the structures that form its boundaries (Fig. 13-1). It extends posteriorly to the point where the third ventricle becomes continuous with the cerebral aqueduct and anteriorly as far as the interventricular foramina (Fig. 13-3). The diencephalon is thus a midline structure with symmetrical right and left halves. Obviously, these subdivisions of the brain are made for convenience, and from a functional point of view nerve fibers freely cross the boundaries.

GROSS FEATURES

The **inferior surface** of the diencephalon is the only area exposed to the surface in the intact brain (Fig. 13-2). It is formed by hypothalamic and other structures, which include, from anterior to posterior: the **optic chiasma,** with the **optic tract** on either side; the **infundibulum,** with the **tuber cinereum;** and the **mammillary bodies.**

The **superior surface** of the diencephalon is concealed by the **fornix,** which is a thick bundle of fibers that originates in the **hippocampus** of the temporal lobe and arches posteriorly over the **thalamus** (Fig. 13-3) to join the **mammillary body.** The actual superior wall of the diencephalon is formed by the **roof of the third ventricle.** This consists of a layer of ependyma, which is continuous with the rest of the ependymal lining of the third ventricle. It is covered superiorly by a vascular fold of pia mater, called the **tela choroidea of the third ventricle.** From the roof of the third ventricle a pair of vascular processes, the **choroid plexuses of the third ventricle,** project downward

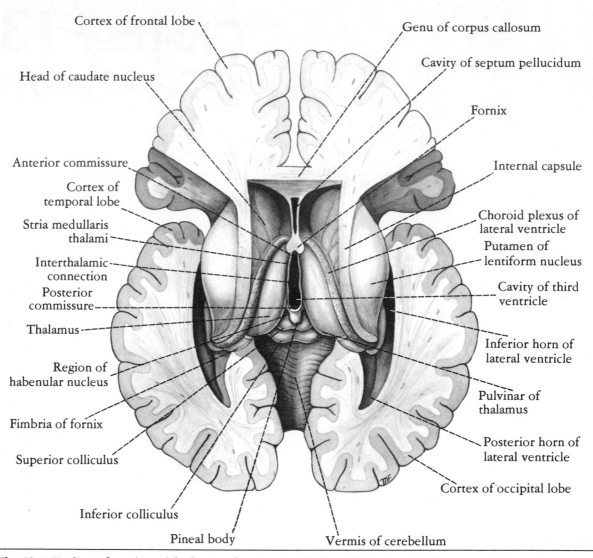

Cortex of frontal lobe

Head of caudate nucleus

Anterior commissure

Cortex of temporal lobe

Stria medullaris thalami

Interthalamic connection

Posterior commissure

Thalamus

Region of habenular nucleus

Fimbria of fornix

Superior colliculus

Inferior colliculus

Pineal body

Genu of corpus callosum

Cavity of septum pellucidum

Fornix

Internal capsule

Choroid plexus of lateral ventricle

Putamen of lentiform nucleus

Cavity of third ventricle

Inferior horn of lateral ventricle

Pulvinar of thalamus

Posterior horn of lateral ventricle

Cortex of occipital lobe

Vermis of cerebellum

Fig. 13-1. Horizontal section of the brain, showing the third and lateral ventricles exposed from above.

from the midline into the cavity of the third ventricle.

The **lateral surface** of the diencephalon is bounded by the **internal capsule** of white matter and consists of nerve fibers that connect the cerebral cortex with other parts of the brainstem and spinal cord (Fig. 13-1).

Since the diencephalon is divided into symmetrical halves by the slitlike third ventricle, it also has a medial surface. The **medial surface** of the diencephalon (i.e., the lateral wall of the third ventricle) is formed in its superior part by the medial surface of the **thalamus** and in its inferior part by the **hypothalamus** (Fig. 13-3). These two areas are separated from one another by a shallow sulcus, the **hypothalamic sulcus.** A bundle of nerve fibers, which are afferent fibers to the habenular nucleus, forms a ridge along the superior margin of the medial surface of the diencephalon and is called the **stria medullaris thalami** (Fig. 13-1).

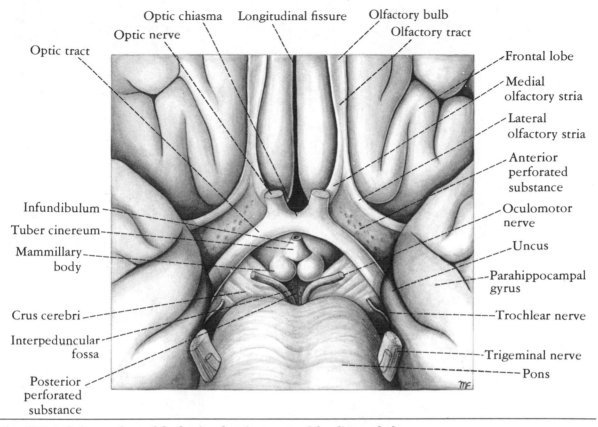

Optic chiasma   Longitudinal fissure   Olfactory bulb
Optic nerve   Olfactory tract
Optic tract   Frontal lobe
Medial olfactory stria
Lateral olfactory stria
Anterior perforated substance
Infundibulum   Oculomotor nerve
Tuber cinereum   Uncus
Mammillary body   Parahippocampal gyrus
Crus cerebri   Trochlear nerve
Interpeduncular fossa   Trigeminal nerve
Pons
Posterior perforated substance

Fig. 13-2. Inferior surface of the brain, showing parts of the diencephalon.

The diencephalon may be divided into four major parts: (1) the thalamus, (2) the subthalamus, (3) the epithalamus, and (4) the hypothalamus.

Thalamus

The thalamus is a large ovoid mass of gray matter that forms the major part of the diencephalon. It is a region of great functional importance and serves as a cell station to all the main sensory systems (except the olfactory pathway). The thalamus is situated on each side of the third ventricle (Fig. 13-3). The anterior end of the thalamus is narrow and rounded and forms the posterior boundary of the interventricular foramen. The posterior end (Fig. 13-4) is expanded to form the **pulvinar,** which overhangs the superior colliculus and the superior brachium. The **lateral geniculate** body

forms a small elevation on the under aspect of the lateral portion of the pulvinar.

The superior surface of the thalamus is covered medially by the tela choroidea and the fornix, and laterally it is covered by ependyma and forms part of the floor of the lateral ventricle; the lateral part is partially hidden by the choroid plexus of the lateral ventricle (Fig. 13-1).

The inferior surface is continuous with the tegmentum of the midbrain (Fig. 13-3).

The medial surface of the thalamus forms the superior part of the lateral wall of the third ventricle and is usually connected to the opposite thalamus by a band of gray matter, the **interthalamic connection** (interthalamic adhesion) (Fig. 13-3).

The lateral surface of the thalamus is separated from the lentiform nucleus by the band of white matter called the **internal capsule** (Fig. 13-1).

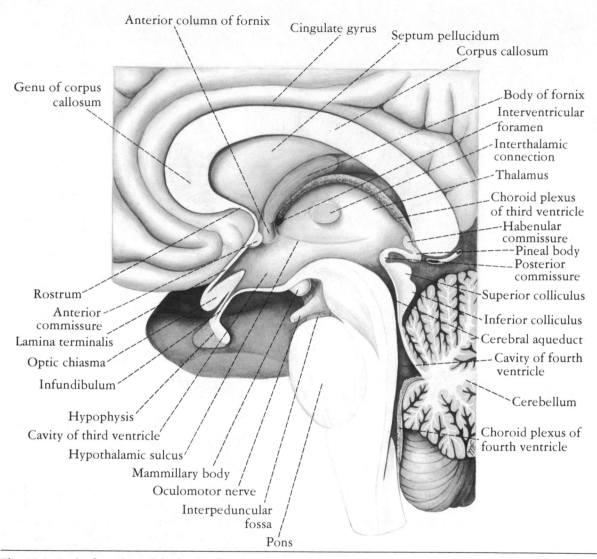

Fig. 13-3. Sagittal section of the brain showing the medial surface of the diencephalon.

Subdivisions of the Thalamus

The thalamus is covered on its superior surface by a thin layer of white matter, called the **stratum zonale,** and on its lateral surface by another layer, the **external medullary lamina** (Fig. 13-4). The gray matter of the thalamus is divided by a vertical sheet of white matter, the **internal medullary lamina,** into medial and lateral halves. Antero-superiorly, the internal medullary lamina splits so

that it is Y shaped (Fig. 13-4). The thalamus is thus subdivided into three main parts; the anterior part lies between the limbs of the Y, and the medial and lateral parts lie on the sides of the stem of the Y.

Each of the three parts of the thalamus contains a group of thalamic nuclei (Fig. 13-4). Moreover, smaller nuclear groups are situated within the internal medullary lamina, and some are located on the medial and lateral surfaces of the thalamus. The detailed description of the thalamic nuclei and

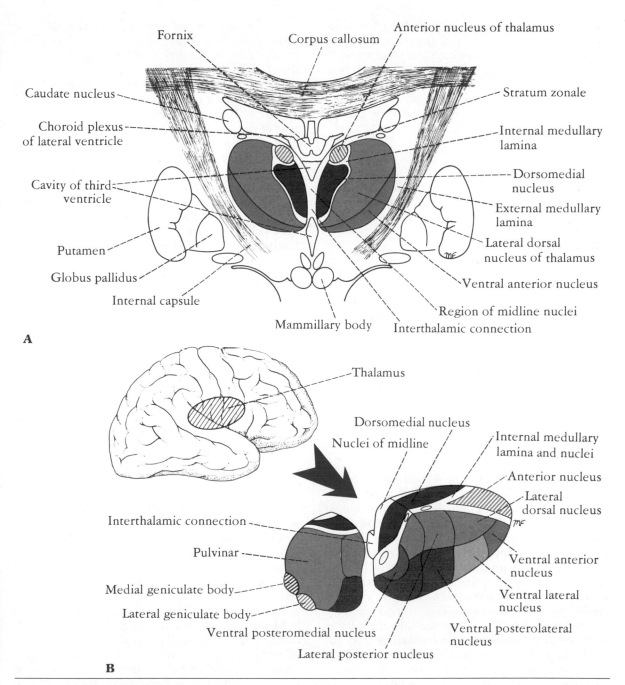

Fig. 13-4. Nuclei of the thalamus.
A. Transverse section through anterior end of thalamus.
B. Diagram showing position of thalamus within right cerebral hemisphere and the relative position of the thalamic nuclei to one another.

their connections is given on page 461. The thalamus is a very important cell station and receives the main sensory tracts (except the olfactory pathway). It should be regarded as a station where much of the information is integrated and relayed to the cerebral cortex and many other subcortical regions. It also plays a key role in the integration of visceral and somatic functions.

Subthalamus

The subthalamus lies inferior to the thalamus and, therefore, is situated between the thalamus and the tegmentum of the midbrain; craniomedially, it is related to the hypothalamus.

The structure of the subthalamus is extremely complex and only a brief description will be given here. Among the collections of nerve cells found in the subthalamus are the cranial ends of the **red nuclei** and the **substantia nigra.** The **subthalamic nucleus** has the shape of a biconvex lens. The nucleus has important connections with the corpus striatum (see p. 327); as a result, it is involved in the control of muscle activity.

The subthalamus also contains many important tracts that pass up from the tegmentum to the thalamic nuclei; the cranial ends of the medial, spinal, and trigeminal lemnisci are examples.

Epithalamus

The epithalamus consists of the habenular nuclei and their connections, and the pineal gland.

The **habenular nucleus** is a small group of nerve cells situated just medial to the posterior surface of the thalamus. Afferent fibers are received from the amygdaloid nucleus in the temporal lobe (see p. 318) through the stria medullaris thalami; other fibers pass from the hippocampal formation through the fornix. Some of the fibers of the stria medullaris thalami cross the midline and reach the habenular nucleus of the opposite side; these latter fibers form the **habenular commissure** (Fig. 13-3). Axons from the habenular nucleus pass to the interpeduncular nucleus in the roof of the interpeduncular fossa, the tectum of the midbrain, the thalamus, and the reticular formation of the midbrain. The habenular nucleus is believed to be a center for integration of olfactory, visceral, and somatic afferent pathways.

The **pineal gland** or **body** is a small, conical structure that is attached by the pineal stalk to the diencephalon. It projects backward so that it lies posterior to the midbrain (Fig. 13-3). The base of the pineal stalk possesses a recess that is continuous with the cavity of the third ventricle (Fig. 13-3). The superior part of the base of the stalk contains the **habenular commissure;** the inferior part of the base of the stalk contains the **posterior commissure.**

On microscopic section, the pineal gland is seen to be incompletely divided into lobules by connective tissue septa that extend into the substance of the gland from the capsule. Two types of cells are found in the gland, the **pinealocytes** and the **glial cells.** Concretions of calcified material called **brain sand** progressively accumulate within the pineal gland with age (Fig. 13-5).

The pineal gland possesses no nerve cells, but adrenergic sympathetic fibers derived from the superior cervical sympathetic ganglia enter the gland and run in association with the blood vessels and the pinealocytes.

The pineal gland, once thought to be of little importance, is now recognized as an endocrine gland capable of influencing the activities of the pituitary gland, the islets of Langerhans, the parathyroids, the adrenals, and the gonads. The pineal secretions reach their target organs via the bloodstream or through the cerebrospinal fluid. Their actions are mainly inhibitory and either directly inhibit the production of hormones or indirectly inhibit the secretion of releasing factors by the hypothalamus.

In animal experiments, it has been shown that pineal activity exhibits a circadian rhythm and this is influenced by light. The gland has been found to be most active during darkness. The probable nervous pathway from the retina runs to the suprachiasmatic nucleus of the hypothalamus, then to the tegmentum of the midbrain, and then via the reticulospinal tract to the sympathetic outflow in the thoracic part of the spinal cord.

Melatonin and **serotonin** are present in high concentrations within the pineal gland. The release of norepinephrine from the sympathetic endings within the gland probably stimulates the release of these substances from the pinealocytes.

Hypothalamus

The **hypothalamus** is that part of the diencephalon that extends from the region of the optic

Groups of pinealocytes

Concretions (brain sand)

Fig. 13-5. Photomicrograph of section of pineal gland stained with hematoxylin and eosin.

chiasma to the caudal border of the mammillary bodies (Fig. 13-2). It lies below the hypothalamic sulcus on the lateral wall of the third ventricle. The hypothalamus controls and integrates the functions of the autonomic nervous system and the endocrine systems and plays a vital role in maintaining body homeostasis. It is involved in such activities as regulation of body temperature, body fluids, drives to eat and drink, sexual behavior, and emotion.

Anterior to the hypothalamus is an area that extends forward from the optic chiasma to the lamina terminalis and the anterior commissure; it is referred to as the **preoptic area.** Caudally, the hypothalamus merges into the tegmentum of the midbrain. Superior to the hypothalamus lies the thalamus and inferolaterally is the subthalamic region.

When observed from below, the hypothalamus is seen to be related to the following structures, from anterior to posterior: (1) the optic chiasma, (2) the tuber cinereum and the infundibulum, and (3) the mammillary bodies.

Optic Chiasma

The optic chiasma is a flattened bundle of nerve fibers situated at the junction of the anterior wall and floor of the third ventricle (Figs. 13-2 and 13-3). The superior surface is attached to the **lamina terminalis,** and inferiorly it is related to the **hypophysis cerebri,** from which it is separated by

the **diaphragma sellae.** The anterolateral corners of the chiasma are continuous with the **optic nerves,** and the posterolateral corners with the **optic tracts.** A small recess, the **optic recess of the third ventricle,** lies on its superior surface.

The origin and destination of the nerve fibers within the optic chiasma are fully described on page 422. It is important to remember that the fibers originating from the nasal half of each retina cross the median plane at the chiasma to enter the optic tract of the opposite side.

Tuber Cinereum

The tuber cinereum is a convex mass of gray matter, as seen from the inferior surface (Figs. 13-2 and 13-3). It is continuous inferiorly with the **infundibulum.** The infundibulum is hollow and becomes continuous with the posterior lobe of the **hypophysis cerebri.** The **median eminence** is a raised part of the tuber cinereum to which is attached the infundibulum. The median eminence, the infundibulum, and the posterior lobe (pars nervosa) of the hypophysis cerebri together form the **neurohypophysis.**

Mammillary Bodies

These are two small hemispherical bodies situated side by side posterior to the tuber cinereum (Figs. 13-2 and 13-3). They possess a central core of gray matter invested by a capsule of myelinated nerve fibers. The nervous connections of these bodies are described on page 321. Posterior to the mammillary bodies lies an area of the brain that is pierced by a number of small apertures and is called the **posterior perforated substance.** (For a discussion of anterior perforated substance, see p. 535.) These apertures transmit the central branches of the posterior cerebral arteries.

It is thus seen that anatomically the hypothalamus is a relatively small area of the brain that is strategically well placed close to the limbic system, the thalamus, the ascending and descending tracts, and the hypophysis. Physiologically, there is hardly any activity in the body that is not influenced by the hypothalamus.

Hypothalamic Nuclei

Microscopically, the hypothalamus is composed of small nerve cells that are arranged in groups or nuclei, many of which are not clearly segregated from one another. In this account, only the principal nuclear groups and their connections will be given. For functional reasons the **preoptic area** is included as part of the hypothalamus. For purposes of description, the nuclei are divided by an imaginary parasagittal plane into medial and lateral zones (Fig. 13-6). The columns of the fornix and the mammillothalamic tract, which serve as markers, lie within the plane.

Medial Zone

In the medial zone, the following hypothalamic nuclei may be recognized, from anterior to posterior: the **preoptic nucleus,** the **paraventricular nucleus,** the **dorsomedial nucleus,** the **ventromedial nucleus,** the **infundibular nucleus,** and the **posterior nucleus** (Fig. 13-6).

Lateral Zone

In the lateral zone, the following hypothalamic nuclei may be recognized, from anterior to posterior: the **supraoptic nucleus,** the large **lateral nucleus,** the **tuberomammillary nucleus,** and the **lateral tuberal nuclei** (Fig. 13-6). Some of the nuclei, for example, the preoptic nucleus, extend into both the medial and lateral zones. The mammillary body, with its medial and lateral mammillary nuclei, overlaps both zones. The **suprachiasmatic nucleus** also overlaps both zones and consists of a small group of neurons lying just above the optic chiasma; it receives nerve fibers from the retina.

The connections of the hypothalamus are described in detail in Chapter 25. In general, the afferent fibers reach the hypothalamus through ascending visceral and somatic sensory pathways and also by fibers that arise in the cerebral cortex, the olfactory pathways, the midbrain, and limbic structures. Efferent fibers descend to lower centers and influence the peripheral parts of the autonomic nervous system. Other fibers pass to the hypophysis cerebri and thus assist in controlling the endocrine glands of the body.

Third Ventricle

The third ventricle, which is derived from the forebrain vesicle, is a slitlike cleft between the two thalami (Figs. 13-1 and 13-3). It communicates anteriorly with the **lateral ventricles** through the **interventricular foramina** and posteriorly with the **fourth ventricle** through the **cerebral aqueduct.** The third ventricle has anterior, posterior, lateral, superior, and inferior walls and is lined with ependyma.

The **anterior wall** is formed by a thin sheet of gray matter, the **lamina terminalis,** across which runs the **anterior commissure** (Fig. 13-3). The anterior commissure is a round bundle of nerve fibers that are situated anterior to the **anterior columns of the fornix;** they connect the right and left temporal lobes.

The **posterior wall** is formed by the opening into the cerebral aqueduct (Fig. 13-3). Superior to this opening is the small **posterior commissure.** Superior to the commissure is the **pineal recess,** which projects into the stalk of the **pineal body.** Superior to the pineal recess is the small **habenular commissure.**

The **lateral wall** is formed by the medial surface of the **thalamus** superiorly and the **hypothalamus** inferiorly (Fig. 13-3). These two structures are separated by the **hypothalamic sulcus.** The lateral wall is limited superiorly by the **stria medullaris thalami.** The lateral walls are joined by the **interthalamic connection.**

Fig. 13-6. The hypothalamic nuclei.
A. Medial zone nuclei lying medial to the plane of the fornix and the mammillothalamic tract.
B. Lateral zone nuclei lying lateral to the plane of the fornix and the mammillothalamic tract.

The **superior wall or roof** is formed by a layer of ependyma that is continuous with the lining of the ventricle. Superior to this layer is a two-layered fold of pia mater called the **tela choroidea of the third ventricle.** The vascular tela choroidea projects downward on each side of the midline, invaginating the ependymal roof to form the **choroid plexuses of the third ventricle.** Within the tela choroidea lie the **internal cerebral veins.** Superi-

orly, the roof of the ventricle is related to the **fornix** and the **corpus callosum.**

The **inferior wall or floor** is formed by the **optic chiasma,** the **tuber cinereum,** the **infundibulum,** with its funnel-shaped recess, and the **mammillary bodies** (Figs. 13-2 and 13-3). The **hypophysis** is attached to the infundibulum. Posterior to these structures lies the **tegmentum of the cerebral peduncles.**

CLINICAL NOTES

The **diencephalon** is a convenient term that encompasses the third ventricle and the structures that surround it. It is an anatomical term and the region has no specific function, since many systems enter and leave the area. It is customary to divide the diencephalon into four major areas: the thalamus, the subthalamus, the epithalamus, and the hypothalamus. Each of these areas and their connections are dealt with in detail in subsequent chapters. Only a brief overview of some important clinical features will be given here.

THALAMUS

The thalamus is a large mass of gray matter that forms the major part of the diencephalon and is a very important sensory relay station. Ascending sensory fibers synapse here and then are projected to the sensory areas of the cerebral cortex. Interference with this pathway causes sensory loss. The many connections that exist between the different nuclei within the thalamus are believed to permit an integration of much of the sensory information received by the thalamus. In this regard, it is interesting to note that the thalamus does not receive olfactory information directly.

The thalamus should be regarded as a primitive sensory center, and one that gives rise to a crude form of consciousness. For example, if the sensory cortex is destroyed, one can still appreciate the presence of a hot object in the hand; however, appreciation of the shape, weight, and exact temperature of the object would be impaired.

The many connections between the frontal cortex, the hypothalamus, and the thalamus indicate

that the thalamus plays a role in the integration of visceral and somatic functions.

LESIONS OF THE THALAMUS

Sensory Loss

These lesions usually result from thrombosis or hemorrhage of one of the arteries that supply the thalamus. Since the thalamus is concerned with receiving sensory impulses from the opposite side of the body, the disability resulting from a lesion within it will be confined to the contralateral side of the body. There may be a major impairment of all forms of sensation, which could include light touch, tactile localization and discrimination, and loss of appreciation of joint movements.

Thalamic Syndrome

This syndrome may occur as the patient is recovering from a thalamic infarct. Spontaneous pain, which is often excessive (thalamic overreaction), occurs on the opposite side of the body. The painful sensation may be aroused by light touch or by cold, and may fail to respond to powerful analgesic drugs.

Abnormal Involuntary Movements

Choreoathetosis with ataxia may follow vascular lesions of the thalamus. It is not certain whether these signs in all cases are due to the loss of function of the thalamus or to involvement of the neighboring caudate and lentiform nuclei. The ataxia may arise as the result of the loss of appreciation of muscle and joint movement owing to a thalamic lesion.

Thalamic Hand

The contralateral hand is held in an abnormal posture in some patients with thalamic lesions. The wrist is pronated and flexed, the metacarpophalangeal joints are flexed, and the interphalangeal joints are extended. The fingers can be moved actively, but the movements are slow. The condition is due to altered muscle tone in the different muscle groups.

Subthalamus

The subthalamus should be regarded as one of the extrapyramidal motor nuclei and has a large connection with the globus pallidus. Lesions of the subthalamus result in sudden, forceful involuntary movements in a contralateral extremity. The movements may be jerky (choreiform) or violent (ballistic).

Epithalamus

The epithalamus is composed largely of the habenular nuclei and their connections, and probably assists in the correlation of olfactory and somatic impulses. The **pineal gland** consists essentially of pinealocytes and glial cells supported by a connective tissue framework. The vascular pattern is that of an endocrine gland. As the result of regressive changes that occur with age, calcareous concretions accumulate within the glial cells and connective tissue of the gland. These deposits are useful to the radiologist, since they serve as a landmark and assist in determining whether the pineal gland has been displaced laterally by a space-occupying lesion within the skull.

The functions of the pineal gland are mainly inhibitory and have been shown to influence the pituitary gland, the islets of Langerhans, the parathyroids, the adrenals, and the gonads.

Although melatonin is present in high concentrations in the pineal gland and has been shown to cause the aggregation of melanin granules in frog melanophores, it apparently has no effect on mammalian melanocytes. Clinical observation of patients with pineal tumors has indicated that the pineal gland has an antigonadotropic function.

HYPOTHALAMUS

The hypothalamus is that area of the brain that forms the floor and lower part of the lateral wall of the third ventricle. Research and clinical observations have revealed that it is an area of the nervous system that is of great functional importance. Not only does it control emotional states, but it assists in the regulation of fat, carbohydrate, and water metabolism. Among its many other activities, it influences body temperature, genital functions, sleep, and food intake. The pituitary and the hypothalamus constitute a closely integrated unit and the hypothalamus plays a role in the release of pituitary hormones. For further clinical notes, see page 479.

SYNDROMES OF THE HYPOTHALAMUS

Lesions of the hypothalamus may result from infection, trauma, or vascular disorders. Tumors, such as a craniopharyngioma or **chromophobe adenoma of the pituitary** and **pineal tumors,** may interfere with the function of the hypothalamus. The most common abnormalities include **genital hypoplasia** or **atrophy, diabetes insipidus, obesity, disturbances of sleep, irregular pyrexia,** and **emaciation.** Some of these disorders may occur together, for example, in the **adiposogenital dystrophy syndrome.**

CLINICAL PROBLEMS

Answers on Page 601

1. A 45-year-old man who had suddenly developed a weakness of the left leg 12 hours previously was admitted to a medical ward. On examination, he was found to have paralysis of the left leg and weakness of the muscles of the left arm. The muscles of the affected limbs showed in-

creased tone and there was an exaggeration of the tendon reflexes on the left side of the body. There was also considerable sensory loss on the left side of the body, involving both the superficial and deep sensations. During the examination the patient would exhibit spontaneous jerking movements of the left leg. When asked to touch the tip of his nose with the left index finger, he demonstrated considerable intention tremor. The same test with the right arm showed nothing abnormal. Three days later, the patient started to complain of agonizing pain down the left leg. The pain would start spontaneously or be initiated by the light touch of the bed sheet. What is your diagnosis? How can you explain the various signs and symptoms?

2. A 53-year-old woman was admitted to an emergency department after she had collapsed in the street. Apart from being confused and disoriented, she exhibited violent, uncoordinated movements of her right arm and right leg and slight spontaneous movements on the right side of her face. The physician was able to ascertain from a friend that the patient had been perfectly fit that morning and had no previous history of this condition. On examination, the involuntary movements of the right limbs were mainly confined to the muscles of the proximal part of the limbs. One week later, the patient died of cardiac failure. What is the medical term used to describe this condition? Which area of the brain is likely to be involved in the production of this condition?

3. A 64-year-old man was admitted to a hospital on the suspicion that he had a cerebral tumor. One of the investigations asked for by the physician was a simple anteroposterior and lateral radiograph of the head. Using your knowledge of neuroanatomy, name the structure that would assist the radiologist in this case in determining whether lateral displacement of the brain had occurred within the skull.

4. During a discussion with a dermatologist that followed the examination of a patient with vitiligo, a fourth-year medical student suggested that excessive production of melatonin by the patient might be responsible for the condition. What is the action of melatonin on melanocytes in the skin? Where is melatonin normally produced?

5. A 12-year-old boy was seen by a pediatrician because his parents were concerned about his excessive weight and lack of development of the external genitalia. On examination, the child was seen to be tall for his age and very obese. The excessive fat was concentrated especially in the lower part of the anterior abdominal wall and the proximal parts of the limbs. His penis and testes were small. Is it possible that disease of the diencephalon might account for this condition?

NATIONAL BOARD TYPE QUESTIONS

Answers on Page 620

In each of the following questions, answer:
  (a) If (1) only is correct
  (b) If (2) only is correct
  (c) If both (1) and (2) are correct, and
  (d) If neither (1) nor (2) is correct

1. Which of the following statements is (are) correct concerning the diencephalon?
   (1) It extends anteriorly as far as the interventricular foramen.
   (2) It is bounded laterally by the internal capsule.

2. Which of the following statements is (are) correct concerning the structures that make up the diencephalon?
   (1) The thalamus is located in the lateral wall of the third ventricle.
   (2) The epithalamus is formed by the cranial end of the substantia nigra and the red nuclei.

3. Which of the following statements is (are) correct concerning the pineal gland?
   (1) It produces a secretion that is opaque to x-rays.
   (2) It contains high concentrations of melatonin and serotonin.

Select the best response:

4. The following statements concerning the thalamus are correct **except**:
   (a) It is the largest part of the diencephalon and serves as a relay station to all the main

sensory tracts (except the olfactory pathway).

(b) It is separated from the lentiform nucleus by the internal capsule.

(c) It forms the anterior boundary of the interventricular foramen.

(d) It may be joined to the thalamus on the opposite side.

(e) The gray matter of the thalamus is divided by a vertical sheet of white matter called the internal medullary lamina.

5. The following statements concerning the hypothalamus are correct **except**:

(a) It is formed by the lower part of the lateral wall and floor of the third ventricle.

(b) Functionally, it is usual to include with the hypothalamus the area between the lamina terminalis and the optic chiasma.

(c) Caudally the hypothalamus merges with the tectum of the midbrain.

(d) The nuclei are divided into medial and lateral zones by the columns of the fornix and the mammillothalamic tract.

(e) The mammillary bodies are part of the hypothalamus.

In the following questions, answer:

(a) IF (1), (2), AND (3) ONLY ARE CORRECT

(b) IF (1) AND (3) ONLY ARE CORRECT

(c) IF (2) AND (4) ONLY ARE CORRECT

(d) IF (4) ONLY IS CORRECT

(e) IF ALL ARE CORRECT

6. Which of the following statements is (are) correct concerning the hypothalamus?

(1) The hypothalamus controls and integrates the activities of the autonomic and endocrine systems.

(2) It receives many afferent visceral and somatic sensory fibers.

(3) It gives off efferent fibers that pass to the sympathetic and parasympathetic outflows in the brain and spinal cord.

(4) It sends no nerve fibers to the hypophysis cerebri.

7. Which of the following statements is (are) correct concerning the third ventricle?

(1) The posterior wall is formed by the opening into the cerebral aqueduct and the pineal recess.

(2) It does not communicate directly with the lateral ventricles.

(3) The vascular tela choroidea projects from the roof to form the choroid plexus.

(4) Lying in the floor of the ventricle from anterior to posterior are the mammillary bodies, the optic chiasma, and the tuber cinereum.

In Figure 13-7, match the numbers listed on the left with the appropriate structures listed on the right. The answers may be used more than once.

8. Number 1
9. Number 2
10. Number 3
11. Number 4
12. Number 5
13. Number 6
14. Number 7

(a) Genu of corpus callosum

(b) Interventricular foramen

(c) Body of fornix

(d) Anterior commissure

(e) None of the above

Fig. 13-7. Sagittal section of the brain showing the medial surface of the diencephalon.

ADDITIONAL READING

Axelrod, J. The pineal gland. *Endeavour* 29:144, 1970.

Haywood, J. N. Functional and morphological aspects of hypothalamic neurons. *Physiol. Rev.* 57:574, 1977.

Kappers, J. A. The mammalian pineal gland: A survey. *Acta Neurochir. Genesskd.* 120:109, 1976.

Kappers, J. A. Short History of Pineal Discovery and Research. In J. A. Kappers and P. Peret (eds.), *The Pineal Gland of Vertebrates Including Man. Proceedings of the First Colloquim of the European Study Group (EPSG), Amsterdam, 1978* (Progress in Brain Research, vol. 52). Amsterdam: Biomedical Press, 1978. P. 3.

Lederis, K., and Veale, W. L. (Eds.). *Current Studies of Hypothalamic Function.* New York: Karger, 1978.

Morgane, P. J., and Panksepp, J. (Eds.). *Handbook of the Hypothalamus.* Vol. 1:*Anatomy of the Hypothalamus.* New York: Dekker, 1979.

Snell, R. S. Effect of melatonin on mammalian epidermal melanocytes. *J. Invest. Dermatol.* 44:273, 1965.

Sowers, J. R. (Ed.). *Hypothalamic Hormones.* Stroudsburg, Pennsylvania: Dowden, Hutchinson & Ross, 1980.

Swanson, L. W., and Sawchenko, P. E. Hypothalamic integration: Organization of the paraventricular and supraoptic nuclei. *Ann. Rev. Neurosci.* 6:269, 1983.

Walton, J. N. *Brain's Diseases of the Nervous System* (8th ed.). New York and London: Oxford University Press, 1977.

Chapter 14
The Cerebral Hemispheres

The cerebral hemispheres are separated by a deep midline sagittal fissure, the **longitudinal cerebral fissure** (Fig. 14-1). The fissure contains the sickle-shaped fold of dura mater, the **falx cerebri,** and the **anterior cerebral arteries.** In the depths of the fissure, the great commissure, the **corpus callosum,** connects the hemispheres across the midline (Fig. 14-1). A second horizontal fold of dura mater separates the cerebral hemispheres from the cerebellum and is called the **tentorium cerebelli.**

In order to increase the surface area of the cerebral cortex maximally, the surface of each cerebral hemisphere is thrown into **folds** or **gyri,** which are separated from each other by **sulci** or **fissures** (Fig. 14-1). For ease of description, it is customary to divide each hemisphere into **lobes,** which are named according to the cranial bones under which they lie. The **central and parieto-occipital sulci** and the **lateral and calcarine sulci** are boundaries used for the division of the cerebral hemisphere into **frontal, parietal, temporal,** and **occipital lobes** (Figs. 14-2 and 14-6).

MAIN SULCI

The **central sulcus** (Fig. 14-2) is of great importance because the gyrus that lies anterior to it contains the motor cells that initiate the movements of the opposite side of the body; posterior to it lies the general sensory cortex that receives sensory information from the opposite side of the body. The central sulcus indents the superior medial border of the hemisphere about 0.4 inch (1 cm) behind the midpoint (Fig. 14-3). It runs downward and forward across the lateral aspect of the hemisphere, and its lower end is separated from the posterior ramus of the lateral sulcus by a narrow bridge of cortex. The central sulcus is the only sulcus of any length on this surface of the hemisphere that indents the supermedial border and lies between two parallel gyri.

The **lateral sulcus** (Fig. 14-2) is a deep cleft found mainly on the inferior and lateral surfaces of the cerebral hemisphere. It consists of a short stem that divides into three rami. The stem arises on the

Fig. 14-1. Superior view of cerebral hemispheres.

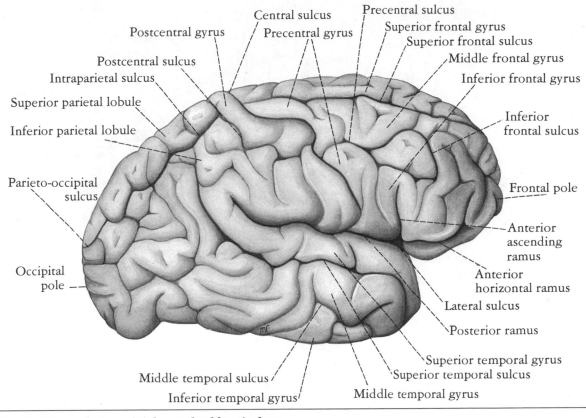

Fig. 14-2. Lateral view of right cerebral hemisphere.

inferior surface and on reaching the lateral surface it divides into the **anterior horizontal ramus** and the **anterior ascending ramus,** and continues as the **posterior ramus** (Figs. 14-2 and 14-5). An area of cortex called the **insula** lies at the bottom of the deep lateral sulcus and cannot be seen from the surface unless the lips of the sulcus are separated (Fig. 14-4).

The **parieto-occipital sulcus** begins on the superior medial margin of the hemisphere about 2 inches (5 cm) anterior to the occipital pole (Figs. 14-3 and 14-5). It passes downward and anteriorly on the medial surface to meet the calcarine sulcus (Fig. 14-3).

The **calcarine sulcus** is found on the medial surface of the hemisphere (Figs. 14-3 and 14-5). It commences under the posterior end of the corpus callosum and arches upward and backward to reach the occipital pole, where it stops. In some

brains, however, it continues for a short distance onto the lateral surface of the hemisphere. The calcarine sulcus is joined at an acute angle by the parieto-occipital sulcus about halfway along its length.

LOBES OF THE CEREBRAL HEMISPHERE

Superolateral Surface of the Hemisphere

The **frontal lobe** occupies the area anterior to the central sulcus and superior to the lateral sulcus (Figs. 14-5 and 14-6). The superolateral surface of the frontal lobe is divided by three sulci into four gyri. The **precentral sulcus** runs parallel to the central sulcus and the **precentral gyrus** lies between them (Figs. 14-2 and 14-5). Extending ante-

Fig. 14-3. Medial view of right cerebral hemisphere.

riorly from the precentral sulcus are the **superior and inferior frontal sulci.** The **superior frontal gyrus** lies superior to the superior frontal sulcus, the **middle frontal gyrus** lies between the superior and inferior frontal sulci, and the **inferior frontal gyrus** lies inferior to the inferior frontal sulcus (Figs. 14-2 and 14-5). The inferior frontal gyrus is invaded by the anterior and ascending rami of the lateral sulcus.

The **parietal lobe** occupies the area posterior to the central sulcus and superior to the lateral sulcus; it extends posteriorly as far as the parieto-occipital sulcus (Figs. 14-2, 14-5, and 14-6). The lateral surface of the parietal lobe is divided by two sulci into three gyri. The **postcentral sulcus** runs parallel to the central sulcus and the **postcentral gyrus** lies

between them. Running posteriorly from the middle of the postcentral sulcus is the **intraparietal sulcus** (Figs. 14-2 and 14-5). The intraparietal sulcus has superior to it the **superior parietal lobule** (gyrus) and inferior to it the **inferior parietal lobule** (gyrus).

The **temporal lobe** occupies the area inferior to the lateral sulcus (Figs. 14-2, 14-5, and 14-6). The lateral surface of the temporal lobe is divided into three gyri by two sulci. The **superior** and **middle temporal sulci** run parallel to the posterior ramus of the lateral sulcus, and divide the temporal lobe into the **superior, middle,** and **inferior temporal gyri;** the inferior temporal gyrus is continued onto the inferior surface of the hemisphere (Figs. 14-2 and 14-5).

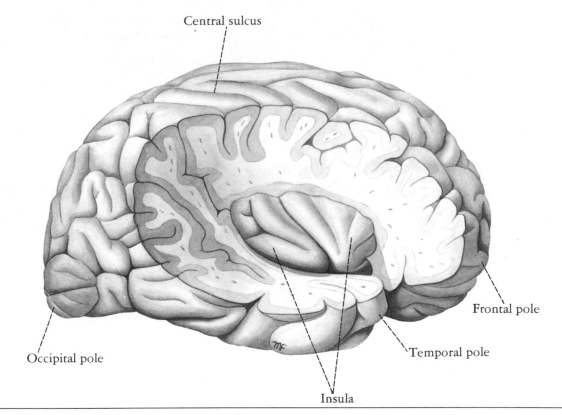

Fig. 14-4. Lateral view of right cerebral hemisphere dissected to reveal the right insula.

The **occipital lobe** occupies the small area behind the parieto-occipital sulcus (Figs. 14-2, 14-5, and 14-6).

Medial and Inferior Surface of the Hemisphere

The lobes of the cerebral hemisphere are not clearly defined on the medial and inferior surfaces. However, there are many important areas that should be recognized. The **corpus callosum,** which is the largest commissure of the brain, forms a striking feature on this surface (Figs. 14-3 and 14-5). The **cingulate gyrus** begins beneath the anterior end of the corpus callosum and continues above the corpus callosum until it reaches its posterior end (Figs. 14-3 and 14-5). The gyrus is separated from the corpus callosum by the **callosal**

sulcus. The cingulate gyrus is separated from the superior frontal gyrus by the **cingulate sulcus** (Fig. 14-5).

The **paracentral lobule** is the area of the cerebral cortex that surrounds the indentation produced by the central sulcus on the superior border (Figs. 14-3 and 14-5). The anterior part of this lobule is a continuation of the precentral gyrus on the superior lateral surface, and the posterior part of the lobule is a continuation of the postcentral gyrus.

The **precuneus** (Figs. 14-3 and 14-5) is an area of cortex bounded anteriorly by the upturned posterior end of the cingulate sulcus and posteriorly by the parieto-occipital sulcus.

The **cuneus** (Figs. 14-3 and 14-5) is a triangular area of cortex bounded above by the parieto-occipital sulcus, inferiorly by the calcarine sulcus, and posteriorly by the superior medial margin.

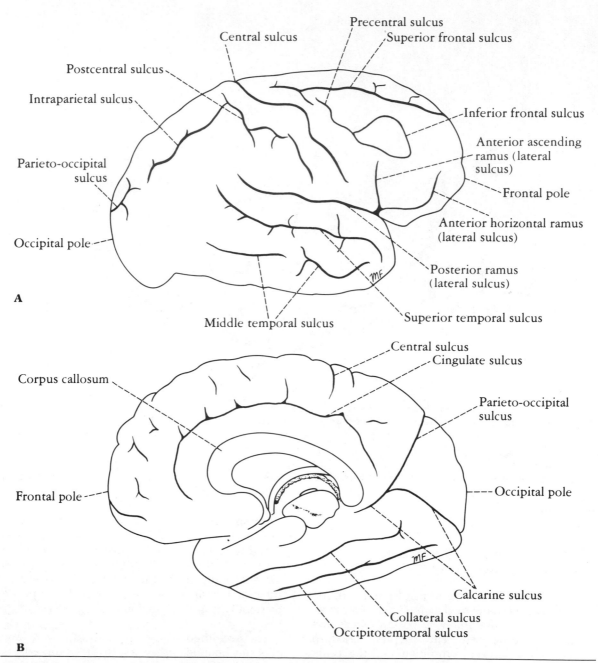

**Fig. 14-5. A. Lateral view of right cerebral hemisphere showing main sulci.
B. Medial view of right cerebral hemisphere showing main sulci.**

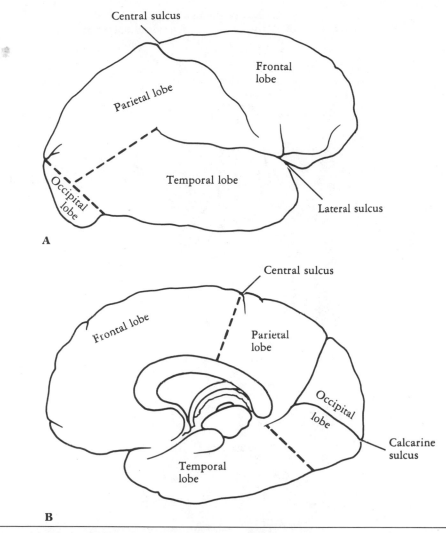

Central sulcus

Frontal lobe

Parietal lobe

Occipital lobe

Temporal lobe

Lateral sulcus

A

Central sulcus

Frontal lobe

Parietal lobe

Occipital lobe

Calcarine sulcus

Temporal lobe

B

**Fig. 14-6. A. Lateral view of right cerebral hemisphere showing lobes.
B. Medial view of right cerebral hemisphere showing lobes. Note that the dashed lines indicate the approximate position of the boundaries where there are no sulci.**

The **collateral sulcus** is situated on the inferior surface of the hemisphere (Figs. 14-3 and 14-7). This runs anteriorly below the calcarine sulcus. Between the collateral sulcus and the **calcarine sulcus** is the **lingual gyrus.** Anterior to the lingual gyrus is the **parahippocampal gyrus;** the latter terminates in front as the hooklike **uncus** (Fig. 14-7).

The **medial occipitotemporal gyrus** extends from the occipital pole to the temporal pole (Fig.

14-7). It is bounded medially by the **collateral** and **rhinal sulci** and laterally by the **occipitotemporal sulcus.** The **occipitotemporal gyrus** lies lateral to the sulcus and is continuous with the inferior temporal gyrus (Fig. 14-7).

On the inferior surface of the frontal lobe, the olfactory bulb and tract overlie a sulcus called the **olfactory sulcus** (Fig. 14-7). Medial to the olfactory sulcus is the **gyrus rectus** and lateral to the sulcus are a number of **orbital gyri.**

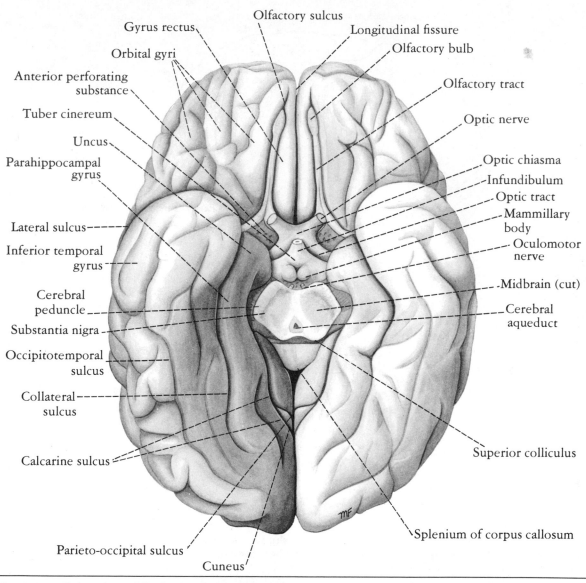

Fig. 14-7. Inferior view of the brain; the medulla oblongata, the pons, and the cerebellum have been removed.

INTERNAL STRUCTURE OF THE CEREBRAL HEMISPHERES

The cerebral hemispheres are covered with a layer of gray matter, the cerebral cortex, the structure and function of which will be dealt with in Chapter 15. Located in the interior of the cerebral hemispheres are the **lateral ventricles,** masses of gray matter, the **basal nuclei,** and nerve fibers. The nerve fibers are embedded in neuroglia and constitute the **white matter** (Fig. 14-9).

Lateral Ventricles

There are two lateral ventricles and one is present in each cerebral hemisphere (Figs. 14-8, 14-9, and 14-10). Each ventricle is a roughly **C**-shaped cavity lined with ependyma and filled with cerebrospinal fluid (Fig. 14-8). The lateral ventricle may be divided into a **body,** which occupies the parietal lobe, and from which **anterior, posterior,** and **inferior horns** extend into the frontal, occipital, and temporal lobes, respectively. The lateral ventricle communicates with the cavity of the third ventricle through the **interventricular foramen** (Figs. 14-3 and 14-8). This opening, which lies in the anterior part of the medial wall of the lateral ventricle, is bounded anteriorly by the anterior column of the fornix and posteriorly by the anterior end of the thalamus.

The **body of the lateral ventricle** extends from the interventricular foramen posteriorly as far as the posterior end of the thalamus. Here it becomes continuous with the posterior and the inferior horns. The body of the lateral ventricle has a roof, a floor, and a medial wall (Fig. 14-10).

The **roof** is formed by the undersurface of the **corpus callosum** (Fig. 14-10). The **floor** is formed by the body of the **caudate nucleus** and the lateral margin of the thalamus. The superior surface of the thalamus is obscured in its medial part by the **body of the fornix.** The **choroid plexus** of the ventricle projects into the body of the ventricle through the slitlike gap between the body of the fornix and the superior surface of the thalamus. This slitlike gap is known as the **choroidal fissure;** through it the blood vessels of the plexus invaginate the pia mater of the tela choroidea and the ependyma of the lateral ventricle. The **medial wall** is formed by the **septum pellucidum** ante-

riorly; posteriorly the roof and the floor come together on the medial wall (Fig. 14-10).

The **anterior horn of the lateral ventricle** extends forward into the frontal lobe (Figs. 14-8 and 14-10). It is continuous posteriorly with the body of the ventricle at the interventricular foramen. The anterior horn has a roof, a floor, and a medial wall. The **roof** is formed by the undersurface of the anterior part of the **corpus callosum;** the **genu of the corpus callosum** limits the anterior horn anteriorly (Fig. 14-10). The **floor** is formed by the rounded **head of the caudate nucleus,** and medially a small portion is formed by the superior surface of the **rostrum of the corpus callosum.** The **medial wall** is formed by the **septum pellucidum** and the **anterior column of the fornix** (Fig. 14-10).

The **posterior horn of the lateral ventricle** extends posteriorly into the occipital lobe (Figs. 14-8 and 14-10). The **roof** and **lateral wall** are formed by the fibers of the **tapetum** of the **corpus callosum.** Lateral to the tapetum are the fibers of the **optic radiation** (Fig. 14-10). The **medial wall** of the posterior horn has two elevations. The superior swelling is caused by the splenial fibers of the corpus callosum, called the **forceps major,** passing posteriorly into the occipital lobe; this superior swelling is referred to as the **bulb of the posterior horn.** The inferior swelling is produced by the **calcarine sulcus** and is called the **calcar avis** (Fig. 14-10).

The **inferior horn of the lateral ventricle** extends anteriorly into the temporal lobe (Fig. 14-8). The inferior horn has a roof and a floor (Fig. 14-10).

The **roof** is formed by the inferior surface of the **tapetum of the corpus callosum** and by the **tail of the caudate nucleus** (see Fig. 16-4). The latter passes anteriorly to end in the **amygdaloid nucleus.** Medial to the tail of the caudate nucleus is the **stria terminalis,** which also ends anteriorly in the amygdaloid nucleus.

The **floor** is formed laterally by the **collateral eminence,** produced by the **collateral** fissure, and medially by the **hippocampus** (see Figs. 16-3 and 16-4). The anterior end of the hippocampus is expanded and slightly furrowed to form the **pes hippocampus.** The hippocampus is composed of gray matter; however, the ventricular surface of the hippocampus is covered by a thin layer of white mat-

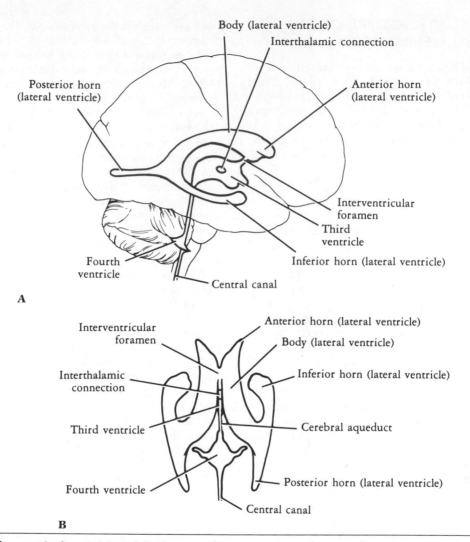

Fig. 14-8. The ventricular cavities of the brain.
A. Lateral view.
B. Superior view.

ter called the **alveus,** which is formed from the axons of the cells of the hippocampus. These axons converge on the medial border of the hippocampus to form a bundle known as the **fimbria.** The fimbria of the hippocampus becomes continuous posteriorly with the **posterior column of the fornix.**

In the interval between the stria terminalis and the fimbria is the temporal part of the choroidal fissure. It is here that the lower part of the **choroid plexus** of the lateral ventricle invaginates the ep-

endyma from the medial side and closes the fissure (see Fig. 16-4).

Basal Nuclei (Basal Ganglia)

The term **basal nuclei** is applied to a collection of masses of gray matter situated within each cerebral hemisphere. They are the corpus striatum, the amygdaloid nucleus, and the claustrum.

Fig. 14-9. Horizontal section of the cerebrum as seen from above, showing the relationship between the lentiform nucleus, the caudate nucleus, the thalamus, and the internal capsule.

Corpus Striatum

The corpus striatum is situated lateral to the thalamus. It is almost completely divided by a band of nerve fibers, the **internal capsule,** into the caudate nucleus and the lentiform nucleus (Figs. 14-9 and 14-14).

The **caudate nucleus,** a large C-shaped mass of gray matter that is closely related to the lateral ventricle, lies lateral to the thalamus (Fig. 14-11). The

lateral surface of the nucleus is related to the internal capsule, which separates it from the lentiform nucleus.

The **lentiform nucleus** is a wedge-shaped mass of gray matter, whose broad convex base is directed laterally and its blade medially (Figs. 14-9 and 14-11). It is buried deep in the white matter of the cerebral hemisphere and is related medially to the internal capsule, which separates it from the caudate nucleus and the thalamus. The lentiform nu-

Fig. 14-10. Coronal sections of brain passing through:
A. The anterior horn of the lateral ventricle.
B. The body of the lateral ventricle.
C. The posterior horn of the lateral ventricle.

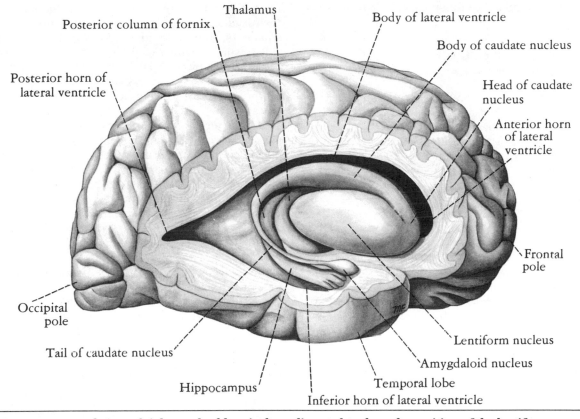

Posterior column of fornix

Thalamus

Body of lateral ventricle

Body of caudate nucleus

Posterior horn of lateral ventricle

Head of caudate nucleus

Anterior horn of lateral ventricle

Frontal pole

Occipital pole

Lentiform nucleus

Tail of caudate nucleus

Amygdaloid nucleus

Temporal lobe

Hippocampus

Inferior horn of lateral ventricle

Fig. 14-11. Lateral view of right cerebral hemisphere dissected to show the position of the lentiform nucleus, the caudate nucleus, the thalamus, and the hippocampus.

cleus is related laterally to a thin sheet of white matter, the **external capsule** (Fig. 14-9), that separates it from a thin sheet of gray matter, called the **claustrum** (Fig. 14-9). The claustrum, in turn, separates the external capsule from the subcortical white matter of the insula. Inferiorly at its anterior end, the lentiform nucleus is continuous with the caudate nucleus.

The detailed structure and connections of the corpus striatum will be considered in Chapter 17. Briefly, it may be stated that the corpus striatum receives afferent fibers from different areas of the cerebral cortex, the thalamus, subthalamus, and brainstem. Efferent fibers then travel back to the same areas of the nervous system. The function of the corpus striatum is concerned with muscular movement, which now is believed to be accom-

plished by controlling the cerebral cortex rather than through direct descending pathways to the brainstem and spinal cord.

Amygdaloid Nucleus

The amygdaloid nucleus is situated in the temporal lobe close to the uncus (Fig. 14-11). The amygdaloid nucleus is considered part of the limbic system and is described in Chapter 16.

Claustrum

The claustrum is a thin sheet of gray matter that is separated from the lateral surface of the lentiform nucleus by the **external capsule** (Fig. 14-9). Lateral to the claustrum is the subcortical white matter of the insula. The function of the claustrum is unknown.

White Matter of the Cerebral Hemispheres

The white matter is composed of myelinated nerve fibers of different diameters supported by neuroglia. The nerve fibers may be classified into three groups according to their connections: (1) commissural fibers, (2) association fibers, and (3) projection fibers.

Commissures

These fibers essentially connect corresponding regions of the two hemispheres. They are as follows: the corpus callosum, the anterior commissure, the posterior commissure, the fornix, and the habenular commissure.

The **corpus callosum,** the largest commissure of the brain, connects the two cerebral hemispheres (Figs. 14-3 and 14-12). It lies at the bottom of the longitudinal fissure. For purposes of description, it is divided into the rostrum, the genu, the body, and the splenium.

The **rostrum** is the thin part of the anterior end of the corpus callosum, which is prolonged posteriorly to be continuous with the upper end of the lamina terminalis (Fig. 14-3).

The **genu** is the curved anterior end of the corpus callosum that bends inferiorly in front of the septum pellucidum (Figs. 14-3 and 14-12).

The **body** of the corpus callosum arches posteriorly and ends as the thickened posterior portion called the **splenium** (Fig. 14-12).

Traced laterally, the fibers of the genu curve forward into the frontal lobes and form the **forceps minor** (Fig. 14-12). The fibers of the body extend laterally as the **radiation of the corpus callosum** (Fig. 14-12). They intersect with bundles of association and projection fibers as they pass to the cerebral cortex. Some of the fibers form the roof and lateral wall of the posterior horn of the lateral ventricle and the lateral wall of the inferior horn of the lateral ventricle; these fibers are referred to as the **tapetum.** Traced laterally, the fibers in the splenium arch backward into the occipital lobe and form the **forceps major** (Fig. 14-12).

The **anterior commissure** is a small bundle of nerve fibers that cross the midline in the **lamina terminalis** (Fig. 14-3). When traced laterally, a smaller or anterior bundle curves forward on each side toward the anterior perforated substance and the olfactory tract. A larger bundle curves posteriorly on each side and grooves the inferior surface of the lentiform nucleus to reach the temporal lobes.

The **posterior commissure** is a bundle of nerve fibers that cross the midline immediately above the opening of the cerebral aqueduct into the third ventricle (see Fig. 13-3); it is related to the inferior part of the stalk of the pineal gland. Various collections of nerve cells are situated along its length. The destinations and functional significance of many of the nerve fibers are not known. However, the fibers from the pretectal nuclei involved in the pupillary light reflex are believed to cross in this commissure on their way to the parasympathetic part of the oculomotor nuclei (see p. 425).

The **fornix** is composed of myelinated nerve fibers and constitutes the efferent system of the hippocampus that passes to the mammillary bodies of the hypothalamus (see p. 321). The nerve fibers first form the **alveus** (see Fig. 16-4), which is a thin layer of white matter covering the ventricular surface of the hippocampus, then converge to form the **fimbria.** The fimbriae of the two sides increase in thickness and, on reaching the posterior end of the hippocampus, they arch forward above the thalamus and below the corpus callosum to form the **posterior columns of the fornix.** The two columns then come together in the midline to form the **body of the fornix** (Fig. 14-13). A more detailed description of the fornix is given on page 321. The **commissure of the fornix** consists of transverse fibers that cross the midline from one column to another just before the formation of the body of the fornix. The function of the commissure of the fornix is to connect the hippocampal formations of the two sides.

The **habenular commissure** is a small bundle of nerve fibers that cross the midline in the superior part of the root of the pineal stalk (see Fig. 13-3). The commissure is associated with the **habenular nuclei,** which are situated on either side of the midline in this region. The habenular nuclei receive many afferents from the amygdaloid nuclei and the hippocampus. These afferent fibers pass to the habenular nuclei in the **stria medullaris thal-**

Fig. 14-12. A. Coronal section of the brain passing through the anterior horn of the lateral ventricle and the optic chiasma.
B. Superior view of the brain dissected to show the fibers of the corpus callosum and the corona radiata.

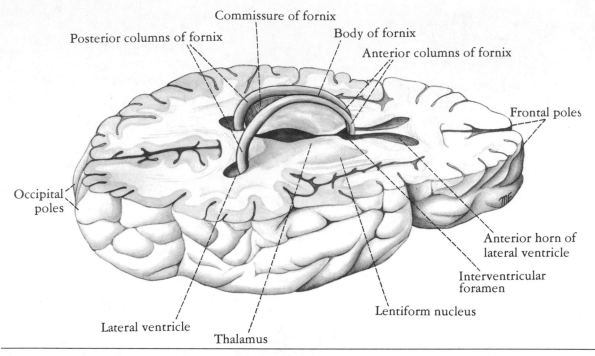

Commissure of fornix

Posterior columns of fornix

Body of fornix

Anterior columns of fornix

Frontal poles

Occipital poles

Anterior horn of lateral ventricle

Interventricular foramen

Lentiform nucleus

Lateral ventricle

Thalamus

Fig. 14-13. Horizontal section of the brain leaving the fornix in position.

ami. Some of the fibers cross the midline to reach the contralateral nucleus through the habenular commissure. The function of the habenular nucleus and its connections in man is unknown.

Association Fibers

These nerve fibers essentially connect various cortical regions within the same hemisphere and may be divided into short and long groups (Fig. 14-15). The **short association fibers** lie immediately beneath the cortex and connect adjacent gyri; these fibers run transversely to the long axis of the sulci (Fig. 14-15). The **long association fibers** are collected into named bundles that can be dissected in a formalin-hardened brain. The **uncinate fasciculus** connects the first motor speech area and the gyri on the inferior surface of the frontal lobe with the cortex of the pole of the temporal lobe. The **cingulum** is a long, curved fasciculus lying within the white matter of the cingulate gyrus (Fig. 14-3). It connects the frontal and parietal lobes with para-

hippocampal and adjacent temporal cortical regions. The **superior longitudinal fasciculus** is the largest bundle of nerve fibers. It connects the anterior part of the frontal lobe to the occipital and temporal lobes. The **inferior longitudinal fasciculus** runs anteriorly from the occipital lobe, passing lateral to the optic radiation, and is distributed to the temporal lobe. The **fronto-occipital fasciculus** connects the frontal lobe to the occipital and temporal lobes. It is situated deep within the cerebral hemisphere and is related to the lateral border of the caudate nucleus.

Projection Fibers

Afferent and efferent nerve fibers passing to and from the brainstem to the entire cerebral cortex must travel between large nuclear masses of gray matter within the cerebral hemisphere. At the upper part of the brainstem these fibers form a compact band known as the **internal capsule,** which is flanked medially by the caudate nucleus and the

Genu of corpus callosum

Head of caudate nucleus

Frontopontine fibers

Thalamocortical fibers
to frontal lobe

Lentiform nucleus

Corticonuclear fibers
(head and neck)

Corticospinal fibers
(upper limb)

Corticospinal fibers
(trunk) and
corticorubral fibers

Corticospinal fibers
(lower limb)

Temporopontine fibers

Auditory radiation

Optic radiation

Anterior horn of
lateral ventricle

Anterior limb of
internal capsule

Genu of internal
capsule

Thalamus

Thalamocortical
fibers to parietal lobe
(general sensation)

Posterior limb of
internal capsule

Splenium of
corpus callosum

Lateral ventricle

Fig. 14-14. Horizontal section of the right cerebral hemisphere showing the relationships and different parts of the internal capsule.

thalamus, and laterally by the lentiform nucleus (Fig. 14-9). Because of the wedge shape of the lentiform nucleus, as seen on horizontal section, the internal capsule is bent to form an **anterior limb** and a **posterior limb,** which are continuous with each other at the **genu** (Figs. 14-14 and 14-16). Once the nerve fibers have emerged superiorly from between the nuclear masses, they radiate in all directions to the cerebral cortex. These radiating projection fibers are known as the **corona radiata** (Fig. 14-16). Most of the projection fibers lie medial to the association fibers, but they intersect the commissural fibers of the corpus callosum and the anterior commissure. The nerve fibers lying within the most posterior part of the posterior limb of the internal capsule radiate toward the calcarine sulcus and are known as the **optic radiation** (Fig. 14-14). The detailed arrangement of the fibers within the internal capsule is shown in Figure 14-14.

Septum Pellucidum

The septum pellucidum is a thin vertical sheet of nervous tissue consisting of white and gray matter covered on either side by ependyma (Figs. 14-3 and 14-9). It stretches between the fornix and the corpus callosum. Anteriorly, it occupies the interval between the body of the corpus callosum and the rostrum. It is essentially a double membrane with a closed, slitlike cavity between the membranes. The septum pellucidum forms a partition between the anterior horns of the lateral ventricles.

Fig. 14-15. Lateral view of the right cerebral hemisphere, which has been dissected to show some of the principal association fibers.

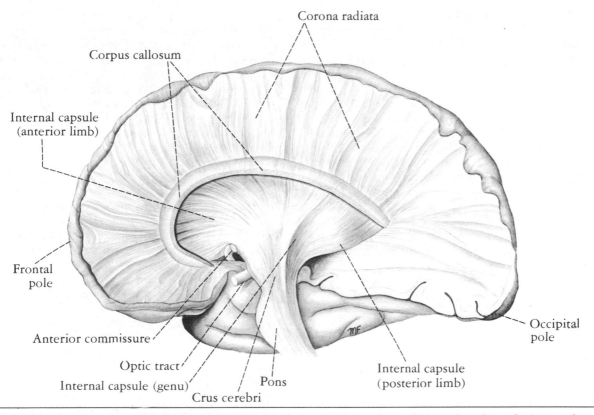

Fig. 14-16. Medial view of the right cerebral hemisphere, which has been dissected to show the internal capsule and the corona radiata. The thalamus has been removed. Note the interdigitation of the horizontally running fibers of the corpus callosum and the vertical fibers of the corona radiata.

Tela Choroidea

The tela choroidea is a two-layered fold of pia mater. It is situated between the fornix superiorly and the roof of the third ventricle and the upper surfaces of the two thalami inferiorly. When seen from above, the anterior end is situated at the interventricular foramina (see Fig. 18-4). Its lateral edges are irregular and project laterally into the body of the lateral ventricles. Here they are covered by ependyma and form the choroid plexuses of the lateral ventricle. Posteriorly, the lateral edges continue into the inferior horn of the lateral ventricle and are covered with ependyma so that the choroid plexus projects through the choroidal fissure.

On either side of the midline the tela choroidea projects down through the roof of the third ventricle to form the choroid plexuses of the third ventricle.

The blood supply of the tela choroidea and, therefore, also the choroid plexuses of the third and lateral ventricle are derived from the **choroidal branches of the internal carotid and basilar arteries.** The venous blood drains into the **internal cerebral veins,** which unite to form the **great cerebral vein.** The great cerebral vein joins the **inferior sagittal sinus** to form the **straight sinus.**

CLINICAL NOTES

CEREBRAL CORTEX, SULCI, AND LOBES OF THE CEREBRAL HEMISPHERE

The cerebral cortex is composed of gray matter. Only about one-third lies on the exposed convexity of the gyri; the remaining two-thirds form the walls of the sulci. The major part of the cortex can be divided into six laminae, which exhibit marked regional differences in structure, as will be described in Chapter 15. Moreover, different areas of the cortex have different functions, and the anatomical division of the cortex into lobes and gyri by sulci enables the physician to localize loss of function or accurately place a brain lesion. For example, focal lesions of the precentral gyrus will produce contralateral hemiparesis, while lesions of the postcentral gyrus will result in contralateral hemisensory loss. More widespread lesions of the frontal lobe might cause symptoms and signs indicative of loss of attention span or change in social behavior. Widespread degeneration of the cerebral cortex gives rise to symptoms of dementia.

LATERAL VENTRICLES

Each lateral ventricle contains about 7 to 10 ml of cerebrospinal fluid. This fluid is produced in the choroid plexus of the lateral ventricle and normally drains into the third ventricle through the interventricular foramen (foramen of Monro). Blockage of the foramen by a cerebral tumor would result in distention of the ventricle, thus producing a type of **hydrocephalus.**

The choroid plexus of the lateral ventricle is continuous with that of the third ventricle through the interventricular foramen. The choroid plexus is largest where the body and posterior and inferior horns join, and it is here that it may become calcified with age. It is important that this calcification, as seen on radiographs, is not confused with that of the pineal gland.

In the past, the size and shape of the lateral ventricle was investigated clinically by pneumoencephalography (Figs. 14-17 through 14-20). In this procedure, small amounts of air were introduced into the subarachnoid space by lumbar puncture with the patient in the sitting position. If the patient already had a raised intracranial pressure, this method was dangerous (see p. 32), and air or radiopaque fluid was injected directly into the lateral ventricles through a burr hole in the skull (this procedure was referred to as **ventriculography**). Although occasionally still used, this procedure has been replaced by CT scans and MRI (Figs. 14-21 through 14-24).

BASAL NUCLEI

The **basal nuclei,** in this discussion, refers to the masses of gray matter that are deeply placed within the cerebrum. They include the caudate nucleus, the lentiform nucleus, the amygdaloid nucleus, and the claustrum.

Because of the close relationship that exists between these nuclei and the internal capsule, tumors of the caudate or lentiform nuclei may cause severe motor or sensory symptoms on the opposite side of the body. Tumors pressing on the anterior limb of the internal capsule will cause progressive spastic hemiplegia, while more posteriorly situated tumors will produce impairment of sensation on the opposite side.

Disorders of function of the basal nuclei will be considered after the connections of these nuclei have been discussed in Chapter 17.

COMMISSURES OF THE CEREBRUM

The major commissure is the large corpus callosum. The majority of the fibers within the corpus callosum interconnect symmetrical areas of the cerebral cortex. Because it transfers information from one hemisphere to another, the corpus callosum is essential for learned discrimination, sensory experience, and memory.

Occasionally the corpus callosum fails to develop and in these individuals no definite signs or symptoms appear. Should the corpus callosum be destroyed by disease in later life, however, each hemisphere becomes isolated and the patient responds as if he has two separate brains. His general intelligence and behavior appear normal, since over the years both hemispheres have been trained to respond to different situations. If a pencil is placed

Fig. 14-17. Anteroposterior pneumoencephalogram of a 28-year-old man.

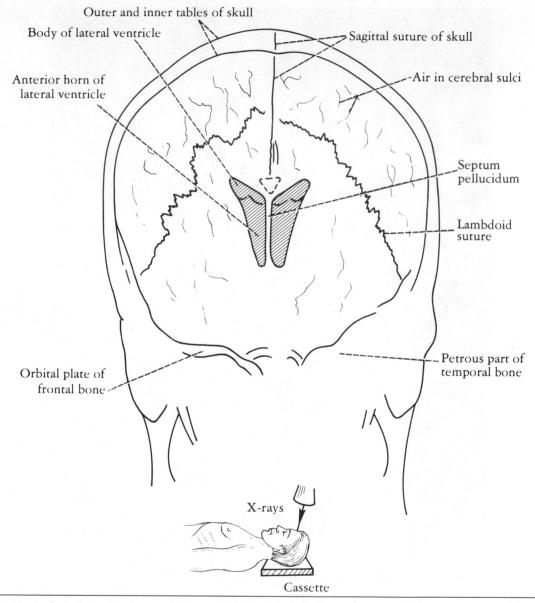

Fig. 14-18. Explanation of radiograph seen in Figure 14-17. Note the position of the x-ray gun relative to the head and the film cassette.

Fig. 14-19. Lateral pneumoencephalogram of a 28-year-old man.

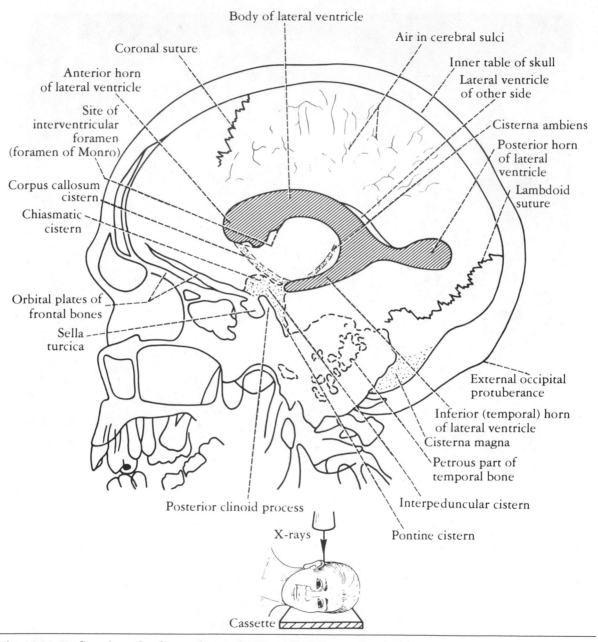

Fig. 14-20. Explanation of radiograph seen in Figure 14-19. Note the position of the x-ray gun relative to the head and the film cassette.

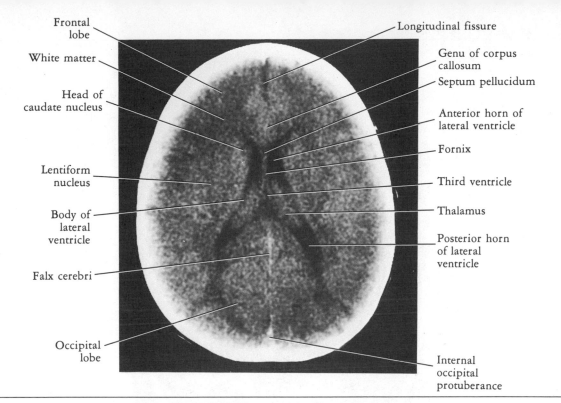

Fig. 14-21. Horizontal (axial) CT scan of the brain.

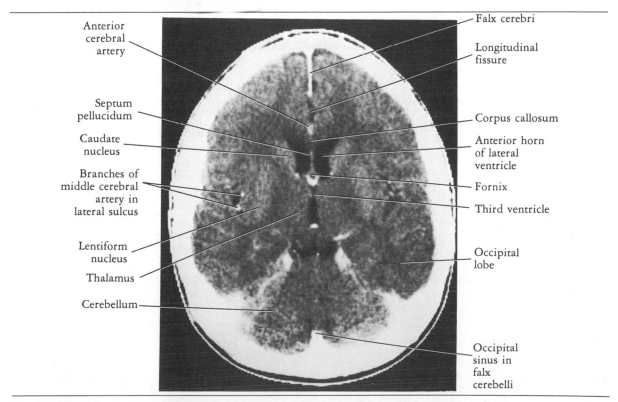

Fig. 14-22. Horizontal (axial) CT scan of the brain (contrast enhanced).

Frontal lobe

Longitudinal fissure

Gray matter

White matter

Genu of corpus callosum

Head of caudate nucleus

Anterior horn of lateral ventricle

Septum pellucidum

Body of lateral ventricle

Body of fornix

Choroid plexus in lateral ventricle

Posterior horn of lateral ventricle

Occipital lobe

Fig. 14-23. Horizontal (axial) MRI scan of the brain.

in his right hand (with his eyes closed) he will recognize the object by touch and be able to describe it. If the pencil is placed in his left hand, the tactile information will pass to his right postcentral gyrus. This information will not be able to travel through the corpus callosum to his speech area in his left hemisphere and, therefore, he will be unable to describe the object in his left hand.

Section of the corpus callosum has been attempted surgically, with some success, in order to prevent the spread of seizures from one hemisphere to the other.

INTERNAL CAPSULE

The internal capsule is an important compact band of white matter. It is composed of ascending and descending nerve fibers that connect the cerebral cortex to the brainstem and spinal cord. The internal capsule is flanked medially by the caudate nucleus and thalamus and laterally by the lentiform nucleus. The arrangement of the nerve fibers within the internal capsule is shown in Figure 14-14.

The internal capsule is frequently involved in vascular disorders of the brain. The blood supply of the internal capsule is described on page 536. The most common cause of arterial hemorrhage is atheromatous degeneration in an artery in a patient with high blood pressure. Because of the high concentration of important nerve fibers within the internal capsule, even a small hemorrhage may cause widespread effects on the contralateral side of the body. Not only is the immediate neural tissue destroyed by the blood, which later clots, but neighboring nerve fibers may be compressed or be edematous.

Fig. 14-24. Coronal MRI scan of the brain.

CLINICAL PROBLEMS

Answers on Page 602

1. A neurosurgeon explained to his residents that he would attempt to remove the glioma located in the right middle frontal gyrus by turning back a flap of the scalp and removing a rectangular piece of the overlying skull. Where exactly is the right middle frontal gyrus in the brain? What are the names of the sulci that lie above and below this gyrus? Which skull bone overlays this gyrus?

2. While performing an autopsy, a pathologist had great difficulty in finding the central sulcus in each cerebral hemisphere. Since finding this sulcus is the key to localizing many other sulci and gyri, what landmarks would you use to identify the central sulcus? Are the sulci and gyri in the two hemispheres similar in size and shape? Are there individual variations in the arrangement of the sulci and gyri?

3. A fourth-year medical student was shown coronal and horizontal MR images of the brain and

was asked to comment on his observations. The patient was a 55-year-old man. The student responded by saying that the left lateral ventricle was larger than normal and that there was an area of low signal intensity close to the left interventricular foramen suggesting the presence of a brain tumor. On looking at a standard lateral radiograph of the skull and brain he noted a small area of "calcification" situated in the region of the posterior part of the left ventricle. Using your knowledge of neuroanatomy, describe the location of the lateral ventricle in the brain. What are the different parts of the lateral ventricle? Where is the cerebrospinal fluid in the lateral ventricle produced and what does it normally drain into? What is responsible for the calcification seen in the left lateral ventricle in this patient?

4. A medical student, while performing an au-

topsy, found that the patient had no corpus callosum. On consulting the patient's clinical notes he was surprised to find no reference to a neurological disorder. Are you surprised that this patient had no recorded neurological signs and symptoms?

5. During a lecture, a distinguished neurologist repeatedly referred to the corpus striatum, the basal ganglia, and the basal nuclei. Are you sure you understand the differences, if any, between these terms?

NATIONAL BOARD TYPE QUESTIONS

Answers on Page 620

IN EACH OF THE FOLLOWING QUESTIONS, ANSWER:
  (a) IF (1) ONLY IS CORRECT
  (b) IF (2) ONLY IS CORRECT
  (c) IF BOTH (1) AND (2) ARE CORRECT, AND
  (d) IF NEITHER (1) NOR (2) IS CORRECT

1. Which of the following statements is (are) correct concerning the longitudinal cerebral fissure?
   (1) The fissure contains the sickle-shaped fold of dura mater, the falx cerebri, and the anterior cerebral blood arteries.
   (2) In the depths of the fissure the corpus callosum crosses the midline.

2. Which of the following statements is (are) correct concerning the central sulcus?
   (1) The frontal lobe lies anterior to it, and the parietal lies posterior.
   (2) The central sulcus extends onto the medial surface of the cerebral hemisphere and reaches the corpus callosum.

3. Which of the following statements is (are) correct concerning the areas of the cerebral hemisphere?
   (1) The cuneus is an area of cortex bounded anteriorly by the upturned posterior end of the cingulate sulcus and posteriorly by the parieto-occipital sulcus.
   (2) The lingual gyrus lies between the collateral sulcus and the calcarine sulcus.

Select the best response:

4. The following statements concerning the lateral ventricle are correct **except**:
   (a) Each ventricle is C-shaped and filled with cerebrospinal fluid.
   (b) It communicates with the third ventricle through the interventricular foramen.
   (c) The body of the ventricle occupies the parietal lobe.
   (d) The choroid plexus projects through the lateral wall of the ventricle.
   (e) The roof of the anterior horn is formed by the corpus callosum.

5. The following structures are closely related to the lateral ventricle in the positions stated **except**:
   (a) The head of the caudate nucleus is related to the floor of the anterior horn.
   (b) The lateral wall of the posterior horn is related to the tapetum.
   (c) The hippocampus forms part of the floor of the inferior horn of the lateral ventricle.
   (d) The genu of the corpus callosum forms the anterior wall of the anterior horn of the lateral ventricle.
   (e) The lentiform nucleus forms part of the floor of the body of the lateral ventricle.

In the following questions, answer:
  (a) IF (1), (2), AND (3) ONLY ARE CORRECT
  (b) IF (1) AND (3) ONLY ARE CORRECT
  (c) IF (2) AND (4) ONLY ARE CORRECT
  (d) IF (4) ONLY IS CORRECT, OR
  (e) IF ALL ARE CORRECT

6. Which of the following statements is (are) correct concerning the corpus callosum?
   (1) The rostrum forms the anterior end.
   (2) It is connected to the fornix by the septum pellucidum.
   (3) Most of the fibers within the corpus callosum interconnect symmetrical areas of the cerebral cortex.
   (4) The fibers of the genu curve forward into the frontal lobes as the forceps major.

7. Which of the following statements is (are) correct concerning the anterior commissure?
   (1) It lies embedded in the superior part of the lamina terminalis.
   (2) The fibers are concerned with the transmission of auditory sensations.
   (3) Some of the fibers are concerned with smell sensations.
   (4) It forms the anterior boundary of the interventricular foramen.
8. Which of the following statements is (are) correct concerning the internal capsule?
   (1) It has an anterior limb, a genu, and a posterior limb.
   (2) The genu and the anterior part of the posterior limb contain the corticobulbar and corticospinal fibers.
   (3) It is related laterally to the lentiform nucleus.
   (4) It is continuous above with the corona radiata.

9. Which of the following statements is (are) correct concerning the basal ganglia?
   (1) The caudate nucleus is not fused with the lentiform nucleus.
   (2) The corpus striatum is concerned with muscular movement.
   (3) The lentiform nucleus is related medially to the external capsule.
   (4) The lentiform nucleus is wedge shaped as seen on horizontal section of the brain.

In Figure 14-25, match the numbers listed on the left with the appropriate structure listed on the right. Any answer may be used more than once.

10. Number 1
11. Number 2
12. Number 3
13. Number 4
14. Number 5

(a) Optic radiation
(b) Lateral sulcus
(c) Lentiform nucleus
(d) Anterior horn of lateral ventricle
(e) None of the above

Fig. 14-25. Horizontal section of cerebrum as seen from above.

Fig. 14-26. Lateral view of left cerebral hemisphere.

In Figure 14-26, match the numbers listed on the left with the appropriate structures listed on the right. Any answer may be used more than once.

15. Number 1
16. Number 2
17. Number 3
18. Number 4
19. Number 5
20. Number 6

(a) Central sulcus
(b) Postcentral gyrus
(c) Superior temporal gyrus
(d) Superior parietal lobule
(e) None of the above

ADDITIONAL READING

Crosby, E. C., Humphrey, T., and Lauer, E. W. *Correlative Anatomy of the Nervous System.* New York: Macmillan, 1962.

Jacobs, E. R. *Medical Imaging: A Concise Textbook.* New York and Tokyo: Igaku-Shoin, 1987.

Sobotta, J. *Atlas of Human Anatomy.* H. Ferner and J. Staubesand (Eds.) (10th Engl. ed.). Baltimore and Munich: Urban and Schwarzenberg, 1983. Vol. I.

Williams, P. L., Warwick, R., Dyson, M., and Bannister, L. H. *Gray's Anatomy* (37th Brit. ed.). Philadelphia: Saunders, 1989.

Chapter 15
The Structure and Functional Localization of the Cerebral Cortex

STRUCTURE OF THE CEREBRAL CORTEX

The cerebral cortex forms a complete covering of the cerebral hemisphere. It is composed of gray matter and has been estimated to contain approximately 10 billion neurons. The surface area of the cortex has been increased by throwing it into convolutions, or gyri, separated by fissures or sulci. The thickness of the cortex varies from 1.5 to 4.5 mm. The cortex is thickest over the crest of a gyrus and thinnest in the depth of a sulcus. The cerebral cortex, like gray matter elsewhere in the central nervous system, consists of a mixture of nerve cells, nerve fibers, neuroglia, and blood vessels. The following types of nerve cells are present in the cerebral cortex: (1) pyramidal cells, (2) stellate cells, (3) fusiform cells, (4) horizontal cells of Cajal, and (5) cells of Martinotti (Fig. 15-1).

Nerve Cells of the Cerebral Cortex

The **pyramidal cells** are named from the shape of their cell bodies (Fig. 15-1). Most of the cell bodies measure 10 to 50 μm long. However, there are giant pyramidal cells, also known as **Betz cells**, whose cell bodies measure as much as 120 μm; these are found in the motor precentral gyrus of the frontal lobe.

The apices of the pyramidal cells are oriented toward the pial surface of the cortex. From the apex of each cell a thick apical dendrite extends upward toward the pia, giving off collateral branches. From the basal angles, several basal dendrites pass laterally into the surrounding neuropil. Each dendrite possesses numerous **dendritic spines** for synaptic junctions with axons of other neurons (Fig. 15-1). The axon arises from the base of the cell body and either terminates in the deeper cortical layers or, more commonly, enters the white matter of the cerebral hemisphere as a projection, association, or commissural fiber.

The **stellate** cells, sometimes called granule cells because of their small size, are polygonal in shape and their cell bodies measure about 8 μm in diameter (Fig. 15-1). These cells have multiple branching dendrites and a relatively short axon, which terminates on a nearby neuron.

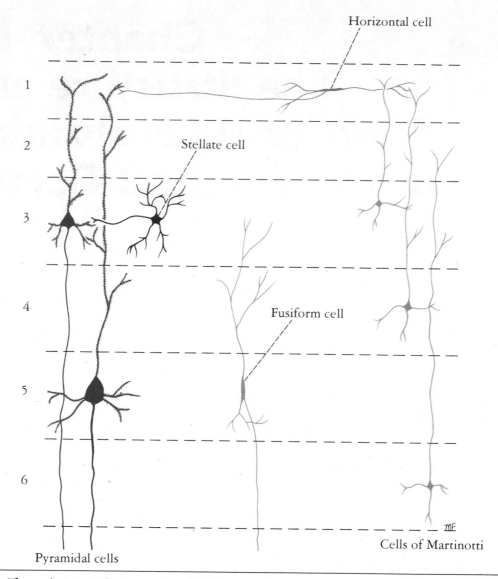

Horizontal cell

Stellate cell

Fusiform cell

Cells of Martinotti

Pyramidal cells

Fig. 15-1. The main types of neurons found in the cerebral cortex.

The **fusiform cells** have their long axis vertical to the surface and are concentrated mainly in the deepest cortical layers (Fig. 15-1). Dendrites arise from each pole of the cell body. The inferior dendrite branches within the same cellular layer, while the superficial dendrite ascends toward the surface of the cortex and branches in the superficial layers. The axon arises from the inferior part of the cell body and enters the white matter as a projection, association, or commissural fiber.

The **horizontal cells of Cajal** are small, fusiform, horizontally oriented cells found in the most superficial layers of the cortex (Fig. 15-1). A dendrite emerges from each end of the cell and an axon runs parallel to the surface of the cortex, making contact with the dendrites of pyramidal cells.

The **cells of Martinotti** are small, multipolar cells that are present throughout the levels of the cortex (Fig. 15-1). The cell has short dendrites, but the axon is directed toward the pial surface of the cortex, where it ends in a more superficial layer, commonly the most superficial layer. The axon gives origin to a few short collateral branches en route.

Nerve Fibers of the Cerebral Cortex

The nerve fibers of the cerebral cortex are arranged both radially and tangentially (Figs. 15-2 and 15-3). The **radial fibers** run at right angles to the cortical surface. They include the afferent entering projection, association, and commissural fibers that terminate within the cortex, and the axons of pyramidal, stellate, and fusiform cells, which leave the cortex to become projection, association, and commissural fibers of the white matter of the cerebral hemisphere.

The **tangential fibers** run parallel to the cortical surface and are, for the most part, collateral and terminal branches of afferent fibers. They include also the axons of horizontal and stellate cells, and collateral branches of pyramidal and fusiform cells. The tangential fibers are most concentrated in layers 4 and 5, where they are referred to as the outer and inner **bands of Baillarger**, respectively (Figs. 15-2 and 15-3). The bands of Baillarger are particularly well developed in the sensory areas due to the high concentration of the terminal parts of the thalamocortical fibers. In the visual cortex, the

outer **band of Baillarger**, which is so thick it can be seen with the naked eye, is known as the **stria of Gennari**. Because of this obvious band, or stria, the visual cortex in the walls of the calcarine sulcus is sometimes called the **striate cortex**.

Layers of the Cerebral Cortex

It is convenient, for descriptive purposes, to divide the cerebral cortex into layers that may be distinguished by the types, density, and arrangement of their cells (Figs. 15-1 and 15-3). The names and characteristic features of the layers are described here; regional differences will be discussed later.

1. **Molecular layer (plexiform layer).** This is the most superficial layer; it consists mainly of a dense network of tangentially oriented nerve fibers (Figs. 15-1 and 15-3). These fibers are derived from the apical dendrites of the pyramidal cells and fusiform cells, the axons of the stellate cells, and the cells of Martinotti. Afferent fibers originating in the thalamus and in association with commissural fibers also are present. Scattered among these nerve fibers are occasional horizontal cells of Cajal. This most superficial layer of the cortex clearly is where large numbers of synapses between different neurons occur.
2. **External granular layer.** This layer contains large numbers of small pyramidal cells and stellate cells (Figs. 15-1 and 15-3). The dendrites of these cells terminate in the molecular layer, and the axons enter deeper layers, where they terminate or pass on to enter the white matter of the cerebral hemisphere.
3. **External pyramidal layer.** This layer is composed of pyramidal cells, whose cell body size increases from the superficial to the deeper borders of the layer (Figs. 15-1 and 15-3). The apical dendrites pass into the molecular layer and the axons enter the white matter as projection, association, or commissural fibers.
4. **Internal granular layer.** This layer is composed of closely packed stellate cells (Figs. 15-1 and 15-3). There is a high concentration of horizontally arranged fibers known collectively as the **external band of Baillarger**.
5. **Ganglionic layer (internal pyramidal layer).** This layer contains very large and medium-sized pyramidal cells (Figs. 15-1 and 15-3). Scattered

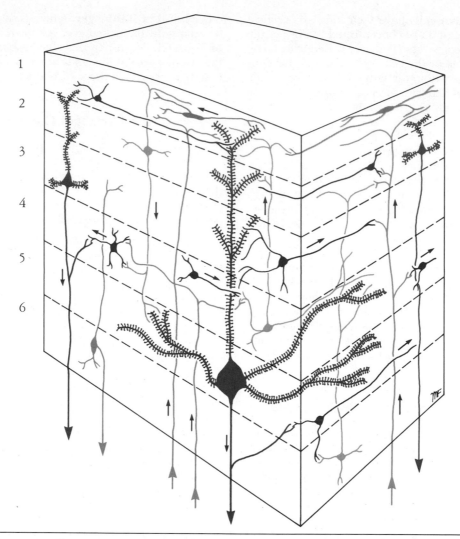

Fig. 15-2. The neuronal connections of the cerebral cortex. Note the presence of the afferent and efferent fibers.

1
Molecular layer

2
External
granular layer

3
External
pyramidal layer

4
Internal
granular layer

5
Ganglionic layer
(internal
pyramidal
layer)

6
Multiform layer
(layer of
polymorphic
cells)

External band
of Baillarger

Inner band
of Baillarger

Efferent cortical fibers   Afferent cortical fibers

Fig. 15-3. The layers of the cerebral cortex, showing the neurons on the left and the nerve fibers on the right.

among the pyramidal cells are stellate cells and cells of Martinotti. In addition, there are a large number of horizontally arranged fibers that form the **inner band of Baillarger** (Fig. 15-3). In the motor cortex of the precentral gyrus, the pyramidal cells of this layer are very large and are known as Betz cells. These cells account for about 3 percent of the projection fibers of the **corticospinal or pyramidal tract**.

6. **Multiform layer (layer of polymorphic cells).** Although the majority of the cells are fusiform, many of the cells are modified pyramidal cells, whose cell bodies are triangular or ovoid (Figs. 15-1 and 15-3). The cells of Martinotti also are conspicuous in this layer. Many nerve fibers are present that are entering or are leaving the underlying white matter.

Variations in Cortical Structure

The system of numbering and nomenclature of the cortical layers used above is similar to that distinguished by Brodmann (1909). It is important, however, to realize that not all areas of the cerebral cortex possess six layers (Fig. 15-3). Those areas of the cortex in which the basic six layers cannot be recognized are referred to as **heterotypical**, as opposed to the majority, which are **homotypical** and possess six layers. Two heterotypical areas will be described: the granular and the agranular type.

In the **granular type**, the granular layers are well developed and contain densely packed stellate cells (Fig. 15-3). Thus, layers 2 and 4 are well developed, and layers 3 and 5 are poorly developed, so that layers 2 through 5 merge into a single layer of predominantly granular cells. It is these cells that receive thalamocortical fibers. The granular type of cortex is found in the postcentral gyrus, the superior temporal gyrus, and in parts of the hippocampal gyrus.

In the **agranular type** of cortex, the granular layers are poorly developed, so that layers 2 and 4 are practically absent (Fig. 15-3). The pyramidal cells in layers 3 and 5 are densely packed and are very large in size. The agranular type of cortex is found in the precentral gyrus and other areas in the frontal lobe. These areas give rise to large numbers of efferent fibers that are associated with motor function.

Mechanisms of the Cerebral Cortex

A study of the histology of the cerebral cortex, combined with the neurophysiological recordings made with microelectrodes, suggests that the cerebral cortex is organized into vertical units of functional activity (Fig. 15-2). Such a functional unit possesses afferent fibers, internuncial neurons, and efferent fibers. An afferent fiber may synapse directly with an efferent neuron or may involve vertical chains of internuncial neurons. A single vertical chain of neurons may be involved or the wave of excitation may spread to adjacent vertical chains through short axon granular cells. The horizontal cells of Cajal permit activation of vertical units that lie some distance away from the incoming afferent fiber (Fig. 15-2).

CORTICAL AREAS

Clinicopathological studies in man and electrophysiological and ablation studies in animals have, over the past century, produced evidence that different areas of the cerebral cortex are functionally specialized. However, the precise division of the cortex into different areas of specialization, as described by Brodmann, oversimplifies and misleads the reader. The simple division of cortical areas into motor and sensory is erroneous, for many of the sensory areas are far more extensive than originally described, and it is known that motor responses can be obtained on stimulation of sensory areas. Until a satisfactory terminology has been devised to describe the various cortical areas, the main cortical areas will be named by their anatomical location.

Frontal Lobe

The **precentral area** is situated in the precentral gyrus and includes the anterior wall of the central sulcus and the posterior parts of the superior, middle, and inferior frontal gyri; it extends over the superomedial border of the hemisphere into the paracentral lobule (Fig. 15-4). Histologically, the characteristic feature of this area is the almost complete absence of the granular layers and the prominence of the pyramidal nerve cells. The giant

Fig. 15-4. Functional localization of the cerebral cortex.
A. Lateral view of left cerebral hemisphere.
B. Medial view of left cerebral hemisphere.

pyramidal cells of Betz, which may measure as much as 120 μm long and 60 μm wide, are concentrated most highly in the superior part of the precentral gyrus and the paracentral lobule; their numbers diminish as one passes anteriorly in the precentral gyrus or inferiorly toward the lateral fissure. The great majority of the corticospinal and corticobulbar fibers originate from the small pyramidal cells in this area. It has been estimated that the number of Betz cells present is between 25,000 and 30,000 and accounts for only about 3 percent of the corticospinal fibers. It is interesting to note that the postcentral gyrus and the second somatosensory areas, as well as the occipital and temporal lobes, give origin to descending tracts also; they are involved in controlling the sensory input to the nervous system and are not involved in muscular movement.

The precentral area may be divided into posterior and anterior regions. The posterior region— referred to as the **motor area**, **primary motor area**, or Brodmann's area 4—occupies the precentral gyrus extending over the superior border into the paracentral lobule (Fig. 15-4). The anterior region is known as the **premotor area**, **secondary motor area**, or Brodmann's area 6 and parts of areas 8, 44, and 45. It occupies the anterior part of the precentral gyrus and the posterior parts of the superior, middle, and inferior frontal gyri.

The primary motor area, if electrically stimulated, produces isolated movements on the opposite side of the body as well as contraction of muscle groups concerned with the performance of a specific movement. Although isolated ipsilateral movements do not occur, bilateral movements of the extraocular muscles, the muscles of the upper part of the face, the tongue and the mandible, and the larynx and the pharynx do occur.

The movement areas of the body are represented in inverted form in the precentral gyrus (Fig. 15-5). Starting from below and passing superiorly are structures involved in swallowing, tongue, jaw, lips, larynx, eyelid, and brow. The next area is an extensive region for movements of the fingers, especially the thumb, hand, wrist, elbow, shoulder, and trunk. The movements of the hip, knee, and ankle are represented in the highest areas of the precentral gyrus; the toes are situated on the medial surface of the cerebral hemisphere in the paracentral lobule. The anal and vesical sphincters are also located in the paracentral lobule. The area of cortex controlling a particular movement is proportional to the skill involved in performing the movement and is unrelated to the mass of muscle participating in the movement.

The function of the primary motor area is thus to carry out the individual movements of different parts of the body. To assist in this function, it receives numerous afferent fibers from the premotor area, the sensory cortex, the thalamus, the cerebellum, and the basal ganglia. The primary motor cortex is not responsible for the design of the pattern of movement but is the final station for conversion of the design into execution of the movement.

The premotor area, which is wider superiorly than below and narrows down to be confined to the anterior part of the precentral gyrus, has no giant pyramidal cells of Betz. Electrical stimulation of the premotor area produces muscular movements similar to those obtained by stimulation of the primary motor area; however, stronger stimulation is necessary to produce the same degree of movement.

The premotor area receives numerous inputs from the sensory cortex, the thalamus and the basal ganglia. The function of the premotor area is to store programs of motor activity assembled as the result of past experience. The premotor area thus programs the activity of the primary motor area. It is particularly involved in controlling coarse postural movements through its connections with the basal ganglia.

The **supplementary motor area** is situated in the medial frontal gyrus on the medial surface of the hemisphere and anterior to the paracentral lobule. Stimulation of this area results in movements of the contralateral limbs, but a stronger stimulus is necessary than when the primary motor area is stimulated. Removal of the supplementary motor area produces no permanent loss of movement.

The **frontal eye field** (Fig. 15-4) extends forward from the facial area of the precentral gyrus into the middle frontal gyrus (parts of Brodmann's areas 6, 8, and 9). Electrical stimulation of this region causes conjugate movements of the eyes, especially toward the opposite side. The exact pathway taken by nerve fibers from this area is not known, but they are thought to pass to the superior colliculus of the midbrain. The superior colliculus

Fig. 15-5. A motor homunculus on the precentral gyrus.

is connected to the nuclei of the extraocular muscles by the reticular formation. The frontal eye field is considered to control voluntary scanning movements of the eye and is independent of visual stimuli. The involuntary following of moving objects by the eyes involves the visual area of the occipital cortex to which the frontal eye field is connected by association fibers.

The **motor speech area of Broca** (Fig. 15-4) is located in the inferior frontal gyrus between the anterior and ascending rami and the ascending and posterior rami of the lateral fissure (Brodmann's areas 44 and 45). In the majority of individuals, this area is important on the left or dominant hemisphere and ablation will result in paralysis of speech. In those individuals in whom the right hemisphere is dominant, the area on the right side is of importance. The ablation of this region in the nondominant hemisphere has no effect on speech.

Broca's speech area brings about the formation of words by its connections with the adjacent primary motor areas; the muscles of the larynx, mouth, tongue, soft palate, and the respiratory muscles are appropriately stimulated.

The **prefrontal cortex** is an extensive area that lies anterior to the precentral area. It includes the greater parts of the superior, middle, and inferior frontal gyri, the orbital gyri, most of the medial frontal gyrus, and the anterior half of the cingulate gyrus (Brodmann's areas 9, 10, 11, and 12). Large numbers of afferent and efferent pathways connect the prefrontal area with other areas of the cerebral cortex, the thalamus, the hypothalamus, and the corpus striatum. The frontopontine fibers also connect this area to the cerebellum through the pontine nuclei. The commissural fibers of the forceps minor and genu of the corpus callosum unite these areas in both cerebral hemispheres.

The prefrontal area is concerned with the makeup of the individual's personality. As the result of the input from many cortical and subcortical sources, this area plays a role as a regulator of the person's depth of feeling. It also exerts its influence in determining the initiative and judgment of an individual.

Parietal Lobe

The **primary somesthetic area** (Fig. 15-4) occupies the postcentral gyrus on the lateral surface of the hemisphere and the posterior part of the paracentral lobule on the medial surface (Brodmann's areas 3, 1, and 2). Histologically, the anterior part of the postcentral gyrus is the area that borders the central sulcus (area 3), is granular in type, and contains only scattered pyramidal cells. The **outer layer of Baillarger** is broad and very obvious. The posterior part of the postcentral gyrus (areas 1 and 2) possesses fewer granular cells. The primary somesthetic areas of the cerebral cortex receive projection fibers from the ventral posterior lateral and ventral posterior medial nuclei of the thalamus. The opposite half of the body is represented as inverted. The pharyngeal region, tongue, and jaws are represented in the most inferior part of the postcentral gyrus; this is followed by the face, fingers, hand, arm, trunk, and thigh. The leg and the foot areas are found on the medial surface of the hemisphere in the posterior part of the paracentral lobule. The anal and genital regions are also found in this latter area. The apportioning of the cortex for a particular part of the body is related to its functional importance rather than to its size. The face, lips, thumb, and index finger have particularly large areas assigned to them.

Although most sensations reach the cortex from the contralateral side of the body, some from the oral region go to the same side, and those from the pharynx, larynx, and perineum go to both sides.

The **secondary somesthetic area** (Fig. 15-4) is in the superior lip of the posterior limb of the lateral fissure. The face area lies most anterior and the leg area is posterior. The body is bilaterally represented with the contralateral side dominant. The detailed connections of this area are unknown, but the spinothalamic tracts are believed to be associated with it. The functional significance of this area is unknown.

The **somesthetic association area** (Fig. 15-4) occupies the superior parietal lobule extending onto the medial surface of the hemisphere (Brodmann's areas 5 and 7). This area has many connections with other sensory areas of the cortex. It is believed that its main function is to receive and integrate different sensory modalities. For example, it enables one to recognize objects placed in the

hand without the help of vision. In other words, it not only receives information concerning the size and shape of an object but relates this to past sensory experiences, so that the information may be interpreted and recognition occurs. A quarter placed in the hand can be distinguished from a dime or a nickel by the size, shape, and feel of the coin without having to use one's eyes.

Occipital Lobe

The **primary visual area** (Brodmann's area 17) is situated in the walls of the posterior part of the calcarine sulcus and occasionally extends around the occipital pole onto the lateral surface of the hemisphere (Fig. 15-4). Macroscopically, this area can be recognized by the thinness of the cortex and the visual stria, and microscopically, it is seen to be a granular type of cortex with only a few pyramidal cells present.

The visual cortex receives afferent fibers from the lateral geniculate body. The fibers first pass forward in the white matter of the temporal lobe and then turn back to the primary visual cortex in the occipital lobe. The visual cortex receives fibers from the temporal half of the ipsilateral retina and the nasal half of the contralateral retina. The right half of the field of vision, therefore, is represented in the visual cortex of the left cerebral hemisphere and vice versa. It is also important to note that the superior retinal quadrants (inferior field of vision) pass to the superior wall of the calcarine sulcus, while the inferior retinal quadrants (superior field of vision) pass to the inferior wall of the calcarine sulcus.

The macula lutea, which is the central area of the retina and the area for most perfect vision, is represented on the cortex in the posterior part of area 17 and accounts for one-third of the visual cortex. The peripheral parts of the retina in the region of the orra serrata are represented in the anterior part of area 17.

The **secondary visual area** (Brodmann's areas 18 and 19) surrounds the primary visual area on the medial and lateral surfaces of the hemisphere (Fig. 15-4). This area receives afferent fibers from area 17 and other cortical areas, as well as from the thalamus. The function of the secondary visual area is to relate the visual information received by the primary visual area to past visual experiences, thus enabling the individual to recognize and appreciate what he is seeing.

The **occipital eye field** is thought to exist in the secondary visual area in man (Fig. 15-4). Stimulation produces conjugate deviation of the eyes, especially to the opposite side. The function of this eye field is believed to be reflex and associated with movements of the eye when it is following an object. The occipital eye fields of both hemispheres are connected by nervous pathways, and also are thought to be connected to the superior colliculus. By contrast, the frontal eye field controls voluntary scanning movements of the eye and is independent of visual stimuli.

Temporal Lobe

The **primary auditory area** (Brodmann's areas 41 and 42) includes the gyrus of Heschl and is situated in the inferior wall of the lateral sulcus (Fig. 15-4). Area 41 is a granular type of cortex; area 42 is homotypical and is mainly an auditory association area.

Projection fibers to the auditory area arise principally in the medial geniculate body and form the **auditory radiation of the internal capsule**. The anterior part of the primary auditory area is concerned with the reception of sounds of low frequency and the posterior part of the area with the sounds of high frequency. A unilateral lesion of the auditory area produces partial deafness in both ears, the greater loss being in the contralateral ear. This can be explained on the basis that the medial geniculate body receives fibers mainly from the organ of Corti of the opposite side as well as some fibers from the same side.

The **secondary auditory area** (auditory association cortex) is situated posterior to the primary auditory area (Fig. 15-4) in the lateral sulcus and in the superior temporal gyrus (Brodmann's area 22). This area is thought to be necessary for the interpretation of sounds.

The **sensory speech area of Wernicke** (Fig. 15-4) is localized in the left dominant hemisphere, mainly in the superior temporal gyrus, with extensions round the posterior end of the lateral sulcus into the parietal region. Wernicke's area is connected to Broca's area by a bundle of nerve fibers called the **arcuate fasciculus**. It receives fibers from the visual cortex in the occipital lobe and the auditory cortex in the superior temporal gyrus. Wernicke's area permits the understanding of the written and spoken language and enables a person to read a sentence, understand it, and say it out loud (Figs. 15-6 and 15-7).

Other Cortical Areas

The **taste area** is situated at the lower end of the postcentral gyrus in the superior wall of the lateral sulcus and in the adjoining area of the insula (Brodmann's area 43). Ascending fibers from the nucleus solitarius probably ascend to the ventral posteromedial nucleus of the thalamus, where they synapse on neurons that send fibers to the cortex.

The **vestibular area** is thought to be situated near the part of the postcentral gyrus concerned with sensations of the face. Its location lies opposite the auditory area in the superior temporal gyrus.

The **insula** is an area of the cortex that is buried within the lateral sulcus and forms its floor (see Fig. 14-4). It can be examined only when the lips of the lateral sulcus are separated widely. Histologically, the posterior part is granular and the anterior part is agranular, thus resembling the adjoining cortical areas. Its fiber connections are incompletely known. It is believed to be associated with visceral functions.

Association Cortex

The primary sensory areas with their granular cortex and the primary motor areas with their agranular cortex form only a small part of the total cortical surface area. The remaining areas have all six cellular layers and therefore are referred to as homotypical cortex. Classically, these large remaining areas were known as association areas, though precisely what they associate is not known. The original concept, that they receive information from the primary sensory areas, to be integrated and analyzed in the association cortex and then fed to the motor areas, has not been established. It has now become apparent, as the result of clinical studies and animal experimentation, that these areas of the cortex have multiple inputs and outputs and are very much concerned with our behavior, discrimination, and interpretation of sensory experiences. Three main association areas are recog-

Primary motor area

Angular gyrus

Broca's area

Visual areas

Wernicke's area

Larynx

Eye

Fig. 15-6. Probable nerve pathways involved in reading a sentence and repeating it out loud.

nized: prefrontal, anterior temporal, and posterior parietal.

The prefrontal cortex is discussed on page 306. The anterior temporal cortex is thought to play a role in the storage of previous sensory experiences. Stimulation may cause the individual to recall objects seen or music heard in the past. In the posterior parietal cortex, the sensory input of touch and pressure and proprioception is integrated into concepts of size, form, and texture. This ability is known as **stereognosis**. An appreciation of the body image is also assembled in the posterior parietal cortex. A person is able to develop a body scheme that he or she is able to appreciate consciously. The right side of the body is represented in the left hemisphere and the left side of the body in the right hemisphere.

CEREBRAL DOMINANCE

An anatomical examination of the two cerebral hemispheres shows that the cortical gyri and fissures are almost identical. Moreover, nervous pathways projecting to the cortex do so largely contralaterally and equally to identical cortical areas. In addition, the cerebral commissures, especially the corpus callosum and the anterior commissure, provide a pathway for information that is received in one hemisphere to be transferred to the other. Nevertheless, we know that certain nervous activity

Fig. 15-7. Probable nerve pathways involved with hearing a question and answering it.

is predominantly performed by one of the two cerebral hemispheres. Handedness, perception of language, and speech are functional areas of behavior that are in most individuals controlled by the dominant hemisphere. By contrast, spatial perception, recognition of faces, and music are interpreted by the nondominant hemisphere (Fig. 15-8).

More than 90 percent of the adult population are right-handed and are therefore left hemisphere-dominant. About 96 percent of the adult population are left hemisphere-dominant for speech.

The work of Yakolev and Rakic on human fetuses and neonates has shown that more descending fibers in the left pyramid cross over the midline in the decussation than vice versa. This would suggest

that, in most individuals, the anterior horn cells on the right side of the spinal cord have a greater corticospinal innervation than those on the left side, which might explain the dominance of the right hand.

Other workers have shown that the speech area of the adult cortex is larger on the left than on the right. It is believed that the two hemispheres of the newborn have equipotential capabilities. During childhood, one hemisphere slowly comes to dominate the other, and it is only after the first decade that the dominance becomes fixed. This would explain why a 5-year-old child with damage to the dominant hemisphere can easily learn to become left-handed and speak well, whereas in the case of the adult this is almost impossible.

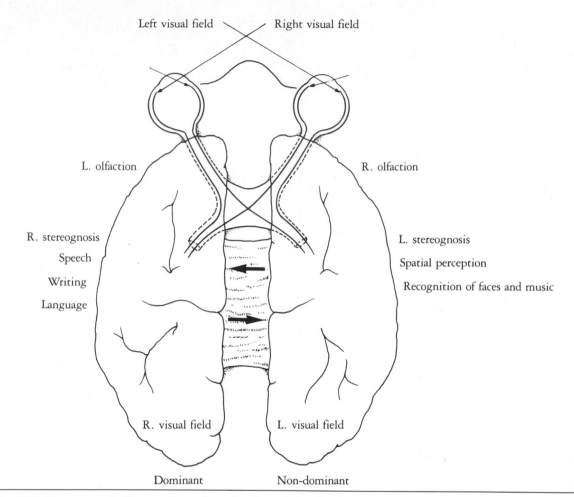

Left visual field   Right visual field

L. olfaction   R. olfaction

R. stereognosis   L. stereognosis

Speech   Spatial perception

Writing   Recognition of faces and music

Language

R. visual field   L. visual field

Dominant   Non-dominant

Fig. 15-8. Nervous activities performed predominantly by dominant and nondominant hemispheres.

CLINICAL NOTES

GENERAL CONSIDERATIONS

The cerebral cortex reaches its greatest degree of development in human beings. Microscopically, most of the cerebral cortex can be seen to be made up of six identifiable layers. Areas of specialization occur, as, for example, in the motor cortex in the precentral gyrus, where there is a relative absence of granular cells in the second and fourth layers, and in the somesthetic cortex in the postcentral gyrus, where there is a relative absence of pyramidal cells in the third and fifth layers.

Four groups of nerve fibers pass out and in to the cerebral cortex. **Corticofugal fibers** project from the cortex to lower areas of the central nervous system, such as the corticonuclear and corticospinal tracts. **Corticopetal fibers** project from the thalamus and other lower nuclei to the cortex. **Association fibers** connect different cortical regions of the same hemisphere. **Commissural fibers** connect identical portions of the two cerebral hemispheres.

Microscopical and electrophysiological research has led to the belief that the cerebral cortex is organized into vertical units of functional activity. The basal dendrites and the apical dendrite of the pyramidal cells run in a vertical direction, the axons of interconnecting neurons are vertically arranged, and most cortical afferents run in a vertical direction. A single vertical chain of neurons initially may be involved in cortical activity or the wave of excitation may spread to involve neighboring vertical chains or vertical chains situated at some distance through horizontally arranged nerve cells.

The cerebral cortex should be regarded as the last receiving station involved along a line of stations receiving information from the eyes and ears and organs of general sensation. The function of the cortex is, in simple terms, to discriminate, and it relates the received information to past memories. The enriched sensory input is then presumably discarded, stored, or translated into action. In this whole process, there is interplay between the cortex and basal nuclei provided by the many cortical and subcortical nervous connections.

LESIONS OF THE CEREBRAL CORTEX

In human beings, the effect of destruction of different areas of the cerebral cortex has been studied by examining patients with lesions resulting from cerebral tumors, vascular accidents, surgery, or head injuries. Moreover, it has been possible to take electrical recordings from different areas of the cortex during surgical exposure of the cerebral cortex, or when stimulating different parts of the cortex in the conscious patient. One thing that has emerged from these studies is that the human cerebral cortex possesses, in a remarkable degree, the ability to reorganize the remaining intact cortex so that a certain amount of cerebral recovery is possible after brain lesions.

LESIONS OF THE MOTOR CORTEX

Lesions of the primary **motor cortex** in one hemisphere result in paralysis of the contralateral extremities, the finer and more skilled movements suffering most. Destruction of the **primary motor area** (area 4) produces more severe paralysis than destruction of the **secondary motor area** (area 6).

Destruction of both areas produces the most complete form of contralateral paralysis.

Lesions of the **secondary motor area** alone produce a difficulty in the performance of skilled movements, with little loss of strength.

The **Jacksonian epileptic seizure** is due to an irritative lesion of the primary motor area (area 4). The convulsion begins in the part of the body represented in the primary motor area that is being irritated. The convulsive movement may be restricted to one part of the body, such as the face or the foot, or it may spread to involve many regions, depending on the spread of irritation of the primary motor area.

MUSCLE SPASTICITY CAUSED BY LESIONS OF THE MOTOR CORTEX

A discrete lesion of the primary motor cortex (area 4) results in little change in the muscle tone. However, larger lesions involving the primary and secondary motor areas (areas 4 and 6), which are the most common, result in muscle spasm. The explanation for this is that the primary motor cortex gives origin to corticospinal and corticonuclear tracts and the secondary motor cortex gives origin to extrapyramidal tracts that pass to the basal ganglia and the reticular formation. The corticospinal and corticonuclear tracts tend to increase muscle tone, but the extrapyramidal fibers transmit inhibitory impulses that lower muscle tone (see p. 396). Destruction of the secondary motor area removes the inhibitory influence and, consequently, the muscles are spastic.

LESIONS OF THE FRONTAL EYE FIELD

Destructive lesions of the frontal eye field of one hemisphere cause the two eyes to deviate to the side of the lesion and an inability to turn the eyes to the opposite side. The involuntary tracking movement of the eyes when following moving objects is unaffected, since the lesion does not involve the visual cortex in the occipital lobe.

Irritative lesions of the frontal eye field of one hemisphere cause the two eyes to periodically deviate to the opposite side of the lesion.

LESIONS OF THE MOTOR SPEECH AREA OF BROCA

Destructive lesions in the left inferior frontal gyrus result in the loss of ability to produce speech, that is, **expressive aphasia**. The patients, however, retain the ability to think the words they wish to say, they can write the words, and they can understand their meaning when they see or hear them.

LESIONS OF THE SENSORY SPEECH AREA OF WERNICKE

Destructive lesions restricted to Wernicke's speech area in the dominant hemisphere produce a loss of ability to understand the spoken and written word, that is, **receptive aphasia**. Since Broca's area is unaffected, speech is unimpaired, and the patient can produce fluent speech. However, he is unaware of the meaning of the words he uses and he uses incorrect words or even nonexistent words. The patient is also unaware of his mistakes.

LESIONS OF THE MOTOR AND SENSORY SPEECH AREAS

Destructive lesions involving both Broca's and Wernicke's speech areas result in loss of the production of speech and the understanding of the spoken and written word, that is, **global aphasia**.

LESIONS OF THE DOMINANT ANGULAR GYRUS

Destructive lesions in the angular gyrus in the posterior parietal lobe (often considered a part of Wernicke's area) divides the pathway between the visual association area and the anterior part of Wernicke's area. This results in the patient being unable to read **(alexia)** or write **(agraphia)**.

LESIONS OF THE PREFRONTAL CORTEX

It is now generally agreed that destruction of the prefrontal region does not produce any marked loss of intelligence. It is an area of the cortex that is capable of associating experiences that are necessary for the production of abstract ideas, judgment, emotional feeling, and personality. Tumors or traumatic destruction of the prefrontal cortex result in the person's losing initiative and judgment. Emotional changes that occur include a tendency to euphoria. The patient no longer conforms to the accepted mode of social behavior and becomes careless of dress and appearance.

Frontal leukotomy (cutting the fiber tracts of the frontal lobe), and **frontal lobectomy** (removal of the frontal lobe) are surgical procedures that have been used to reduce the emotional responsiveness of patients with obsessive emotional states and intractable pain. The surgical technique was developed to remove the frontal association activity, so that past experience is not recalled and the possibilities of the future are not considered; thus introspection is lessened.

A patient suffering severe pain, such as may be experienced in the terminal stages of cancer, will still feel the pain following frontal lobectomy, but he will no longer worry about the pain and therefore will not suffer. It should be pointed out that the introduction of effective tranquilizing and mood-elevating drugs has made these operative procedures largely obsolete.

LESIONS OF THE SENSORY CORTEX

The lower centers of the brain, principally the thalamus, relay a large part of the sensory signals to the cerebral cortex for analysis. The sensory cortex is necessary for the appreciation of spatial recognition, recognition of relative intensity, and recognition of similarity and difference.

Lesions of the **primary somesthetic area** of the cortex result in contralateral sensory disturbances, which are most severe in the distal parts of the limbs. Crude painful, tactile, and thermal stimuli often return, but this is believed to be due to the function of the thalamus. The patient remains unable to judge degrees of warmth, unable to localize tactile stimuli accurately, and unable to judge weights of objects. Loss of muscle tone may also be a symptom of lesions of the sensory cortex.

Lesions of the secondary somesthetic area of the cortex do not cause recognizable sensory defects.

LESIONS OF THE SOMESTHETIC ASSOCIATION AREA

Lesions of the superior parietal lobule interfere with the patient's ability to combine touch, pressure, and proprioceptive impulses, so he is unable to appreciate texture, size, and form. This loss of integration of sensory impulses is called **astereognosis**. For example, with the eyes closed, the individual would be unable to recognize a key placed in his hand.

Destruction of the posterior part of the parietal lobe, which integrates somatic and visual sensations, will interfere with the appreciation of body image on the opposite side of the body. The individual may fail to recognize the opposite side of the body as his own. He may fail to wash it or dress it, or to shave that side of his face.

LESIONS OF THE PRIMARY VISUAL AREA

Lesions involving the walls of the posterior part of one calcarine sulcus result in a loss of sight in the opposite visual field, that is, **crossed homonymous hemianopia**. It is interesting to note that the central part of the visual field, when tested, apparently is normal. This so-called macular sparing is probably due to the patient's shifting his eyes very slightly while the visual fields are being examined. The following clinical defects should be understood. Lesions of the upper half of one primary visual area, that is, the area above the calcarine sulcus, result in **inferior quadrantic hemianopia**, whereas lesions involving one visual area below the calcarine sulcus results in **superior quadrantic hemianopia**. Lesions of the occipital pole produce central scotomas. The most common causes of these lesions are vascular disorders, tumors, and injuries from gunshot wounds.

LESIONS OF THE SECONDARY VISUAL AREA

Lesions of the secondary visual area result in a loss of ability to recognize objects seen in the opposite field of vision. The reason for this is that the area of cortex that stores past visual experiences has been lost.

LESIONS OF THE PRIMARY AUDITORY AREA

Because the primary auditory area in the inferior wall of the lateral sulcus receives nerve fibers from both cochleae, a lesion of one cortical area will produce slight bilateral loss of hearing, but the loss will be greater in the opposite ear. The main defect noted is a loss of ability to locate the source of the sound. Bilateral destruction of the primary auditory areas causes complete deafness.

LESIONS OF THE SECONDARY AUDITORY AREA

Lesions of the cortex posterior to the primary auditory area in the lateral sulcus and in the superior temporal gyrus result in an inability to interpret sounds. The patient may experience **word deafness (acoustic verbal agnosia)**.

CEREBRAL DOMINANCE

Although both hemispheres are almost identical in structure, we know that in the majority of the adult population, handedness, perception of language, speech, spatial judgment, and areas of behavior are controlled by one hemisphere and not the other. About 90 percent of people are right-handed, and the control resides in the left hemisphere. The remainder are left-handed, and a few individuals are ambidextrous. In 90 percent of individuals, speech and understanding of spoken and written language are controlled by the left hemisphere. Thus, in most adults, the left cerebral hemisphere is dominant.

From a clinical point of view, the age at which cerebral dominance comes into effect is important. For example, when cerebral damage occurs before the child has learned to speak, speech usually develops and is maintained in the remaining intact hemisphere. This transference of speech control is much more difficult in older persons.

CEREBRAL CORTICAL POTENTIALS

Electrical recordings taken from inside neurons of the cerebral cortex show a negative resting potential of about 60 mV. The action potentials overshoot the zero potential. It is interesting to know that the resting potential shows marked fluctuation, which is probably due to the continuous but variable reception of afferent impulses from other neurons. Spontaneous electrical activity can be recorded from the cortical surface rather than intracellularly; such recordings are known as **electrocorticograms**. Similar recordings can be made by placing the electrodes on the scalp. The result of this latter procedure is referred to as the **electroencephalogram (EEG)**. The changes of electrical potential recorded usually are very small and in the order of 50 μV. Characteristically, three frequency bands may be recognized in the normal individual; they are referred to as **alpha**, **beta**, and **delta rhythms**. Abnormalities of the electroencephalogram may be of great value clinically in helping to diagnose cerebral tumors, epilepsy, and cerebral abscess. An electrically silent cortex indicates cerebral death.

CONSCIOUSNESS

A conscious patient is one who is aware of himself and his surroundings. The brain is receiving an inflow of sensory information from the sensory nerves and special senses and the patient is responding by normal speech and normal voluntary motor activity, and his eyes are open and their movements are normal. Recent research has indicated that the reticular formation of the brainstem, through the thalamocortical projections, activates the cerebral cortex and maintains consciousness. It is suggested that drugs, such as anesthetics that produce unconsciousness, selectively depress the **reticular alerting mechanism**, while those that cause wakefulness have a stimulating effect on this mechanism.

It is important that a physician be able to recognize the different signs and symptoms associated with different stages of consciousness, namely, **lethargy**, **stupor**, and **coma** (unconsciousness). In a lethargic individual, the speech is slow and voluntary movement is diminished and slow. The movement of the eyes is slow. A stuporized patient will speak only if stimulated with painful stimuli. The voluntary movements are nearly absent, the eyes are closed, and there is very little spontaneous eye movement. A deeply stuporized patient will not

speak; there will be mass movements of different parts of the body in response to severe pain. The eyes will show even less spontaneous movement.

An unconscious patient will not speak and will respond only reflexly to painful stimuli, or not at all; the eyes are closed and do not move.

Clinically, it is not uncommon to observe a patient with, for example, intracranial bleeding pass progressively from consciousness to lethargy, stupor, and coma, and then, if recovery occurs, pass in the reverse direction. For these altered states of unconsciousness to occur, the thalamocortical system and the reticular formation must be either directly involved bilaterally or indirectly affected by distortion or pressure.

Sleep

Sleep is a changed state of consciousness. The pulse rate, respiratory rate, and blood pressure fall, the eyes deviate upward, the pupils contract but react to light, the tendon reflexes are lost, and the plantar reflex may become extensor. A sleeping person is not, however, unconscious, because he may be awakened quickly by the cry of a child, for example, even though he has slept through the background noise of an air-conditioner.

Sleep is facilitated by reducing the sensory input and by fatigue. This results in decreased activity of the reticular formation and the thalamocortical activating mechanism. Whether this decreased activity is a passive phenomenon, or whether the reticular formation is actively inhibited, is not known.

EPILEPSY

Epilepsy is a symptom in which there is a sudden transitory disturbance of the normal physiology of the brain, usually the cerebral cortex, which ceases spontaneously and tends to recur. The condition is usually associated with a disturbance of normal electrical activity and in its most typical form is accompanied by seizures. In partial seizures, the abnormality occurs in only one part of the brain and the patient does not lose consciousness. In generalized seizures, the abnormal activity involves large areas of the brain bilaterally and the individual loses consciousness.

In some patients with generalized seizures, there

may be nonconvulsive attacks, in which the patient suddenly stares blankly into space. This syndrome is referred to as *petit mal*. In the majority of patients with generalized seizures, there is a sudden loss of consciousness and there are tonic spasm and clonic contractions of the muscles. There are transient apnea and often loss of bowel and bladder control. The convulsions usually last from a few seconds to a few minutes.

In most patients with epilepsy the cause is unknown; in some there appears to be a hereditary predisposition; in a few, a local lesion, such as a cerebral tumor or scarring of the cortex following trauma, is the cause.

CLINICAL PROBLEMS

Answers on Page 602

1. During a practical class in pathology, a student was shown a slide illustrating a particular form of cerebral tumor. At the edge of the section there was present a small area of the cerebral cortex. The instructor asked the student whether the tissue had been removed from a motor or sensory area of the cortex. What is the main difference in structure between the motor and sensory areas of the cerebral cortex?

2. A 43-year-old man was examined by a neurologist for a suspected brain tumor. The patient was tested for stereognosis, that is, the appreciation of form in three dimensions. With the patient's eyes closed, a hairbrush was placed in his right hand and he was asked to recognize the object. He was unable to recognize the brush even after the neurologist moved the brush about in the patient's hand. On opening his eyes, the patient immediately recognized the brush. (a) Name the area of the cerebral cortex likely to be diseased in this patient. (b) Do you think that it is necessary for the object to be moved around in the patient's hand?

3. A 65-year-old man attended his physician because he noticed that for the past three weeks he had been dragging his right foot when walking. On physical examination, he was found to have an increase in tone of the flexor muscles of the right arm, and when he walked he tended to hold his right arm adducted and flexed. He also held his right fist tightly clenched. On study of the patient's gait, he was seen to have difficulty in flexing his right hip and knee. There was slight but definite weakness and increased tone of the muscles of the right leg. As the patient walked, he was noted to move his right leg in a semicircle and to place the forefoot on the ground before the heel. Examination of the right shoe showed evidence of increased wear beneath the right toes. Given that this patient had a cerebrovascular lesion involving the cerebral cortex, which area of the cortex was involved to cause these symptoms?

4. While examining an unconscious patient, a physician noted that when the patient's head was gently rotated to the right the two eyes deviated to the left. On rotation of the patient's head to the left, the patient's eyes still looked to the left. Which area of the cortex is likely to be damaged in this patient?

5. A 25-year-old soldier was wounded in Vietnam by an antipersonnel bomb. A small piece of shrapnel entered the right side of his skull over the precentral gyrus. Five years later, he was examined by a physician during a routine physical checkup and was found to have weakness of the left leg. The physician could not detect any increase in muscle tone in his left leg. Can you explain why it is that most patients with damage to the motor area of the cerebral cortex have spastic muscle paralysis while in a few the muscle tone remains normal?

6. A 22-year-old woman was involved in an automobile accident. She was thrown from the car and suffered severe head injuries. Although she was unconscious for 5 hours, she made a remarkable recovery and left the hospital one month later with very slight weakness of her right leg. Nothing else abnormal was noted. Four months later she was seen by a neurologist because she was experiencing sudden attacks of jerking movements of her right leg and foot. The attacks lasted only a few minutes. One week later the patient had a very severe attack, which involved her right leg and then spread to her right arm. On this occasion, she lost consciousness during the attack. What is the nature of

these attacks? Using your knowledge of neuro-anatomy, do you think this patient's present condition is related to her automobile accident? Which area of the cerebral cortex is involved?

7. A distinguished neurobiologist gave a lecture on the physiology of the cerebral cortex to the freshman medical student class. Having reviewed the structure of the different areas of the cerebral cortex and the functional localization of the cerebral cortex, he stated that our knowledge of the cytoarchitecture of the human cerebral cortex has contributed very little to our understanding of the normal functional activity of the cerebral cortex. Do you agree with his statement? What do you understand by the term, "the vertical chain theory"?

8. An 18-year-old boy received a gunshot wound that severely damaged his left precentral gyrus. On recovering from the incident, he left the hospital with a spastic paralysis of the right arm and leg. The patient, however, still possessed some coarse voluntary movements of the right shoulder, hip, and knee. How can you explain the presence of these residual movements on the right side?

9. A 53-year-old professor and chairman of a department of anatomy received a severe head injury while rock climbing. During the ascent of a crevasse, his companion's ice axe fell from his belt and struck the professor's head, causing a depressed fracture of the frontal bone. After convalescing from his accident, the professor returned to his position in the medical school. It quickly became obvious to the faculty and the student body that the professor's social behavior had changed dramatically. His lectures, although amusing, no longer had direction. Although previously a smartly dressed man, he now had an unkempt appearance. The organization of the department started to deteriorate rapidly. Finally, he was removed from office after being found one morning urinating into the trash basket in one of the classrooms. Using your knowledge of neuroanatomy, can you explain the professor's altered behavior?

10. A 50-year-old woman with a cerebrovascular lesion, on questioning, was found to experience difficulty in understanding spoken speech, although she fully understood written speech. Which area of the cerebral cortex was damaged?

11. A 62-year-old man, on recovering from a stroke, was found to have difficulty in understanding written speech (alexia) but could easily understand spoken speech and written symbols. Which area of the cerebral cortex is damaged in this patient?

12. What is understood by the following terms: (a) *coma*, (b) *sleep*, and (c) *electroencephalogram?* Name three neurological conditions in which the diagnosis may be assisted by the use of an electroencephalogram.

NATIONAL BOARD TYPE QUESTIONS

Answers on Page 620

IN EACH OF THE FOLLOWING QUESTIONS, ANSWER:
  (a) IF (1) ONLY IS CORRECT
  (b) IF (2) ONLY IS CORRECT
  (c) IF BOTH (1) AND (2) ARE CORRECT, AND
  (d) IF NEITHER (1) NOR (2) IS CORRECT

1. Which of the following statements is (are) correct?
  (1) The cerebral cortex is thickest over the crest of a gyrus and thinnest in the depth of a sulcus.
  (2) The largest giant pyramidal cells are found in the precentral gyrus.

2. Which of the following statements is (are) correct?

  (1) In the visual cortex, the outer band of Baillarger is so thick it can be seen with the naked eye.
  (2) The molecular layer is the most superficial layer of the cerebral cortex and is composed of the small cell bodies of the granular cells.

3. Which of the following statements is (are) correct?
  (1) Those areas of the cortex in which there are only five basic layers are known as homotypical areas.
  (2) From the functional point of view the cerebral cortex is organized into vertical units of activity.

Select the best response:

4. The following statements concerning the precentral area of the frontal lobe of the cerebral cortex are true **except**:
   (a) The posterior region is known as the primary motor area.
   (b) The primary motor area is responsible for skilled movements on the opposite side of the body.
   (c) The function of the premotor area is to store programs of motor activity which are conveyed to the primary motor area for the execution of movements.
   (d) Individual muscles are represented in the primary motor area.
   (e) The area of cortex controlling a particular movement is proportional to the skill involved.

5. The following statements concerning the motor speech area of Broca are true **except**:
   (a) In most individuals this area is important on the left or dominant hemisphere.
   (b) Broca's speech area brings about the formation of words by its connections with the primary motor area.
   (c) It is not connected to the sensory speech area of Wernicke.
   (d) It is located in the inferior frontal gyrus between the anterior and ascending rami and the ascending and posterior rami of the lateral fissure.
   (e) Brodmann's areas 44 and 45 represent the motor speech area.

6. The following statements concerning the primary somesthetic area are true **except**:
   (a) It occupies the postcentral gyrus.
   (b) Histologically, it contains large numbers of granular cells and few pyramidal cells.
   (c) The opposite half of the body is represented inverted.
   (d) Although most sensations reach the cortex from the contralateral side of the body, sensations from the hand and mouth go to both sides.
   (e) The area extends onto the posterior part of the paracentral lobule.

7. The following statements concerning the visual areas of the cortex are true **except**:
   (a) The primary visual area is located in the walls of the parieto-occipital sulcus.

   (b) The visual cortex receives afferent fibers from the lateral geniculate body.
   (c) The right half of the visual field is represented in the visual cortex of the left cerebral hemisphere.
   (d) The superior retinal quadrants pass to the inferior portion of the visual cortex.
   (e) The secondary visual area (Brodmann's areas 18 and 19) surrounds the primary visual area on the medial and lateral surfaces of the hemisphere.

In the following questions, answer:
   (a) IF (1), (2), AND (3) ONLY ARE CORRECT
   (b) IF (1) AND (3) ONLY ARE CORRECT
   (c) IF (2) AND (4) ONLY ARE CORRECT
   (d) IF (4) ONLY IS CORRECT, OR
   (e) IF ALL ARE CORRECT.

8. Which of the following statements is (are) correct concerning the superior temporal gyrus?
   (1) The primary auditory area is situated in the inferior wall of the lateral sulcus.
   (2) The main projection fibers to the primary auditory area arise from the thalamus.
   (3) The sensory speech area of Wernicke is localized in the superior temporal gyrus in the dominant hemisphere.
   (4) A unilateral lesion of the auditory area produces no effect on the hearing from the opposite ear.

9. Which of the following statements is (are) correct concerning the association areas of the cortex?
   (1) They form a large area of the cortical surface.
   (2) The prefrontal area is concerned with the make-up of the individual's personality.
   (3) They are concerned with the interpretation of sensory experiences.
   (4) An appreciation of the body image is assembled in the posterior parietal cortex and the right side of the body is represented in the left hemisphere.

10. Which of the following statements is (are) correct concerning cerebral dominance?
   (1) The cortical gyri of the dominant and nondominant hemispheres are arranged differently.
   (2) More than 90 percent of the adult popula-

Fig. 15-9. Lateral view of left cerebral hemisphere.

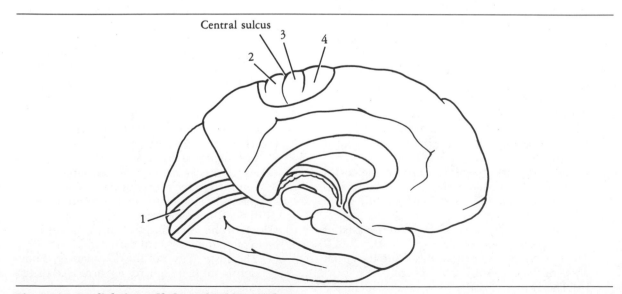

Fig. 15-10. Medial view of left cerebral hemisphere.

tion are right-handed and are therefore left hemisphere-dominant.

(3) About 50 percent of the adult population are right hemisphere-dominant for speech.

(4) The nondominant hemisphere interprets spatial perception, recognition of faces, and music.

In Figure 15-9, match the numbers listed on the left with the most likely functional areas of the cerebral cortex listed on the right.

11. Number 1
12. Number 2
13. Number 3
14. Number 4

(a) Primary motor area
(b) Secondary auditory area
(c) Frontal eye field
(d) Primary somesthetic area
(e) None of the above

In Figure 15-10, match the numbers listed on the left with the most likely functional area of the cerebral cortex listed on the right.

15. Number 1
16. Number 2
17. Number 3
18. Number 4

(a) Premotor area
(b) Primary somesthetic area
(c) Primary visual area
(d) Primary motor area
(e) None of the above

ADDITIONAL READING

Benson, D. F. *Aphasia, Alexia, and Agraphia.* New York: Churchill Livingstone, 1979.

Begleiter, H. (ed.). *Evoked Brain Potentials and Behavior.* New York: Plenum, 1979.

Berlucchi, G. Cerebral dominance and interhemispheric communication in normal man. In *The Neurosciences, Third Study Program.* Cambridge, Massachusetts: MIT Press, 1974. P. 65.

Bindman, L. *The Neurophysiology of the Cerebral Cortex.* Austin: University of Texas Press, 1981.

Bloodstein, O. *Speech Pathology: An Introduction.* Boston: Houghton Mifflin, 1979.

Broadbent, D. E. Division of function and integration of behavior. In *The Neurosciences, Third Study Program.* Cambridge, Massachusetts: MIT Press, 1974. P. 31.

Brodmann, K. *Vergleichende Lokalisationslebre der Grossbirnrinde.* Leipzig: Barth, 1909.

Campbell, A. W. *Histological Studies on the Localization of Cerebral Function.* Cambridge, Massachusetts: Harvard University Press, 1905.

Cartwright, R. D. *A Primer on Sleep and Dreaming.* Reading, Massachusetts: Addison-Wesley, 1978.

Chow, K. L., and Leiman, A. L. The structural and functional organization of the neocortex. *Neurosci. Res. Prog. Bull.* 8:153, 1970.

Damasio, A. R., and Geschwind, N. The neural basis of language. *Annu. Rev. Neurosci.* 7:127, 1984.

von Economo, C., and Koskinas, G. N. *The Cytoarchitec-* *tonics of the Human Cerebral Cortex.* New York and London: Oxford University Press, 1929.

Foerster, O. The cerebral cortex in man. *Lancet* 2:309, 1931.

Fois, A., and Low, N. *The Electroencephalogram of the Normal Child.* Springfield, Illinois: Thomas, 1961.

Geschwind, N. Language and the brain. *Sci. Am.* 226:76, 1972.

Guyton, A. C. *Textbook of Medical Physiology* (7th ed.). Philadelphia: Saunders, 1986.

Hubel, T. H., and Wiesel, T. N. Functional architecture of macaque monkey visual cortex. *Proc. R. Soc. Lond. [Biol.].* 198:1, 1977.

Jackson, J. H. Selected writings of John Hughlings Jackson. In J. Taylor (ed.), *On Epilepsy and Epileptiform Convulsions.* London: Hodder & Stoughton, 1931. Vol. 1.

Jasper, H. H., Ward, A. A., and Pope, A. (eds.). *Basic Mechanisms of the Epilepsies.* Boston: Little, Brown, 1969.

Klass, D. W., and Daly, D. C. (eds.). *Current Practice of Clinical Electroencephalography.* New York: Raven, 1979.

Milner, B. Hemispheric specialization: Scope and limits. In *The Neurosciences, Third Study Program.* Cambridge, Massachusetts: MIT Press, 1974. P. 75.

Nieuwenhuys, R. *Chemoarchitecture of the Brain.* Berlin: Springer-Verlag, 1985.

Penfield, W., and Boldrey, E. Somatic motor and sensory representation in the cerebral cortex of man as studied by electrical stimulation. *Brain* 60:389, 1937.

Penfield, W., and Rasmussen, T. *The Cerebral Cortex of Man: A Clinical Study of Localization of Function.* New York and London: Macmillan, 1950.

Penfield, W., and Roberts, L. *Speech and Brain Mechanisms.* Princeton, New Jersey: Princeton University Press, 1959.

Plum, F., and Posner, J. B. *The Diagnosis of Stupor and Coma* (3rd ed.). Philadelphia: Davis, 1980.

Porter, R. The cerebral cortex and control of movement performance. In M. Swash and C. Kennard (eds.), *Scientific Basis of Clinical Neurology.* Edinburgh: Churchill Livingstone, 1985. P. 19.

Powell, T. P. S. Certain aspects of the intrinsic organisation of the cerebral cortex. In O. Pompeiano and C. A. Marsan (eds.), *Brain Mechanisms of Perpetual Awareness and Purposeful Behavior.* New York: Raven Press, 1981. Pp. 1.

Sholl, D. A. *Organization of the Cerebral Cortex.* London: Methuen, 1956.

Sperry, R. W. Lateral specialization in the surgically separated hemispheres. In *The Neurosciences, Third Study Program.* Cambridge, Massachusetts: MIT Press, 1974. P. 5.

Sutherland, J. M., and Tait, H. *The Epilepsies: Modern Diagnosis and Treatment.* Edinburgh: Livingstone, 1969.

Teuber, H. L. Why two brains. In *The Neurosciences, Third Study Program.* Cambridge, Massachusetts: MIT Press, 1974. P. 71.

Trevarthen, C. Hemispheric specialization. In I. Darian-Smith (ed.), *Handbook of Physiology.* Sec. 1, Vol. III. Bethesda: American Physiological Society, 1984. P. 1129.

Walton, J. N. *Brain's Diseases of the Nervous System* (8th ed.). New York and London: Oxford University Press, 1977.

Williams, P. L., Warwick, R., Dyson, M., and Bannister, L. H. *Gray's Anatomy* (37th Brit. ed.). Philadelphia: Saunders, 1989.

Woolsey, C. N. Cortical localization as defined by evoked potential and electrical stimulation studies. In G. Shaltenbrand and C. N. Woolsey (eds.), *Cerebral Localization and Organization.* Madison, Wisconsin: University of Wisconsin Press, 1964. P. 17.

Ziberman, A. M. The specialization of the language hemisphere. In *The Neurosciences, Third Study Program.* Cambridge, Massachusetts: MIT Press, 1974. P. 43.

Chapter 16
The Reticular Formation and the Limbic System

RETICULAR FORMATION

The reticular formation, as its name would suggest, resembles a net (reticular) that is made up of nerve cells and nerve fibers. The net extends up through the axis of the central nervous system from the spinal cord to the cerebrum. It receives input from most of the sensory systems and has efferent fibers that descend and influence nerve cells at all levels of the central nervous system. The exceptionally long dendrites of the neurons of the reticular formation permit input from widely placed ascending and descending pathways. Through its many connections it can influence skeletal muscle activity, somatic and visceral sensations, the autonomic and endocrine systems, and even the level of consciousness.

GENERAL ARRANGEMENT

The reticular formation consists of a deeply placed continuous network of nerve cells and fibers that extend from the spinal cord, through the medulla, the pons, the midbrain, the subthalamus, the hypothalamus, and the thalamus. The diffuse network may be divided into three longitudinal columns, the first occupying the median plane, called the **median column**, and consisting of intermediate-sized neurons, the second called the **medial column** containing large neurons, and the third or **lateral column** containing mainly small neurons (Fig. 16-1).

The groups of neurons are poorly defined and it is difficult to trace an anatomical pathway through the network. Nevertheless, experiments have shown that polysynaptic pathways exist and that both crossed and uncrossed ascending and descending pathways are present, involving many neurons that serve both somatic and visceral functions.

Inferiorly, the reticular formation is continuous with the interneurons of the gray matter of the spinal cord, while superiorly impulses are relayed to the cerebral cortex; a substantial projection of fibers also leaves the reticular formation to enter the cerebellum.

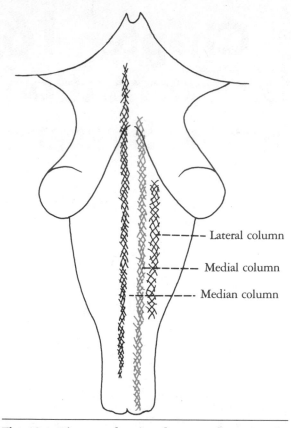

Fig. 16-1. Diagram showing the approximate positions of the median, medial, and lateral columns of the reticular formation in the brainstem.

AFFERENT PROJECTIONS

Many different afferent pathways project onto the reticular formation from most parts of the central nervous system. From the spinal cord there are the spinoreticular tracts, the spinothalamic tracts, and the medial lemniscus. From the cranial nerve nuclei there are ascending afferent tracts which will include the vestibular, acoustic, and visual pathways. From the cerebellum, there is the cerebelloreticular pathway. From the subthalamic, hypothalamic, and thalamic nuclei and from the corpus striatum and the limbic system there are further afferent tracts. Other important afferent fibers arise in the primary motor cortex of the frontal lobe and from the somesthetic cortex of the parietal lobe.

EFFERENT PROJECTIONS

Multiple efferent pathways extend down to the brainstem and spinal cord through the reticulobulbar and reticulospinal tracts to neurons in the motor nuclei of the cranial nerves and the anterior horn cells of the spinal cord. Other descending pathways extend to the sympathetic outflow and the craniosacral parasympathetic outflow of the autonomic nervous system. Additional pathways extend to the corpus striatum, the cerebellum, the red nucleus, the substantia nigra, the tectum, and the nuclei of the thalamus, subthalamus, and hypothalamus. Most regions of the cerebral cortex receive efferent fibers as well.

FUNCTIONS OF THE RETICULAR FORMATION

From the previous description of the vast number of connections of the reticular formation to all parts of the nervous system, it is not surprising to find that the functions are many. A few of the more important functions will be considered here.

1. **Control of skeletal muscle.** Through the reticulospinal and reticulobulbar tracts, the reticular formation can influence the activity of the alpha and gamma motor neurons. Thus the reticular formation can modulate muscle tone and reflex activity. It can also bring about reciprocal inhibition; for example, when the flexor muscles contract, the antagonistic extensors relax. The reticular formation, assisted by the vestibular apparatus of the inner ear and the vestibular spinal tract, plays an important role in maintaining the tone of the antigravity muscles when standing. The so-called respiratory centers of the brainstem, described by neurophysiologists as being in the control of the respiratory muscles, are now considered part of the reticular formation.

2. **Control of somatic and visceral sensations.** By virtue of its central location in the cerebrospinal axis, the reticular formation can influence all ascending pathways that pass to supraspinal levels. The influence may be facilitative or inhibitory. In particular, the reticular formation may have a key role in the "gating mechanism" for the control of pain perception (see p. 368).

3. **Control of the autonomic nervous system.** Higher control of the autonomic nervous system, from the cerebral cortex, hypothalamus, and other subcortical nuclei, can be exerted by the reticulobulbar and reticulospinal tracts, which descend to the sympathetic outflow and the parasympathetic craniosacral outflow.

4. **Control of the endocrine nervous system.** Either directly or indirectly through the hypothalamic nuclei, the reticular formation can influence the synthesis or release of releasing or release-inhibiting factors and thereby control the activity of the hypophysis cerebri.

5. **Influence on the biological clocks.** By means of its multiple afferent and efferent pathways to the hypothalamus, the reticular formation probably influences the biological rhythms.

6. **The reticular activating system.** Multiple ascending pathways carrying sensory information to higher centers are channeled through the reticular formation, which in turn projects this information to different parts of the cerebral cortex, causing a sleeping person to awaken. In fact, it has been suggested that the state of consciousness is dependent on the continuous projection of sensory information to the cortex. Different degrees of wakefulness seem to depend on the degree of activity of the reticular formation.

From the above description it must be apparent that in the network of neurons in the cerebrospinal axis, almost totally ignored in the past, is now being shown to influence practically all activities of the body.

LIMBIC SYSTEM

The word *limbic* means border or margin and the term *limbic system* was loosely used to include a group of structures that lie in the border zone between the cerebral cortex and the hypothalamus. Now it is recognized, as the result of research, that the limbic system is involved with many other structures beyond the border zone in the control of emotion, behavior, and drive; it also appears to be important to memory.

Anatomically, the limbic structures include the subcallosal, the cingulate, and the parahippocam-
pal gyri, the hippocampal formation, the amygdaloid nucleus, the mammillary bodies, and the anterior thalamic nucleus (Fig. 16-2). The alveus, the fimbria, the fornix, the mammillothalamic tract, and the stria terminalis constitute the connecting pathways of this system.

HIPPOCAMPAL FORMATION

The hippocampal formation consists of the hippocampus, the dentate gyrus, and the parahippocampal gyrus.

The **hippocampus** is a curved elevation of gray matter that extends throughout the entire length of the floor of the inferior horn of the lateral ventricle (Fig. 16-3). Its anterior end is expanded to form the **pes hippocampus**. It is named hippocampus because it resembles a sea horse in coronal section. The convex ventricular surface is covered with ependyma, beneath which lies a thin layer of white matter called the **alveus** (Fig. 16-4). The alveus consists of nerve fibers that have originated in the hippocampus and these converge medially to form a bundle called the **fimbria** (Figs. 16-3 and 16-4). The fimbria in turn becomes continuous with the crus of the fornix (Fig. 16-3). The hippocampus terminates posteriorly beneath the splenium of the corpus callosum.

The **dentate gyrus** is a narrow, notched band of gray matter that lies between the fimbria of the hippocampus and the parahippocampal gyrus (Fig. 16-3). Posteriorly, the gyrus accompanies the fimbria almost to the splenium of the corpus callosum and becomes continuous with the **indusium griseum**. The indusium griseum is a thin, vestigial layer of gray matter that covers the superior surface of the corpus callosum (Fig. 16-5). Embedded in the superior surface of the indusium griseum are two slender bundles of white fibers on each side called the **medial and lateral longitudinal striae**. The striae are the remains of the white matter of the vestigial indusium griseum. Anteriorly, the dentate gyrus is continued into the **uncus**.

The **parahippocampal gyrus** lies between the hippocampal fissure and the collateral sulcus and is continuous with the hippocampus along the medial edge of the temporal lobe (Figs. 16-3 and 16-4).

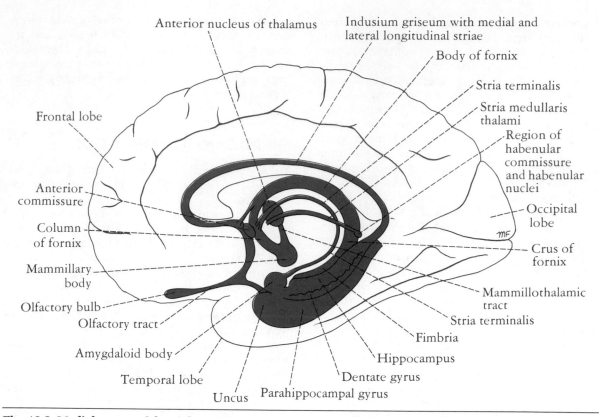

Fig. 16-2. Medial aspect of the right cerebral hemisphere, showing structures that form the limbic system.

AMYGDALOID NUCLEUS

The amygdaloid nucleus is so named because it resembles an almond. It is situated partly anterior and partly superior to the tip of the inferior horn of the lateral ventricle (see Fig. 14-11). It is fused with the tip of the tail of the caudate nucleus, which has passed anteriorly in the roof of the inferior horn of the lateral ventricle. The stria terminalis emerges from its posterior aspect.

The mammillary bodies and the anterior nucleus of the thalamus are considered elsewhere in this text.

CONNECTING PATHWAYS OF THE LIMBIC SYSTEM

These pathways are the alveus, the fimbria, the fornix, the mammillothalamic tract, and the stria terminalis.

The **alveus** consists of a thin layer of white matter that lies on the superior or ventricular surface of the hippocampus (Fig. 16-4). It is composed of nerve fibers that originate in the hippocampal cortex. The fibers converge on the medial border of the hippocampus to form a bundle called the **fimbria**.

The fimbria now leaves the posterior end of the hippocampus as the **crus of the fornix** (Fig. 16-3). The crus from each side curves posteriorly and superiorly beneath the splenium of the corpus callosum and around the posterior surface of the thalamus. The two crura now converge to form the **body of the fornix,** which is applied closely to the undersurface of the corpus callosum (Fig. 16-2). As the two crura come together they are connected by transverse fibers called the **commissure of the fornix** (Fig. 14-13). These fibers decussate and join the hippocampi of the two sides.

Anteriorly, the body of the fornix is connected to the undersurface of the corpus callosum by the

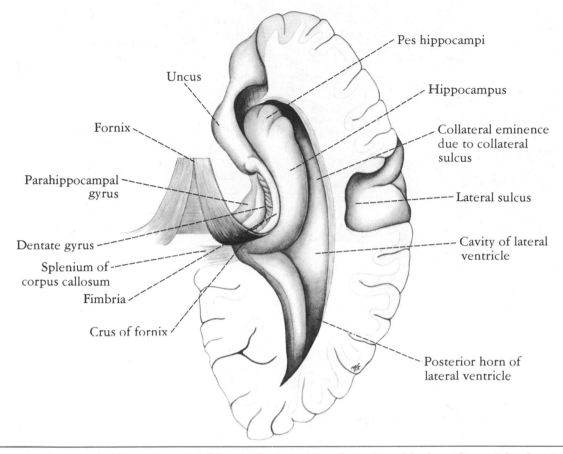

Fig. 16-3. Dissection of the right cerebral hemisphere exposing the cavity of the lateral ventricle, showing the hippocampus, the dentate gyrus, and the fornix.

septum pellucidum. Inferiorly, the body of the fornix is related to the tela choroidea and the ependymal roof of the third ventricle.

The body of the fornix splits anteriorly into two anterior **columns of the fornix**, each of which curves anteriorly and inferiorly over the interventricular foramen (foramen of Monro). Then each column disappears into the lateral wall of the third ventricle to reach the **mammillary body** (Fig. 16-2).

The **mammillothalamic tract** provides important connections between the mammillary body and the anterior nuclear group of the thalamus.

The **stria terminalis** emerges from the posterior aspect of the amygdaloid nucleus and runs as a bundle of nerve fibers posteriorly in the roof of the

inferior horn of the lateral ventricle on the medial side of the tail of the caudate nucleus (Fig. 16-2). It follows the curve of the caudate nucleus and comes to lie in the floor of the body of the lateral ventricle.

STRUCTURE OF THE HIPPOCAMPUS AND THE DENTATE GYRUS

The cortical structure of the parahippocampal gyrus is six-layered (Fig. 16-4). As the cortex is traced into the hippocampus there is a gradual transition from a six- to a three-layered arrangement. These three layers are the superficial **molecular layer**,

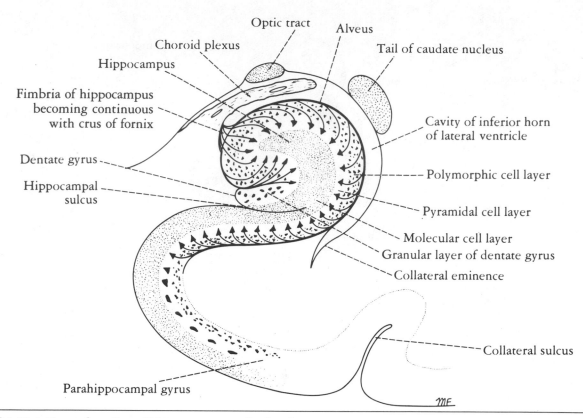

Fig. 16-4. Coronal section of hippocampus and related structures.

consisting of nerve fibers and scattered small neurons; the **pyramidal layer**, consisting of many large pyramidal shaped neurons; and the inner **polymorphic layer**, which is similar in structure to the polymorphic layer of the cortex seen elsewhere.

The dentate gyrus also has three layers but the pyramidal layer is replaced by the granular layer (Fig. 16-4). The granular layer is composed of densely arranged rounded or oval neurons that give rise to axons that terminate upon the dendrites of the pyramidal cells in the hippocampus. A few of the axons join the fimbria and enter the fornix.

Afferent Connections of the Hippocampus

Afferent connections of the hippocampus may be divided into six groups (Fig. 16-6):

1. Fibers arising in the cingulate gyrus passing to the hippocampus.
2. Fibers arising from the septal nuclei (nuclei lying within the midline close to the anterior commissure) pass posterior in the fornix to the hippocampus.
3. Fibers arising from one hippocampus pass across the midline to the opposite hippocampus in the commissure of the fornix.
4. Fibers from the indusium griseum pass posteriorly in the longitudinal striae to the hippocampus.
5. Fibers from the entorhinal area or olfactory associated cortex pass to the hippocampus.
6. Fibers arising from the dentate and parahippocampal gyri travel to the hippocampus.

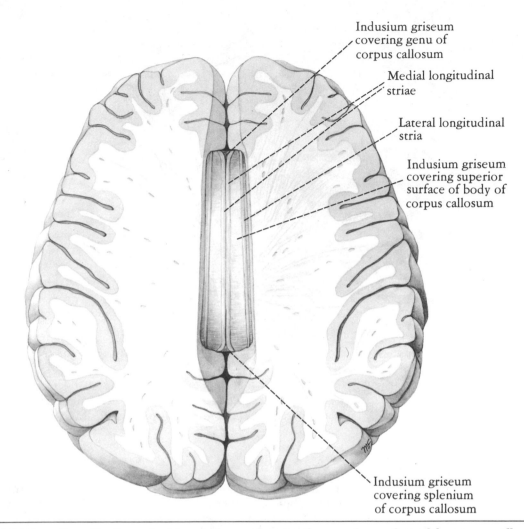

Indusium griseum
covering genu of
corpus callosum

Medial longitudinal
striae

Lateral longitudinal
stria

Indusium griseum
covering superior
surface of body of
corpus callosum

Indusium griseum
covering splenium
of corpus callosum

Fig. 16-5. Dissection of both cerebral hemispheres, showing the superior surface of the corpus callosum.

Efferent Connections of the Hippocampus

Axons of the large pyramidal cells of the hippocampus emerge to form the alveus and the fimbria. The fimbria continues as the crus of the fornix. The two crura converge to form the body of the fornix. The body of the fornix splits into the two columns of the fornix, which curve downward and forward in front of the interventricular foramina. The fibers within the fornix are distributed to the following regions (Fig. 16-6):

1. Fibers pass posterior to the anterior commissure to enter the mammillary body, where they end in the medial nucleus.
2. Fibers pass posterior to the anterior commissure to end in the anterior nuclei of the thalamus.
3. Fibers pass posterior to the anterior commissure to enter the tegmentum of the midbrain.
4. Fibers pass anterior to the anterior commissure to end in the septal nuclei, the lateral preoptic area, and the anterior part of the hypothalamus.
5. Fibers join the stria medullaris thalami to reach the habenular nuclei.

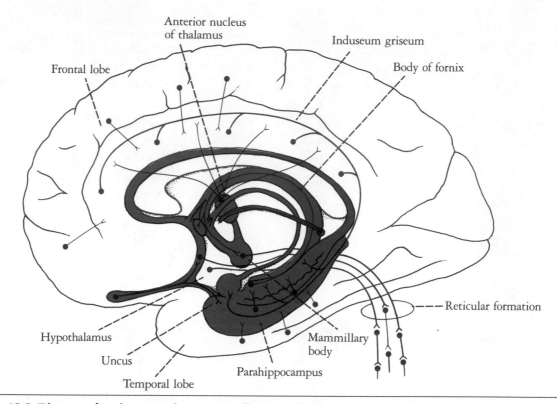

Fig. 16-6. Diagram showing some important afferent and efferent connections of the limbic system.

Consideration of the above complex anatomical pathways indicates that the structures composing the limbic system are not only interconnected, but also send projection fibers to many different parts of the nervous system. Physiologists now recognize the importance of the hypothalamus as being the major output pathway of the limbic system.

FUNCTIONS OF THE LIMBIC SYSTEM

The limbic system, via the hypothalamus and its connections with the outflow of the autonomic nervous system and its control of the endocrine system, is able to influence many aspects of emotional behavior. These include particularly the reactions of fear and anger and the emotions associated with sexual behavior.

There is also evidence that the hippocampus is concerned with recent memory. Memory for remote past events usually is unaffected by lesions of this structure. There is no evidence that the limbic system has an olfactory function. The various afferent and efferent connections of the limbic system provide pathways for the integration and effective homeostatic responses to a wide variety of environmental stimuli.

CLINICAL NOTES

GENERAL CONSIDERATIONS

Reticular Formation

The **reticular formation** has been described as consisting of a continuous network of nerve cells and fibers that extend through the neuroaxis from the spinal cord to the cerebral cortex. The functional significance of these neurons is becoming increasingly apparent as neurobiological research continues. The reticular formation not only modulates the control of motor systems but influences sensory systems as well. By means of its multiple ascending pathways, which project to different parts of the cerebral cortex, it is believed to influence the state of consciousness.

LOSS OF CONSCIOUSNESS

In experimental animals it has been shown that damage to the reticular formation, which spares the ascending sensory pathways, causes persistent unconsciousness. Pathological lesions of the reticular formation in man may result in loss of consciousness and even coma. It has been suggested that loss of consciousness that occurs in epilepsy may be due to inhibition of the activity of the reticular formation in the upper part of the diencephalon.

Limbic System

The anatomical connections of the limbic system are extremely complex and, since their significance is not fully understood, it is unnecessary for a student of medicine to commit all of them to memory. The results of neurophysiological experiments, which have included stimulation and ablation of different parts of the limbic system in animals, are not entirely clear. Nevertheless, certain important roles have been inferred: (1) The limbic structures are involved in the development of sensations of emotion and with the visceral responses accompanying those emotions, and (2) the hippocampus is concerned with recent memory.

Destruction of the Amygdaloid Complex

Unilateral or bilateral destruction of the amygdaloid nucleus and the paraamygdaloid area in patients suffering from aggressive behavior in many cases results in a decrease in aggressiveness, emotional instability, and restlessness, increased interest in food, and hypersexuality. There is no disturbance in memory. Monkeys that have been subjected to bilateral removal of the temporal lobes demonstrate what is known as the **Klüver-Bucy syndrome**. They become docile and show no evidence of fear or anger and are unable to appreciate objects visually. They have an increased appetite and increased sexual activity. Moreover, the animals indiscriminately seek partnerships with male and female animals.

Precise stereotactic lesions in the amygdaloid complex in man reduce emotional excitability and bring about normalization of behavior in patients with severe disturbances. No loss of memory occurs.

Temporal Lobe Dysfunction

Temporal lobe epilepsy may be preceded by an aura of acoustic or olfactory experience. The olfactory aura is usually an unpleasant odor. The patient is often confused, anxious, and docile and may perform automatic and complicated movements, such as undressing in public or driving a car, and then, following the seizure, may have no memory of what occurred previously.

CLINICAL PROBLEMS   *Answers on Page 604*

1. While discussing the neurological basis of emotions during a ward round, a neurologist asked a third-year medical student what he knew about the Klüver-Bucy syndrome. Can you answer that question? Does it ever occur in the human subject?

2. A 23-year-old woman visited her neurologist with a four-year history of epileptic attacks. A

friend of hers vividly described one of her attacks. For a few seconds before the convulsions began the patient would complain of an unpleasant odor, similar to that encountered in a cow shed. This was followed by a shrill cry as she fell to the floor unconscious. Her whole body immediately became involved in generalized tonic and clonic movements. Clearly, this patient had a generalized form of epileptic seizure. Using your knowledge of neuroanatomy, could you suggest which lobe of the brain was initially involved in the epileptic discharge?

3. A 54-year-old man died in the hospital with a cerebral tumor. He had always been intellectually very bright and could easily recall events in his childhood. For the past six months his family had noticed that he had difficulty in recalling where he had placed things, such as his pipe. He also had difficulty in recalling recent news events and, just before he died, he could not remember that his brother had visited him the day before. Using your knowledge of neuroanatomy, could you suggest which part of the brain was being affected by the expanding and highly invasive tumor?

NATIONAL BOARD TYPE QUESTIONS

Answers on Page 620

IN EACH OF THE FOLLOWING QUESTIONS, ANSWER:
   (a) IF (1) ONLY IS CORRECT
   (b) IF (2) ONLY IS CORRECT
   (c) IF BOTH (1) AND (2) ARE CORRECT, AND
   (d) IF NEITHER (1) NOR (2) IS CORRECT

1. Which of the following statements is (are) correct?
   (1) The reticular formation is a diffuse network of nerve fibers, without nerve cell bodies, that extend through the neuroaxis from the spinal cord to the thalamus.
   (2) The main pathways through the reticular formation may easily be traced from one part of the central nervous system to another.
2. Which of the following statements is (are) correct?
   (1) Superiorly the reticular formation is relayed to the cerebral cortex.
   (2) Afferent pathways project into the reticular formation from most parts of the central nervous system.
3. Which of the following statements is (are) correct?
   (1) Reticulobulbar and reticulospinal tracts form the efferent pathways from the reticular formation to the motor nuclei of the cranial nerves and the anterior horn cells of the spinal cord, respectively.
   (2) The cerebral cortex does not receive efferent fibers from the reticular formation.

In the following questions, answer:
   (a) IF (1), (2), AND (3) ONLY ARE CORRECT
   (b) IF (1) AND (3) ONLY ARE CORRECT
   (c) IF (2) AND (4) ONLY ARE CORRECT
   (d) IF (4) ONLY IS CORRECT, OR
   (e) IF ALL ARE CORRECT

4. Which of the following statements is (are) correct concerning the functions of the reticular formation?
   (1) It influences the activity of the alpha and gamma motor neurons.
   (2) It brings about reciprocal inhibition during contraction of the prime mover muscles.
   (3) It helps maintain the tone of the antigravity muscles.
   (4) It opposes the actions of the vestibular spinal tract.
5. Which of the following statements is (are) correct concerning the functions of the reticular formation?
   (1) It can influence all ascending pathways to the supraspinal levels.
   (2) It may control the reception of pain.
   (3) By means of its reticulobulbar and reticulospinal tracts it can control the parasympathetic and sympathetic outflows.
   (4) It can affect the biological rhythms.
6. Which of the following structure(s) collectively form(s) the limbic system?
   (1) Amygdaloid nucleus
   (2) Pulvinar of thalamus

Fig. 16-7. Medial aspect of the right cerebral hemisphere, showing structures that form the limbic system.

(3) Hippocampal formation
(4) Genu of the corpus callosum

7. Which of the following statements is (are) correct concerning the efferent connections of the hippocampus?
   (1) They arise from the large pyramidal cells of the cortex.
   (2) They travel through the fornix.
   (3) Some of the fibers enter the mammillary body.
   (4) Some of the fibers end in the anterior nuclei of the thalamus.

8. Which of the following statements is (are) correct concerning the functions of the limbic system?
   (1) It is concerned with the reactions of fear and anger.
   (2) It is concerned with visual experiences.
   (3) The hippocampus is concerned with recent memory.
   (4) The limbic system plays an important role in olfactory function.

In Figure 16-7, match the numbers listed on the left with the appropriate structures listed on the right. Any answer may be used more than once.

9. Number 1
10. Number 2
11. Number 3
12. Number 4

(a) Uncus
(b) Body of fornix
(c) Parahippocampal gyrus
(d) Dentate gyrus
(e) None of the above

ADDITIONAL READING

Amaral, D. G., and Cowan, W. M. Subcortical afferents to the hippocampal formation in the monkey. *J. Comp. Neurol.* 189:573, 1980.

Braitenberg, V., and Schüz, A. Some anatomical comments on the hippocampus. In W. Seifert (ed.), *Neu-robiology of the Hippocampus*. London and New York: Academic, 1983. P. 21.

Breathnach, C. S. The limbic system. *J. Irish Med. Assoc.* 73:331, 1980.

Gerstenbrand, F., Poewe, W., Aichner, F., and Sultuari, L.

Klüver-Bucy syndrome in man: Experience with post traumatic cases. *Neurosci. Behav. Rev.* 7:413, 1983.

Horel, J. A. The neuroanatomy of amnesia. A critique of the hippocampal memory hypothesis. *Brain* 101:403, 1978.

Isaacson, R. L. *The Limbic System* (2nd ed.). New York and London: Plenum, 1982.

Klemm, W. R. Ascending and descending excitatory influences in the brain stem reticulum: A re-examination. *Brain Res.* 36:444, 1972.

Loftus, G. R., and Loftus, E. F. *Human Memory: The Processing of Information.* Hillsdale, New Jersey: Lawrence Erlbaum Associates, 1976.

Lopes de Silva, F. H., and Arnolds, D. E. A. T. Physiology of the hippocampus and related structures. *Annu. Rev. Physiol.* 40:185, 1978.

Mishkin, M., and Appenzeller, F. Anatomy of memory. *Sci. Am.,* June 1987. P. 80.

Moore, R. Y. The reticular formation: Monoamine neuron systems. In J. A. Hobson and M. A. B. Brazier (eds.), *The Reticular Formation Revisited.* New York: Raven, 1980. P. 67.

Price, J. L., and Amaral, D. G. An autoradiographic study of the projections of the central nucleus of the monkey amygdala. *J. Neurosci.* 1:1242, 1981.

Willis, W. D. The raphe-spinal system. In *Brainstem Control of Spinal Function.* New York: Academic, 1984. P. 141.

Willis, W. D., Gerhart, K. D., Willcockson, W. S., *et al.* Primate raphe- and reticulospinal neurons: Effects of stimulation in periaqueductal gray or VPL thalamic nucleus. *J. Neurophysiol.* 51:467, 1984.

Zola-Morgan, S., Squire, L. R., and Mishkin, M. The neuroanatomy of amnesia: amygdala-hippocampus versus temporal stem. *Science* 218:1337, 1982.

Chapter 17
The Basal Nuclei (Basal Ganglia) and Their Connections

The term **basal nuclei** is applied to a collection of masses of gray matter situated within each cerebral hemisphere. They are the corpus striatum, the amygdaloid nucleus, and the claustrum. The basal nuclei play an important role in the control of posture and voluntary movement.

In this chapter the basal nuclei, their connections, and their functions will be briefly described.

CORPUS STRIATUM

The corpus striatum is situated lateral to the thalamus and is almost completely divided by a band of nerve fibers, the **internal capsule**, into the caudate nucleus and the lentiform nucleus (Fig. 17-1).

CAUDATE NUCLEUS

The caudate nucleus is a large C-shaped mass of gray matter that is closely related to the lateral ventricle and lies lateral to the thalamus (Fig. 17-1). The lateral surface of the nucleus is related to the internal capsule, which separates it from the lentiform nucleus (Fig. 17-2). For purposes of descrip-

tion, it may be divided up into a head, a body, and a tail.

The **head** of the caudate nucleus is large and rounded and forms the lateral wall of the anterior horn of the lateral ventricle (Fig. 17-2). The head is continuous inferiorly with the putamen of the lentiform nucleus (the caudate nucleus and the putamen are sometimes referred to as the **neostriatum**). Just superior to this point of union, strands of gray matter pass through the internal capsule, giving the region a striated appearance; hence the term **corpus striatum**.

The **body** of the caudate nucleus is long and narrow and is continuous with the head in the region of the interventricular foramen. The body of the caudate nucleus forms part of the floor of the body of the lateral ventricle.

The **tail** of the caudate nucleus is long and slender and is continuous with the body in the region of the posterior end of the thalamus. It follows the contour of the lateral ventricle and continues forward in the roof of the inferior horn of the lateral ventricle. It terminates anteriorly in the **amygdaloid nucleus** (Fig. 17-1).

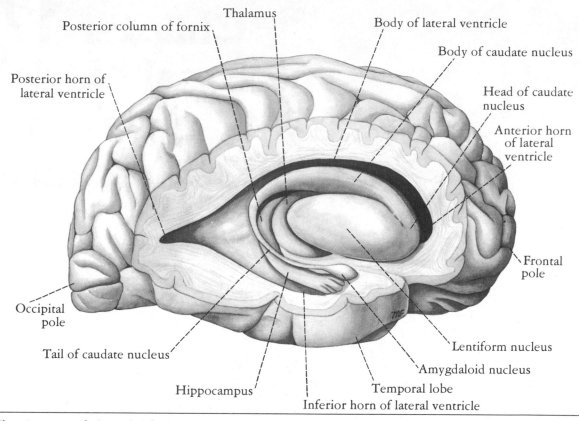

Posterior column of fornix

Thalamus

Body of lateral ventricle

Body of caudate nucleus

Posterior horn of lateral ventricle

Head of caudate nucleus

Anterior horn of lateral ventricle

Frontal pole

Occipital pole

Tail of caudate nucleus

Lentiform nucleus

Amygdaloid nucleus

Hippocampus

Temporal lobe

Inferior horn of lateral ventricle

Fig. 17-1. Lateral view of right cerebral hemisphere dissected to show the position of the different basal nuclei.

LENTIFORM NUCLEUS

The lentiform nucleus is a wedge-shaped mass of gray matter, whose broad convex base is directed laterally and its blade medially (Fig. 17-2). It is buried deep in the white matter of the cerebral hemisphere and is related medially to the internal capsule, which separates it from the caudate nucleus and the thalamus. The lentiform nucleus is related laterally to a thin sheet of white matter, the **external capsule** (Fig. 17-2), which separates it from a thin sheet of gray matter, called the **claustrum**. The claustrum, in turn, separates the external capsule from the subcortical white matter of the insula. A vertical plate of white matter divides the nucleus into a larger, darker lateral portion, the **putamen**, and an inner lighter portion, the **globus pallidus** (Fig. 17-2). Inferiorly at its anterior end,

the putamen is continuous with the head of the caudate nucleus (Fig. 17-1).

AMYGDALOID NUCLEUS

The amygdaloid nucleus is situated in the temporal lobe close to the uncus (Fig. 17-1). The amygdaloid nucleus is considered to be part of the limbic system and is described in Chapter 16.

CLAUSTRUM

The claustrum is a thin sheet of gray matter that is separated from the lateral surface of the lentiform nucleus by the external capsule (Fig. 17-2). Lateral to the claustrum is the subcortical white matter of the insula. The function of the claustrum is unknown.

Fig. 17-2. Horizontal section of the cerebrum as seen from above, showing the relationships of the different basal nuclei.

CONNECTIONS OF THE CORPUS STRIATUM

Afferent Fibers

Corticostriate Fibers

All parts of the cerebral cortex send axons to the caudate nucleus and the putamen (Fig. 17-3). Each part of the cerebral cortex projects to a specific part of the caudate-putamen complex. Most of the pro-jections are from the cortex of the same side. The largest input is from the sensory-motor cortex. Glutamate is the neurotransmitter of the corticostriate fibers.

Thalamostriate Fibers

The intralaminar nuclei of the thalamus send large numbers of axons to the caudate nucleus and the putamen (Fig. 17-3).

Fig. 17-3. Some of the main connections between the cerebral cortex, the basal nuclei, the thalamic nuclei, and the brainstem.

Nigrostriate Fibers

Neurons in the substantia nigra send axons to the caudate nucleus and the putamen (Fig. 17-3) and liberate dopamine at their terminals as the neurotransmitter. It is believed that these fibers are inhibitory in function.

Brainstem Striatal Fibers

Ascending fibers from the brainstem end in the caudate nucleus and putamen (Fig. 17-3) and liberate serotonin at their terminals as the neurotransmitter. It is thought that these fibers are inhibitory in function.

Efferent Fibers

Striatopallidal Fibers

These fibers pass from the caudate nucleus and putamen to the globus pallidus (Fig. 17-3). They have gamma-aminobutyric acid (GABA) as their neurotransmitter.

Striatonigral Fibers

Fibers pass from the caudate nucleus and putamen to the substantia nigra (Fig. 17-3). Some of the fibers use GABA or acetylcholine as the neurotransmitter while others use substance P.

CONNECTIONS OF THE GLOBUS PALLIDUS

Afferent Fibers

Striatopallidal Fibers

These fibers pass from the caudate nucleus and putamen to the globus pallidus. As noted previously, these fibers have GABA as their neurotransmitter.

Efferent Fibers

Pallidofugal Fibers

These complicated fibers may be divided into groups: (1) the **ansa lenticularis**, which pass to the thalamic nuclei, (2) the **fasciculus lenticu-**laris, which pass to the subthalamus, (3) the **pallidotegmental** fibers, which terminate in the caudal tegmentum of the midbrain, and (4) the **pallidosubthalamic fibers**, which pass to the subthalamic nuclei.

FUNCTIONS OF THE BASAL NUCLEI

The basal nuclei are joined together and connected with many different regions of the nervous system by a very complex number of neurons.

Basically, the corpus striatum receives afferent information from most of the cerebral cortex, the thalamus, the subthalamus, and the brainstem, including the substantia nigra. The information is integrated within the corpus striatum and the outflow passes back to the areas listed above. This circular pathway is believed to function as follows:

The activity of the basal nuclei is initiated by information received from the sensory cortex, the thalamus and the brainstem. The outflow from the basal nuclei is channeled through the globus pallidus, which then influences the activities of the motor areas of the cerebral cortex or other motor centers in the brainstem. Thus the basal nuclei can control muscular movements by influencing the cerebral cortex rather than through direct descending pathways to the brainstem and spinal cord.

Destruction of the motor cerebral cortex prevents the individual from performing fine discrete movements of the hands and feet on the opposite side of the body (see pp. 305 and 395). However, the individual is still capable of performing gross crude movements of the opposite limbs. If destruction of the corpus striatum then takes place, paralysis of the remaining movements of the opposite side of the body occurs.

It has been shown that the globus pallidus plays a role in controlling the axial and girdle movements of the body and the positioning of the proximal parts of the limbs. The activity in the neurons of the globus pallidus increases before active movements take place in the distal limb muscles. This important function enables the trunk and limbs to be placed in appropriate positions before the motor part of the cerebral cortex activates discrete movements in the hands and feet.

CLINICAL NOTES

COMMON CLINICAL SYNDROMES ASSOCIATED WITH DISEASE OF THE BASAL NUCLEI

Chorea

In this syndrome the patient exhibits quick, jerky, irregular movements that are nonrepetitive. Swift grimaces and sudden movements of the head or limbs are good examples. In **Huntington's chorea** there is a degeneration of the GABA-secreting, P substance–secreting, and the acetylcholine-secreting neurons of the striatonigral inhibiting pathway. This results in the dopamine-secreting neurons of the substantia nigra becoming overactive so that the nigrostriatal pathway inhibits the caudate nucleus and the putamen. This inhibition produces the abnormal movements seen in this disease.

Athetosis

This consists of slow, sinuous, writhing movements that most commonly involve the distal segments of the limbs. Degeneration of the globus pallidus occurs with a breakdown of the circuitry involving the basal nuclei and the cerebral cortex.

Hemiballismus

This is a form of involuntary movement confined to one side of the body. It usually involves the proximal extremity musculature and the limb suddenly flies about in all directions out of control. The lesion occurs in the opposite subthalamic nucleus or its connections; it is in the subthalamic nucleus that smooth movements of different parts of the body are integrated.

Parkinson's Disease

This disease is associated with neuronal degeneration in the substantia nigra and to a lesser extent in the globus pallidus, putamen, and caudate nucleus. The degeneration of the inhibitory nigrostriate fibers results in a reduction in the release of the neurotransmitter dopamine within the corpus striatum. This leads to hypersensitivity of the dopamine receptors in the postsynaptic neurons in the corpus striatum, which become overactive. The signs and symptoms of the disease include tremor, cogwheel rigidity, and bradykinesis (see also p. 399).

CLINICAL PROBLEMS

Answers on Page 604

1. A 10-year-old girl was seen by a neurologist because of the gradual development of involuntary movements. To begin with, the movements were regarded by her parents as general restlessness, but later abnormal facial grimacing and jerking movements of the arms and legs began to occur. The child was now having difficulty in performing normal movements of the arms and walking was becoming increasingly difficult. The abnormal movements appeared to be worse in the upper limbs and were more exaggerated on the right side of body. The movements were made worse when the child became excited but disappeared completely when she slept. The child was recently treated for rheumatic fever. Is there any possible connection between this child's symptoms and the basal nuclei in the cerebral hemispheres?

2. A 40-year-old man was seen by his physician complaining of rapid and jerky involuntary movements involving the upper and lower limbs. The condition started about 6 months ago and was getting progressively worse. He said that he was extremely worried about his health because his father had developed similar symptoms 20 years ago and had died in a mental institution. His wife told the physician that he also suffered from episodes of extreme depression and that she had noticed that he had periods of irritability and impulsive behaviour. The physician made

the diagnosis of Huntington's chorea. Using your knowledge of neuroanatomy try and explain how this disease involves the basal nuclei.

3. A 61-year-old man suddenly developed uncoordinated movements of the trunk and right arm. The right upper limb would suddenly, vigorously, and aimlessly be thrown about, knocking over anything in its path. The patient was recovering from a right-sided hemiplegia, secondary to a cerebral hemorrhage. What is the name given to this clinical sign? Does this condition involve the basal nuclei?

NATIONAL BOARD TYPE QUESTIONS

Answers on Page 620

IN EACH OF THE FOLLOWING QUESTIONS, ANSWER:
- (a) IF (1), (2), AND (3) ONLY ARE CORRECT
- (b) IF (1) AND (3) ONLY ARE CORRECT
- (c) IF (2) AND (4) ONLY ARE CORRECT
- (d) IF (4) ONLY IS CORRECT
- (e) IF ALL ARE CORRECT

1. Which of the following statements concerning the basal nuclei (ganglia) is (are) correct?
   (1) The caudate nucleus and the putamen form the neostriatum.
   (2) The head of the caudate nucleus is connected to the putamen.
   (3) The internal capsule lies medial to the globus pallidus.
   (4) The tegmentum forms part of the basal nuclei.

2. Which of the following statements concerning the basal nuclei (ganglia) is (are) correct?
   (1) The amygdaloid nucleus is connected to the caudate nucleus.
   (2) The claustrum does not form part of the basal nuclei.
   (3) The corpus striatum lies lateral to the thalamus.
   (4) The lentiform nucleus is completely divided by the external capsule into the globus pallidus and the putamen.

3. Which of the following statements concerning the basal nuclei (ganglia) is (are) correct?
   (1) The corpus striatum is made up of the caudate nucleus and the lentiform nucleus.
   (2) The head of the caudate nucleus lies medial to the internal capsule.
   (3) The insula does not form part of the basal nuclei.
   (4) The tail of the caudate nucleus lies in the roof of the lateral ventricle.

4. Which of the following statements concerning the caudate nucleus is (are) correct?
   (1) It is divided up into a head, body, and tail.
   (2) It is a **C**-shaped mass of gray matter.
   (3) The body of the caudate nucleus forms part of the floor of the body of the lateral ventricle.
   (4) The head lies medial to the anterior horn of the lateral ventricle.

5. Which of the following statements concerning the afferent corticostriate fibers to the corpus striatum is (are) correct?
   (1) Glutamate is the neurotransmitter substance.
   (2) All parts of the cerebral cortex send fibers to the caudate nucleus and the putamen.
   (3) The largest input is from the sensory-motor part of the cerebral cortex.
   (4) Each part of the cerebral cortex is randomly projected to different parts of the corpus striatum.

6. Which of the following statements concerning the nigrostriate fibers is (are) correct?
   (1) The cells in the substantia nigra send nerve fibers to the putamen.
   (2) Dopamine is the neurotransmitter substance.
   (3) The nigrostriate fibers are inhibitory in function.
   (4) The caudate nucleus receives nerve fibers from the substantia nigra.

7. Which of the following statements concerning the efferent fibers of the corpus striatum is (are) correct?
   (1) None of the efferent fibers descend directly to the motor nuclei of the cranial nerves.
   (2) Some of the striatopallidal fibers have GABA as the neurotransmitter.
   (3) The striatonigral fibers pass from the caudate nucleus to the substantia nigra.
   (4) Many of the efferent fibers pass directly to the cerebellum.

Fig. 17-4. Horizontal section of the cerebrum.

8. Which of the following statements concerning the functions of the basal ganglia is (are) correct?
   (1) The corpus striatum integrates information received directly from the cerebellar cortex.
   (2) The outflow of the basal nuclei is channeled through the globus pallidus to the motor areas of the cerebral cortex, thus influencing muscular activities.
   (3) The globus pallidus only influences the movements of the axial part of the body.
   (4) The activities of the globus pallidus precede the activities of the motor cortex concerned with discrete movements of the hands and the feet.

Match the numbered structures shown in Figure 17-4 with the appropriate lettered structure listed below on the right.

9. Structure 1
10. Structure 2
11. Structure 3
12. Structure 4
13. Structure 5
14. Structure 6

(a) Anterior horn of lateral ventricle
(b) Internal capsule
(c) Claustrum
(d) Putamen
(e) External capsule
(f) Globus pallidus

ADDITIONAL READING

Aron, A. M., Freeman, J. M., and Carter, S. The natural history of Sydenham's chorea. *Am. J. Med.* 38:83, 1965.

Bird, E. D. Chemical pathology of Huntington's disease. *Annu. Rev. Pharmacol. Toxicol.* 20:533, 1980.

Carpenter, M. B. Anatomy of the Corpus Striatum and Brain Stem Integrating Systems. In V. B. Brooks (ed.), *Handbook of Physiology.* Sec. 1, Vol. II. Bethesda: American Physiological Society, 1981. P. 947.

DeLong, M., and Georgopoulos, A. P. Motor Functions of the Basal Ganglia. In V. B. Brooks (ed.), *Handbook of Physiology.* Sec. 1, Vol. II. Bethesda: American Physiological Society, 1981. P. 1017.

Di Chiara, G. (ed.). *GABA and the Basal Ganglia.* New York: Raven, 1981.

Duvoisin, R. C. *Parkinson's Disease.* New York: Raven, 1978.

Hayden, M. R. *Huntington's Chorea.* New York: Springer-Verlag, 1981.

Klawans, H. L., Moses, H., Nausieda, P. A., Bergen, D., and Weiner, W. J. Treatment and prognosis of hemiballismus. *N. Engl. J. Med.* 295:1348, 1976.

Penney, J. B., Jr., and Young, A. B. Speculations on the functional anatomy of the basal ganglia disorders. *Annu. Rev. Neurosci.* 6:73, 1983.

Shoulson, I., and Fahn, S. Huntington's disease: Clinical care and evaluation. *Neurology* (Minneap.) 29:1, 1979.

Chapter 18
The Ventricular System and the Formation and Fate of the Cerebrospinal Fluid

VENTRICULAR SYSTEM

The ventricles of the brain are the lateral ventricles, the third ventricle, and the fourth ventricle (Fig. 18-1). The two **lateral ventricles** communicate through the **interventricular foramina** (of Monro) with the **third ventricle**. The third ventricle is connected to the **fourth ventricle** by the **cerebral aqueduct (aqueduct of Sylvius)**. The fourth ventricle in turn is continuous with the narrow **central canal** of the spinal cord and, through the three foramina in its roof, with the subarachnoid space. The central canal has a small dilatation at its inferior end, referred to as the **terminal ventricle** (Fig. 18-1).

The ventricles are developmentally derived from the cavity of the neural tube. They are lined throughout with **ependyma** and are filled with **cerebrospinal fluid**.

Lateral Ventricles

There are two lateral ventricles and one is present in each cerebral hemisphere (Fig. 18-2). The ventricle is a roughly C-shaped cavity and may be divided into a **body**, which occupies the parietal lobe and from which **anterior**, **posterior**, and **inferior horns** extend into the frontal, occipital, and temporal lobes, respectively. The lateral ventricle communicates with the cavity of the third ventricle through the **interventricular foramen** (Figs. 18-2 and 18-3). This opening, which lies in the anterior part of the medial wall of the ventricle, is bounded anteriorly by the anterior column of the fornix and posteriorly by the anterior end of the thalamus.

A detailed description of the different parts of the lateral ventricles is given on page 269.

The **choroid plexus of the lateral ventricle** projects into the ventricle on its medial aspect and is a vascular fringe composed of pia mater covered with the ependymal lining of the ventricular cavity (Fig. 18-4). The choroid plexus is, in fact, the irregular lateral edge of the tela choroidea, which is a two-layered fold of pia mater situated between the fornix superiorly and the upper surface of the thalamus (Fig. 18-6). At the junction of the body of the lateral ventricle and the inferior horn the choroid

Superior sagittal venous sinus
Arachnoid granulation
Dura mater
Arachnoid mater
Subarachnoid space filled with cerebrospinal fluid
Pia mater
Choroid plexus of lateral ventricle
Lateral ventricle
Interventricular foramen
Third ventricle
Cerebral aqueduct
Tentorium cerebelli
Fourth ventricle
Lateral opening of the fourth ventricle (foramen of Luschka)
Median opening of the fourth ventricle (foramen of Magendie)
Central canal of spinal cord
Choroid plexus of third ventricle
Choroid plexus of fourth ventricle
Subarachnoid space filled with cerebrospinal fluid
Terminal ventricle
Inferior end of spinal cord (level of lower border of first lumbar vertebra in adult)
Inferior end of subarachnoid space (level of lower border of second sacral vertebra)
Filum terminale

Fig. 18-1. The origin and circulation of the cerebrospinal fluid.

Fig. 18-2. A cast of the ventricular cavities of the brain as seen from:
A. Lateral view.
B. Anterior view.
C. Superior view.

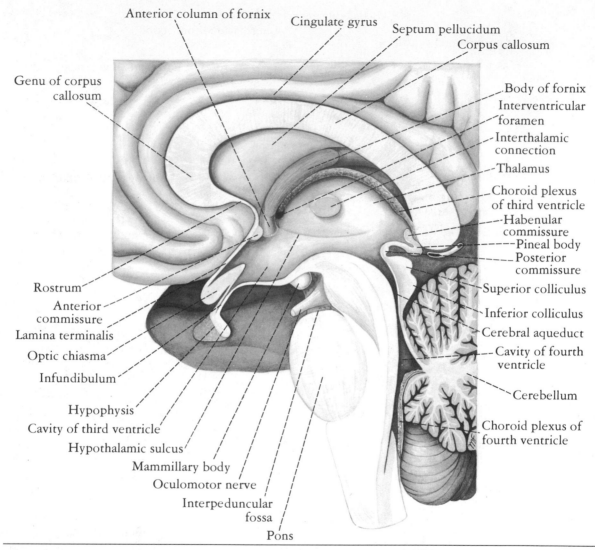

Fig. 18-3. Sagittal section of the brain, showing the third ventricle, the cerebral aqueduct, and the fourth ventricle.

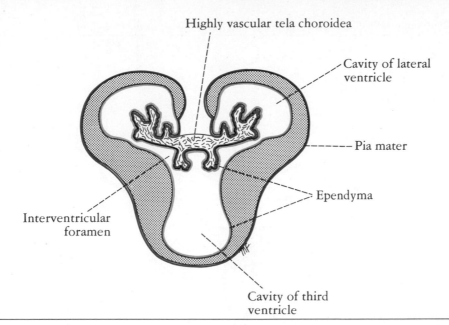

Fig. 18-4. Schematic diagram of coronal section of the third and lateral ventricles at the site of the interventricular foramina. Shows the structure of the tela choroidea and its relationship with the ependyma and pia mater.

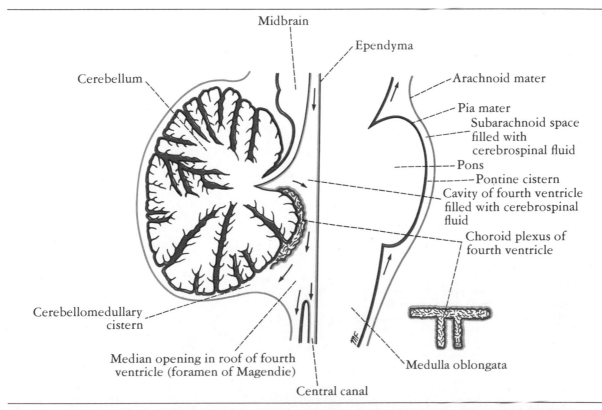

Fig. 18-5. Sagittal section of fourth ventricle, showing origin and circulation of cerebrospinal fluid. Note the position of the foramen of Magendie.

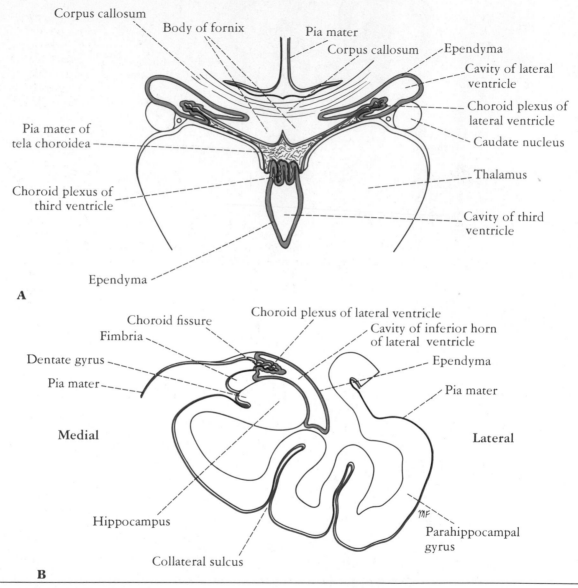

Fig. 18-6. Coronal section of:
A. Cavities of third and lateral ventricles.
B. Cavity of inferior horn of lateral ventricle.

plexus is continued into the inferior horn and projects through the choroidal fissure.

Third Ventricle

The third ventricle is a slitlike cleft between the two thalami. It communicates anteriorly with the lateral ventricles through the interventricular foramina (of Monro) and posteriorly with the fourth ventricle through the cerebral aqueduct (of Sylvius) (Fig. 18-3). The walls of the third ventricle are described on page 254.

The **choroid plexuses of the third ventricle** are formed from the tela choroidea situated above the roof of the ventricle (Fig. 18-4). The vascular tela choroidea projects downward on each side of the midline, invaginating the ependymal roof of the ventricle. The two vascular ridges or fringes that hang from the roof of the third ventricle are referred to as the choroid plexuses of that ventricle.

The blood supply of the tela choroidea and therefore also of the choroid plexuses of the third and lateral ventricles is derived from the **choroidal branches of the internal carotid and basilar arteries.** The venous blood drains into the internal cerebral veins, which unite to form the great cerebral vein. The great cerebral vein joins the inferior sagittal sinus to form the straight sinus.

Cerebral Aqueduct (Aqueduct of Sylvius)

The cerebral aqueduct, a narrow channel about ¾-inch (1.8 cm) long, connects the third with the fourth ventricle (Fig. 18-3). It is lined with ependyma and is surrounded by a layer of gray matter called the **central gray.** The direction of flow of cerebrospinal fluid is from the third to the fourth ventricle. There is no choroid plexus in the cerebral aqueduct.

Fourth Ventricle

The fourth ventricle is a cavity situated anterior to the cerebellum and posterior to the pons and the superior half of the medulla oblongata (Fig. 18-5). It is continuous above with the cerebral aqueduct and below with the central canal of the spinal cord.

The fourth ventricle possesses lateral boundaries, a roof, and a rhomboid-shaped floor. The details of these boundaries are fully described on page 229.

The tent-shaped roof projects into the cerebellum. The lateral recesses extend laterally around the sides of the medulla and open anteriorly as the **lateral openings of the fourth ventricle**, or the **foramina of Luschka** (see Fig. 1-14). A median aperture in the roof of the fourth ventricle, the **foramen of Magendie**, also is present (Fig. 18-5). It is through these three openings that the cerebrospinal fluid enters the subarachnoid space.

The **choroid plexus of the fourth ventricle** has a T shape; the vertical part of the T is double (Fig. 18-5). It is suspended from the inferior half of the roof of the ventricle and is formed from the highly vascular tela choroidea. The tela choroidea is a two-layered fold of pia mater that projects through the roof of the ventricle and is covered by ependyma. The horizontal part of the T extends into the lateral recesses of the ventricle on each side. The blood supply to the plexus is from the **posterior inferior cerebellar arteries**.

Central Canal of the Spinal Cord and Medulla Oblongata

The central canal opens superiorly into the fourth ventricle. Inferiorly, it extends through the inferior half of the medulla oblongata and through the entire length of the spinal cord. In the conus medullaris of the spinal cord, it expands to form the **terminal ventricle** (Fig. 18-1). The central canal is closed at its lower end, is filled with cerebrospinal fluid, and is lined with ependyma. The central canal is surrounded by gray matter, **the gray commissure**. There is no choroid plexus in the central canal.

Subarachnoid Space

The subarachnoid space is the interval between the arachnoid mater and pia mater and therefore is present where these meninges envelop the brain and spinal cord (Fig. 18-1). The space is filled with cerebrospinal fluid and contains the large blood vessels of the brain (Fig. 18-7). It is traversed by a network of fine trabeculae formed of delicate connective tissue. The subarachnoid space completely

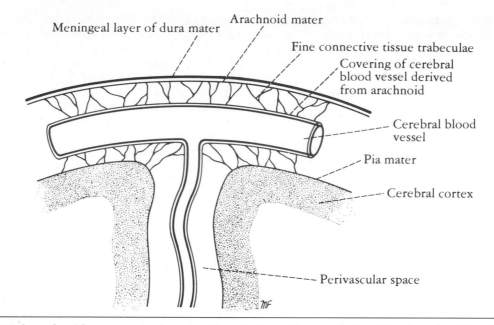

Meningeal layer of dura mater

Arachnoid mater

Fine connective tissue trabeculae

Covering of cerebral blood vessel derived from arachnoid

Cerebral blood vessel

Pia mater

Cerebral cortex

Perivascular space

Fig. 18-7. Subarachnoid space around cerebral hemisphere. Shows relationship of cerebral blood vessel to meninges and cerebral cortex.

surrounds the brain and extends along the olfactory nerves to the mucoperiosteum of the nose. The subarachnoid space also extends along the cerebral blood vessels as they enter and leave the substance of the brain and stops where the vessels become an arteriole or a venule.

In certain situations around the base of the brain, the arachnoid does not closely follow the surface of the brain so that the subarachnoid space expands to form **subarachnoid cisterns**. The descriptions of the **cerebellomedullary cistern**, the **pontine cistern**, and the **interpeduncular cistern**, which are the largest cisterns, are on page 527.

Inferiorly, the subarachnoid space extends beyond the lower end of the spinal cord and invests the **cauda equina** (see Fig. 1-27). The subarachnoid space ends below at the level of the interval between the second and third sacral vertebrae.

The subarachnoid space surrounds the cranial and spinal nerves and follows them to the point where they leave the skull and vertebral canal. Here the arachnoid mater and pia mater fuse with the perineurium of each nerve.

CEREBROSPINAL FLUID

The cerebrospinal fluid is a clear, colorless fluid. It possesses, in solution, inorganic salts similar to those in the blood plasma. The glucose content is about half that of blood and there is only a trace of protein. Only a few cells are present and these are lymphocytes. The normal lymphocyte count is 0 to 3 cells/mm^3. In the lateral recumbent position the cerebrospinal fluid pressure, as measured by lumbar puncture, is about 60 to 150 mm water. This pressure may be easily raised by straining or coughing or compressing the internal jugular veins in the neck (see p. 33). The total volume of cerebrospinal fluid in the subarachnoid space and within the ventricles is about 130 ml.

Functions of the Cerebrospinal Fluid

The cerebrospinal fluid, which bathes the external and internal surfaces of the brain and spinal cord, serves as a cushion between the central nervous system and the surrounding bones, thus protecting it against mechanical trauma. The close relationship of the fluid to the nervous tissue and the blood enables it to serve as a reservoir and assist in the regulation of the contents of the skull. For example, if the brain volume or the blood volume increases the cerebrospinal fluid volume decreases. Since the cerebrospinal fluid is an ideal physiological substrate, it probably plays an active part in the nourishment of the nervous tissue; it almost certainly assists in the removal of products of neuronal metabolism. It is possible that the secretions of the pineal gland influence the activities of the pituitary gland by circulating through the cerebrospinal fluid in the third ventricle (see p. 252).

Formation of Cerebrospinal Fluid

The cerebrospinal fluid is formed mainly in the choroid plexuses of the lateral, third, and fourth ventricles; some originates from the ependymal cells lining the ventricles and from the brain substance through the perivascular spaces.

The choroid plexuses have a much folded surface and each fold consists of a core of vascular connective tissue covered with cuboidal epithelium of the ependyma (Fig. 18-8). Electron-microscopic examination of the epithelial cells shows that their free surfaces are covered with microvilli. The blood of the capillaries is separated from the ventricular lumen by endothelium, a basement membrane, and the surface epithelium. The epithelial cells are fenestrated and permeable to large molecules.

There is considerable evidence that the choroid plexuses actively secrete cerebrospinal fluid. It has been shown experimentally in animals, for example, that the passage of Na is stopped when a carbonic anhydrase inhibitor is applied to the choroid plexus. Furthermore, it has been shown that the

Fig. 18-8. Microscopic structure of choroid plexus. Shows path taken by fluids in the formation of cerebrospinal fluid.

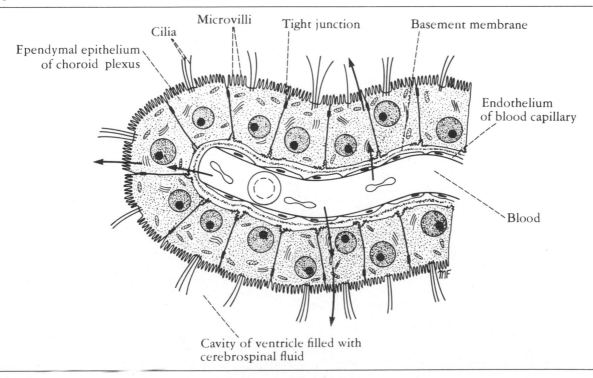

Ependymal epithelium of choroid plexus — Cilia — Microvilli — Tight junction — Basement membrane — Endothelium of blood capillary — Blood — Cavity of ventricle filled with cerebrospinal fluid

concentrations of electrolytes—particularly K, Ca, and Mg—differ in the cerebrospinal fluid as compared with the blood plasma.

Circulation of Cerebrospinal Fluid

The circulation begins with its secretion from the choroid plexuses in the ventricles and its production from the brain surface. The fluid passes from the lateral ventricles into the third ventricle through the interventricular foramina (Figs. 18-1 and 18-9). It then passes into the fourth ventricle through the cerebral aqueduct. The circulation is aided by the arterial pulsations of the choroid plexuses.

From the fourth ventricle, the fluid passes through the median aperture and the lateral foramina of the lateral recesses of the fourth ventricle and enters the subarachoid space. The fluid slowly moves through the cerebellomedullary cistern and pontine cisterns and flows superiorly through the

interval in the tentorium cerebelli to reach the inferior surface of the cerebrum (Figs. 18-1 and 18-9). It now moves superiorly over the lateral aspect of each cerebral hemisphere. Some of the cerebrospinal fluid moves inferiorly in the subarachnoid space around the spinal cord and cauda equina. It is believed that the pulsations of the cerebral and spinal arteries and the movements of the vertebral column facilitate this gradual flow of fluid.

Absorption of Cerebrospinal Fluid

The main sites for the absorption of the cerebrospinal fluid are the **arachnoid villi** that project into the dural venous sinuses, especially the **superior sagittal sinus** (Fig. 18-10). The arachnoid villi tend to be grouped together to form elevations known as **arachnoid granulations**. Structurally, each arachnoid villus is a diverticulum of the subarachnoid space that pierces the dura mater. The arachnoid diverticulum is capped by a thin cellular

Fig. 18-9. Circulation of cerebrospinal fluid. Dashed line indicates course taken by fluid within the cavities of the central nervous system.

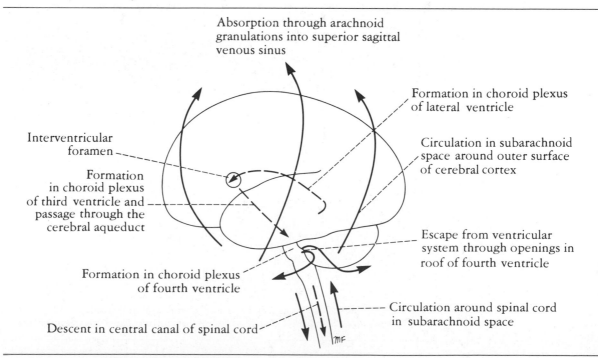

Absorption through arachnoid granulations into superior sagittal venous sinus

Formation in choroid plexus of lateral ventricle

Interventricular foramen

Circulation in subarachnoid space around outer surface of cerebral cortex

Formation in choroid plexus of third ventricle and passage through the cerebral aqueduct

Escape from ventricular system through openings in roof of fourth ventricle

Formation in choroid plexus of fourth ventricle

Circulation around spinal cord in subarachnoid space

Descent in central canal of spinal cord

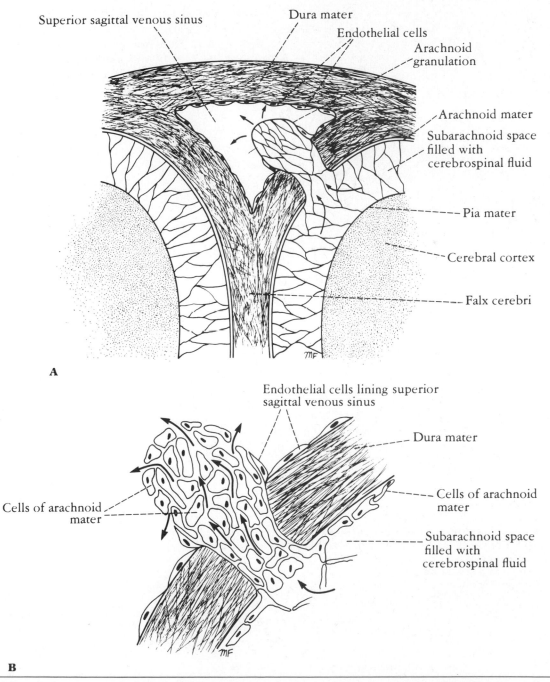

**Fig. 18-10. A. Coronal section of superior sagittal sinus, showing an arachnoid granulation.
B. Magnified view of arachnoid granulation, showing path taken by cerebrospinal fluid into venous system.**

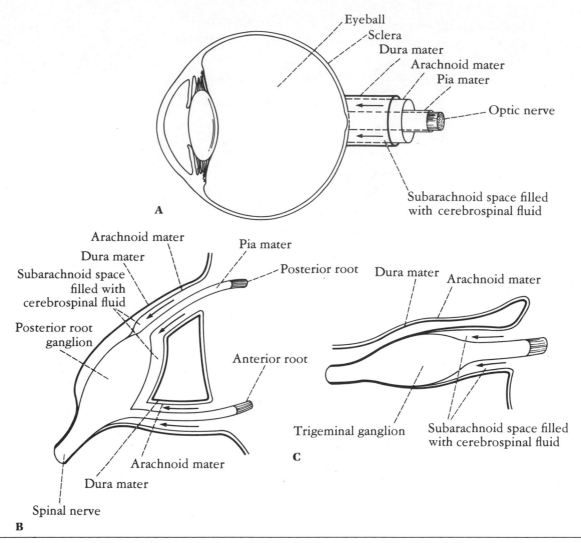

Fig. 18-11. Course taken by cerebrospinal fluid around:
A. The optic nerve.
B. The roots of a spinal nerve.
C. The trigeminal nerve.

layer, which in turn is covered by the endothelium of the venous sinus. The arachnoid granulations increase in number and size with age and tend to become calcified with advanced age.

The absorption of cerebrospinal fluid into the venous sinuses occurs when the cerebrospinal fluid pressure exceeds that in the sinus. Electron-microscopic studies of the arachnoid villi seem to indicate that fine tubules lined with endothelium permit a direct flow of fluid from the subarachnoid space into the lumen of the venous sinuses. Should the venous pressure rise and exceed the cerebrospinal fluid pressure, compression of the tips of the villi closes the tubules and prevents the reflux of blood into the subarachnoid space.

Some of the cerebrospinal fluid probably is absorbed directly into the veins in the subarachnoid space and some possibly escapes through the perineural lymph vessels of the cranial and spinal nerves.

Because the production of cerebrospinal fluid from the choroid plexuses is constant, the rate of absorption of cerebrospinal fluid through the arachnoid villi controls the cerebrospinal fluid pressure.

Extensions of the Subarachnoid Space

A sleeve of the subarachnoid space extends around the optic nerve to the back of the eyeball (Fig. 18-11). Here the arachnoid mater and pia mater fuse with the sclera. The central artery and vein of the retina cross this extension of the subarachnoid space to enter the optic nerve and they may be compressed in patients with raised cerebrospinal fluid pressure.

Small extensions of the subarachnoid space also occur around the other cranial and spinal nerves (Fig. 18-11). It is here that some communication may occur between the subarachnoid space and the perineural lymph vessels.

The subarachnoid space also extends around the arteries and veins of the brain and spinal cord at points where they penetrate the nervous tissue (Fig. 18-7). The pia mater, however, quickly fuses with the outer coat of the blood vessel below the surface of the brain and spinal cord, thus closing off the subarachnoid space.

CLINICAL NOTES

GENERAL CONSIDERATIONS

The cerebrospinal fluid is a clear, colorless fluid that fills the ventricles of the brain and bathes the external surface of the brain and spinal cord. It is formed from the choroid plexuses within the ventricles and circulates through the three openings in the roof of the fourth ventricle to reach the subarachnoid space. The fluid is produced continuously at a rate of about 0.5 ml/min and with a total volume of about 130 ml; this corresponds to a turnover time of about 5 hours.

Once the cerebrospinal fluid has escaped from the fourth ventricle it flows upward through the tentorial notch of the tentorium cerebelli and slowly spreads over the surface of the cerebral hemisphere to the arachnoid granulations of the venous sinuses. This diffuse spread over the hemi-spheres is assisted by the pulsations of the brain and the cerebral arteries. It is important to realize that the cerebrospinal fluid not only bathes the ependymal and pial surfaces of the brain and spinal cord but penetrates the nervous tissue along the blood vessels.

There does not appear to be a substantial flow of fluid, either up or down, around the spinal cord and cauda equina. Here a slow process of mixing occurs that depends on the movements of the vertebral column, respiration, coughing, and the changing positions of the body.

The functions of the cerebrospinal fluid are protection of the central nervous system from trauma, regulation of the intracranial pressure, nourishment of the nervous tissue, and removal of waste products.

THE OPTIC NERVE, RAISED CEREBROSPINAL FLUID PRESSURE, AND PAPILLEDEMA

The optic nerves are surrounded by sheaths derived from the pia mater, arachnoid mater, and dura mater. There is an extension of the intracranial subarachnoid space forward around the optic nerve to the back of the eyeball (Fig. 18-11). A rise of cerebrospinal fluid pressure caused by an intracranial tumor will compress the thin walls of the retinal vein as it crosses the extension of the subarachnoid space to enter the optic nerve. This will result in congestion of the retinal vein, bulging forward of the optic disc, and edema of the disc; the last condition is referred to as **papilledema**. Since both subarachnoid extensions are continuous with the intracranial subarachnoid space, both eyes will exhibit papilledema. Persistent papilledema leads to optic atrophy and blindness.

HYDROCEPHALUS

Hydrocephalus is an abnormal increase in the volume of the cerebrospinal fluid within the skull. If the hydrocephalus is accompanied by a raised cerebrospinal fluid pressure, then it is due to either (1) an abnormal increase in the formation of the fluid, (2) a blockage of the circulation of the fluid, or (3) a diminished absorption of the fluid. Rarely, hydrocephalus occurs with a normal cerebrospinal fluid pressure and in these patients there is a compensatory hypoplasia or atrophy of the brain substance.

HYDROCEPHALUS RESULTING FROM EXCESSIVE FORMATION OF CEREBROSPINAL FLUID

This condition is rare and may occur when there is a tumor of the choroid plexuses.

HYDROCEPHALUS RESULTING FROM BLOCKAGE OF THE CIRCULATION OF CEREBROSPINAL FLUID

An obstruction of the interventricular foramen by a tumor will block the drainage of the lateral ventricle on that side. The continued production of cerebrospinal fluid by the choroid plexus of that ventricle will cause distention of that ventricle and atrophy of the surrounding neural tissue.

An obstruction in the cerebral aqueduct may be congenital or result from inflammation or pressure from a tumor. This causes a symmetrical distention of both lateral ventricles and distention of the third ventricle.

Obstruction of the median aperture (foramen of Magendie) in the roof of the fourth ventricle and the two lateral apertures (foramina of Luschka) in the lateral recesses of the fourth ventricle by inflammatory exudate, or by tumor growth, will produce symmetrical dilatation of both lateral ventricles and the third and fourth ventricle.

Sometimes inflammatory exudate secondary to meningitis will block the subarachnoid space and obstruct the flow of cerebrospinal fluid over the outer surface of the cerebral hemispheres. Here, again, the entire ventricular system of the brain will become distended.

HYDROCEPHALUS RESULTING FROM DIMINISHED ABSORPTION OF CEREBROSPINAL FLUID

Interference with the absorption of cerebrospinal fluid at the arachnoid granulations may be caused by inflammatory exudate, venous thrombosis or pressure on the venous sinuses, or obstruction of the internal jugular vein.

CLINICAL INVESTIGATION OF THE CEREBRAL VENTRICLES

The size of the cerebral ventricles may be investigated clinically by the use of (1) CT scans and MRIs and, if necessary, (2) intracranial pneumography.

Computed tomography and **magnetic resonance imaging** are safe and easy to perform. The outline of the ventricles may be demonstrated by using these methods. Apart from ventricular distention or distortion, the cerebral tumor causing the condition also may be demonstrated.

Intracranial pneumography is essentially the replacement of cerebrospinal fluid within the ventricles and subarachnoid space with air or oxygen. Because the air or gas is less dense than the fluid or neural tissue, the ventricles and cerebral gyri can be visualized. In an **encephalogram**, the air or oxygen is introduced through a lumbar puncture. The skull is then radiographed. In a **ventriculogram**, the air or oxygen is introduced into the lateral ventricle through a needle inserted through a hole in the skull (in a young child the needle may be inserted through a suture). The skull then is radiographed. In ventriculography, only the ventricles will be visualized.

CEREBROSPINAL FLUID PRESSURE AND COMPOSITION

The clinical measurement of cerebrospinal fluid pressure by means of a lumbar puncture is described on page 32. The normal composition of cerebrospinal fluid is described on page 176.

CLINICAL PROBLEMS

Answers on Page 604

1. Using your knowledge of the anatomical pathways along which the cerebrospinal fluid flows, name the sites at which pathological blockage is most likely to occur.
2. During the examination of a patient who had just been admitted to the emergency room following an automobile accident, the resident asked the student what role the cerebrospinal fluid plays in protecting the brain from trauma.
3. A 55-year-old man was being investigated for signs and symptoms that suggested the presence of a cerebral tumor. Examination of the CT scan showed gross enlargement and distortion of the left lateral ventricle. What other investigation might be carried out in this patient to display the ventricles of the brain? Using your knowledge of neuroanatomy, can you accurately position the tumor in this case?
4. A 3-year-old child had been referred to the children's hospital because the circumference of his head greatly exceeded the normal limit for his age. After a careful history had been taken and a detailed physical examination had been performed, a diagnosis of hydrocephalus was made. What is your definition of hydrocephalus? Name three common causes of hydrocephalus in young children.
5. A 50-year-old man was found on ophthalmoscopic examination to have edema of both optic discs (bilateral papilledema) and congestion of the retinal veins. The cause of the condition was found to be a rapidly growing intracranial tumor. Using your knowledge of neuroanatomy, explain the papilledema. Why does the patient exhibit bilateral papilledema?

NATIONAL BOARD TYPE QUESTIONS

Answers on Page 620

In each of the following questions, answer:
   (a) If (1) only is correct
   (b) If (2) only is correct
   (c) If both (1) and (2) are correct, and
   (d) If neither (1) nor (2) is correct

1. Which of the following statements is (are) correct?
   (1) The two lateral ventricles communicate directly with one another through the foramen of Monro.
   (2) The aqueduct of Sylvius connects the fourth ventricle with the central canal of the spinal cord.

2. Which of the following statements is (are) correct?
   (1) The ventricles are developed from the neural tube in the embryo.
   (2) The ventricular system is lined throughout with tela choroidea.

3. Which of the following statements is (are) correct?
   (1) The choroid plexuses are found in the lateral ventricles and the third and the fourth ventricles.
   (2) The choroid plexus of the lateral ventricle projects into the cavity on its medial side through the choroidal fissure.

Select the best response:

4. The following statements concerning the third ventricle are true **except**:
   (a) It is situated between the thalami.
   (b) It communicates with the lateral ventricles through the interventricular foramina.
   (c) It is continuous with the fourth ventricle through the cerebral aqueduct.
   (d) The choroid plexus is located in the floor.
   (e) The choroid plexus receives its arterial supply through the internal carotid and basilar arteries.

5. The following statements concerning the subarachnoid space are true **except**:
   (a) The space is the interval between the arachnoid mater and the pia mater.
   (b) The space contains cerebrospinal fluid and the cerebral arteries, but not the cerebral veins.
   (c) In certain situations the space is expanded to form cisterns.
   (d) The fourth ventricle drains into it through three foramina.
   (e) The space surrounds the cranial and spinal nerves to the point where they leave the skull and the vertebral canal.

In the following questions, answer:
   (a) IF (1), (2), AND (3) ONLY ARE CORRECT
   (b) IF (1) AND (3) ONLY ARE CORRECT
   (c) IF (2) AND (4) ONLY ARE CORRECT
   (d) IF (4) ONLY IS CORRECT, OR
   (e) IF ALL ARE CORRECT

6. Which of the following statements is (are) correct concerning the formation of the cerebrospinal fluid?
   (1) It is largely formed by the choroid plexuses.
   (2) Some of the fluid may originate from the brain substance.
   (3) It is actively secreted by the ependymal cells covering the choroid plexus.
   (4) The fluid is produced continuously at a rate of about 0.5 ml/min.

7. Which of the following statements is (are) correct concerning the cerebrospinal fluid?
   (1) Its circulation through the ventricles is aided by the arterial pulsations of the choroid plexuses.

   (2) Its circulation in the subarachnoid space is aided by the pulsations of the cerebral and spinal arteries and the movements of the vertebral column.
   (3) It exits from the ventricular system through the foramen of Magendie and the foramina of Luschka.
   (4) It extends inferiorly in the subarachnoid space to the level of the fifth sacral vertebra.

8. Which of the following statements is (are) correct concerning the absorption of the cerebrospinal fluid?
   (1) The minor sites for the absorption of the cerebrospinal fluid are into the veins in the subarachnoid space and the perineural lymph vessels.
   (2) The arachnoid villi play an important role in the absorption of cerebrospinal fluid.
   (3) The fine tubules found within the arachnoid villi permit direct flow of cerebrospinal fluid into the venous sinuses.
   (4) The cerebrospinal fluid is passed into the blood by active transport through the cells forming the arachnoid villi.

Fig. 18-12. Lateral view of brain showing outline of ventricular cavities.

In Figure 18-12, match the numbers listed on the left with the appropriate structures listed on the right. An answer may be used more than once.

9. Number 1
10. Number 2
11. Number 3
12. Number 4

(a) Cerebral aqueduct
(b) Body of lateral ventricle
(c) Third ventricle
(d) Fourth ventricle
(e) None of the above

ADDITIONAL READING

Alksne, J. F., and Lovings, E. T. Functional ultrastructure of the arachnoid villus. *Arch. Neurol.* 27:371, 1972.

Bowsher, D. *Cerebrospinal Fluid Dynamics in Health and Disease.* Springfield, Illinois: Thomas, 1960.

Cserr, H. F. Physiology of the choroid plexus. *Physiol. Rev.* 51:273, 1971.

Cserr, H. F. Relationship between cerebrospinal fluid and interstitial fluid of brain. *Fed. Proc.* 33:2075, 1974.

Davson, H. Formation and drainage of the cerebrospinal fluid. In K. Shapiro, A. Marmarov, and H. Portnoy (eds.), *Hydrocephalus.* New York: Raven, 1984. P. 3.

Davson, H. *Physiology of the Cerebrospinal Fluid.* London: Churchill Livingstone, 1970.

Fishman, R. A. *Cerebrospinal Fluids in Diseases of the Nervous System.* Philadelphia: Saunders, 1982.

Gaab, M. R., and Koos, W. T. Hydrocephalus in infancy and childhood: Diagnosis and indication for operation. *Neuropediatrics* 15:173, 1984.

Millen, J. W., and Woollam, D. H. M. *The Anatomy of the Cerebrospinal Fluid.* New York and London: Oxford University Press, 1962.

Pollay, M. Research into human hydrocephalus: A review. In K. Shapiro, A. Marmarov, and H. Portnoy (eds.), *Hydrocephalus.* New York: Raven, 1984. P. 301.

Pollay, M. Transport mechanisms in the choroid plexus. *Fed. Proc.* 33:2064, 1974.

Porliskock, J. T., and Levine, J. E. Cerebrospinal fluid absorption. In J. P. Kapp and H. H. Schmidek (eds.), *Cerebral Venous System and Its Disorders.* New York: Grune & Stratton, 1984. P. 251.

Wright, E. M. Transport processes in the formation of cerebrospinal fluid. *Rev. Physiol. Biochem. Pharmacol.* 83:1, 1978.

Chapter 19
Blood-Brain and Blood-Cerebrospinal Fluid Barriers

The central nervous system requires a very stable environment in order to function normally. This stability is provided by isolating the nervous system from the blood by the existence of the so-called blood-brain barrier and the blood–cerebrospinal fluid barrier.

BLOOD-BRAIN BARRIER

The experiments of Paul Ehrlich in 1882 showed that living animals injected intravascularly with vital dyes, such as trypan blue, demonstrated staining of all the tissues of the body except the brain and spinal cord. Later, it was demonstrated that although most of the brain is not stained by the intravenous injection of trypan blue the following areas do in fact become stained: the pineal gland, the posterior lobe of the pituitary, the tuber cinereum, the wall of the optic recess, and the vascular area postrema* at the lower end of the fourth ven-

*Area of medulla on floor of fourth ventricle just rostral to the opening into the central canal.

tricle. These observations led to the concept of a blood-brain barrier (for which blood-brain spinal cord barrier would be a more accurate name).

It has been shown that the permeability of the blood-brain barrier is inversely related to the size of the molecules and directly related to their lipid solubility. Gases and water pass readily through the barrier, whereas glucose and electrolytes pass more slowly. The barrier is almost impermeable to plasma proteins and other large organic molecules. This would explain why in the early experiments with trypan blue, which quickly binds to the plasma protein albumin, that the dye did not pass into the neural tissue in the greater part of the brain.

Structure of the Blood-Brain Barrier

Examination of an electron micrograph of the central nervous system shows that the lumen of a blood capillary is separated from the extracellular spaces about the neurons and neuroglia by the following structures: (1) the endothelial cells in the wall of the capillary, (2) a continuous basement membrane surrounding the capillary outside the endothelial cells, and (3) the foot processes of the astrocytes that adhere to the outer surface of the capillary wall (Fig. 19-1).

The use of electron-dense markers such as lanthanum and horseradish peroxidase (Brightman and Reese, 1969) has shown that these substances do not penetrate between the endothelial cells of the capillaries because of the presence of tight junctions that form belts around the cells. When the dense markers are introduced into the extracellular spaces of the neuropil they pass between the perivascular foot processes of the astrocytes as far as the endothelial lining of the capillary. On the basis of this evidence, it is believed that the tight junctions between the endothelial cells of the blood capillaries are largely responsible for the blood-brain barrier* (Fig. 19-1).

Although the blood-brain barrier exists in the newborn, there is evidence that it is more permeable to certain substances than it is in the adult.

The structure of the blood-brain barrier is not identical in all regions of the central nervous system. In fact, in those areas where the blood-brain barrier appears to be absent, the capillary endothelium contains fenestrations across which proteins and small organic molecules may pass from the blood to the nervous tissue (Fig. 19-2). It has been suggested that areas such as the area postrema of the floor of the fourth ventricle and the hypothalamus may serve as sites at which neuronal receptors may sample the chemical content of the plasma directly. The hypothalamus, which is involved in the regulation of the metabolic activity of the body, might bring about appropriate modifications of activity, thereby protecting the nervous tissue.

BLOOD–CEREBROSPINAL FLUID BARRIER

There is free passage of water, gases, and lipid-soluble substances from the blood to the cerebrospinal fluid. Macromolecules such as proteins and most hexoses other than glucose are unable to enter the cerebrospinal fluid. It has been suggested that a barrier similar to the blood-brain barrier exists in the choroid plexuses.

Structure of the Blood–Cerebrospinal Fluid Barrier

Electron-microscopic examination of a villus of a choroid plexus shows that the lumen of a blood capillary is separated from the lumen of the ventricle by the following structures: (1) the endothelial cells, which are fenestrated and have very thin walls (the fenestrations are not true perforations but are filled by a thin diaphragm), (2) a continuous basement membrane surrounding the capillary outside the endothelial cells, (3) scattered pale cells with flattened processes, and (4) a continuous basement membrane, upon which rest (5) the choroidal epithelial cells (Fig. 19-3). The use of electron-dense markers has not been entirely successful in localizing the barrier precisely. Horseradish peroxidase injected intravenously appears as a coating on the luminal surface of the endothelial cells and in many areas examined it did pass between the endothelial cells. It is probable that the tight junctions between the choroidal epithelial cells serve as the barrier (Fig. 19-3).

CEREBROSPINAL FLUID– BRAIN INTERFACE

Although vital dyes given by intravenous injection do not gain access to most brain tissues, if the dyes are injected into the subarachnoid space or into the ventricles they soon enter the extracellular spaces around the neurons and glial cells. Thus there is no comparable physiological barrier between the cerebrospinal fluid and the extracellular compartment of the central nervous system. It is inter-

---

*It is interesting to note that peripheral nerves are isolated from the blood in the same manner as the central nervous system. The endothelial cells of the blood capillaries in the endoneurium have tight junctions, so that there is a blood-nerve barrier.

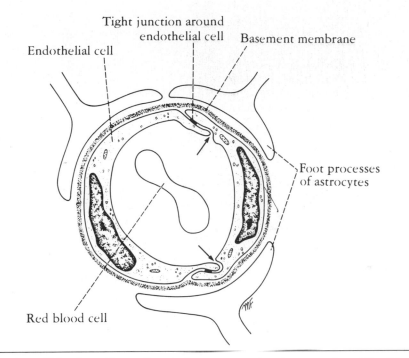

Tight junction around endothelial cell

Endothelial cell

Basement membrane

Foot processes of astrocytes

Red blood cell

Fig. 19-1. Cross section of blood capillary of central nervous system in area where blood-brain barrier exists.

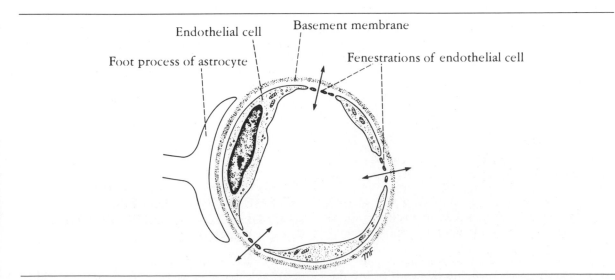

Endothelial cell

Basement membrane

Foot process of astrocyte

Fenestrations of endothelial cell

Fig. 19-2. Cross section of blood capillary of central nervous system where blood-brain barrier appears to be absent. Note presence of fenestrations in endothelial cells.

Fig. 19-3. Section of villus of choroid plexus.

esting, however, to consider the structures that separate the cerebrospinal fluid from the nervous tissue. Three sites must be examined: (1) the pia-covered surface of the brain and spinal cord, (2) the perivascular extensions of the subarachnoid space into the nervous tissue, and (3) the ependymal surface of the ventricles (Fig. 19-4).

The pia-covered surface of the brain consists of a loosely arranged layer of pial cells resting on a basement membrane (Fig. 19-4). Beneath the basement membrane are the astrocytic foot processes. No intercellular junctions exist between adjacent pial cells or between adjacent astrocytes, so that the extracellular spaces of the nervous tissue are in almost direct continuity with the subarachnoid space.

The prolongation of the subarachnoid space into the central nervous tissue quickly ends below the surface of the brain, where the fusion of the outer covering of the blood vessel with the pial covering of the nervous tissue occurs.

The ventricular surface of the brain is covered with columnar ependymal cells with localized tight junctions (Fig. 19-4). Intercellular channels exist that permit free communication between the ventricular cavity and the extracellular neuronal space. The ependyma does not have a basement membrane and there are no specialized astrocytic foot processes because the neuroglial cells are loosely arranged.

FUNCTIONAL SIGNIFICANCE OF THE BLOOD-BRAIN AND BLOOD–CEREBROSPINAL FLUID BARRIERS

In normal conditions, these two important semipermeable barriers protect the brain and spinal cord from potentially harmful substances while permitting gases and nutriments to enter the nervous tissue.

Fig. 19-4. Section of cerebrospinal fluid–brain interface.
A. Outer surface of brain.
B. Ventricular surface of brain.

CLINICAL NOTES

In no other organ is the regulation of the composition of the extracellular fluid between fine limits as important as in the brain and spinal cord. The functions of the blood-brain and blood–cerebrospinal fluid barriers are to protect the brain from variations in blood composition and especially from toxic compounds. In the newborn child or premature infant, where these barriers are not fully developed, toxic substances such as bilirubin can readily enter the central nervous system and produce yellowing of the brain and kernicterus. This is not possible in the adult.

BRAIN TRAUMA AND THE BLOOD-BRAIN BARRIER

Any injury to the brain, whether it be due to direct trauma or to inflammatory or chemical toxins, causes a breakdown of the blood-brain barrier, allowing the free diffusion of large molecules into the nervous tissue. It is believed that this is brought about by actual destruction of the vascular endothelial cells or disruption of their tight junctions.

DRUGS AND THE BLOOD-BRAIN BARRIER

The systemic administration of **penicillin** results in only a small amount entering the central nervous system. This is fortunate, because penicillin in high concentrations is toxic to nervous tissue. In the presence of meningitis, however, the meninges become more permeable locally, at the site of inflammation, thus permitting sufficient antibiotic to reach the infection. **Chloramphenicol** and the **tetracyclines** readily cross the blood-brain barrier and enter the nervous tissue. The **sulfonamide**

drugs also easily pass through the blood-brain barrier.

Lipid-soluble substances such as the anesthetic agent **thiopentone** rapidly enter the brain after intravenous injection. On the other hand, water-soluble substances such as exogenous **norepinephrine** cannot cross the blood-brain barrier. **Phenylbutazone** is a drug that becomes bound to plasma protein and the large drug protein molecule is unable to cross the barrier. Most tertiary amines are lipid-soluble, such as **atropine**, and quickly enter the brain, whereas the quaternary compounds, such as **atropine methylnitrate**, do not.

In Parkinson's disease there is a deficiency of the neurotransmitter dopamine in the corpus striatum. Unfortunately, dopamine cannot be used in the treatment, as it will not cross the blood-brain barrier. L-Dopa readily crosses the barrier and has been used with great success.

CLINICAL PROBLEMS

Answers on Page 605

1. A 5-year-old girl was admitted to the children's hospital with symptoms of headache, general malaise, and vomiting. On examination, the body temperature was found to be 104°F and the pulse rate was rapid. Attempts to flex the neck produced pain and resulted in the patient's flexing her hip and knee joints. A lumbar puncture was performed and the cerebrospinal fluid was seen to be cloudy, and the pressure was raised to 190 mm of water. Microscopic examination of the fluid showed a large number of polymorphonuclear leukocytes. A diagnosis of meningitis was made. Subsequent culture revealed the infection to be a meningococcal meningitis. The resident vaguely remembered reading in a textbook the importance of the blood-brain barrier in the use of antibiotics for the treatment of meningitis. What is the blood-brain barrier? Does the presence of the blood-brain barrier influence your choice and dose of antibiotics to be used in this patient?

2. During a ward round in the children's hospital, the pediatrician informed the students that the 4-day-old baby with jaundice had a serum indi-

rect bilirubin level of 45 mg/100 ml and that by now the bile pigment was staining the brain a yellow color (kernicterus). The neuronal damage was revealed clinically by lethargy and poor feeding habits and by occasional muscle spasms. He said the prognosis was very poor. One of the students observed that he could not understand why the bile pigment was having such a dramatic effect on the baby. Recently he had examined a patient who was dying of inoperable carcinoma of the head of the pancreas with total obstruction of the common bile duct. In that patient the skin was a deep yellow color but, apart from complaints of the intense skin irritation owing to the high concentration of bile salts in the blood, and loss of weight, the patient had no symptoms and no neurological abnormalities. Can you explain why the baby had neuronal damage and the adult did not?

3. Name five areas of the brain where the blood-brain barrier appears to be absent. What do you think is the significance of the fact that in a few areas of the brain the barrier is absent?

NATIONAL BOARD TYPE QUESTIONS

Answers on Page 621

IN EACH OF THE FOLLOWING QUESTIONS, ANSWER:

(a) IF (1) ONLY IS CORRECT
(b) IF (2) ONLY IS CORRECT
(c) IF BOTH (1) AND (2) ARE CORRECT, AND
(d) IF NEITHER (1) NOR (2) IS CORRECT

1. Which of the following statements is (are) correct?
   (1) The blood-brain barrier protects the brain from toxic compounds of high molecular weight.
   (2) The blood-brain barrier is absent from the pineal gland.

2. Which of the following statements is (are) correct concerning the structure of the blood-brain barrier?
   (1) The endothelial cells of the blood capillaries are nonfenestrated.
   (2) The endothelial cells of the blood capillaries are held together by localized tight junctions.

3. Which of the following statements is (are) correct concerning the passage of drugs through the blood-brain barrier?
   (1) Dopamine readily passes through the barrier in the treatment of Parkinson's disease.

   (2) Chloramphenicol and the tetracyclines cannot cross the barrier.

4. Which of the following statements is (are) correct concerning the blood–cerebrospinal fluid barrier?
   (1) The beltlike tight junctions between the choroidal ependymal cells form the barrier.
   (2) Proteins and most hexoses, other than glucose, are unable to cross the barrier.

5. Which of the following statements is (are) correct concerning the cerebrospinal fluid–brain interface?
   (1) The ventricular surface of the brain is covered with columnar ependymal cells with extensive beltlike tight junctions.
   (2) In the pia-covered surface of the brain, no tight junctions exist between adjacent pial cells.

6. Which of the following statements is (are) correct concerning the blood-brain barrier?
   (1) In the newborn child the blood-brain barrier is not fully developed.
   (2) Cerebral trauma or inflammation has no effect on the integrity of the blood-brain barrier.

ADDITIONAL READING

Bradbury, M. W. B. The structure and function of the blood-brain barrier. *Fed. Proc.* 43:186, 1984.

Brightman, M. W. The distribution within the brain of ferritin injected into cerebrospinal fluid compartments: II. Parenchymal distribution. *Am. J. Anat.* 117:193, 1965.

Brightman, M. W., and Reese, T. W. Junctions between intimately apposed cell membranes in the vertebrate brain. *J. Cell. Biol.* 40:648, 1969.

Broadwell, R. D., and Brightman, M. W. Entry of peroxidase into neurons of the central and peripheral nervous systems from extracerebral and cerebral blood. *J. Comp. Neurol.* 166:257, 1976.

Cervos-Navarro, J., Artigas, J., and Mesulja, B. J. Morphofunctional aspects of the normal and pathological blood-brain barrier. *Acta Neuropathol. (Berl.)* 7 (suppl):1, 1983.

Davson, H. The blood-brain barrier. In G. H. Bourne (ed.), *The Structure and Function of the Nervous System.* New York: Academic, 1972. Vol. 4, p. 548.

Eisenberg, H. M. New ways of looking at the blood-brain barrier. In H. M. Eisenberg and R. L. Suddith (eds.), *Concepts in Pediatric Neurosurgery.* New York: Plenum, 1983. Vol. 2, p. 127.

Klatzo, I. Disturbances of the blood-brain barrier in cerebrovascular disorders. *Acta Neuropathol. (Berl.)* 8 (suppl):81, 1983.

Lewis, A. J. *Mechanisms of Neurological Disease.* Boston: Little, Brown, 1976.

Oldendorf, W. H. Some clinical aspects of the blood-brain barrier. *Hosp. Pract.* 17(2):143, 1982.

Saunders, N. R., and Milgard, K. Development of the blood brain barrier. *J. Dev. Physiol.* 6:45, 1984.

Woodbury, D. M. Blood-cerebrospinal fluid-brain fluid relations. In T. C. Ruch and H. D. Patton (eds.), *Physiology and Biophysics.* Philadelphia: Saunders, 1965. P. 942.

Chapter 20
The Ascending Tracts of the Spinal Cord

On entering the spinal cord, the sensory nerve fibers of different sizes and functions are sorted out and segregated into nerve bundles or **tracts** (Fig. 20-1). Some of the nerve fibers serve to link different segments of the spinal cord, while others ascend from the spinal cord to higher centers and, thus, connect the spinal cord with the brain. It is the bundles of the ascending fibers that are referred to as the **ascending tracts**. The white matter of the spinal cord is composed of ascending and descending tracts embedded in neuroglia.

The ascending tracts conduct afferent information, which may or may not reach consciousness. The information may be divided into two main groups: (1) **exteroceptive** information, which originates from outside the body, such as pain, temperature, and touch, and (2) **proprioceptive** information, which originates from inside the body, for example, from muscles and joints.

ANATOMICAL ORGANIZATION

General information from the peripheral sensory endings is conducted through the nervous system by a series of neurons. In its simplest form, the ascending pathway to consciousness consists of three neurons (Fig. 20-1). The first neuron, the **first-order neuron**, has its cell body in the **posterior root ganglion** of the spinal nerve. A peripheral process connects with a sensory receptor ending (see Chapter 5), whereas a central process enters the spinal cord through the posterior root to synapse on the **second-order neuron**. The second-order neuron gives rise to an axon that decussates (crosses to the opposite side) and ascends to a higher level of the central nervous system, where it synapses with the **third-order neuron** (Fig. 20-1). The third-order neuron is usually in the thalamus and gives rise to a projection fiber that passes to a sensory region of the cerebral cortex (Fig. 20-1). The three-neuron chain described is the most common arrangement, but some afferent pathways use more or fewer neurons. Many of the neurons in the ascending pathways branch and give a major input into the reticular formation, which in turn activates the cerebral cortex, maintaining wakefulness (see p. 317). Other branches pass to motor neurons and participate in reflex muscular activity.

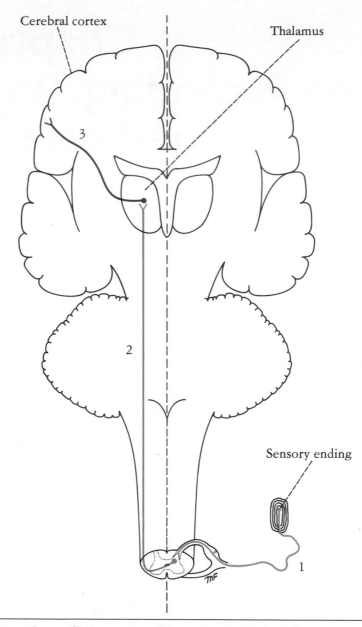

Fig. 20-1. Simplest form of ascending sensory pathway from the sensory nerve ending to the cerebral cortex. Note the three neurons involved.

Functions of the Ascending Tracts

Painful and thermal sensations ascend in the lateral spinothalamic tract; light touch and pressure ascend in the anterior spinothalamic tract (Fig. 20-2). Discriminative touch, that is, the ability to localize accurately the area of the body touched and also to be aware that two points are touched simultaneously, even though they are close together (two-point discrimination), ascends in the posterior white columns (Fig. 20-2). Also ascending in the posterior white columns is information from muscles and joints pertaining to movement and position of different parts of the body. In addition, vibratory sensations ascend in the posterior white column. Unconscious information from muscles, joints, the skin, and subcutaneous tissue reaches the cerebellum by way of the anterior and posterior

spinocerebellar tracts and by the cuneocerebellar tract (Fig. 20-2). Pain, thermal, and tactile information is passed to the superior colliculus of the midbrain through the spinotectal tract for the purpose of spinovisual reflexes (Fig. 20-2). The spinoreticular tract provides a pathway from the muscles, joints, and skin to the reticular formation, while the spino-olivary tract provides an indirect pathway for further afferent information to reach the cerebellum (Fig. 20-2).

Pain and Temperature Pathways

LATERAL SPINOTHALAMIC TRACT

The pain and thermal receptors in the skin and other tissues are free nerve endings. The pain impulses are transmitted to the spinal cord in fast-

Fig. 20-2. Transverse section of spinal cord, showing origin of main ascending sensory tracts. Note that sensations of pain and temperature ascend in the lateral spinothalamic tract and light touch and pressure ascend in the anterior spinothalamic tract.

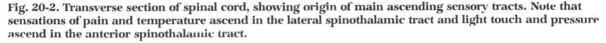

conducting delta A type fibers and slow-conducting C-type fibers. The fast-conducting fibers alert the individual to initial sharp pain, and the slow-conducting fibers are responsible for prolonged burning aching pain. The sensations of heat and cold also travel by delta A and C fibers.

The axons entering the spinal cord from the posterior root ganglion proceed to the tip of the posterior gray column and divide into ascending and descending branches (Fig. 20-3). These branches travel for a distance of one or two segments of the spinal cord and form the **posterolateral tract of Lissauer** (Fig. 20-3). These fibers of the first-order neuron terminate by synapsing with cells in the posterior gray column, including cells in the substantia gelatinosa. Substance P, a peptide, is thought to be the neurotransmitter at these synapses.

The axons of the second-order neurons now cross obliquely to the opposite side in the anterior gray and white commissures within one spinal segment of the cord, ascending in the contralateral white column as the lateral spinothalamic tract (Fig. 20-3). The lateral spinothalamic tract lies medial to the anterior spinocerebellar tract. As the lateral spinothalamic tract ascends through the spinal cord, new fibers are added to the anteromedial aspect of the tract, so that in the upper cervical segments of the cord the sacral fibers are posterolateral and the cervical segments are anteromedial. The fibers carrying pain are situated slightly anterior to those conducting temperature.

As the lateral spinothalamic tract ascends through the medulla oblongata, it lies near the lateral surface and between the inferior olivary nucleus and the nucleus of the spinal tract of the trigeminal nerve. It is now accompanied by the anterior spinothalamic tract and the spinotectal tract; together they form the **spinal lemniscus** (Fig. 20-3).

The spinal lemniscus continues to ascend through the posterior part of the pons (Fig. 20-3). In the midbrain it lies in the tegmentum lateral to the medial lemniscus. Many of the fibers of the lateral spinothalamic tract end by synapsing with the third-order neuron in the ventral posterolateral nucleus of the thalamus (Fig. 20-3). It is believed that here crude pain and temperature sensations are appreciated and emotional reactions are initiated.

The axons of the third-order neurons in the ventral posterolateral nucleus of the thalamus now pass through the posterior limb of the internal capsule and the corona radiata to reach the somesthetic area in the postcentral gyrus of the cerebral cortex (Fig. 20-3). The contralateral half of the body is represented as inverted, with the hand and mouth situated inferiorly and the leg situated superiorly, and with the foot and anogenital region on the medial surface of the hemisphere. (For details, see p. 295.) From here, the information is transmitted to other regions of the cerebral cortex to be used by motor areas and the parietal association area. The role of the cerebral cortex is interpreting the quality of the sensory information at the level of consciousness.

OTHER TERMINATIONS OF THE LATERAL SPINOTHALAMIC TRACT

It is now generally agreed that pain impulses ascending through the lateral spinothalamic tract travel in two pathways. The initial sharp, pricking pain terminates in the ventral posterolateral nucleus of the thalamus and is then relayed to the cerebral cortex.

The burning pain terminates in the reticular formation, which then activates the entire nervous system. It is these impulses that alert the individual to an injury, and although the site of the injury is poorly localized, nevertheless they arouse the nervous system and create a sense of urgency.

Pain Control in the Central Nervous System

THE ANALGESIA SYSTEM

It has been shown experimentally that stimulation of certain areas of the brainstem can reduce or block sensations of pain. These areas include the periventricular area of the diencephalon, the periaqueductal gray matter of the midbrain, and midline nuclei of the brainstem. It is believed that fibers of the reticulospinal tract pass down to the spinal cord and synapse on cells concerned with pain sensation in the posterior gray column. The analgesic system can suppress both sharp pricking pain and burning pain sensations.

Recently two compounds with morphinelike actions, called the **enkephalins** and the **endorphins**, have been isolated in the central nervous

Fig. 20-3. Pain and temperature pathways.

system. It has been suggested that these compounds serve as neurotransmitter substances in the analgesic system of the brain and that they may inhibit the release of substance P in the posterior gray column.

THE GATING THEORY

It has long been known that massage and the application of liniments to painful areas in the body can be very effective in relieving pain. The technique of acupuncture, which was discovered several thousand years ago in China, is also beneficial in relieving pain. Low-frequency electrical stimulation of the skin has been reported to produce pain relief in certain cases. Although the precise mechanism for these phenomena is not understood, the gating theory was proposed some years ago. It was suggested that at the site where the pain fiber enters the central nervous system, inhibition could occur by means of connector neurons excited by large, myelinated afferent fibers carrying nonpainful information of touch and pressure. The excess tactile stimulation, produced by massage, for example, "closed the gate" for pain. Once the nonpainful tactile stimulation ceased, however, "the gate was opened" and the painful stimuli ascended the lateral spinothalamic tract. While the gate theory may partially explain the phenomena, it is probable that the analgesia system is also involved with the liberation of enkephalins and endorphins in the posterior gray columns.

Light Touch and Pressure Pathways

ANTERIOR SPINOTHALAMIC TRACT

The axons enter the spinal cord from the posterior root ganglion and proceed to the tip of the posterior gray column, where they divide into ascending and descending branches (Fig. 20-4). These branches travel for a distance of one or two segments of the spinal cord, contributing to the **posterolateral tract of Lissauer**. It is believed that these fibers of the first-order neuron terminate by synapsing with cells in the substantia gelatinosa group in the posterior gray column (Fig. 20-4).

The axons of the second-order neuron now cross very obliquely to the opposite side in the anterior gray and white commissures within several spinal segments, and ascend in the opposite anterolateral white column as the anterior spinothalamic tract (Fig. 20-4). As the anterior spinothalamic tract ascends through the spinal cord, new fibers are added to the medial aspect of the tract, so that in the upper cervical segments of the cord the sacral fibers are mostly lateral and the cervical segments are mostly medial.

As the anterior spinothalamic tract ascends through the medulla oblongata, it accompanies the lateral spinothalamic tract and the spinotectal tract, all of which form the **spinal lemniscus** (Fig. 20-4).

The spinal lemniscus continues to ascend through the posterior part of the pons, and the tegmentum of the midbrain and the fibers of the anterior spinothalamic tract terminate by synapsing with the third-order neuron in the ventral posterolateral nucleus of the thalamus (Fig. 20-4). Crude awareness of touch and pressure is believed to be appreciated here.

The axons of the third-order neurons in the ventral posterolateral nucleus of the thalamus pass through the posterior limb of the **internal capsule** (Fig. 20-4) and the **corona radiata** to reach the somesthetic area in the postcentral gyrus of the cerebral cortex. The contralateral half of the body is represented inverted, with the hand and mouth situated inferiorly, as described previously. (For details, see p. 300.) The conscious appreciation of touch and pressure depends on the activity of the cerebral cortex. It should be emphasized that the sensations can be only crudely localized, and very little discrimination of intensity is possible.

Discriminative Touch, Vibratory Sense, and Conscious Muscle Joint Sense

POSTERIOR WHITE COLUMN: FASCICULUS GRACILIS AND FASCICULUS CUNEATUS

The axons enter the spinal cord from the posterior root ganglion and pass directly to the posterior white column of the same side (Fig. 20-5). Here the fibers divide into long ascending and short descending branches. The descending branches pass down a variable number of segments, giving off collateral branches that synapse with cells in the posterior gray horn, with internuncial neurons,

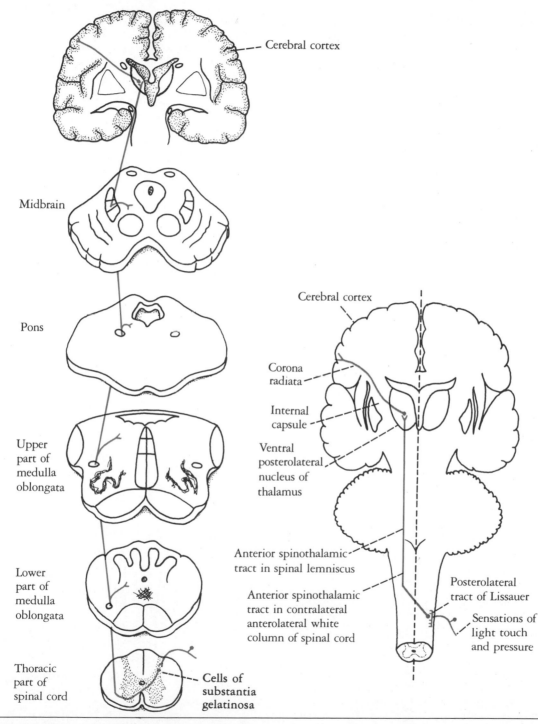

Fig. 20-4. Light touch and pressure pathways.

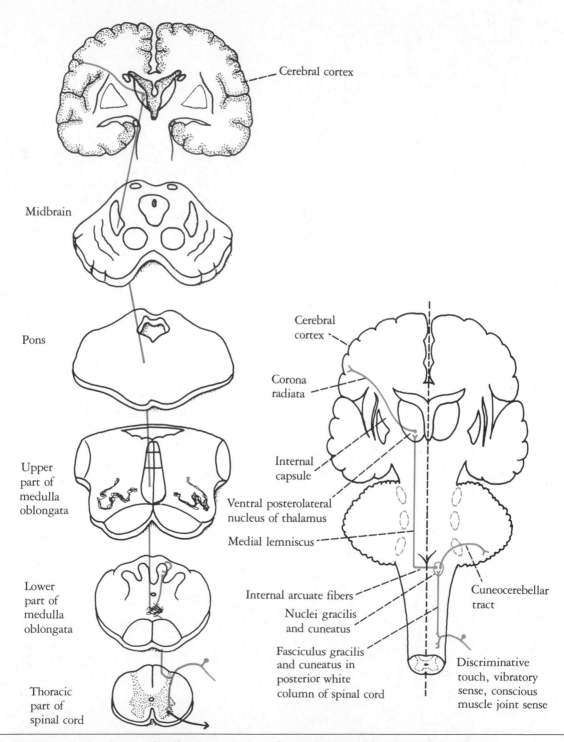

Cerebral cortex

Midbrain

Pons

Upper
part of
medulla
oblongata

Lower
part of
medulla
oblongata

Thoracic
part of
spinal cord

Cerebral
cortex

Corona
radiata

Internal
capsule

Ventral posterolateral
nucleus of thalamus

Medial lemniscus

Internal arcuate fibers

Nuclei gracilis
and cuneatus

Fasciculus gracilis
and cuneatus in
posterior white
column of spinal cord

Cuneocerebellar
tract

Discriminative
touch, vibratory
sense, conscious
muscle joint sense

Fig. 20-5. Discriminative touch, vibratory sense, and conscious muscle joint sense pathways.

and with anterior horn cells (Fig. 20-5). It is clear that these short descending fibers are involved with intersegmental reflexes.

The long ascending fibers may also end by synapsing with cells in the posterior gray horn, with internuncial neurons, and with anterior horn cells. This distribution may extend over numerous segments of the spinal cord (Fig. 20-5). As in the case of the short descending fibers, they are involved with intersegmental reflexes.

Many of the long ascending fibers travel upward in the posterior white column as the **fasciculus gracilis** and **fasciculus cuneatus** (Fig. 20-5). The fasciculus gracilis is present throughout the length of the spinal cord and contains the long ascending fibers from the sacral, lumbar, and lower six thoracic spinal nerves. The fasciculus cuneatus is situated laterally in the upper thoracic and cervical segments of the spinal cord and is separated from the fasciculus gracilis by a septum. The fasciculus cuneatus contains the long ascending fibers from the upper six thoracic and all the cervical spinal nerves.

The fibers of the fasciculus gracilis and cuneatus ascend ipsilaterally and terminate by synapsing on the second-order neurons in the **nuclei gracilis and cuneatus** of the medulla oblongata (Fig. 20-5). The axons of the second-order neurons, called the **internal arcuate fibers**, sweep anteromedially around the central gray matter and cross the median plane, decussating with the corresponding fibers of the opposite side in the **sensory decussation** (Fig. 20-5). The fibers then ascend as a single compact bundle, the **medial lemniscus**, through the medulla oblongata, the pons, and the midbrain (Fig. 20-5). The fibers terminate by synapsing on the third-order neurons in the ventral posterolateral nucleus of the thalamus.

The axons of the third-order neuron leave and pass through the posterior limb of the **internal capsule** and **corona radiata** to reach the somesthetic area in the postcentral gyrus of the cerebral cortex (Fig. 20-5). The contralateral half of the body is represented inverted, with the hand and mouth situated inferiorly, as described previously. (For details, see p. 300.) In this manner, the impressions of touch with fine gradations of intensity, exact localization, and two-point discrimination can be appreciated. Vibratory sense and the position of the different parts of the body can be consciously recognized.

It should be mentioned that a number of fibers in the fasciculus cuneatus from the cervical and upper thoracic segments, having terminated on the second-order neuron of the nucleus cuneatus, are relayed and travel as the axons of the second-order neurons to enter the cerebellum through the inferior cerebellar peduncle of the same side (Fig. 20-5). The pathway is referred to as the **cuneocerebellar tract** and the fibers are known as the **posterior external arcuate fibers**. The function of these fibers is to convey information of muscle joint sense to the cerebellum.

Muscle Joint Sense Pathways to the Cerebellum

POSTERIOR SPINOCEREBELLAR TRACT

The axons entering the spinal cord from the posterior root ganglion enter the posterior gray column and terminate by synapsing on the second-order neurons at the base of the posterior gray column (Fig. 20-6). These neurons are known collectively as the **nucleus dorsalis (Clark's column)**. The axons of the second-order neurons enter the posterolateral part of the lateral white column on the same side and ascend as the posterior spinocerebellar tract to the medulla oblongata. Here the tract joins the inferior cerebellar peduncle and terminates in the cerebellar cortex (Fig. 20-6). Note that it does not ascend to the cerebral cortex. Since the nucleus dorsalis (Clark's column) extends only from the eighth cervical segment caudally to the third or fourth lumbar segments, axons entering the spinal cord from the posterior roots of the lower lumbar and sacral segments ascend in the posterior white column until they reach the third or fourth lumbar segments, where they enter the nucleus dorsalis.

The posterior spinocerebellar fibers receive muscle joint information, from the muscle spindles, tendon organs, and joint receptors of the trunk and lower limbs. This information concerning tension of muscle tendons and the movements of muscles and joints is used by the cerebellum in the coordination of limb movements and the maintenance of posture.

Fig. 20-6. Muscle joint sense pathways to cerebellum.

ANTERIOR SPINOCEREBELLAR TRACT

The axons entering the spinal cord from the posterior root ganglion terminate by synapsing with the second-order neurons in the **nucleus dorsalis** at the base of the posterior gray column (Fig. 20-6). The majority of the axons of the second-order neurons cross to the opposite side and ascend as the anterior spinocerebellar tract in the contralateral white column; the minority of the axons ascend as the anterior spinocerebellar tract in the lateral white column of the same side (Fig. 20-6). The fibers, having ascended through the medulla oblongata and pons, enter the cerebellum through the superior cerebellar peduncle and terminate in the cerebellar cortex. It is believed that those fibers that crossed over to the opposite side in the spinal cord cross back within the cerebellum (Fig. 20-6). The anterior spinocerebellar tract conveys muscle joint information from the muscle spindles, tendon organs, and joint receptors of the trunk and the upper and lower limbs. It is also believed that the cerebellum receives information from the skin and superficial fascia by this tract.

CUNEOCEREBELLAR TRACT

These fibers have already been described on page 371. They originate in the nucleus cuneatus and enter the cerebellum through the inferior cerebellar peduncle of the same side (Fig. 20-5). The fibers are known as the **posterior external arcuate fibers** and their function is to convey information of muscle joint sense to the cerebellum.

Other Ascending Pathways

SPINOTECTAL TRACTS

The axons enter the spinal cord from the posterior root ganglion and travel to the gray matter where they synapse on unknown second-order neurons (Fig. 20-7). The axons of the second-order neurons cross the median plane and ascend as the spinotectal tract in the anterolateral white column lying close to the lateral spinothalamic tract. After passing through the medulla oblongata and pons, they terminate by synapsing with neurons in the superior colliculus of the midbrain (Fig. 20-7). This pathway provides afferent information for spino-

visual reflexes and brings about movements of the eyes and head toward the source of the stimulation.

SPINORETICULAR TRACT

The axons enter the spinal cord from the posterior root ganglion and terminate on unknown second-order neurons in the gray matter (Fig. 20-7). The axons from these second-order neurons ascend the spinal cord as the spinoreticular tract in the lateral white column mixed with the lateral spinothalamic tract. The majority of the fibers are uncrossed and terminate by synapsing with neurons of the reticular formation in the medulla oblongata, pons, and midbrain (Fig. 20-7). The spinoreticular tract provides an afferent pathway for the reticular formation, which plays an important role in influencing levels of consciousness. (For details, see pp. 308 and 315.)

SPINO-OLIVARY TRACT

The axons enter the spinal cord from the posterior root ganglion and terminate on unknown second-order neurons in the posterior gray column (Fig. 20-7). The axons from the second-order neurons cross the midline and ascend as the spino-olivary tract in the white matter at the junction of the anterior and lateral columns. The axons end by synapsing on third-order neurons in the inferior olivary nuclei in the medulla oblongata (Fig. 20-7). The axons of the third-order neurons cross the midline and enter the cerebellum through the inferior cerebellar peduncle. The spino-olivary tract conveys information to the cerebellum from cutaneous and proprioceptive organs.

Visceral Sensory Tracts

Sensations that arise in viscera located in the thorax and abdomen enter the spinal cord through the posterior roots. The cell bodies of the first-order neuron are situated in the posterior root ganglia. The peripheral processes of these cells receive nerve impulses from pain* and stretch receptor endings in the viscera. The central processes, having en-

---

*The causes of visceral pain include ischemia, chemical damage, spasm of smooth muscle, and distention.

Superior colliculus

Midbrain

Pons

Spinoreticular tract
passing to reticular
formation

Inferior
cerebellar peduncle

Inferior olivary nucleus

Medulla oblongata

Spinoreticular tract in
lateral white column
of spinal cord

Spinotectal tract in
anterolateral white column
of spinal cord

Spino-olivary tract in
anterolateral white column
of spinal cord

Afferent information for
spinovisual reflexes

From cutaneous and
proprioceptive organs

Afferent information
that influences consciousness

Fig. 20-7. Spinotectal, spinoreticular, and spino-olivary tracts.

tered the spinal cord, synapse with second-order neurons in the gray matter, probably in the posterior or lateral gray columns.

The axons of the second-order neurons are believed to join the spinothalamic tracts and ascend and terminate on the third-order neurons in the ventral posterolateral nucleus of the thalamus. The final destination of the axons of the third-order neurons is probably in the postcentral gyrus of the cerebral cortex.

Many of the visceral afferent fibers that enter the spinal cord branch and participate in reflex activity.

CLINICAL NOTES

GENERAL CONSIDERATIONS

Two main types of sensory information enter the spinal cord through the posterior roots: (1) conscious sensory information, which is conveyed to the cerebral cortex for interpretation through the thalamus, and (2) unconscious sensory information, which is conveyed to the cerebellum and assists in coordinating muscle activity. Other sensory information is conducted to the midbrain for the purpose of activating visual reflexes and to the reticular formation to activate this system. Some of the unconscious sensory information takes part in local spinal reflex activity.

SUMMARY OF THE PRINCIPAL SENSORY PATHWAYS

CONSCIOUS SENSORY INFORMATION

The pain and temperature sensations ascend in the lateral spinal thalamic tract on the contralateral side of the spinal cord and eventually reach the postcentral gyrus of the cerebral cortex on the opposite side of the body (Fig. 20-3).

Discriminative touch, vibratory sense, and muscle joint sense ascend in the fasciculus gracilis and the fasciculus cuneatus on the ipsilateral side of the spinal cord and eventually reach the postcentral gyrus on the opposite side of the body, the pathway having crossed the midline in the medulla oblongata (Fig. 20-5).

Light touch and pressure sensations ascend in the anterior spinothalamic tract on the contralateral side of the spinal cord and eventually reach the postcentral gyrus on the opposite side of the body (Fig. 20-4).

UNCONSCIOUS SENSORY INFORMATION

Sensations from the muscles, tendons, and joints ascend in the posterior spinocerebellar tracts on the ipsilateral side of the spinal cord and in the anterior spinocerebellar tracts on both sides of the cord (Fig. 20-6). Although most of the fibers in the anterior spinocerebellar tracts have crossed from the opposite side, there is clinical evidence to suggest that the fibers cross back to their original side within the cerebellum. Thus, the above proprioceptive information is conveyed ultimately to the cerebellar hemisphere of the same side of the body. Additional proprioceptive information is carried to the cerebellar cortex of the same side through the cuneocerebellar tracts (Fig. 20-5) and indirectly through the spino-olivary tract (Fig. 20-7).

The spinotectal tract carries afferent information from the opposite side of the body to the superior colliculus of the midbrain for spinovisual reflexes (Fig. 20-7). Other afferent information is conveyed to the reticular formation in the brainstem for the purpose of alerting this system.

Neurons of the Sensory Pathways

It is interesting to note that those pathways that travel the farthest, that is, from the spinal cord to the cerebral cortex, have three orders of neurons. The first-order neuron has its cell body in the posterior root ganglion; the second-order neuron has its cell body either in the posterior gray column of the spinal cord or in the nucleus gracilis or nucleus cuneatus in the medulla oblongata; the third-order neuron has its cell body in the ventral posterolateral nucleus of the thalamus.

Those pathways that ascend from the spinal

cord to the cerebellum or midbrain have two orders of neurons. The first-order neuron has its cell body in the posterior root ganglion. The second-order neuron has its cell body in the gray matter of the spinal cord or in the nucleus cuneatus (cuneocerebellar tract).

INJURY TO THE ASCENDING TRACTS WITHIN THE SPINAL CORD

LATERAL SPINOTHALAMIC TRACT

Destruction of this tract produces contralateral loss of pain and thermal sensibilities below the level of the lesion. The patient will not, therefore, respond to pinprick or recognize hot and cold objects placed in contact with the skin.

ANTERIOR SPINOTHALAMIC TRACT

Destruction of this tract produces contralateral loss of light touch and pressure sensibilities below the level of the lesion. Remember that discriminative touch will still be present, because this information is conducted through the fasciculus gracilis and fasciculus cuneatus. The patient will not feel the light touch of a piece of cotton placed against the skin or feel pressure from a blunt object placed against the skin.

FASCICULUS GRACILIS AND FASCICULUS CUNEATUS

Destruction of these tracts cuts off the supply of information from the muscles and joints to consciousness; thus, the individual does not know about the position and movements of his ipsilateral limbs below the level of the lesion. With the patient's eyes closed, he is unable to tell you where his limb or part of his limb is in space. For example, if you passively dorsiflex his big toe, he is unable to tell you whether the toe is pointing upward or downward. The patient has impaired muscular control and his movements are jerky or ataxic.

The patient also has loss of vibration sense below the level of the lesion on the same side. This is easily tested by applying a vibrating tuning fork to a bony prominence such as the lateral malleolus of the fibula or the styloid process of the radius.

There will also be a loss of tactile discrimination on the side of the lesion. This is tested most easily by gradually separating the two points of a compass until the patient can appreciate them as two separate points, not as one, when they are applied to the skin surface. Tactile discrimination varies from one part of the body to another. In a normal individual, the points have to be separated by about 3 to 4 mm before they are recognized as separate points on the tips of the fingers. On the back, however, the points have to be separated by 65 mm or more before they can be recognized as separate points.

The sense of general light touch would be unaffected, because these impulses ascend in the anterior spinothalamic tracts.

It should be pointed out that it is extremely rare for a lesion of the spinal cord to be so localized as to affect one sensory tract only. It is more usual to have several ascending and descending tracts involved.

SOMATIC AND VISCERAL PAIN

Somatic pain has been considered extensively in this chapter. The sense organs for somatic pain are the naked nerve endings. The initial sharp pain is transmitted by fast-conducting fibers and the more prolonged burning pain travels in the slow-conducting nerve fibers (see p. 366).

In the viscera, there are special receptors, chemoreceptors, baroreceptors, osmoreceptors, and stretch receptors that are sensitive to a variety of stimuli including ischemia, stretching, and chemical damage. Afferent fibers from the visceral receptors reach the central nervous system via the sympathetic and parasympathetic parts of the autonomic nervous system (see pp. 487 and 489). Once within the central nervous system, the pain impulses travel by the same ascending tracts as does the somatic pain and ultimately reach the postcentral gyrus.

Visceral pain is poorly localized and often associated with salivation, nausea, vomiting, tachycardia, and sweating. Visceral pain may be referred from the organ involved to a distant area of the body (**referred pain**).

TREATMENT OF CHRONIC PAIN

New techniques, such as acupuncture and electrical stimulation of the skin, are now being used with success. Relief of pain can be achieved by the use of placebos in a few patients. The anticipation of the relief of pain is thought to stimulate the release of endorphins, which inhibit the normal pain pathway.

RELIEF OF PAIN BY RHIZOTOMY OR CORDOTOMY

Surgical relief of pain has been used extensively in patients with terminal cancer. Posterior rhizotomy or division of the posterior root of a spinal nerve effectively severs the conduction of pain into the central nervous system. It is a relatively simple procedure, but, unfortunately, the operation deprives the patient of other sensations besides pain. Moreover, if the pain sensation is entering the spinal cord through more than one spinal nerve, it may be necessary to divide several posterior roots.

Thoracic cordotomy has been performed with success in patients with severe pain originating from the lower abdomen or pelvis. Essentially, the operation consists of dividing the lateral spinothalamic tracts by inserting a knife into the anterolateral quadrant of the spinal cord. It is important to remember that the lateral spinothalamic fibers have originated in cells of the substantia gelatinosa in the opposite posterior gray column, and that they cross the spinal cord obliquely and reach their tract in the white column three or four segments higher than their posterior root of entry. Cervical cordotomy has been performed successfully in patients with intractable pain in the neck or thorax.

TABES DORSALIS

Tabes dorsalis is caused by syphilis. The organism causes a selective destruction of nerve fibers at the point of entrance of the posterior root into the spinal cord, especially in the lower thoracic and lumbosacral regions (Fig. 20-8). The following symptoms and signs may be present: (1) stabbing pains in the lower limbs, which may be very severe; (2) paresthesia, with numbness in the lower limbs; (3) hypersensitivity of skin to touch, heat, and cold; (4)

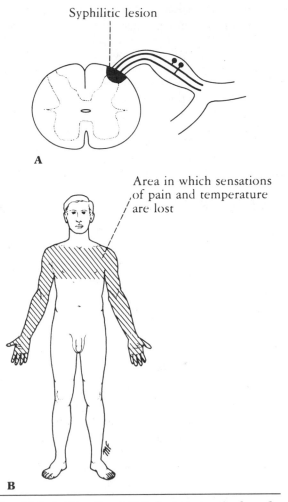

Fig. 20-8. A. Site of syphilitic lesion on spinal cord. B. Skin area in which sensations of pain and temperature are lost in syringomyelia.

loss of sensation in the skin of parts of the trunk and lower limbs; loss of awareness that the urinary bladder is full; (5) loss of appreciation of posture or passive movements of the limbs, especially the legs; (6) loss of deep pain sensation, such as when the muscles are forcibly compressed or when the tendo Achillis is compressed between the finger and thumb; (7) loss of pain sensation in the skin in certain areas of the body, such as the side of the nose or the medial border of the forearm, or the thoracic wall between the nipples, or the lateral border of the leg; (8) ataxia of the lower limbs as the result of loss of proprioceptive sensibility (the unsteadiness in gait is compensated to some extent by vision; however, in the dark, or if the eyes are closed, the ataxia becomes worse and the person may fall); (9) hypotonia as the result of loss of proprioceptive information that arises from the muscles and joints; and (10) loss of tendon reflexes, owing to degeneration of the afferent fiber component of the reflex arc (the knee and ankle tendon jerks are lost early in the disease).

SYRINGOMYELIA

This disease is due to a developmental abnormality in the formation of the central canal of the spinal cord. It is accompanied by gliosis and cavitation of the cervical segments of the spinal cord and brainstem (Fig. 20-8). It occasionally occurs at other lev-els of the spinal cord. The condition interrupts the lateral and anterior spinothalamic tracts as they cross the spinal cord in the anterior gray and white commissures. The patient has segmental losses of pain and thermal sensibility, which are often bilateral, and some impairment of touch sensation. These result in injuries, especially burns. As the cavitation expands, other tracts and nerve cells become involved. Atrophy of the anterior horn cells in the lower cervical and upper thoracic regions may lead to wasting and weakness of the muscles of the upper limb.

PERNICIOUS ANEMIA AND MULTIPLE SCLEROSIS

These diseases may also produce extensive sensory losses owing to involvement of the ascending tracts of the spinal cord.

CLINICAL PROBLEMS

Answers on Page 605

1. A 20-year-old male student celebrated the passing of an examination by drinking several beers at a party. On the way home, he drove his car head-on into a bridge abutment. On examination in the emergency room, he was found to have a fracture dislocation of the ninth thoracic vertebra with signs and symptoms of severe damage to the spinal cord. On physical examination, he had an upper motor neuron paralysis of the left leg. He also had loss of muscle joint sense of the left leg. On testing of cutaneous sensibility, he had a band of cutaneous hyperesthesia extending around the abdominal wall on the left side at the level of the umbilicus. Just below this, he had a narrow band of anesthesia and analgesia. On the right side, there was total analgesia, thermoanesthesia, and partial loss of tactile sense of the skin of the abdominal wall below the level of the umbilicus and involving the whole of the right leg. Using your knowledge of neuroanatomy, state the level at which the spinal cord was damaged. Was the spinal cord completely sectioned? If not, on which side did the hemisection occur? Explain the sensory losses found on examination in this patient.

2. A 35-year-old woman was admitted to the hospital for investigation. She had symptoms of analgesia and thermoanesthesia on the medial side of the left hand of six months' duration. Three weeks prior to her admittance, she had severely burned the little finger of her left hand on a hot stove, and was unaware that the burn had occurred until she smelled the burning skin. On physical examination, she was found to have considerably reduced pain and temperature sense involving the eighth cervical and first thoracic dermatomes of the left hand. However, her sense of tactile discrimination was perfectly normal in these areas. Examination of the right arm showed a similar but much less severe dissociated sensory loss involving the same areas. No further abnormal signs were discovered. Using your knowledge of neuroanatomy, can you state which tract or tracts were involved in this pathological process? Do you know the name of this disease?

3. A 60-year-old man walked into the neurology clinic and the physician paid particular attention to his gait. The patient raised his feet unnecessarily high and brought them to the ground in a stamping manner. While he was waiting for the physician, it was noticed that he stood with his feet wide apart. On questioning, the patient said that he was finding it increasingly difficult to walk and was starting to use a stick, especially when he went out for walks in the dark. The physician asked the patient to stand with his toes and heels together and to close his eyes. The patient immediately started to sway and the nurse had to steady him to prevent him from falling. On further examination, the patient was found to have loss of muscle joint sense of both legs and was unable to detect any feeling of vibration when a vibrating tuning fork was placed on the medial malleolus of either leg. No other sensory losses were noted. Using your knowledge of neuroanatomy, name the ascending pathways that are involved, by disease, in this patient. Can you name a disease that could be responsible for these findings?

4. A 68-year-old man had an advanced inoperable carcinoma of the prostate with multiple metastases in the lumbar vertebrae and innominate bones. Apart from the severe intractable pain, the patient was still able to enjoy life among his family. After a full discussion of the prognosis with the patient and his wife she turned to the physician and said, "Can't you do something to stop this terrible pain, so that my husband can die happy?" What can a physician do to help his patient under these circumstances?

NATIONAL BOARD TYPE QUESTIONS

Answers on Page 621

Match the tracts listed below on the left with the probable cell of origin listed below on the right. An answer may be used more than once.

1. Fasciculus cuneatus
2. Anterior spinothalamic
3. Fasciculus gracilis
4. Anterior spinocerebellar

   (a) Substantia gelatinosa
   (b) Clarke's column
   (c) Posterior root ganglion
   (d) Cells of lateral gray column
   (e) None of the above.

Match the tracts listed below on the left with the statement listed below on the right. An answer may be used more than once.

5. Fasciculus gracilis
6. Spinotectal tract
7. Lateral spinothalamic
8. Posterior spinocerebellar

   (a) It does not cross to opposite side
   (b) It crosses to opposite side in spinal cord
   (c) It crosses to opposite side in medulla oblongata
   (d) It both crosses and remains uncrossed
   (e) None of the above

Match the tracts listed below on the left with the appropriate nucleus of termination listed below on the right. An answer may be used more than once.

9. Anterior spinothalamic tract
10. Posterior white column tracts
11. Spinotectal tract
12. Spinoreticular tract
13. Anterior spinocerebellar tract

   (a) Inferior colliculus
   (b) Ventral posterolateral nucleus of thalamus
   (c) Superior colliculus
   (d) Olive
   (e) None of the above

Match the sensations listed below on the left with the appropriate nervous pathway listed below on the right.

14. Two-point tactile discrimination
15. Pain
16. Unconscious muscle joint sense
17. Pressure
18. Vibration

   (a) Anterior spinocerebellar tract
   (b) Lateral spinothalamic tract
   (c) Fasciculus cuneatus
   (d) Anterior spinothalamic tract
   (e) None of the above

In the following questions, answer:
   (a) IF (1), (2), AND (3) ONLY ARE CORRECT
   (b) IF (1) AND (3) ONLY ARE CORRECT
   (c) IF (2) AND (4) ONLY ARE CORRECT
   (d) IF (4) ONLY IS CORRECT, OR
   (e) IF ALL ARE CORRECT

19. Which of the following statements is (are) consistent with the "gate" theory of pain?
   (1) Stimulation of large non-pain-conducting fibers increases pain sensitivity.
   (2) Massage applied to the skin over the painful joint increases the pain sensitivity.
   (3) Stimulation of delta A- and C-type fibers decreases pain sensitivity.
   (4) Degeneration of large non-pain-conducting fibers increases pain sensitivity.

20. Are the following statements correct concerning the reception of pain?
   (1) The slow-conducting C-type fibers are responsible for prolonged, burning pain.
   (2) Substance P, a peptide, is thought to be the neurotransmitter at the synapses where the first-order neuron terminates on the cells in the posterior gray column.
   (3) The enkephalins and endorphins may serve to inhibit the release of substance P in the posterior gray column.
   (4) Many of the tracts conducting the initial sharp, pricking pain terminate in the ventral posterolateral nucleus of the thalamus.

ADDITIONAL READING

Bannister, R. *Brain's Clinical Neurology* (6th ed.). London and Toronto: Oxford University Press, 1985.

Bashbaum, A. I., and Fields, H. L. Endogenous pain control systems: Brain stem spinal pathways and endorphin circuitry. *Annu. Rev. Neurosci.* 7:309, 1984.

Beaumont, A., and Hughes, J. Biology of opioid peptides. *Annu. Rev. Pharmacol. Toxicol.* 19:245, 1979.

Bond, M. R. *Pain—Its Nature, Analysis and Treatment.* New York: Churchill Livingstone, 1984.

Bonica, J. J., et al. (eds.) *Proceedings of the Second World Congress on Pain.* New York: Raven, 1979.

Carr, D. B. Endorphins in contemporary medicine. *Compr. Ther.* 9:40, 1983.

Fairley, P. *The Conquest of Pain.* New York: Scribner, 1979.

Guttmann, L. *Spinal Cord Injuries* (2nd ed.). Oxford: Blackwell, 1976.

Jennett, W. B. *An Introduction to Neurosurgery* (2nd ed.). St. Louis: Mosby, 1970.

Jessell, T. M. Neurotransmitters and CNS disease: Pain. *Lancet* 2:1084, 1982.

Mann, F. Treatment of intractable pain by acupuncture. *Lancet* 2:57, 1973.

Melzack, R., and Wall, P. D. Pain mechanisms: A new theory. *Science* 150:971, 1973.

Roberts, H. H. T., and Llewelyn, M. B. The supraspinal control of pain. *Bioscience* 32:587, 1982.

Walton, J. N. *Brain's Diseases of the Nervous System* (8th ed.). New York and London: Oxford University Press, 1977.

Williams, P. L., Warwick, R., Dyson, M., and Bannister, L. H. *Gray's Anatomy* (37th Brit. ed.). Philadelphia: Saunders, 1989.

Youmans, J. R. *Neurological Surgery.* Philadelphia: Saunders, 1973. Vol. 3.

Chapter 21
The Descending Tracts of the Spinal Cord and Skeletal Muscle Activity

The motor neurons situated in the anterior gray columns of the spinal cord send axons to innervate skeletal muscle through the anterior roots of the spinal nerves. These motor neurons are sometimes referred to as the **lower motor neurons** and constitute the final common pathway to the muscles (Fig. 21-1).

The lower motor neurons are constantly bombarded by nervous impulses that descend from the medulla, pons, midbrain, and cerebral cortex, as well as those that enter along sensory fibers from the posterior roots. The nerve fibers that descend in the white matter from different supraspinal nerve centers are segregated into nerve bundles called the **descending tracts**. These supraspinal neurons and their tracts are sometimes referred to as the **upper motor neurons** and they provide numerous separate pathways that can influence motor activity.

ANATOMICAL ORGANIZATION

Control of skeletal muscle activity from the cerebral cortex and other higher centers is conducted through the nervous system by a series of neurons (Fig. 21-1). The descending pathway from the cerebral cortex is often made up of three neurons. The first neuron, the **first-order neuron**, has its cell body in the cerebral cortex. Its axon descends to synapse on the **second-order neuron**, an internuncial neuron, situated in the anterior gray column of the spinal cord (Fig. 21-1). The axon of the second-order neuron is short and synapses with the **third-order neuron**, the lower motor neuron, in the anterior gray column (Fig. 21-1). The axon of the third-order neuron innervates the skeletal muscle through the anterior root and spinal nerve. In some instances, the axon of the first-order neuron terminates directly on the third-order neuron (as in reflex arcs).

FUNCTIONS OF THE DESCENDING TRACTS

The corticospinal tracts (Fig. 21-2) are the pathways concerned with voluntary, discrete, skilled movements, especially those of the distal parts of

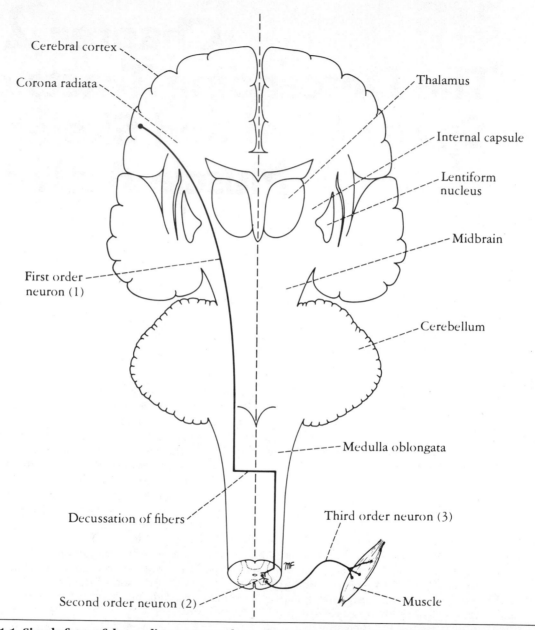

Fig. 21-1. Simple form of descending motor pathway from the cerebral cortex to the skeletal muscle. Note the three neurons involved.

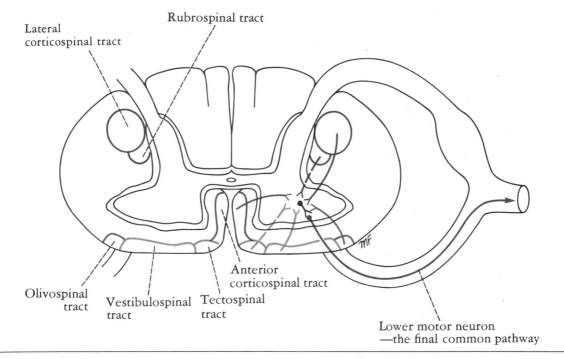

Fig. 21-2. Transverse section of spinal cord, showing termination of descending motor tracts. Note that there is now considerable doubt as to the existence of the olivospinal tract as a separate pathway.

the limbs. The **reticulospinal tracts** may facilitate or inhibit the activity of the alpha and gamma motor neurons in the anterior gray columns and may, therefore, facilitate or inhibit voluntary movement or reflex activity. The **tectospinal tract** (Fig. 21-2) is concerned with reflex postural movements in response to visual stimuli. Those fibers that are associated with the sympathetic neurons in the lateral gray column are concerned with the pupillo-dilation reflex in response to darkness. The **rubrospinal tract** (Fig. 21-2) acts on both the alpha and gamma motor neurons in the anterior gray columns and facilitates the activity of flexor muscles and inhibits the activity of extensor or antigravity muscles. The **vestibulospinal tract** (Fig. 21-2), by acting on the motor neurons in the anterior gray columns, facilitates the activity of the extensor muscles, inhibits the activity of the flexor muscles, and is concerned with the postural activity associated with balance. The **olivospinal tract** (Fig. 21-2) may play a role in muscular activity, but there is doubt that it exists. The **descending autonomic**

fibers are concerned with the control of visceral activity.

CORTICOSPINAL TRACTS

Fibers of the corticospinal tract arise as axons of pyramidal cells situated in the fifth layer of the cerebral cortex (Fig. 21-3). About one-third of the fibers originate from the primary motor cortex (area 4), one-third from the secondary motor cortex (area 6), and one-third from the parietal lobe (areas 3, 1, and 2); thus, two-thirds of the fibers arise from the precentral gyrus and one-third from the postcentral gyrus.* Since electrical stimulation of different parts of the precentral gyrus produces movements of different parts of the opposite side of the body, we can represent the parts of the body in this area of the cortex. Such a homunculus is shown in Figure 21-3. Note that the region control-

*These fibers do not control motor activity but influence sensory input to the nervous system.

Fig. 21-3. Corticospinal tracts.

ling the face is situated inferiorly and the lower limb is situated superiorly and on the medial surface of the hemisphere. The homunculus is a distorted picture of the body, with the various parts having a size proportional to the area of the cerebral cortex devoted to their control. It is interesting to find that the majority of the corticospinal fibers are myelinated and are relatively slow-conducting, small fibers.

The descending fibers converge in the **corona radiata** and then pass through the posterior limb of the **internal capsule** (Fig. 21-3). Here, the fibers are organized so that those closest to the genu are concerned with cervical portions of the body, while those situated more posteriorly are concerned with the lower extremity. The tract then continues through the middle three-fifths of the **basis pedunculi of the midbrain** (Fig. 21-3). Here, the fibers concerned with cervical portions of the body are situated medially, while those concerned with the leg are placed laterally.

On entering the pons, the tract is broken into many bundles by the **transverse pontocerebellar fibers** (see Figs. 9-3, 9-5, and 9-6). In the medulla oblongata, the bundles become grouped together along the anterior border to form a swelling known as the *pyramid* (hence the alternative name, **pyramidal tract**) (see Fig. 8-1). At the junction of the medulla oblongata and the spinal cord, most of the fibers cross the midline at the **decussation of the pyramids** (Fig. 21-3) and enter the lateral white column of the spinal cord to form the **lateral corticospinal tract** (Fig. 21-2). The remaining fibers do not cross in the decussation, but descend in the anterior white column of the spinal cord as the **anterior corticospinal tract** (Figs. 21-2 and 21-3). These fibers eventually cross the midline and terminate in the anterior gray column of the spinal cord segments in the cervical and upper thoracic regions.

The lateral corticospinal tract descends the length of the spinal cord; its fibers terminate in the anterior gray column of all the spinal cord segments.

Most corticospinal fibers synapse with internuncial neurons, which in turn synapse with alpha motor neurons and some gamma motor neurons. Only the largest corticospinal fibers synapse directly with the motor neurons.

It is important to understand that the cortico-spinal tracts are not the sole pathway for serving voluntary movement. Rather, they form the pathway that confers speed and agility to voluntary movements and is thus used in performing rapid skilled movements. Many of the simple, basic voluntary movements are believed to be mediated by other descending tracts.

BRANCHES OF CORTICOSPINAL TRACTS

1. Branches are given off early in their descent and return to the cerebral cortex to inhibit activity in adjacent regions of the cortex.
2. Branches pass to the caudate and lentiform nuclei, the red nuclei, and the olivary nuclei and the reticular formation. These branches keep the subcortical regions informed about the cortical motor activity. Once alerted, the subcortical regions may react and send their own nervous impulses to the alpha and gamma motor neurons by other descending pathways.

RETICULOSPINAL TRACTS

Throughout the midbrain, pons, and medulla oblongata groups of scattered nerve cells and nerve fibers exist that are collectively known as the **reticular formation**. (See p. 315.) From the pons, these neurons send axons, which are mostly uncrossed, down into the spinal cord and form the **pontine reticulospinal tract** (Fig. 21-4). From the medulla, similar neurons send axons, which are crossed and uncrossed, to the spinal cord and form the **medullary reticulospinal tract**.

The reticulospinal fibers from the pons descend through the anterior white column, while those from the medulla oblongata descend in the lateral white column (Fig. 21-4). Both sets of fibers enter the anterior gray columns of the spinal cord and may facilitate or inhibit the activity of the alpha and gamma motor neurons. By this means the reticulospinal tracts influence voluntary movements and reflex activity. The reticulospinal fibers are also now thought to include the descending autonomic fibers. The reticulospinal tracts thus provide a pathway by which the hypothalamus can control the sympathetic outflow and the sacral parasympathetic outflow.

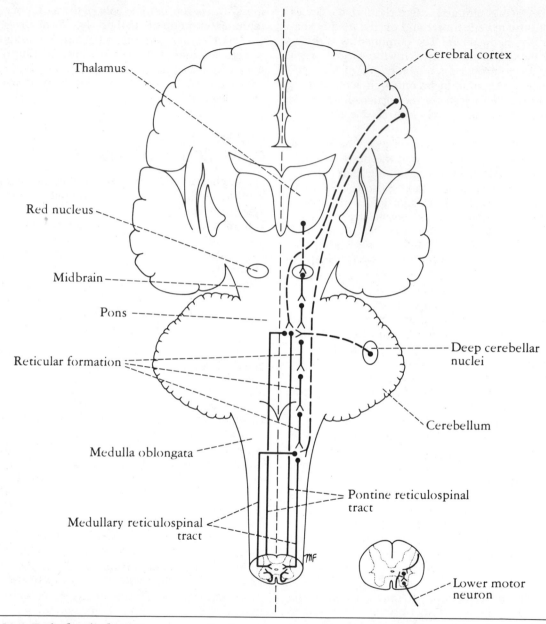

Fig. 21-4. Reticulospinal tracts.

TECTOSPINAL TRACT

Fibers of this tract arise from nerve cells in the **superior colliculus** of the midbrain (Fig. 21-5). Most of the fibers cross the midline soon after their origin and descend through the brainstem close to the **medial longitudinal fasciculus**. The tectospinal tract descends through the anterior white column of the spinal cord close to the anterior median fissure (Figs. 21-2 and 21-5). The majority of the fibers terminate in the anterior gray column in the upper cervical segments of the spinal cord by synapsing with internuncial neurons. These fibers are believed to be concerned with reflex postural movements in response to visual stimuli.

RUBROSPINAL TRACT

The **red nucleus** is situated in the tegmentum of the midbrain at the level of the superior colliculus (Fig. 21-6). The axons of neurons in this nucleus cross the midline at the level of the nucleus and descend as the rubrospinal tract through the pons and medulla oblongata to enter the lateral white column of the spinal cord (Figs. 21-2 and 21-6). The fibers terminate by synapsing with internuncial neurons in the anterior gray column of the cord.

The neurons of the red nucleus receive afferent impulses through connections with the cerebral cortex and the cerebellum. This is believed to be an important indirect pathway by which the cerebral cortex and the cerebellum can influence the activity of the alpha and gamma motor neurons of the spinal cord. The tract facilitates the activity of the flexor muscles and inhibits the activity of the extensor or antigravity muscles.

VESTIBULOSPINAL TRACT

The **vestibular nuclei** are situated in the pons and medulla oblongata beneath the floor of the fourth ventricle (Fig. 21-7). The vestibular nuclei receive afferent fibers from the inner ear through the vestibular nerve and from the cerebellum. The neurons of the lateral vestibular nucleus give rise to the axons that form the vestibulospinal tract. The tract descends uncrossed through the medulla and through the length of the spinal cord in the anterior white column (Figs. 21-2 and 21-7). The fibers terminate by synapsing with internuncial neurons of the anterior gray column of the spinal cord.

The inner ear and the cerebellum, by means of this tract, facilitate the activity of the extensor muscles and inhibit the activity of the flexor muscles in association with the maintenance of balance.

OLIVOSPINAL TRACT

The olivospinal tract was thought to arise from the inferior olivary nucleus and to descend in the lateral white column of the spinal cord (Fig. 21-8), to influence the activity of the motor neurons in the anterior gray column. There is now considerable doubt that it exists.

Descending Autonomic Fibers

The higher centers of the central nervous system associated with the control of autonomic activity are situated in the cerebral cortex, hypothalamus, amygdaloid complex, and reticular formation. Although distinct tracts have not been recognized, investigation of spinal cord lesions has demonstrated that descending autonomic tracts do exist and probably form part of the reticulospinal tract.

The fibers arise from neurons in the higher centers and cross the midline in the brainstem. They are believed to descend in the lateral white column of the spinal cord and to terminate by synapsing on the autonomic motor cells in the lateral gray columns in the thoracic and upper lumbar (sympathetic outflow) and midsacral (parasympathetic) levels of the spinal cord.

INTERSEGMENTAL TRACTS

Short ascending and descending tracts, which originate and end within the spinal cord, exist in the anterior, lateral, and posterior white columns. The function of these pathways is to interconnect the neurons of different segmental levels, and they are particularly important in intersegmental spinal reflexes.

Fig. 21-5. Tectospinal tract.

Fig. 21-6. Rubrospinal tract.

Fig. 21-7. Vestibulospinal tract.

Fig. 21-8. Olivospinal tract. There is now considerable doubt as to the existence of this tract as a separate pathway.

REFLEX ARC

A **reflex** may be defined as an involuntary response to a stimulus. It depends on the integrity of the reflex arc (Fig. 21-9). In its simplest form, a reflex arc consists of the following anatomical structures: (1) a receptor organ, (2) an afferent neuron, (3) an effector neuron, and (4) an effector organ. Such a reflex arc involving only one synapse is referred to as a **monosynaptic reflex arc**. Interruption of the reflex arc at any point along its course would abolish the response.

In the spinal cord, reflex arcs play an important role in maintaining muscle tone, which is the basis for body posture. The receptor organ is situated in the skin, muscle, or tendon. The cell body of the afferent neuron is located in the posterior root ganglion, and the central axon of this first-order neuron terminates by synapsing on the effector neuron. Since the afferent fibers are of large diameter and are rapidly conducting, and because of the presence of only one synapse, a very quick response is possible.

Physiological study of the electrical activity of the effector neuron shows that following the very quick monosynaptic discharge there is a prolonged asynchronous discharge. The reason for this later discharge is that the afferent fibers entering the spinal cord frequently branch, and the branches synapse with many internuncial neurons, which ultimately synapse with the effector neuron (Fig. 21-10). These additional neuronal circuits prolong the bombardment of the effector neurons after the initial stimulation by the afferent neuron has ceased. The presence of internuncial neurons also results in the spread of the afferent stimulus to neurons at different segmental levels of the spinal cord.

In considering reflex skeletal muscle activity it is important to understand the **law of reciprocal innervation** (Fig. 21-10). Simply stated, it means that the flexor and extensor reflexes of the same limb cannot be made to contract simultaneously. For this law to work, the afferent nerve fibers responsible for flexor reflex muscle action must have branches that synapse with the extensor motor neurons of the same limb, causing them to be inhibited.

Another interesting property of spinal reflexes should be pointed out. The evocation of a reflex on one side of the body causes opposite effects on the limb of the other side of the body. This **crossed extensor reflex** (Fig. 21-10) may be demonstrated as follows. Afferent stimulation of the reflex arc that causes the ipsilateral limb to flex results in the contralateral limb being extended.

Influence of Higher Neuronal Centers on the Activities of Spinal Reflexes

The spinal segmental reflex arc involving motor activity is greatly influenced by higher centers in the brain. These influences are mediated through the corticospinal, reticulospinal, tectospinal, rubrospinal, and vestibulospinal tracts. In the clinical condition known as spinal shock, which follows the sudden removal of these influences by severance of the spinal cord, the segmental spinal reflexes are depressed. When the so-called spinal shock disappears in a few weeks, the segmental spinal reflexes return and the muscle tone is increased. This so-called **decerebrate rigidity** is due to the overactivity of the gamma efferent nerve fibers to the muscle spindles, which results from the release of these neurons from the higher centers (see p. 153). The next stage may be **paraplegia in extension** with domination of the increased tone of the extensor muscles over the flexor muscles. Some neurologists believe that this condition is due to incomplete severance of all the descending tracts with persistence of the vestibulospinal tract. Should all the descending tracts be severed, the condition of **paraplegia in flexion** occurs. In this condition, the reflex responses are flexor in nature and the tone of the extensor muscles is diminished.

RENSHAW CELLS AND LOWER MOTOR NEURON INHIBITION

Lower motor neuron axons give off collateral branches as they pass through the white matter to reach the anterior roots of the spinal nerve. These collaterals synapse on neurons described by Renshaw, which in turn synapse on the lower motor neurons (Fig. 21-9). These internuncial neurons are believed to provide feedback on the lower motor neurons, inhibiting their activity.

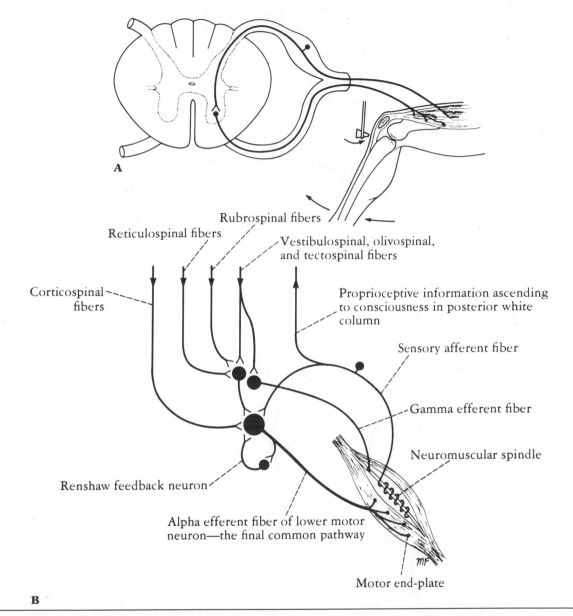

Fig. 21-9. A. A monosynaptic reflex arc.
B. Multiple neurons synapsing with the lower motor neuron.
Note the presence of the Renshaw feedback neuron.

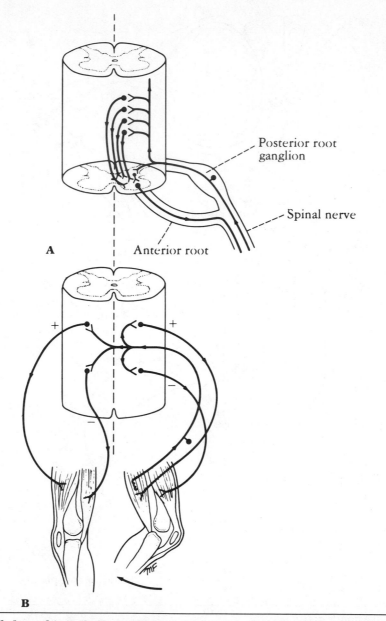

**Fig. 21-10. A. Multiple branching of afferent fibers entering spinal cord and the presence of many internuncial neurons that synapse with the effector neuron.
B. Law of reciprocal innervation and the crossed extensor reflex.**

CLINICAL NOTES

GENERAL CONSIDERATIONS

Muscle Tone

Muscle tone is a state of continuous partial contraction of a muscle and is dependent on the integrity of a monosynaptic reflex arc (see description on p. 152). The receptor organs are the muscle spindles. The afferent neuron enters the spinal cord through the posterior root and synapses with the effector neuron or lower motor neuron in the anterior gray column. The lower motor neuron supplies the muscle fibers by traveling through the anterior roots, the spinal nerves, and peripheral nerves. Muscle tone is abolished if any part of that simple reflex arc is destroyed. An atonic muscle feels soft and flabby and atrophies rapidly.

Normal muscle tone exhibits a certain resilience or elasticity, and when a muscle is passively stretched by moving a joint, a certain degree of resistance is felt. Normal muscle tone depends on the integrity of the monosynaptic reflex arc described above, and the control superimposed on it by impulses received through the descending tracts from supraspinal levels. Note that muscle spindles are excitatory to muscle tone, whereas neurotendinous receptors are inhibitory to muscle tone.

Voluntary Movement

Voluntary movement is initiated by the individual. A series of different muscles are made to contract for the purpose of reaching a goal. This would suggest that the descending tracts that influence the activity of the lower motor neurons are driven by information received by the sensory systems, the eyes, the ears, and the muscles themselves, and are affected further by past afferent information that has been stored in the memory. Moreover, the whole process may be colored by past and present emotional input. The limbic structures appear to play a role in emotion, motivation, and memory and they may influence the initiation process of voluntary movement by their projections to the cerebral cortex.

The descending pathways from the cerebral cortex and the brainstem, that is, the upper motor neurons, influence the activity of the lower motor neurons either directly or through internuncial neurons. Most of the tracts originating in the brainstem that descend to the spinal cord also are receiving input from the cerebral cortex.

The corticospinal tracts are believed to control the prime mover muscles, especially those responsible for the highly skilled movements of the distal parts of the limbs. The other supraspinal descending tracts play a major role in the simple basic voluntary movements, and in addition bring about an adjustment of the muscle tone, so that easy and rapid movements of the joints can take place.

It is interesting to note that the basal ganglia and the cerebellum do not give rise directly to descending tracts that influence the activities of the lower motor neuron, and yet we know that these parts of the nervous system greatly influence voluntary movements. This influence is accomplished indirectly by fibers that project to the cerebral cortex and brainstem nuclei that are the sites of origin of the descending tracts.

Pyramidal and Extrapyramidal Tracts

The term **pyramidal tract** is used commonly by clinicians and refers specifically to the corticospinal tracts. The term came into common usage when it was learned that the corticospinal fibers become concentrated on the anterior part of the medulla oblongata in an area referred to as the **pyramids**.

The term **extrapyramidal tracts** refers to all the descending tracts other than the corticospinal tracts.

UPPER MOTOR NEURON LESIONS

Lesions of the Corticospinal Tracts (Pyramidal Tracts)

Lesions restricted to the corticospinal tracts produce the following clinical signs:

1. The **Babinski sign** is present. The great toe becomes dorsally flexed and the other toes fan out-

ward in response to scratching the skin along the lateral aspect of the sole of the foot. The normal response is plantar flexion of all the toes. Remember that the Babinski sign normally is present during the first year of life, because the corticospinal tract is not myelinated until the end of the first year of life.

The explanation for the Babinski response is thought to be the following. Normally, the corticospinal tracts produce plantar flexion of the toes in response to sensory stimulation of the skin of the sole. When the corticospinal tracts are nonfunctional, the influence of the other descending tracts on the toes becomes apparent, and a kind of withdrawal reflex takes place in response to stimulation of the sole, with the great toe being dorsally flexed and the other toes fanning out.

2. The **superficial abdominal reflexes** are absent. The abdominal muscles fail to contract when the skin of the abdomen is scratched. This reflex is dependent on the integrity of the corticospinal tracts, which exert a tonic excitatory influence on the internuncial neurons.
3. The **cremasteric reflex** is absent. The cremaster muscle fails to contract when the skin on the medial side of the thigh is stroked. This reflex arc passes through the first lumbar segment of the spinal cord. This reflex is dependent on the integrity of the corticospinal tracts, which exert a tonic excitatory influence on the internuncial neurons.
4. There is **loss of performance of fine skilled voluntary movements**. This occurs especially at the distal end of the limbs.

Lesions of the Descending Tracts Other than the Corticospinal Tracts (Extrapyramidal Tracts)

The following clinical signs are present in lesions restricted to the other descending tracts:

1. **Severe paralysis** with little or no muscle atrophy (except secondary to disuse).
2. **Spasticity or hypertonicity** of the muscles. The lower limb is maintained in extension and the upper limb is maintained in flexion.
3. **Exaggerated deep muscle reflexes** and clonus

may be present in the flexors of the fingers, the quadriceps femoris, and the calf muscles.
4. **Clasp-knife reaction**. When passive movement of a joint is attempted there is resistance owing to spasticity of the muscles. The muscles, on stretching, suddenly give way due to organ mediated inhibition.

It should be pointed out that in clinical practice it is rare to have an organic lesion that is restricted only to the pyramidal tracts, or only to the extrapyramidal tracts. Usually, both sets of tracts are affected to a variable extent, producing both groups of clinical signs. As the pyramidal tracts normally tend to increase muscle tone and the extrapyramidal tracts inhibit muscle tone, the balance between these opposing effects will be altered, producing different degrees of muscle tone.

Lesions of the Lower Motor Neuron

Trauma, infection (poliomyelitis), vascular disorders, degenerative diseases, and neoplasms may all produce a lesion of the lower motor neuron by destroying the cell body in the anterior gray column or its axon in the anterior root or spinal nerve. The following clinical signs are present in the lower motor neuron lesions:

1. **Flaccid paralysis** of muscles supplied.
2. **Atrophy** of muscles supplied.
3. **Loss of reflexes** of muscles supplied.
4. **Muscular fasciculation**. This is twitching of muscles seen only when there is slow destruction of the lower motor neuron cell.
5. **Muscular contracture**. This is a shortening of the paralyzed muscles. It occurs more often in the antagonist muscles whose action is no longer opposed by the paralyzed muscles.
6. **Reaction of degeneration**. Normally innervated muscles respond to stimulation by the application of faradic (interrupted) current and the contraction continues as long as the current is passing. Galvanic or direct current causes contraction only when the current is turned on or turned off. When the lower motor neuron is cut, a muscle will no longer respond to interrupted electrical stimulation seven days after nerve section, although it still will respond to direct current. After ten days, the response to direct cur-

rent also ceases. This change in muscle response to electrical stimulation is known as the **reaction of degeneration**.

Types of Paralysis

Hemiplegia is a paralysis of one side of the body and includes the upper limb, one side of the trunk, and the lower limb.

Monoplegia is a paralysis of one limb only.

Diplegia is a paralysis of two corresponding limbs (i.e., arms or legs).

Paraplegia is a paralysis of the two lower limbs.

Quadriplegia is a paralysis of all four limbs.

RELATIONSHIP OF MUSCULAR SIGNS AND SYMPTOMS TO LESIONS OF THE NERVOUS SYSTEM

Abnormal Muscle Tone

Hypotonia

This condition exists when the muscle tone is diminished or absent. It occurs when any part of the monosynaptic stretch reflex arc is interrupted. It also occurs in cerebellar disease as the result of diminished influence on the gamma motor neurons from the cerebellum.

Hypertonia (Spasticity, Rigidity)

This condition exists when the muscle tone is increased. It occurs when lesions exist that involve supraspinal centers or their descending tracts but **not** the corticospinal tract. It also may occur at the local spinal segmental level and be produced by local excitation of the stretch reflex by sensory irritation (e.g., spasm of back muscles secondary to prolapsed intervertebral disc, spasm of abdominal muscles secondary to peritonitis).

Tremors

Tremors are rhythmic involuntary movements that result from the contraction of opposing muscle groups. These may be slow, as in **parkinsonism**, or fast, as in toxic tremors from thyrotoxicosis.

They may occur at rest, as in parkinsonism, or with action, the so-called intention tremor, as seen in cerebellar disease.

Spasms

Spasms are sudden involuntary contractions of large groups of muscles. Examples of spasms are seen in paraplegia and are due to lesions involving the descending tracts but not the corticospinal tract.

Athetosis

Athetosis means continuous, slow, involuntary, dysrhythmic movements that are always the same in the same patient and disappear during sleep. They impede voluntary movement. Athetosis occurs in lesions of the corpus striatum.

Chorea

Chorea consists of a series of continuous, rapid, involuntary, jerky, coarse, purposeless movements, which may occur during sleep. Chorea occurs in lesions of the corpus striatum.

Dystonia

Dystonia consists of frequent, maintained contractions of hypertonic muscles, leading to bizarre postures. It occurs in lesions of the lentiform nucleus.

Myoclonus

Myoclonus is a sudden contraction of an isolated muscle or part of a muscle. It occurs irregularly and commonly involves a muscle of a limb. It may be present in diseases that involve the reticular formation and the cerebellum. Normal myoclonic jerks sometimes occur in individuals as they are falling asleep and are believed to be due to a sudden temporary reactivation of the reticular formation.

Hemiballismus

Hemiballismus is a rare form of involuntary movement confined to one side of the body. It usually involves the proximal extremity musculature and the limb involved is made to fly about in all directions. The lesion responsible occurs in the opposite subthalamic nucleus.

COMMON CLINICAL SYNDROMES AFFECTING THE MOTOR SYSTEMS

Hemisection of the Spinal Cord (Brown-Séquard Syndrome)

Hemisection of the spinal cord may be caused by bullet or stab wounds, or by an expanding tumor. Incomplete hemisection is common; complete hemisection is rare. The following characteristic clinical features (Fig. 21-11) will be seen in patients with a complete hemisection of the cord after the period of spinal shock has ended:

1. Ipsilateral lower motor neuron paralysis in the segment of the lesion and muscular atrophy: These signs are caused by damage to the neurons in the anterior gray column and possibly by damage to the nerve roots of the same segment.

2. Ipsilateral spastic paralysis below the level of the lesion: There is an ipsilateral Babinski sign present and, depending on the segment of the cord damaged, there are an ipsilateral loss of superficial abdominal reflexes and an ipsilateral loss of the cremasteric reflex. All these signs are due to loss of the corticospinal tracts on the side of the lesion. The spastic paralysis is produced by the interruption of the descending tracts other than the corticospinal tracts.

3. Ipsilateral band of cutaneous anesthesia in the segment of the lesion: This is due to the destruction of the posterior root and its entrance into the spinal cord at the level of the lesion.

4. Ipsilateral loss of tactile discrimination and of vibratory and proprioceptive sense below the level of the lesion: These signs are caused by the destruction of the ascending tracts in the posterior white column on the same side of the lesion.

5. Contralateral loss of pain and temperature sense below the lesion: This is due to destruction of the crossed lateral spinothalamic tracts on the same side of the lesion. Because the tracts cross obliquely, the sensory loss occurs two or three segments below the lesion distally.

Fig. 21-11. Brown-Séquard syndrome with spinal cord lesion at right tenth thoracic level.

Lesion on this side

Total loss of all sensations
—hypotonic paralysis

Loss of tactile discrimination, vibratory and proprioceptive sensations—spastic paralysis

Loss of pain and temperature sensations
Impaired tactile sense

6. Contralateral but not complete loss of tactile sense below the lesions: This condition is brought about by the destruction of the crossed anterior spinothalamic tracts on the side of the lesion. Here again, because the tracts cross obliquely, the sensory impairment occurs two or three segments below the lesion distally.

Complete Transection of the Spinal Cord

This transection results in complete loss of all sensibility and voluntary movement below the level of the lesion. It may be caused by fracture dislocation of the vertebral column, by a bullet or stab wound, or by an expanding tumor. The following characteristic clinical features will be seen after the period of spinal shock has ended:

1. Bilateral lower motor neuron paralysis in the segment of the lesion and muscular atrophy: This is due to damage to the neurons in the anterior gray columns and possibly to damage to the nerve roots of the same segment.
2. Bilateral spastic paralysis below the level of the lesion: A bilateral Babinski sign is present and, depending on the level of the segment of the spinal cord damaged, there is bilateral loss of the superficial abdominal and cremaster reflexes. All these signs are caused by an interruption of the corticospinal tracts on both sides of the cord. The bilateral spastic paralysis is produced by the cutting of the descending tracts other than the corticospinal tracts.
3. Bilateral loss of all sensation below the level of the lesion: The loss of tactile discrimination and vibratory and proprioceptive sense is due to bilateral destruction of the ascending tracts in the posterior white columns. The loss of pain, temperature, and light touch is caused by the section of the lateral and anterior spinothalamic tracts on both sides. Because these tracts cross obliquely, the loss of thermal sensations and light touch occurs two or three segments below the lesion distally.
4. Bladder and bowel functions are not under voluntary control, which causes serious difficulties in the management of these patients.

Parkinson's Disease

This disease commences between the ages of 45 and 55 and is associated with neuronal degeneration in the **substantia nigra** and to a lesser extent in the **globus pallidus**, **putamen**, and **caudate nucleus**.

The degeneration of the neurons of the substantia nigra that send their axons to the corpus striatum results in a reduction in the release of the neurotransmitter dopamine within the corpus striatum. This leads to hypersensitivity of the dopamine receptors in the postsynaptic neurons in the striatum.

Patients have the following characteristic signs and symptoms:

1. **Tremor.** This is the result of the alternating contraction of agonists and antagonists. The tremor is slow and occurs most obviously when the limbs are at rest. It disappears during sleep.
2. **Rigidity.** This differs from the rigidity caused by lesions of the upper motor neurons in that it is present to an equal extent in opposing muscle groups. If the tremor is absent, the rigidity is felt as resistance to passive movement and is sometimes referred to as **plastic rigidity**. If the tremor is present, the muscle resistance is overcome as a series of jerks, called **cogwheel rigidity**.
3. **Bradykinesis.** There is a difficulty in initiating and performing new movements. The movements are slow, the face is expressionless, and the voice is slurred and unmodulated. Swinging of the arms in walking is lost.
4. **Postural disturbances.** The patient stands with a stoop and his arms are flexed. He walks by taking short steps and often is unable to stop. In fact, he may break into a shuffling run to maintain his balance.
5. There is no loss of muscle power and no loss of sensibility. Since the corticospinal tracts are normal, the superficial abdominal reflexes are normal and there is no Babinski response. The deep tendon reflexes are normal. The signs and symptoms are due to disease of those supraspinal centers, especially the substantia nigra, that influence the neurons that give origin to descending tracts other than the corticospinal tracts.

Syringomyelia

This condition, which is due to a developmental abnormality in the formation of the central canal, most often affects the brainstem and cervical region of the spinal cord. At the site of the lesion there is cavitation and gliosis in the central region of the neuroaxis. The following characteristic signs and symptoms are found:

1. Loss of pain and temperature sensations in dermatomes on both sides of the body related to the affected segments of the cord. This loss commonly has a shawl-like distribution, caused by the interruption of the lateral spinothalamic tracts as they cross the midline in the anterior gray and white commissures.
2. Tactile discrimination, vibratory sense, and proprioceptive sense are normal. The reason is that the ascending tracts in the posterior white column are unaffected.
3. Lower motor neuron weakness is present in the small muscles of the hand. It may be bilateral or one hand may suffer before the other. As the lesion expands in the lower cervical and upper thoracic region it destroys the anterior horn cells of these segments. Later, the other muscles of the arm and shoulder girdles undergo atrophy.
4. Bilateral spastic paralysis of both legs may occur, with exaggerated deep tendon reflexes and the presence of a positive Babinski response. These signs are produced by the further expansion of the lesion laterally into the white column to involve the descending tracts.
5. A Horner's syndrome (for details, see p. 510) may be present. This is caused by the interruption of the descending autonomic fibers in amongst the reticulospinal tracts in the lateral white column by the expanding lesion.

CLINICAL PROBLEMS

Answers on Page 606

1. During the first physiology lecture to the freshman medical class on the functions of the spinal cord, the professor repeatedly referred to the *lower motor neurons, internuncial neurons,* the *final common pathway,* and the *upper motor neurons.* This is basic terminology. Do you understand what is meant by these terms?
2. A third-year medical student attended a lecture on the effects of trauma on the vertebral column. The orthopedic surgeon described very superficially the different neurological deficits that may follow injury to the spinal cord. At the end of the lecture, the student said he did not understand what was meant by the term *spinal shock.* He could not understand what was the underlying mechanism for this condition. He also asked the surgeon to explain what was meant by paraplegia in extension and paraplegia in flexion. Could the surgeon explain why one condition sometimes passes into the other? These are good questions. Can you answer them?
3. The terms *pyramidal* and *extrapyramidal tracts* are commonly used clinically. Why are students now being urged not to use these terms?
4. While examining a patient with a right-sided hemiplegia caused by a cerebrovascular accident, the neurologist asked the student which clinical signs could be attributed to an interruption of the corticospinal tracts and which signs could be attributed to damage to other descending tracts. Using your knowledge of neuroanatomy, how would you have answered this question?
5. A large civilian aircraft was forced to abort its takeoff because three tires had burst as the plane sped along the runway. The pilot miraculously managed to halt the plane as it veered off the runway and came to an abrupt halt in a ditch. All the passengers escaped injury, but one of the stewardesses was admitted to the emergency room with suspected spinal cord injury. On questioning, the 25-year-old patient said that although she had her seatbelt fastened she was thrown violently forward on impact. She said she could not feel anything in either leg and could not move her legs. On examination, there was complete motor and sensory loss of both legs below the inguinal ligament and absence of all deep tendon reflexes of both legs. Twelve hours later, it was noted that she could move the

toes and ankle of her left lower limb and she had a return of sensations to her right leg except for loss of tactile discrimination, vibratory sense, and proprioceptive sense. She had a band of complete anesthesia over her right inguinal ligament. Her left leg showed a total analgesia, thermoanesthesia, and partial loss of tactile sense. Her right leg was totally paralyzed and the muscles were spastic. There was a right-sided Babinski response, and it was possible to demonstrate right-sided ankle clonus. The right knee jerk was exaggerated. Using your knowledge of neuroanatomy, explain the symptoms and signs found in this patient. Which vertebra was damaged?

6. Why is it dangerous to move a patient who is suspected of having a fracture or dislocation of the vertebral column?

7. An 18-year-old man was admitted to the hospital following a severe automobile accident. After a complete neurological investigation, his family was told that he would be paralyzed from the waist downward for the rest of his life. The neurologist outlined to the medical personnel the importance of preventing complications in these cases. The common complications are the following: (a) urinary infection, (b) bedsores, (c) nutritional deficiency, (d) muscular spasms, and (e) pain. Using your knowledge of neuroanatomy, explain the underlying reasons for these complications. How long after the accident do you think it would be possible to give an accurate prognosis in this case?

8. A 68-year-old man was brought to the neurology clinic by his daughter because she had noticed that his right arm had a tremor. Apparently this had started about six months previously and was becoming steadily worse. When questioned, the patient said he noticed that the muscles of his limbs sometimes felt stiff but he had put this down to old age. While talking, it was noticed, the patient rarely smiled and then only with difficulty. It was also noted that he infrequently blinked his eyes. The patient tended to speak in a low, faint voice.

When asked to walk, the patient was seen to have normal posture and gait, although he tended to hold his right arm flexed at the elbow joint. When he was sitting, it was noted that the fingers of the right hand were alternately contracting and relaxing and there was a fine tremor involving the wrist and elbow on the right side. It was particularly noticed that the tremor was worse when the arm was at rest. When he was asked to hold a book in his right hand, the tremor stopped momentarily, but it started again immediately after the book was placed on the table. The daughter said that when her father falls asleep the tremor stops immediately. On examination, it was found that the passive movements of the right elbow and wrist showed an increase in tone and there was some cogwheel rigidity. There was no sensory loss, either cutaneous or deep sensibility, and the reflexes were normal. Using your knowledge of neuroanatomy, can you make a diagnosis? Which regions of the brain are diseased?

9. Name a center in the central nervous system that may be responsible for the following clinical signs: (a) intention tremor, (b) athetosis, (c) chorea, (d) dystonia, and (e) hemiballismus.

NATIONAL BOARD TYPE QUESTIONS

Answers on Page 621

IN EACH OF THE FOLLOWING QUESTIONS, ANSWER:
  (a) IF (1) ONLY IS CORRECT
  (b) IF (2) ONLY IS CORRECT
  (c) IF BOTH (1) AND (2) ARE CORRECT, AND
  (d) IF NEITHER (1) NOR (2) IS CORRECT

1. Which of the following statements is (are) correct concerning the descending pathways from the cerebral cortex?
  (1) They are usually made up of three neurons.
  (2) The third-order neuron usually supplies striated voluntary muscle fibers.

2. Which of the following statements is (are) correct concerning the corticospinal tracts?
  (1) They arise as axons of the pyramidal cells in the fifth layer of the cerebral cortex.
  (2) They are mainly responsible for controlling the voluntary movements in the proximal muscles of the limbs.

3. Which of the following statements is (are) correct concerning the route taken by the corticospinal tracts?
   (1) They run between the transverse pontocerebellar fibers in the pons.
   (2) They occupy the genu and posterior limb of the internal capsule.
4. Which of the following statements is (are) correct concerning the function of the different corticospinal tracts?
   (1) The corticospinal tracts concerned with movements of the upper limb originate in the precentral gyrus on the medial side of the cerebral hemisphere.
   (2) The corticospinal tracts concerned with movements of the lower limb are located in the medial area of the middle three-fifths of the basis pedunculi.
5. Which of the following statements is (are) correct concerning the reticulospinal tracts?
   (1) They descend in the anterior and lateral white columns of the spinal cord.
   (2) The descending autonomic fibers from higher autonomic centers lie within the reticulospinal tracts.
6. Which of the following statements is (are) correct concerning muscle tone?
   (1) Muscle tone depends on the integrity of at least four neurons.
   (2) An atonic muscle atrophies rapidly.

In the following questions, answer:
   (a) IF (1), (2), AND (3) ONLY ARE CORRECT
   (b) IF (1) AND (3) ONLY ARE CORRECT
   (c) IF (2) AND (4) ONLY ARE CORRECT
   (d) IF (4) ONLY IS CORRECT, OR
   (e) IF ALL ARE CORRECT
7. Which of the following statements is (are) true?
   (1) Hyperactive ankle-jerk reflexes and ankle clonus indicate a release of the lower motor neurons from supraspinal inhibition.
   (2) Muscle spindle afferent nerve fibers send information to the brain as well as to the spinal cord.
   (3) In Parkinson's disease there is a degeneration of dopamine-secreting neurons that originate in the substantia nigra.
   (4) Brain neuronal activity preceding a voluntary movement is limited to the precentral gyrus (area 4).

8. After a hemorrhage into the left internal capsule in a right-handed person, the signs or symptoms might be:
   (1) Right homonymous hemianopia
   (2) Right astereognosis
   (3) Aphasia
   (4) Right hemiplegia
9. After a traumatic lesion of the left half of the spinal cord at the level of the eighth cervical segment, the patient presents the following signs and symptoms:
   (1) Loss of pain and temperature sensations on the left below the level of the lesion
   (2) Loss of position sense of the left leg
   (3) Right hemiplegia
   (4) Left positive Babinski sign
10. Which of the signs or symptoms listed below are indicative of a cerebellar lesion?
    (1) Cogwheel rigidity
    (2) Hemiballismus
    (3) Chorea
    (4) Intention tremor
11. Which of the following regions of white matter would **not** contain corticospinal fibers?
    (1) Pyramid of medulla oblongata
    (2) Lateral white column of spinal cord
    (3) Cerebral peduncle of midbrain
    (4) Anterior limb of internal capsule

Match the tracts listed on the left with the appropriate statement listed on the right. An answer may be used more than once.

12. Rubrospinal
13. Tectospinal
14. Lateral corticospinal
15. Vestibulospinal
16. Anterior corticospinal

(a) Crosses in the spinal cord
(b) Crosses in the medulla oblongata
(c) Uncrossed
(d) None of the above

Match the tracts listed on the left with the cells of origin listed on the right. An answer may be used more than once.

17. Vestibulospinal tract
18. Tectospinal
19. Lateral corticospinal
20. Rubrospinal

(a) Cells in area 4 of cerebral cortex
(b) Cells in inferior colliculus
(c) Cells in red nucleus
(d) None of the above

ADDITIONAL READING

Austin, G. *The Spinal Cord, Basic Aspects and Surgical Considerations* (2nd ed.). Springfield, Illinois: Thomas, 1972.

Brazis, P. W., Masden, J. C., and Biller, J. *Localization in Clinical Neurology.* Boston: Little, Brown, 1990.

Brodal, A. *Neurological Anatomy in Relation to Clinical Medicine* (3rd ed.). Oxford: Oxford University Press, 1981.

Coulter, J. D., Bowker, R. M., Wise, S. P., et al. Cortical, tectal and medullary descending pathways to the cervical spinal cord. *Prog. Brain Res.* 50:263, 1979.

Dawnay, N. A. H., and Glees, F. P. Mapping the primate corticospinal pathway. *J. Anat.* 133:124, 1981.

Dray, A. The physiology and pharmacology of mammalian basal ganglia. *Prog. Neurobiol.* 14:221, 1980.

Freund, H. J. Motor unit and muscle activity in voluntary motor control. *Physiol. Rev.* 63:387, 1983.

Guttmann, L. *Spinal Cord Injuries* (2nd ed.). Oxford: Blackwell, 1976.

Koehler, P. J., and Endtz, L. J. The Brown-Séquard syndrome—true or false? *Arch. Neurol.* 43:921, 1986.

Lagerbäck, P. A. *On α Motor Neuron Collateral Boutons and Renshaw Cells.* Stockholm: Karolinska Institutet, 1982.

Pierce, D. S., and Nickel, V. H. *The Total Care of Spinal Cord Injuries.* Boston: Little, Brown, 1977.

Walton, J. N. *Brain's Diseases of the Nervous System* (8th ed.). New York and Oxford: Oxford University Press, 1977.

Williams, P. L., Warwick, R., Dyson, M., and Bannister, L. H. *Gray's Anatomy* (37th Brit. ed.). Philadelphia: Saunders, 1990.

Chapter 22
Connections of
the Cerebellum

In Chapter 10, the gross anatomy and microscopic structure of the cerebellum were described and the function of the cerebellum was discussed briefly. In this chapter, the detailed connections of the cerebellum to other parts of the nervous system will be considered and the functional significance of this organ in relation to posture and voluntary movement will be discussed.

ORGANIZATION OF THE CEREBELLUM

Essentially, the cerebellum consists of two **cerebellar hemispheres** joined by a **median vermis** (Fig. 22-1). The gray matter of the cerebellum forms the **cerebellar cortex** and the **intracerebellar nuclei**. The white matter is made up of the **intrinsic fibers**, which never leave the cerebellum, the **afferent fibers**, which bring information to the cerebellum, and the **efferent fibers**, which pass to other parts of the central nervous system. The afferent and efferent fibers are grouped together on each side into three large **cerebellar peduncles**.

The afferent fibers to the cerebellum enter the cerebellar cortex, lose their myelin sheath, and end as either **climbing** or **mossy fibers** (Fig. 22-2). The efferent fibers commence as the axons of the Purkinje cells of the cerebellar cortex. Most of these axons synapse with the neurons of the cerebellar nuclei. The axons of these neurons then leave the cerebellum. A few Purkinje cell axons bypass the nuclei and leave the cerebellum without synapsing.

INTERCONNECTIONS OF THE NEURONS OF THE CEREBELLAR CORTEX

Two types of afferent fibers enter the cerebellar cortex, the **climbing fibers** and the **mossy fibers**. The climbing fibers are the terminal fibers of the olivocerebellar tracts (Fig. 22-2). They enter the molecular layer of the cortex, where they branch and make multiple synaptic contacts with one Purkinje cell. A few side branches leave each climbing fiber and synapse with adjacent stellate and basket cells.

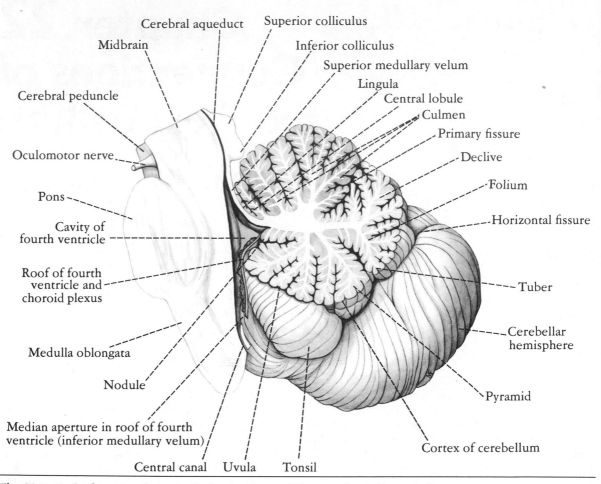

Fig. 22-1. Sagittal section through the brainstem and the vermis of the cerebellum.

The mossy fibers are the terminal fibers of all other cerebellar afferent tracts. They have multiple branches, so a single mossy fiber may stimulate thousands of Purkinje cells through the granule cells (Fig. 22-2). For further details concerning the cerebellar cortical mechanisms, see page 219.

Cerebellar Afferent Fibers from the Cerebral Cortex

The cerebral cortex sends information to the cerebellum by three pathways: (1) the corticopontocerebellar pathway, (2) the cerebro-olivocerebellar pathway, and (3) the cerebroreticulocerebellar pathway.

CORTICOPONTOCEREBELLAR PATHWAY

The corticopontine fibers arise from nerve cells in the frontal, parietal, temporal, and occipital lobes of the cerebral cortex and descend through the corona radiata and internal capsule and terminate upon the pontine nuclei (Fig. 22-3). The pontine nuclei give rise to the **transverse fibers of the pons**, which cross the midline and

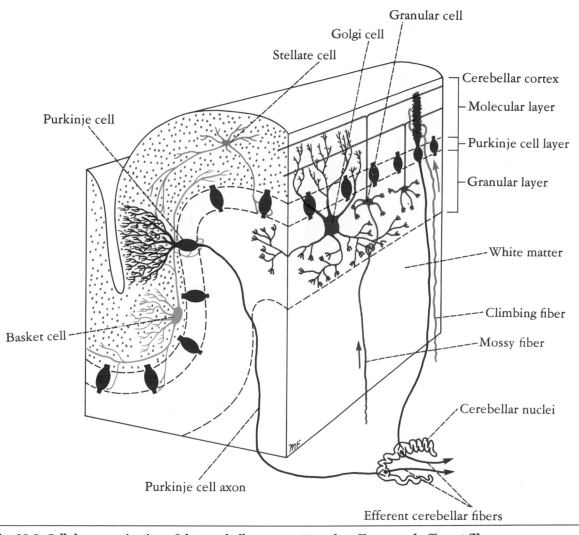

Fig. 22-2. Cellular organization of the cerebellar cortex. Note the afferent and efferent fibers.

enter the opposite cerebellar hemisphere as the middle cerebellar peduncle (see Figs. 9-4, 9-5, and 9-6).

CEREBRO-OLIVOCEREBELLAR PATHWAY

The cortico-olivary fibers arise from nerve cells in the frontal, parietal, temporal, and occipital lobes of the cerebral cortex and descend through the corona radiata and internal capsule to terminate bilaterally upon the inferior olivary nu-

clei (Fig. 22-3). The inferior olivary nuclei give rise to fibers that cross the midline and enter the opposite cerebellar hemisphere through the inferior cerebellar peduncle. These fibers terminate as the climbing fibers in the cerebellar cortex.

CEREBRORETICULOCEREBELLAR PATHWAY

The corticoreticular fibers arise from nerve cells from many areas of the cerebral cortex, particularly the sensorimotor areas. They descend to

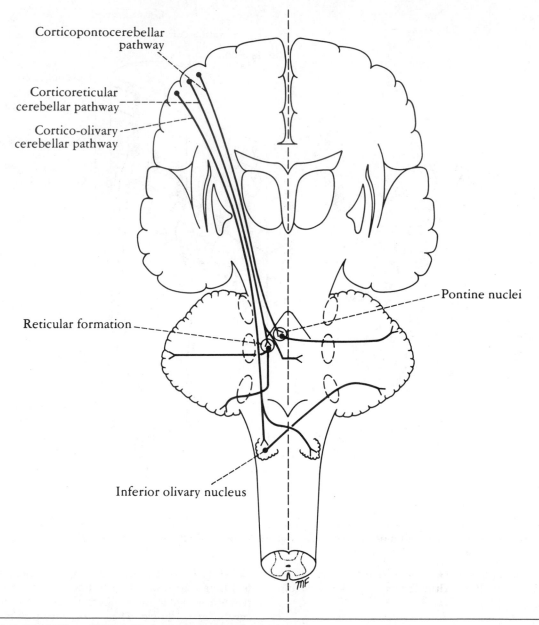

Corticopontocerebellar pathway

Corticoreticular cerebellar pathway

Cortico-olivary cerebellar pathway

Reticular formation

Pontine nuclei

Inferior olivary nucleus

Fig. 22-3. Cerebellar afferent fibers from the cerebral cortex.

terminate in the reticular formation on the same side and on the opposite side in the pons and medulla (Fig. 22-3). The cells in the reticular formation give rise to the reticulocerebellar fibers that enter the cerebellar hemisphere on the same side through the inferior and middle cerebellar peduncles.

This connection between the cerebrum and the cerebellum is important in the control of voluntary movement. Information regarding the initiation of movement in the cerebral cortex is probably transmitted to the cerebellum so that the movement can be monitored and appropriate adjustments in the muscle activity can be made.

Cerebellar Afferent Fibers from the Spinal Cord

The spinal cord sends information to the cerebellum by three pathways: (1) the anterior spinocerebellar tract, (2) the posterior spinocerebellar tract, and (3) the cuneocerebellar tract.

ANTERIOR SPINOCEREBELLAR TRACT

The axons entering the spinal cord from the posterior root ganglion terminate by synapsing with the neurons in the **nucleus dorsalis** (Clark's column) at the base of the posterior gray column. Most of the axons of these neurons cross to the opposite side and ascend as the **anterior spinocerebellar tract** in the contralateral white column; some of the axons ascend as the anterior spinocerebellar tract in the lateral white column of the same side (Fig. 22-4). The fibers enter the cerebellum through the superior cerebellar peduncle and terminate as mossy fibers in the cerebellar cortex. Collateral branches that end in the deep cerebellar nuclei are also given off. It is believed that those fibers that crossed over to the opposite side in the spinal cord cross back within the cerebellum.

The anterior spinocerebellar tract is found at all segments of the spinal cord and its fibers convey muscle joint information from the muscle spindles, tendon organs, and joint receptors of the upper and lower limbs. It is also believed that the cerebellum receives information from the skin and superficial fascia by this tract.

POSTERIOR SPINOCEREBELLAR TRACT

The axons entering the spinal cord from the posterior root ganglion enter the posterior gray column and terminate by synapsing on the neurons at the base of the posterior gray column. These neurons are known collectively as the nucleus dorsalis (Clark's column). The axons of these neurons enter the posterolateral part of the lateral white column on the same side and ascend as the **posterior spinocerebellar tract** to the medulla oblongata (Fig. 22-4). Here the tract enters the cerebellum through the inferior cerebellar peduncle and terminates as mossy fibers in the cerebellar cortex. Collateral branches that end in the deep cerebellar nuclei are also given off. The posterior spinocerebellar tract receives muscle joint information from the muscle spindles, tendon organs, and joint receptors of the trunk and lower limbs.

CUNEOCEREBELLAR TRACT

These fibers originate in the nucleus cuneatus of the medulla oblongata and enter the cerebellar hemisphere on the same side through the inferior cerebellar peduncle (Fig. 22-4). The fibers terminate as mossy fibers in the cerebellar cortex. Collateral branches that end in the deep cerebellar nuclei are also given off. The cuneocerebellar tract receives muscle joint information from the muscle spindles, tendon organs, and joint receptors of the upper limb and upper part of the thorax.

Cerebellar Afferent Fibers from the Vestibular Nerve

The vestibular nerve sends many afferent fibers directly to the cerebellum through the inferior cerebellar peduncle on the same side. Other vestibular afferent fibers pass first to the vestibular nuclei in the brainstem, where they synapse and are relayed to the cerebellum (Fig. 22-4). They enter the cerebellum through the inferior cerebellar peduncle on the same side. All the afferent fibers from the inner ear terminate as mossy fibers in the flocculonodular lobe of the cerebellum.

Superior cerebellar peduncle

Middle cerebellar peduncle

Cerebellum

Inferior cerebellar peduncle

Medulla oblongata

Anterior spinocerebellar tract (majority of fibers)

Spinal cord

Vestibular nuclei

Dentate nucleus

Nucleus cuneatus

Vestibular nerve

Posterior spinocerebellar tract

Anterior spinocerebellar tract (minority of fibers)

Fig. 22-4. Cerebellar afferent fibers from the spinal cord and internal ear.

Other Afferent Fibers

In addition, the cerebellum receives small bundles of afferent fibers from the red nucleus and the tectum.

Cerebellar Efferent Fibers

The entire output of the cerebellar cortex is through the axons of the Purkinje cells. Most of the axons of the Purkinje cells end by synapsing on the neurons of the deep cerebellar nuclei (Fig. 22-2). The axons of the neurons that form the cerebellar nuclei constitute the efferent outflow from the cerebellum. A few Purkinje cell axons pass directly out of the cerebellum to the lateral vestibular nucleus. The efferent fibers from the cerebellum connect with the red nucleus, thalamus, vestibular complex, and reticular formation.

GLOBOSE-EMBOLIFORM-RUBRAL PATHWAY

Axons of neurons in the globose and emboliform nuclei travel through the superior cerebellar peduncle and cross the midline to the opposite side in the **decussation of the superior cerebellar peduncles** (Fig. 22-5). The fibers end by synapsing with cells of the contralateral red nucleus, which give rise to axons of the **rubrospinal tract** (Fig. 22-5). Thus it is seen that this pathway crosses twice, once in the decussation of the superior cerebellar peduncle, and again in the rubrospinal tract close to its origin. By this means, the globose and emboliform nuclei influence motor activity on the same side of the body.

DENTOTHALAMIC PATHWAY

Axons of neurons in the dentate nucleus travel through the superior cerebellar peduncle and cross the midline to the opposite side in the **decussation of the superior cerebellar peduncle** (Fig. 22-5). The fibers end by synapsing with cells in the contralateral **ventrolateral nucleus of the thalamus**. The axons of the thalamic neurons ascend through the internal capsule and corona radiata and terminate in the primary motor area of the cerebral cortex. By this pathway, the dentate nucleus can influence motor activity by acting upon the motor

neurons of the opposite cerebral cortex; impulses from the motor cortex are transmitted to spinal segmental levels through the corticospinal tract. It will be remembered that most of the fibers of the corticospinal tract cross to the opposite side in the decussation of the pyramids or later at the spinal segmental levels. The dentate nucleus thus is able to coordinate muscle activity on the same side of the body.

FASTIGIAL VESTIBULAR PATHWAY

The axons of neurons in the fastigial nucleus travel though the inferior cerebellar peduncle and end by projecting on the neurons of the **lateral vestibular nucleus** on both sides (Fig. 22-5). It will be remembered that some Purkinje cell axons project directly to the lateral vestibular nucleus. The neurons of the lateral vestibular nucleus form the **vestibulospinal tract**. The fastigial nucleus exerts a facilitatory influence mainly on the ipsilateral extensor muscle tone.

FASTIGIAL RETICULAR PATHWAY

The axons of neurons in the fastigial nucleus travel through the inferior cerebellar peduncle and end by synapsing with neurons of the reticular formation (Fig. 22-5). Axons of these neurons influence spinal segmental motor activity through the reticulospinal tract.

Functions of the Cerebellum

The cerebellum receives afferent information concerning voluntary movement from the cerebral cortex and from the muscles, tendons, and joints. It also receives information concerning balance from the vestibular nerve and possibly concerning sight through the tectocerebellar tract. All this information is fed into the cerebellar cortical circuitry by the mossy fibers and the climbing fibers (see Fig. 10-9). After several synaptic relays in the cerebellar cortex, the afferent impulses converge on the Purkinje cells. The axons of the Purkinje cells project with few exceptions on the deep cerebellar nuclei. The output of the lateral cerebellar hemisphere projects to the dentate nucleus, the vermis projects to the fastigial nucleus, and the intermediate re-

Fig. 22-5. Cerebellar efferent fibers.

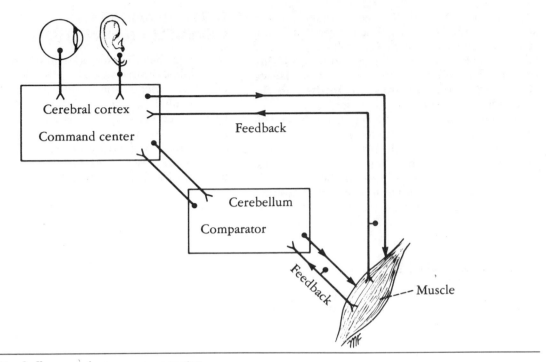

Fig. 22-6. Cerebellum serving as a comparator.

gions of the cortex project to the globose and emboliform nuclei. A few Purkinje cell axons pass directly out of the cerebellum and end on the lateral vestibular nucleus in the brainstem. It is now generally believed that the Purkinje axons exert an inhibitory influence on the neurons of the cerebellar nuclei and the lateral vestibular nuclei.

The cerebellar output is conducted to the sites of origin of the descending pathways that influence motor activity at the segmental spinal level. In this respect, it is interesting to note that the cerebellum has no direct neuronal connections with the lower motor neurons, but exerts its influence indirectly through the cerebral cortex and brainstem.

Physiologists have postulated that the cerebellum functions as a coordinator of precise move-

ments by continually comparing the output of the motor area of the cerebral cortex with the proprioceptive information received from the site of muscle action; it is then able to bring about the necessary adjustments by influencing the activity of the lower motor neurons (Fig. 22-6). This is accomplished by controlling the sequence of firing of the alpha and gamma motor neurons. It is also believed that the cerebellum can send back information to the motor cerebral cortex, to inhibit the agonist muscles and stimulate the antagonist muscles, thus limiting the extent of voluntary movement.

The function of the cerebellum in relation to its phylogenetic development is discussed on page 221.

CLINICAL NOTES

GENERAL CONSIDERATIONS

The cortex of the cerebellum, unlike that of the cerebrum, has a uniform microscopic structure and

physiological investigations show that the activities that occur are identical in all regions. The only fibers that leave the cerebellar cortex are the axons of Purkinje cells and they exert an inhibitory influence on the neurons of the deep cerebellar nuclei and the vestibular nuclei. Each cerebellar hemisphere is connected principally with the same side of the body by nervous pathways, so that **a lesion in one cerebellar hemisphere gives rise to signs and symptoms that are limited to the same side of the body**.

The cerebellum, unlike the cerebrum, has no direct pathway to the lower motor neurons in the spinal cord. It exerts its influence on motor activity indirectly through connections with the cerebral cortex and with nerve centers in the brainstem. The cerebellum regulates muscle tone and postural reflexes. It assists in the performance of smoothly coordinated muscle actions such as walking.

DISTURBANCES OF CEREBELLAR FUNCTION

Cerebellar disorders include tumors, multiple sclerosis, alcoholism, vascular disorders, poisoning with heavy metals and hereditary degeneration.

A detailed description of the signs and symptoms of cerebellar disease is given in Chapter 10, page 222. The many manifestations of cerebellar disease may be reduced to two basic defects: hypotonia, and loss of influence of the cerebellum on the activities of the cerebral cortex.

CLINICAL PROBLEM

Answer on Page 608

1. A 10-year-old girl was taken to a neurologist because her parents had noticed that her gait was becoming awkward. Six months previously, the child had complained that she felt her right arm was clumsy and she had inadvertently knocked a teapot off the table. More recently, her family had noticed that her hand movements were becoming jerky and awkward; this was particularly obvious when she was eating with a knife and fork. The mother commented that her daughter had had problems with her right foot since birth and that she had a clubfoot. She also had scoliosis and was attending an orthopedic surgeon for treatment. The mother said she was particularly worried about her daughter because two other members of the family had similar signs and symptoms.

On physical examination, the child was found to have a lurching gait with a tendency to reel over to the right. Intention tremor was present in the right arm and the right leg. When the strength of the limb muscles was tested, those of the right leg were found to be weaker than those of the left leg. The muscles of the right arm and right lower leg were also hypotonic. She had severe pes cavus of the right foot and a slight pes cavus of the left foot. Kyphoscoliosis of the upper part of the thoracic vertebral column also was present.

On examination of her sensory system, she was found to have loss of muscle joint sense and vibratory sense of both legs. She also had loss of two-point discrimination of the skin of both legs. Her knee jerks were found to be exaggerated, but her ankle jerks were absent. The biceps and triceps jerks of both arms were normal. She had bilateral Babinski responses. Slight nystagmus was present in both eyes. Using your knowledge of neuroanatomy, can you explain the symptoms and signs listed above? Did the disease process involve more than one area of the central nervous system?

Now review the Clinical Problems at the end of Chapter 10.

NATIONAL BOARD TYPE QUESTIONS

Answers on Page 621

IN EACH OF THE FOLLOWING QUESTIONS, ANSWER:
   (a) IF (1) ONLY IS CORRECT
   (b) IF (2) ONLY IS CORRECT
   (c) IF BOTH (1) AND (2) ARE CORRECT, AND
   (d) IF NEITHER (1) NOR (2) IS CORRECT

1. Which of the following statements is (are) correct concerning the afferent fibers entering the cerebellar cortex?
   (1) The climbing fibers make multiple synaptic contacts with a single Purkinje cell.

(2) The mossy fibers may stimulate many Purkinje cells by first stimulating the granular cells.

2. Which of the following statements is (are) correct concerning the intracerebellar nuclei?
   (1) The nuclei send nerve fibers without interruption to the motor cortex of the opposite cerebral hemisphere.
   (2) The output of the cerebellar nuclei influence muscle activity so that movements can progress in an orderly sequence from one movement to the next.

3. Which of the following statements is (are) correct concerning abnormalities of cerebellar function?
   (1) Past pointing is caused by the failure of the cerebellum to inhibit the cerebral cortex after the movement has begun.
   (2) Dysdiadochokinesia is caused by loss of cerebellar function on the opposite side of the body.

In each of the following questions, answer:
   (a) If (1), (2), AND (3) ONLY ARE CORRECT
   (b) If (1) AND (2) ONLY ARE CORRECT
   (c) If (2) AND (4) ONLY ARE CORRECT
   (d) If (4) ONLY IS CORRECT, OR
   (e) If ALL ARE CORRECT

4. Which of the following ascending tracts have cells of origin in the nucleus dorsalis (Clark's column)?
   (1) Fasciculus gracilis
   (2) Anterior spinocerebellar
   (3) Lateral spinothalamic
   (4) Posterior spinocerebellar

5. The superior cerebellar peduncle conveys the following:
   (1) Nerve impulses regulating skilled motor movements
   (2) Fibers that synapse in the ventral lateral nucleus of the thalamus
   (3) Axons that originate in the dentate nucleus
   (4) Axons that run in the medial longitudinal fasciculus

6. The following pathways may be classified as cerebellar efferent:
   (1) Globose-emboliform-rubral
   (2) Fastigial vestibular

(3) Fastigial reticular
(4) Pontocerebellar

Select the best response:

7. The following statements concerning the cerebellum are correct **except**:
   (a) The cortex of different parts of the cerebellum has the same uniform microscopic structure.
   (b) The axons of the Purkinje cells exert a stimulatory influence on the neurons of the deep cerebellar nuclei.
   (c) Each cerebellar hemisphere principally influences movement on the same side of the body.
   (d) Intention tremor is a sign of cerebellar disease.
   (e) The part of the cerebellum that lies in the midline is called the vermis.

Following thrombosis of the posterior inferior cerebellar artery, a patient presents the signs and symptoms listed on the left; match the signs and symptoms with the appropriate structures involved listed on the right.

8. Loss of pain and temperature on the left side of the body
9. Nystagmus
10. Hypotonicity of the muscles on the right with a tendency to fall to the right

   (a) Right reticulospinal tract
   (b) Right inferior cerebellar peduncle
   (c) None of the above

The following important nerve tracts listed on the left enter or leave the cerebellum. Indicate which pathways on the right conduct these tracts.

11. Corticopontocerebellar
12. Cuneocerebellar
13. Cerebellar reticular
14. Cerebellar rubral

   (a) Superior cerebellar peduncle
   (b) Corpus callosum
   (c) Striae medullaris
   (d) Inferior cerebellar peduncle
   (e) Middle cerebellar peduncle

ADDITIONAL READING

Angevine, J. B., Mancall, E. L., and Yakovlev, P. I. *The Human Cerebellum.* Boston: Little, Brown, 1961.

Arshavsky, Y. I., Gelfand, I. M., and Olovsky, G. N. The cerebellum and control of rhythmical movements. *Trends Neurosci.* 6:417, 1983.

Bloedel, J. R., and Courville, J. Cerebellar Afferent Systems. In V. B. Brooks (ed.), *Handbook of Physiology.* Sec. 1, Vol. II. Bethesda: American Physiological Society, 1981. P. 735.

Bloomfield, S., and Marr, D. How the cerebellum may be used. *Nature (Lond.)* 227:1224, 1970.

Brodal, A. *Neurological Anatomy in Relation to Clinical Medicine* (3rd ed.). New York: Oxford University Press, 1981.

Chan-Palay, V. *Cerebellar Dentate Nucleus: Organization, Cytology and Transmitters.* Berlin: Springer-Verlag, 1977.

Colin, F., Manil, J., and Desclin, J. C. The olivocerebellar system. 1. Delayed and slow inhibitory effects: An overlooked salient feature of cerebellar climbing fibers. *Brain Res.* 187:3, 1980.

Eccles, J. C., Ito, M., and Szentagothai, J. *The Cerebellum as a Neuronal Machine.* Berlin and Vienna: Springer, 1967.

Fields, W. D., and Willis, W. D., Jr. *The Cerebellum in Health and Disease.* St. Louis: Warren H. Green, 1970.

Gilman, S. The mechanisms of cerebellar hypotonia. *Brain* 92:621, 1969.

Gilman, S., Bloedal, J. R., and Lechtenberg, R. *Disorders of the Cerebellum.* Philadelphia: Davis, 1981.

Gilman, S. The Cerebellum: Its Role in Posture and Movement. In M. Swash, and C. Kennard (eds.), *Scientific Basis of Clinical Neurology.* Edinburgh: Churchill Livingstone, 1985. P. 36.

Guyton, A. C. *Textbook of Medical Physiology* (7th ed.). Philadelphia: Saunders, 1986.

Ito, M. *The Cerebellum and Neural Control.* New York: Raven, 1984.

Kennedy, P. R., Ross, H. G., and Brooks, V. B. Participation of the principal olivary nucleus in neurocerebellar control. *Exp. Brain Res.* 47:95, 1982.

Lewis, A. J. *Mechanisms of Neurological Disease.* Boston: Little, Brown, 1976.

Llinas, R. R. The cortex of the cerebellum. *Sci. Am.* 232:56, 1975.

Llinas, R. R. Electrophysiology of the Cerebellar Networks. In V. B. Brooks (ed.), *Handbook of Physiology.* Sec. 1, Vol. II. Bethesda: American Physiological Society, 1981. P. 831.

Napper, R. M. A., and Harvey, R. J. Number of parallel fiber synapses on an individual Purkinje cell in the cerebellum of the rat. *J. Comp. Neurol.* 274:168, 1988.

Palay, S. L., and Chan-Palay, V. Cortex and Organization. In *Cerebellar Cortex.* Berlin and Vienna: Springer, 1974.

Chapter 23
The Cranial Nerve Nuclei and Their Central Connections

There are 12 pairs of cranial nerves, which leave the brain and pass through foramina and fissures in the skull. All the nerves are distributed in the head and neck except the tenth, which also supplies structures in the thorax and abdomen. The cranial nerves are named as follows:

1. Olfactory
2. Optic
3. Oculomotor
4. Trochlear
5. Trigeminal
6. Abducent
7. Facial
8. Vestibulocochlear
9. Glossopharyngeal
10. Vagus
11. Accessory
12. Hypoglossal

ORGANIZATION OF THE CRANIAL NERVES

The olfactory, optic, and ventibulocochlear nerves are entirely sensory. The oculomotor, trochlear, ab-ducent, accessory, and hypoglossal nerves are entirely motor. The trigeminal, facial, glossopharyngeal, and vagus nerves are both sensory and motor nerves. The cranial nerves have central motor and/or sensory nuclei within the brain and peripheral nerve fibers that emerge from the brain and exit from the skull to reach their effector or sensory organs.

The different components of the cranial nerves, their functions, and the openings in the skull through which the nerves leave the cranial cavity are summarized in Table 23-1.

MOTOR NUCLEI OF THE CRANIAL NERVES

Somatic Motor and Branchomotor Nuclei

The somatic motor and branchomotor nerve fibers of a cranial nerve are the axons of nerve cells situated within the brain. These nerve cell groups form motor nuclei and they innervate striated muscle.

Table 23-1. Cranial Nerves

Number	Name	Components	Function	Opening in skull
I	Olfactory	Sensory	Smell	Openings in cribriform plate of ethmoid
II	Optic	Sensory	Vision	Optic canal
III	Oculomotor	Motor	Raises upper eyelid, turns eyeball upward, downward, and medially; constricts pupil; accommodates eye	Superior orbital fissure
IV	Trochlear	Motor	Assists in turning eyeball downward and laterally	Superior orbital fissure
V	Trigeminal[a]			
	Ophthalmic division	Sensory	Cornea, skin of forehead, scalp, eyelids, and nose; also mucous membrane of paranasal sinuses and nasal cavity	Superior orbital fissure
	Maxillary division	Sensory	Skin of face over maxilla; teeth of upper jaw; mucous membrane of nose, the maxillary sinus, and palate	Foramen rotundum
	Mandibular division	Motor	Muscles of mastication, mylohyoid, anterior belly of digastric, tensor veli palatini, and tensor tympani	Foramen ovale
		Sensory	Skin of cheek, skin over mandible and side of head, teeth of lower jaw and temporomandibular joint; mucous membrane of mouth and anterior part of tongue	
VI	Abducent	Motor	Lateral rectus muscle turns eyeball laterally	Superior orbital fissure
VII	Facial	Motor	Muscles of face and scalp, stapedius muscle, posterior belly of digastric and stylohyoid muscles	Internal acoustic meatus, facial canal, stylomastoid foramen
		Sensory	Taste from anterior two-thirds of tongue, from floor of mouth and palate	
		Secretomotor parasympathetic	Submandibular and sublingual salivary glands, the lacrimal gland, and glands of nose and palate	
VIII	Vestibulocochlear			Internal acoustic meatus
	Vestibular	Sensory	From utricle and saccule and semicircular canals—position and movement of head	
	Cochlear	Sensory	Organ of Corti—hearing	

Table 23-1. (continued)

Number	Name	Components	Function	Opening in skull
IX	Glossopharyngeal	Motor	Stylopharyngeus muscle—assists swallowing	Jugular foramen
		Secretomotor parasympathetic	Parotid salivary gland	
		Sensory	General sensation and taste from posterior one-third of tongue and pharynx; carotid sinus (baroreceptor), and carotid body (chemoreceptor)	
X	Vagus	Motor and sensory	Heart and great thoracic blood vessels; larynx, trachea, bronchi, and lungs; alimentary tract from pharynx to splenic flexure of colon; liver, kidneys, and pancreas	Jugular foramen
XI	Accessory Cranial root	Motor	Muscles of soft palate (except tensor veli palatini), pharynx (except stylopharyngcus), and larynx (except cricothyroid) in branches of vagus	Jugular foramen
	Spinal root	Motor	Sternocleidomastoid and trapezius muscles	
XII	Hypoglossal	Motor	Muscles of tongue (except palatoglossus) controlling its shape and movement	Hypoglossal canal

ªThe trigeminal nerve also carries proprioceptive impulses from the muscles of mastication and the facial and extraocular muscles.

Each nerve cell with its processes is referred to as a **lower motor neuron**. Such a nerve cell is, therefore, equivalent to the motor cells in the anterior gray columns of the spinal cord.

The motor nuclei of the cranial nerves receive impulses from the cerebral cortex through the corticonuclear (corticobulbar) fibers. These fibers originate from the pyramidal cells in the inferior part of the precentral gyrus (area 4) and from the adjacent part of the postcentral gyrus. The corticonuclear fibers descend through the **corona radiata** and the **genu of the internal capsule**. They pass through the midbrain just medial to the corticospinal fibers in the **basis pedunculi** and end by synapsing either directly with the lower motor neurons within the cranial nerve nuclei or indirectly through the **internuncial neurons**. The corticonuclear fibers thus constitute the **first-order neuron** of the descending pathway, the internuncial neuron constitutes the **second-order neuron**, and the lower motor neuron constitutes the **third-order neuron**.

The majority of the corticonuclear fibers to the motor cranial nerve nuclei cross the median plane before reaching the nuclei. Bilateral connections are present for all the cranial motor nuclei except for part of the facial nucleus that supplies the muscles of the lower part of the face and a part of the hypoglossal nucleus that supplies the genioglossus muscle.

General Visceral Motor Nuclei

The general visceral motor nuclei form the cranial outflow of the parasympathetic portion of the autonomic nervous system. They are the **Edinger-Westphal nucleus** of the oculomotor nerve, the **superior salivatory and lacrimal nuclei** of the facial nerve, the **inferior salivatory nucleus** of the glossopharyngeal nerve, and the **dorsal motor nucleus** of the vagus. These nuclei receive numerous afferent fibers including descending pathways from the hypothalamus.

SENSORY NUCLEI OF THE CRANIAL NERVES

These include somatic and visceral afferent nuclei. The sensory or afferent parts of a cranial nerve are the axons of nerve cells outside the brain and are situated in ganglia on the nerve trunks (equivalent to posterior root ganglion of a spinal nerve) or may be situated in a sensory organ such as the nose, eye, or ear. These cells and their processes form the **first-order neuron**. The central processes of these cells enter the brain and terminate by synapsing with cells forming the sensory nuclei. These cells and their processes form the **second-order neuron**. Axons from these nuclear cells now cross the midline and ascend to other sensory nuclei, such as the thalamus, where they synapse. The nerve cells of these nuclei form the **third-order neuron** and their axons terminate in the cerebral cortex.

OLFACTORY NERVES (CRANIAL NERVE I)

The olfactory nerves arise from the olfactory receptor nerve cells in the olfactory mucous membrane located in the upper part of the nasal cavity above the level of the superior concha (Fig. 23-1). The **olfactory receptor cells** are scattered amongst supporting cells. Each receptor cell consists of a small bipolar nerve cell with a coarse peripheral process that passes to the surface of the membrane and a fine central process. From the coarse peripheral process a number of short cilia arise, the **olfactory hairs,** which project into the mucus covering the surface of the mucous membrane. These projecting hairs react to odors in the air and stimulate the olfactory cells.

The fine central processes form the **olfactory nerve fibers** (Fig. 23-1). Bundles of these nerve fibers pass through the openings of the cribriform plate of the ethmoid bone to enter the olfactory bulb. The olfactory nerve fibers are unmyelinated and are covered with Schwann cells.

OLFACTORY BULB

This ovoid structure possesses several types of nerve cells, the largest of which is the **mitral cell** (Fig. 23-1). The incoming olfactory nerve fibers synapse with the dendrites of the mitral cells and form rounded areas known as **synaptic glomeruli**. Smaller nerve cells called **tufted cells** and **granular cells** also synapse with the mitral cells. The olfactory bulb, in addition, receives axons from the contralateral olfactory bulb through the olfactory tract.

OLFACTORY TRACT

This narrow band of white matter runs from the posterior end of the olfactory bulb beneath the inferior surface of the frontal lobe of the brain (Fig. 23-1). It consists of the central axons of the mitral and tufted cells of the bulb and some centrifugal fibers from the opposite olfactory bulb.

As the olfactory tract reaches the **anterior perforated substance**, it divides into **medial and lateral olfactory striae**. The lateral stria carries the axons to the **olfactory area of the cerebral cortex**, namely, the **periamygdaloid** and **prepiriform areas** (Fig. 23-1). The medial olfactory stria carries the fibers that cross the median plane in the anterior commissure to pass to the olfactory bulb of the opposite side.

The periamygdaloid and prepiriform areas of the cerebral cortex are often known as the **primary olfactory cortex**. The **entorrhinal area (area 28)** of the parahippocampal gyrus, which receives numerous connections from the primary olfactory cortex, is called the **secondary olfactory cortex**. These areas of the cortex are responsible for the appreciation of olfactory sensations (Fig. 23-1). Note that, in contrast to all other sensory pathways, the olfactory afferent pathway has only two neurons and reaches the cerebral cortex without synapsing in one of the thalamic nuclei.

It should also be noted that the primary olfactory

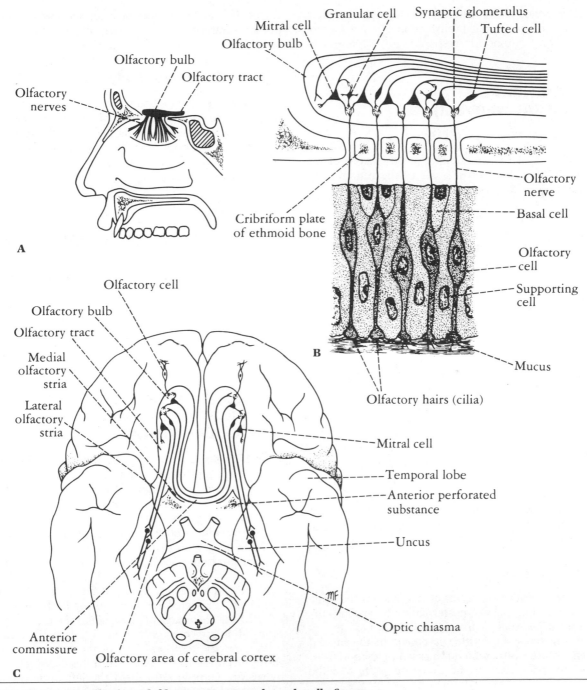

**Fig. 23-1. A. Distribution of olfactory nerves on lateral wall of nose.
B. Connections between olfactory cells and neurons of olfactory bulb.
C. Connections between the olfactory cell and the rest of the olfactory system.**

cortex sends nerve fibers to many other centers within the brain to establish connections for emotional and autonomic responses to olfactory sensations.

OPTIC NERVE (CRANIAL NERVE II)

Origin of the Optic Nerve

The fibers of the optic nerve are the axons of the cells in the **ganglionic layer** of the retina. They converge on the **optic disc** and exit from the eye, about 3 or 4 mm to the nasal side of its center, as the optic nerve (Fig. 23-2). The fibers of the optic nerve are myelinated, but the sheaths are formed from oligodendrocytes rather than Schwann cells, since the optic nerve is comparable to a tract within the central nervous system (CNS).

The optic nerve leaves the orbital cavity through the optic canal and unites with the optic nerve of the opposite side to form the **optic chiasma**.

Optic Chiasma

The optic chiasma is situated at the junction of the anterior wall and floor of the third ventricle. Its anterolateral angles are continuous with the optic nerves and the posterolateral angles are continuous with the optic tracts (Fig. 23-2). In the chiasma, the fibers from the nasal (medial) half of each retina, including the nasal half of the **macula**,* cross the midline and enter the optic tract of the opposite side, while the fibers from the temporal (lateral) half of each retina, including the temporal half of the **macula**, pass posteriorly in the optic tract of the same side.

Optic Tract

The optic tract (Fig. 23-2) emerges from the optic chiasma and passes posterolaterally around the cerebral peduncle. Most of the fibers now terminate by synapsing with nerve cells in the **lateral geniculate body**, which is a small projection from the posterior part of the thalamus. A few of the

*The macula or macula lutea, found at the posterior pole of the eye, is the area of the retina for the most distinct vision. Here the retina is thinned, so that light has greater access to the cones.

fibers pass to the **pretectal nucleus** and the **superior colliculus** of the midbrain and are concerned with light reflexes (Fig. 23-3).

Lateral Geniculate Body

The lateral geniculate body is a small, oval swelling projecting from the **pulvinar of the thalamus**. It consists of six layers of cells upon which synapse the axons of the optic tract. The axons of the nerve cells within the geniculate body leave it to form the **optic radiation** (Fig. 23-2).

Optic Radiation

The fibers of the optic radiation are the axons of the nerve cells of the lateral geniculate body. The tract passes posteriorly through the retrolenticular part of the **internal capsule** and terminates in the **visual cortex (area 17)**, which occupies the upper and lower lips of the calcarine sulcus on the medial surface of the cerebral hemisphere (Fig. 23-2). The visual association cortex (areas 18 and 19) is responsible for recognition of objects and perception of color.

NEURONS OF THE VISUAL PATHWAY AND BINOCULAR VISION

Four neurons are involved in the conduction of visual impulses to the visual cortex: (1) **rods and cones**, which are specialized receptor neurons in the retina; (2) **bipolar neurons**, which connect the rods and cones to the ganglion cells; (3) the **ganglion cells**, whose axons pass to the lateral geniculate body; and (4) the **neurons of the lateral geniculate body**, whose axons pass to the cerebral cortex.

In binocular vision, the right and left fields of vision are projected on portions of both retinae (Fig. 23-2). The image of an object in the right field of vision is projected on the nasal half of the right retina and the temporal half of the left retina. In the optic chiasma, the axons from these two retinal halves are combined to form the left optic tract. The lateral geniculate body neurons now project the complete right field of vision upon the visual cortex of the left hemisphere, and the left visual field on the visual cortex of the right hemisphere

Fig. 23-2. The optic pathway.

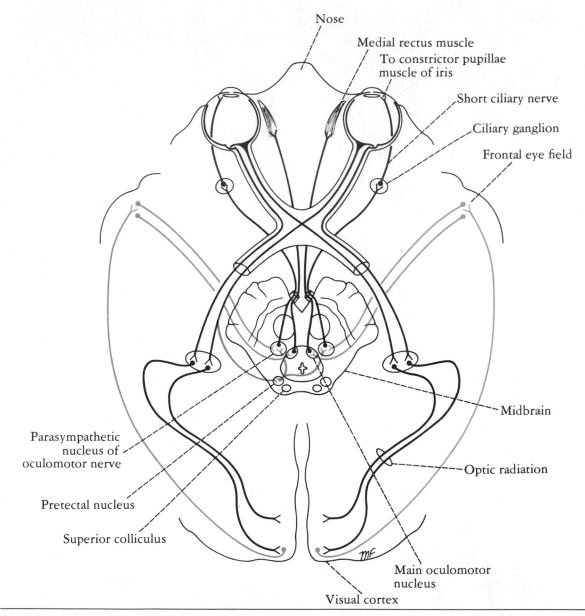

Fig. 23-3. The optic pathway and the visual reflexes.

(Fig. 23-2). The lower retinal quadrants (upper field of vision) project on the lower wall of the calcarine sulcus, while the upper retinal quadrants (lower field of vision) project on the upper wall of the sulcus. Note also that the **macula lutea** is represented on the posterior part of area 17, and the periphery of the retina is represented anteriorly.

VISUAL REFLEXES

Direct and Consensual Light Reflexes

If a light is shone into one eye, the pupils of both eyes normally constrict. The constriction of the pupil upon which the light is shone is called the **direct light reflex**; the constriction of the opposite pupil even though no light fell upon that eye is called the **consensual light reflex** (Fig. 23-3).

The afferent impulses travel through the optic nerve, optic chiasma, and optic tract (Fig. 23-3). Here a small number of fibers leave the optic tract and synapse on nerve cells in the **pretectal nucleus**, which lies close to the superior colliculus. The impulses are passed by axons of the pretectal nerve cells to the parasympathetic nuclei **(Edinger-Westphal nuclei)** of the third cranial nerve on both sides. Here the fibers synapse and the parasympathetic nerves travel through the third cranial nerve to the **ciliary ganglion** in the orbit (Fig. 23-3). Finally, postganglionic parasympathetic fibers pass through the **short ciliary nerves** to the eyeball and the **constrictor pupillae muscle** of the iris. Both pupils constrict in the consensual light reflex because the pretectal nucleus sends fibers to the parasympathetic nuclei on both sides of the midbrain (Fig. 23-3). The fibers that cross the median plane do so close to the cerebral aqueduct in the posterior commissure.

Accommodation Reflex

When the eyes are directed from a distant to a near object, contraction of the medial recti brings about convergence of the ocular axes, the lens thickens to increase its refractive power by contraction of the ciliary muscle, and the pupils constrict to restrict the light waves to the thickest central part of the lens. The afferent impulses travel through the optic nerve, the optic chiasma, the optic tract, the lateral geniculate body, and the optic radiation to the visual cortex. The visual cortex is connected to the eye field of the frontal cortex (Fig. 23-3). From here, cortical fibers descend through the internal capsule to the oculomotor nuclei in the midbrain. The oculomotor nerve travels to the medial recti muscles. Some of the descending cortical fibers synapse with the parasympathetic nuclei (Edinger-Westphal nuclei) of the third cranial nerve on both sides. Here the fibers synapse and the parasympathetic nerves travel through the third cranial nerve to the ciliary ganglion in the orbit. Finally, postganglionic parasympathetic fibers pass through the short ciliary nerves to the **ciliary muscle** and the **constrictor pupillae muscle** of the iris (Fig. 23-3).

Corneal Reflex

Light touching of the cornea or conjunctiva results in blinking of the eyelids. Afferent impulses from the cornea or conjunctiva travel through the ophthalmic division of the trigeminal nerve to the sensory nucleus of the trigeminal nerve (Fig. 23-4A). Internuncial neurons connect with the motor nucleus of the facial nerve on both sides through the medial longitudinal fasciculus. The facial nerve and its branches supply the orbicularis oculi muscle, which causes closure of the eyelids.

Visual Body Reflexes

The automatic scanning movements of the eyes and head made when reading, the automatic movement of the eyes, head, and neck toward the source of the visual stimulus, and the protective closing of the eyes and even the raising of the arm for protection are reflex actions that involve the following reflex arcs (Fig. 23-4B). The visual impulses follow the optic nerves, optic chiasma, and optic tracts to the superior colliculi. Here the impulses are relayed to the tectospinal and tectobulbar (tectonuclear) tracts and to the neurons of the anterior gray columns of the spinal cord and cranial motor nuclei.

Pupillary Skin Reflex

The pupil will dilate if the skin is painfully stimulated by pinching. The afferent sensory fibers are believed to have connections with the efferent pre-

**Fig. 23-4. A. Corneal reflex.
B. Visual body reflex.**

ganglionic sympathetic neurons in the lateral gray columns of the first and second thoracic segments of the spinal cord. The **white rami communicantes** of these segments pass to the sympathetic trunk and the preganglionic fibers ascend to the superior **cervical sympathetic ganglion**. The postganglionic fibers pass through the **internal carotid plexus** and the **long ciliary nerves** to the dilator pupillae muscle of the iris.

OCULOMOTOR NERVE (CRANIAL NERVE III)

The oculomotor nerve is entirely motor in function.

Oculomotor Nuclei

The oculomotor nerve has two motor nuclei: (1) the main motor nucleus and (2) the accessory parasympathetic nucleus.

The **main oculomotor nucleus** is situated in the anterior part of the gray matter that surrounds the **cerebral aqueduct of the midbrain** (Fig. 23-5). It lies at the level of the **superior colliculus**. The nucleus consists of groups of nerve cells that supply all the extrinsic muscles of the eye except the superior oblique and the lateral rectus. The outgoing nerve fibers pass anteriorly through the red nucleus and emerge on the anterior surface of the midbrain in the **interpeduncular fossa**. The main oculomotor nucleus receives corticonuclear fibers from both cerebral hemispheres. It receives tectobulbar fibers from the superior colliculus and through this route receives information from the visual cortex. It also receives fibers from the medial longitudinal fasciculus, by which it is connected to the nuclei of the fourth, sixth, and eighth cranial nerves.

The **accessory parasympathetic nucleus (Edinger-Westphal nucleus)** is situated posterior to the main oculomotor nucleus (Fig. 23-5). The axons of the nerve cells, which are preganglionic, accompany the other oculomotor fibers to the orbit. Here they synapse in the **ciliary ganglion** and postganglionic fibers pass through the **short ciliary nerves** to the constrictor pupillae of the iris and the ciliary muscles. The accessory parasympathetic nucleus receives corticonuclear fibers for the accommodation reflex and fibers from the pre-

tectal nucleus for the direct and consensual light reflexes (Fig. 23-3).

Course of the Oculomotor Nerve

The oculomotor nerve emerges on the anterior surface of the midbrain (Fig. 23-5). It passes forward between the posterior cerebral and the superior cerebellar arteries. It then continues into the middle cranial fossa in the lateral wall of the cavernous sinus. Here, it divides into a superior and an inferior ramus, which enter the orbital cavity through the superior orbital fissure.

The oculomotor nerve supplies the following extrinsic muscles of the eye: the levator palpebrae superioris, superior rectus, medial rectus, inferior rectus, and inferior oblique. It also supplies through its branch to the ciliary ganglion and the short ciliary nerves parasympathetic nerve fibers to the following intrinsic muscles: the constrictor pupillae of the iris and ciliary muscles.

The oculomotor nerve is therefore entirely motor and is responsible for lifting the upper eyelid, turning the eye upward, downward, and medially, constricting the pupil, and accommodating the eye.

TROCHLEAR NERVE (CRANIAL NERVE IV)

The trochlear nerve is entirely motor in function.

Trochlear Nucleus

The trochlear nucleus is situated in the anterior part of the gray matter that surrounds the **cerebral aqueduct of the midbrain** (Fig. 23-6). It lies inferior to the oculomotor nucleus at the level of the **inferior colliculus**. The nerve fibers, after leaving the nucleus, pass posteriorly around the central gray matter to reach the posterior surface of the midbrain.

The trochlear nucleus receives corticonuclear fibers from both cerebral hemispheres. It receives the tectobulbar fibers, which connect it to the visual cortex through the superior colliculus (Fig. 23-6). It also receives fibers from the **medial longitudinal fasciculus**, by which it is connected to the nuclei of the third, sixth, and eighth cranial nerves.

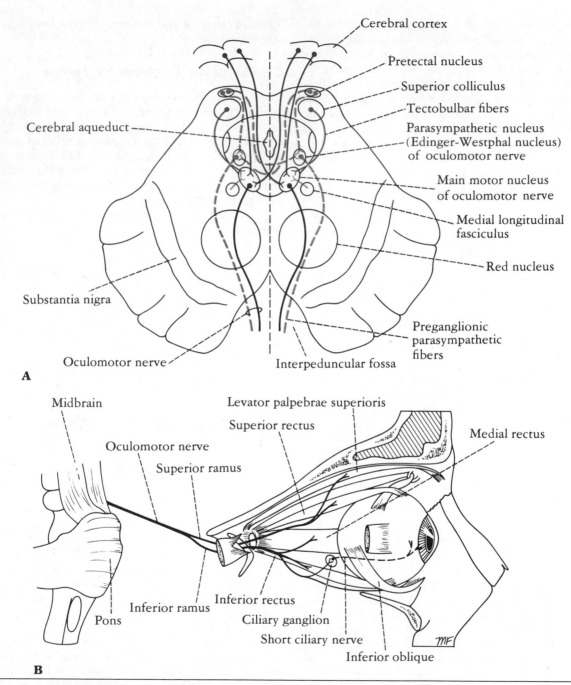

Fig. 23-5. A. Oculomotor nerve nuclei and their central connections.
B. The distribution of the oculomotor nerve.

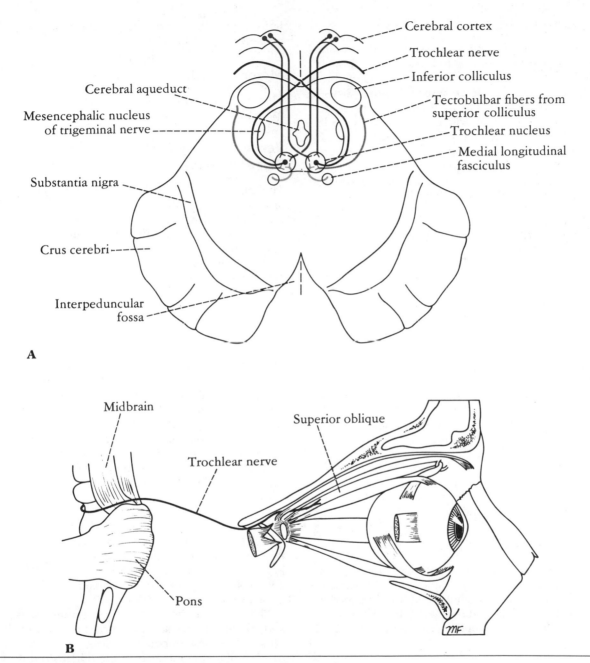

Fig. 23-6. A. Trochlear nerve nucleus and its central connections.
B. Distribution of the trochlear nerve.

Course of the Trochlear Nerve

The trochlear nerve, the most slender of the cranial nerves, and the only one to leave the posterior surface of the brainstem, emerges from the midbrain and **immediately decussates with the nerve of the opposite side**. The trochlear nerve passes forward through the middle cranial fossa in the lateral wall of the cavernous sinus and enters the orbit through the superior orbital fissure. The nerve supplies the superior oblique muscle of the eyeball. The trochlear nerve is entirely motor and assists in turning the eye downward and laterally.

TRIGEMINAL NERVE (CRANIAL NERVE V)

The trigeminal nerve is the largest cranial nerve and contains both sensory and motor fibers. It is the sensory nerve to the greater part of the head and the motor nerve to several muscles, including the muscles of mastication (Fig. 23-8).

Trigeminal Nerve Nuclei

The trigeminal nerve has four nuclei: (1) the main sensory nucleus, (2) the spinal nucleus, (3) the mesencephalic nucleus, and (4) the motor nucleus.

Main Sensory Nucleus

This nucleus lies in the posterior part of the pons, lateral to the motor nucleus (Fig. 23-7A). It is continuous below with the spinal nucleus.

Spinal Nucleus

This nucleus is continuous superiorly with the main sensory nucleus in the pons and extends inferiorly through the whole length of the medulla oblongata and into the upper part of the spinal cord as far as the second cervical segment (Fig. 23-7B).

Mesencephalic Nucleus

This nucleus is composed of a column of unipolar nerve cells situated in the lateral part of the gray matter around the cerebral aqueduct. It extends in-feriorly into the pons as far as the main sensory nucleus (Fig. 23-7).

Motor Nucleus

This nucleus is situated in the pons medial to the main sensory nucleus (Fig. 23-7).

Sensory Components of the Trigeminal Nerve

The sensations of pain and temperature and touch and pressure from the skin of the face and mucous membranes travel along axons whose cell bodies are situated in the **semilunar or trigeminal sensory ganglion** (Fig. 23-7B). The central processes of these cells form the large sensory root of the trigeminal nerve. About half the fibers divide into ascending and descending branches when they enter the pons; the remainder ascend or descend without division (Fig. 23-7B). The ascending branches terminate in the main sensory nucleus and the descending branches terminate in the spinal nucleus. The sensations of touch and pressure are conveyed by nerve fibers that terminate in the main sensory nucleus. The sensations of pain and temperature pass to the spinal nucleus (Fig. 23-7B). The sensory fibers from the ophthalmic division of the trigeminal nerve terminate in the inferior part of the spinal nucleus; fibers from the maxillary division terminate in the middle of the spinal nucleus; and fibers from the mandibular division end in the superior part of the spinal nucleus.

Proprioceptive impulses from the muscles of mastication and from the facial and extraocular muscles are carried by fibers in the sensory root of the trigeminal nerve that have bypassed the semilunar or trigeminal ganglion (Fig. 23-7B). The fibers' cells of origin are the unipolar cells of the mesencephalic nucleus (Fig. 23-7).

The axons of the neurons in the main sensory and spinal nuclei, and the central processes of the cells in the mesencephalic nucleus, now cross the median plane and ascend as the **trigeminal lemniscus** to terminate on the nerve cells of the **ventral posteromedial nucleus of the thalamus**. The axons of these cells now travel through the internal capsule to the postcentral gyrus (areas 3, 1, and 2) of the cerebral cortex.

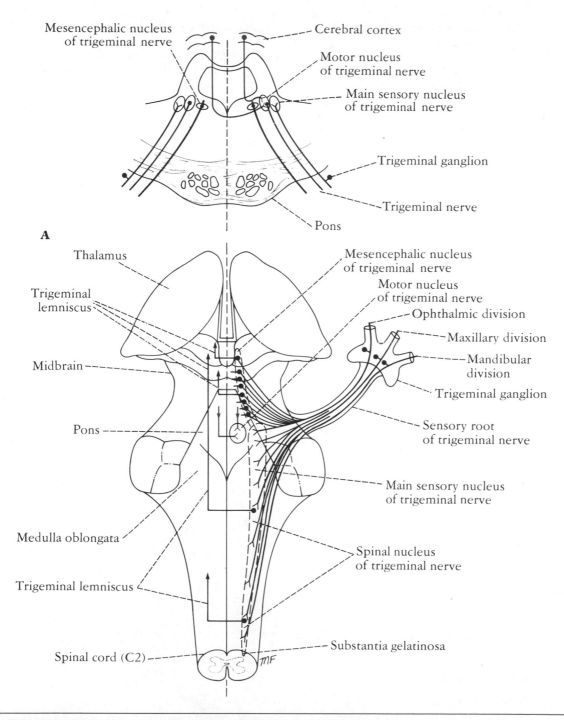

**Fig. 23-7. A. Trigeminal nerve nuclei seen in coronal section of pons.
B. Trigeminal nerve nuclei in the brainstem and their central connections.**

Motor Component of the Trigeminal Nerve

The motor nucleus receives corticonuclear fibers from both cerebral hemispheres (Fig. 23-7). It also receives fibers from the reticular formation, the red nucleus, the tectum, and the medial longitudinal fasciculus. In addition, it receives fibers from the mesencephalic nucleus, thereby forming a monosynaptic reflex arc.

The cells of the motor nucleus give rise to the axons that form the motor root. The motor nucleus supplies the **muscles of mastication**, the **tensor tympani**, the **tensor veli palatini**, and the **mylohyoid** and the **anterior belly of the digastric muscle**.

Course of the Trigeminal Nerve

The trigeminal nerve leaves the anterior aspect of the pons as a small motor root and a large sensory root. The nerve passes forward out of the posterior cranial fossa and rests on the upper surface of the apex of the petrous part of the temporal bone in the middle cranial fossa. The large sensory root now expands to form the crescent-shaped **trigeminal ganglion**, which lies within a pouch of dura mater called the **trigeminal or Meckel's cave**. The ophthalmic, maxillary, and mandibular nerves arise from the anterior border of the ganglion (Fig. 23-8). The ophthalmic nerve (V1) contains only sensory fibers and leaves the skull through the superior orbital fissure to enter the orbital cavity. The

Fig. 23-8. Distribution of trigeminal nerve.

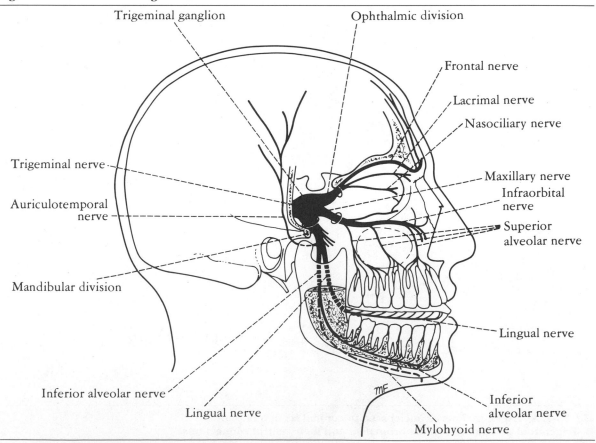

maxillary nerve (V2) also contains only sensory fibers and leaves the skull through the foramen rotundum. The mandibular nerve (V3) contains both sensory and motor fibers and leaves the skull through the foramen ovale.

The sensory fibers to the skin of the face from each division supply a distinct zone (Fig. 23-9), there being little or no overlap of the dermatomes. (Compare with the overlap of the dermatomes of the spinal nerves.) As noted previously, the motor fibers in the mandibular division are mainly distributed to muscles of mastication.

ABDUCENT NERVE (CRANIAL NERVE VI)

The abducent nerve is a small motor nerve that supplies the **lateral rectus muscle** of the eyeball.

Abducent Nerve Nucleus

The small motor nucleus is situated beneath the floor of the upper part of the fourth ventricle, close to the midline and beneath the **colliculus facialis** (Fig. 23-10A). The nucleus receives afferent corticonuclear fibers from both cerebral hemispheres. It receives the tectobulbar tract from the superior colliculus, by which the visual cortex is connected to the nucleus. It also receives fibers from the medial longitudinal fasciculus, by which it is connected to the nuclei of the third, fourth, and eighth cranial nerves (Fig. 23-9A).

Course of the Abducent Nerve

The fibers of the abducent nerve pass anteriorly through the pons and emerge in the groove between the lower border of the pons and the medulla oblongata (Fig. 23-10B). It passes forward through the cavernous sinus, lying below and lateral to the internal carotid artery. The nerve then enters the orbit through the superior orbital fissure. The abducent nerve is entirely a motor nerve and supplies the lateral rectus muscle and is, therefore, responsible for turning the eye laterally.

Fig. 23-9. Sensory nerve supply to the skin of the head and neck. Note that the skin over the angle of the jaw is supplied by the great auricular nerve (C2 and 3) and not by branches of the trigeminal nerve.

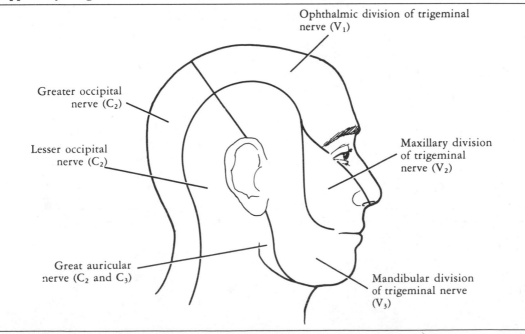

Ophthalmic division of trigeminal nerve (V_1)

Greater occipital nerve (C_2)

Lesser occipital nerve (C_2)

Maxillary division of trigeminal nerve (V_2)

Great auricular nerve (C_2 and C_3)

Mandibular division of trigeminal nerve (V_3)

Fig. 23-10. A. Abducent nerve nucleus and its central connections. B. Distribution of the abducent nerve.

FACIAL NERVE (CRANIAL NERVE VII)

The facial nerve is both a motor and a sensory nerve.

Facial Nerve Nuclei

The facial nerve has three nuclei: (1) the main motor nucleus, (2) the parasympathetic nuclei, and (3) the sensory nucleus.

Main Motor Nucleus

This lies deep in the reticular formation of the lower part of the pons (Fig. 23-11). The part of the nucleus that supplies the muscles of the upper part of the face receives corticonuclear fibers from both cerebral hemispheres. The part of the nucleus that supplies the muscles of the lower part of the face receives only corticonuclear fibers from the opposite cerebral hemisphere.

These pathways explain the voluntary control of facial muscles. However, another involuntary pathway exists, which is separate and controls **mimetic or emotional changes in facial expression**. The origin and course of this upper motor neuron pathway is unknown.

Parasympathetic Nuclei

These lie posterolateral to the main motor nucleus. They are the **superior salivatory** and **lacrimal nuclei** (Fig. 23-11). The superior salivatory nucleus receives afferent fibers from the hypothalamus through the **descending autonomic pathways**. Information concerning taste also is received from the **nucleus of the solitary tract** from the mouth cavity.

The lacrimal nucleus receives afferent fibers from the hypothalamus for emotional responses and from the sensory nuclei of the trigeminal nerve for reflex lacrimation secondary to irritation of the cornea or conjunctiva.

Fig. 23-11. Facial nerve nuclei and their central connections.

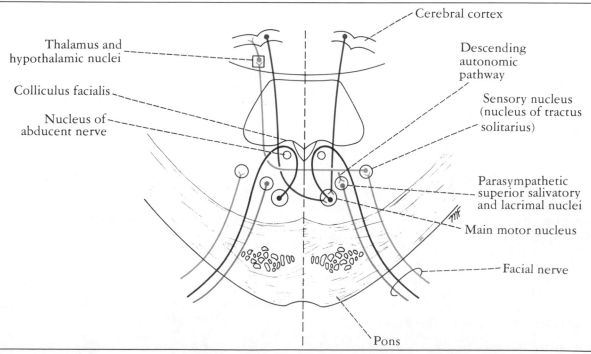

Sensory Nucleus

This is the upper part of the **nucleus of the tractus solitarius** and lies close to the motor nucleus (Fig. 23-11). Sensations of taste travel through the peripheral axons of nerve cells situated in the **geniculate ganglion** on the seventh cranial nerve. The central processes of these cells synapse on nerve cells in the nucleus. Efferent fibers cross the median plane and ascend to the ventral posterior medial nucleus of the opposite thalamus and also a number of hypothalamic nuclei. From the thalamus, the axons of the thalamic cells pass through the internal capsule and corona radiata to end in the taste area of the cortex in the lower part of the postcentral gyrus (Fig. 23-11).

Course of the Facial Nerve

The facial nerve consists of a motor and a sensory root. The fibers of the motor root first travel posteriorly around the medial side of the abducent nucleus (Fig. 23-11). Then they pass around the nucleus beneath the **colliculus facialis** in the floor of the fourth ventricle and finally pass anteriorly to emerge from the brainstem (Fig. 23-11).

The sensory root (**nervus intermedius**) is formed of the central processes of the unipolar cells of the geniculate ganglion. It also contains the efferent preganglionic parasympathetic fibers from the parasympathetic nuclei.

The two roots of the facial nerve emerge from the anterior surface of the brain between the pons and the medulla oblongata. They pass laterally in the posterior cranial fossa with the vestibulocochlear nerve and enter the internal acoustic meatus in the petrous part of the temporal bone. At the bottom of the meatus, the nerve enters the facial canal and runs laterally through the inner ear. On reaching the medial wall of the tympanic cavity, the nerve expands to form the sensory **geniculate ganglion** (Fig. 23-12) and turns sharply backward above the promontory. At the posterior wall of the tympanic cavity the facial nerve turns downward on the medial side of the aditus of the mastoid antrum, descends behind the pyramid, and emerges from the stylomastoid foramen.

Distribution of the Facial Nerve

The **motor nucleus** supplies the muscles of facial expression, the auricular muscles, the stapedius, the posterior belly of the digastric, and the stylohyoid muscles (Fig. 23-12).

The **superior salivatory nucleus** supplies the submandibular and sublingual salivary glands and the nasal and palatine glands. The **lacrimal nucleus** supplies the lacrimal gland.

The **sensory nucleus** receives taste fibers from the anterior two-thirds of the tongue, the floor of the mouth, and the palate.

VESTIBULOCOCHLEAR NERVE (CRANIAL NERVE VIII)

This nerve consists of two distinct parts, the **vestibular nerve** and the **cochlear nerve**, which are concerned with the transmission of afferent information from the internal ear to the central nervous system (Fig. 23-13 and 23-14).

Vestibular Nerve

The vestibular nerve conducts nerve impulses from the utricle and saccule that provide information concerning the position of the head; the nerve also conducts impulses from the semicircular canals that provide information concerning movements of the head.

The nerve fibers of the vestibular nerve are the central processes of nerve cells located in the **vestibular ganglion**, which is situated in the **internal acoustic meatus**. They enter the anterior surface of the brainstem in a groove between the lower border of the pons and the upper part of the medulla oblongata (Fig. 23-13). When they enter the vestibular nuclear complex, the fibers divide into short ascending and long descending fibers; a small number of fibers pass directly to the cerebellum through the inferior cerebellar peduncle, bypassing the vestibular nuclei.

THE VESTIBULAR NUCLEAR COMPLEX

This complex consists of a group of nuclei situated beneath the floor of the fourth ventricle (Fig. 23-13). Four nuclei may be recognized: (1) the **lateral vestibular nucleus**, (2) the **superior vestibular nucleus**, (3) the **medial vestibular nucleus**, and (4) the **inferior vestibular nucleus** (see Fig. 8-6).

The vestibular nuclei receive afferent fibers from the **utricle** and **saccule** and the **semicircular ca-**

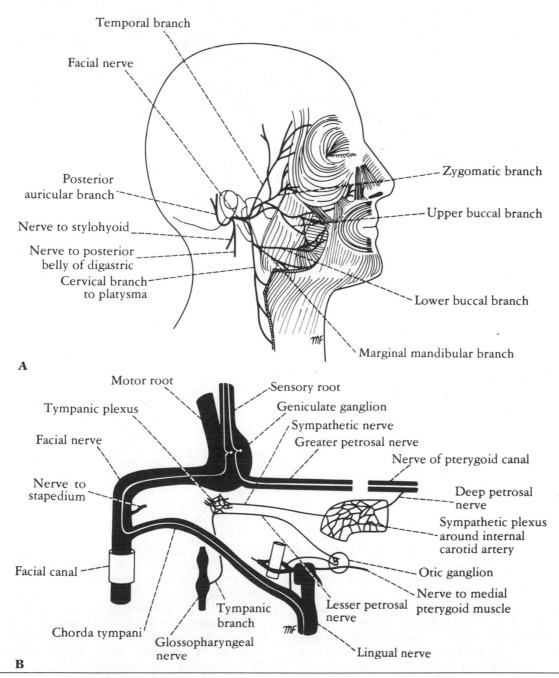

Fig. 23-12. A. Distribution of facial nerve.
B. Branches of facial nerve within petrous part of the temporal bone; the taste fibers are shown in white. The glossopharyngeal nerve is also shown.

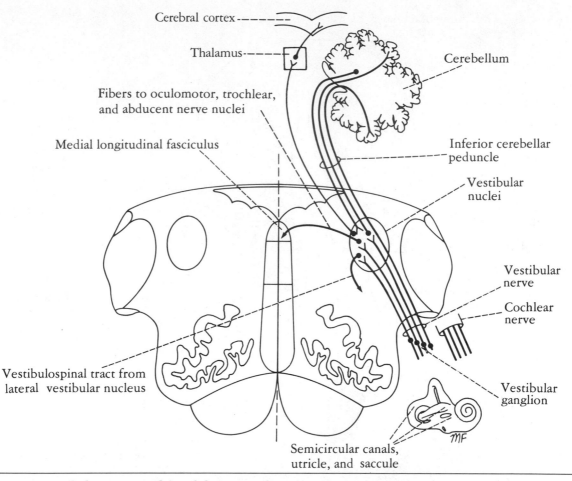

Fig. 23-13. Vestibular nerve nuclei and their central connections.

nals through the vestibular nerve, and fibers from the cerebellum through the inferior cerebellar peduncle (Fig. 23-13). Efferent fibers from the nuclei pass to the cerebellum through the inferior cerebellar peduncle. Efferent fibers also descend uncrossed to the spinal cord from the lateral vestibular nucleus and form the **vestibulospinal tract** (Fig. 23-13). In addition, efferent fibers pass to the nuclei of the oculomotor, trochlear, and abducent nerves through the medial longitudinal fasciculus.

These connections enable the movements of the head and the eyes to be coordinated so that visual fixation on an object can be maintained. In addition, information received from the internal ear can assist in maintaining balance by influencing the muscle tone of the limbs and trunk.

Ascending fibers also pass upward from the vestibular nuclei to the cerebral cortex, to the vestibular area in the postcentral gyrus, just above the lateral fissure. These fibers are thought to relay in the ventral posterior nuclei of the thalamus. The cerebral cortex probably serves to orient the individual consciously in space.

Cochlear Nerve

The cochlear nerve conducts nerve impulses concerned with sound from the organ of Corti in the

Fig. 23-14. Cochlear nerve nuclei and their central connections. The descending pathways have been omitted.

cochlea. The fibers of the cochlear nerve are the central processes of nerve cells located in the **spiral ganglion of the cochlea** (Fig. 23-15). They enter the anterior surface of the brainstem at the lower border of the pons on the lateral side of the emerging facial nerve and are separated from it by the vestibular nerve (Fig. 23-14). On entering the pons the nerve fibers divide, one branch entering the **posterior cochlear nucleus** and the other branch entering the **anterior cochlear nucleus**.

COCHLEAR NUCLEI

The anterior and posterior cochlear nuclei are situated on the surface of the inferior cerebellar peduncle (Fig. 23-14). They receive afferent fibers from the cochlea through the cochlear nerve. The cochlear nuclei send axons (second-order neuron fibers) that run medially through the pons to end in the **trapezoid body** and the olivary nucleus. Here they are relayed in the **posterior nucleus of the trapezoid body** and the superior olivary nucleus on the same or the opposite side. The axons now ascend through the posterior part of the pons and midbrain and form a tract known as the **lateral lemniscus** (Fig. 23-14). Each lateral lemniscus, therefore, consists of third-order neurons from

both sides. As these fibers ascend, some of them relay in small groups of nerve cells, collectively known as the **nucleus of the lateral lemniscus** (Fig. 23-14).

On reaching the midbrain, the fibers of the lateral lemniscus either terminate in the **nucleus of the inferior colliculus** or are relayed in the **medial geniculate body** and pass to the **auditory cortex** of the cerebral hemisphere through the **acoustic radiation of the internal capsule** (Fig. 23-14).

The primary auditory cortex (areas 41 and 42) includes the gyrus of Heschl on the upper surface of the superior temporal gyrus. The recognition and interpretation of sounds on the basis of past experience takes place in the secondary auditory area.

It should be pointed out that nerve impulses from the ear are transmitted along auditory pathways on both sides of the brainstem, with more being projected along the contralateral pathway. Many collateral branches are given off to the reticular activating system of the brainstem (see p. 317). The tonotopic organization present in the organ of Corti is preserved within the cochlear nuclei, the inferior colliculi, and in the primary auditory area.

Fig. 23-15. Distribution of the vestibulocochlear nerve.

DESCENDING AUDITORY PATHWAYS

Descending fibers originating in the auditory cortex and in other nuclei in the auditory pathway accompany the ascending pathway. These fibers are bilateral and end on nerve cells at different levels of the auditory pathway and on the hair cells of the organ of Corti. It is believed that these fibers serve as a feedback mechanism and inhibit the reception of sound. They may also have a role in the process of auditory sharpening, suppressing some signals and enhancing others.

Course of the Vestibulocochlear Nerve

The vestibular and cochlear parts of the nerve leave the anterior surface of the brain between the lower border of the pons and the medulla oblongata (Fig. 23-15). They run laterally in the posterior cranial fossa and enter the internal acoustic meatus with the facial nerve. The fibers are then distributed to the different parts of the internal ear (Fig. 23-15).

GLOSSOPHARYNGEAL NERVE (CRANIAL NERVE IX)

The glossopharyngeal nerve is a motor and a sensory nerve.

Glossopharyngeal Nerve Nuclei

The glossopharyngeal nerve has three nuclei: (1) the main motor nucleus, (2) the parasympathetic nucleus, and (3) the sensory nucleus.

Main Motor Nucleus

This nucleus lies deep in the reticular formation of the medulla oblongata and is formed by the superior end of the nucleus ambiguus (Fig. 23-16). It receives corticonuclear fibers from both cerebral hemispheres. The efferent fibers supply the **stylopharyngeus muscle**.

Parasympathetic Nucleus

This nucleus is also called the **inferior salivatory nucleus** (Fig. 23-16). It receives afferent fibers from the hypothalamus through the **descending autonomic pathways**. It also is thought to receive information from the olfactory system through the reticular formation. Information concerning taste also is received from the nucleus of the solitary tract from the mouth cavity.

The efferent preganglionic parasympathetic fibers reach the otic ganglion through the **tympanic branch of the glossopharyngeal nerve**, the **tympanic plexus**, and the **lesser petrosal nerve** (Fig. 23-17). The postganglionic fibers pass to the **parotid salivary gland**.

Sensory Nucleus

This is part of the **nucleus of the tractus solitarius** (Fig. 23-16). Sensations of taste travel through the peripheral axons of nerve cells situated in the **ganglion** on the glossopharyngeal nerve. The central processes of these cells synapse on nerve cells in the nucleus. Efferent fibers cross the median plane and ascend to the ventral group of nuclei of the opposite thalamus, and also a number of hypothalamic nuclei. From the thalamus, the axons of the thalamic cells pass through the internal capsule and corona radiata to end in the lower part of the postcentral gyrus.

It is interesting to note that afferent information that concerns common sensation enters the brainstem through the superior ganglion of the glossopharyngeal nerve, but ends in the **spinal nucleus of the trigeminal nerve**. Afferent impulses from the **carotid sinus**, a baroreceptor situated at the bifurcation of the common carotid artery, also travel with the glossopharyngeal nerve. They terminate in the **nucleus of the tractus solitarius** and are connected to the **dorsal motor nucleus of the vagus nerve**. The carotid sinus reflex that involves the glossopharyngeal and vagus nerves assists in the regulation of arterial blood pressure.

Course of the Glossopharyngeal Nerve

The glossopharyngeal nerve leaves the anterolateral surface of the upper part of the medulla oblongata as a series of rootlets in a groove between the olive and the inferior cerebellar peduncle (Fig. 23-16). It passes laterally in the posterior cranial fossa and leaves the skull through the jugular fo-

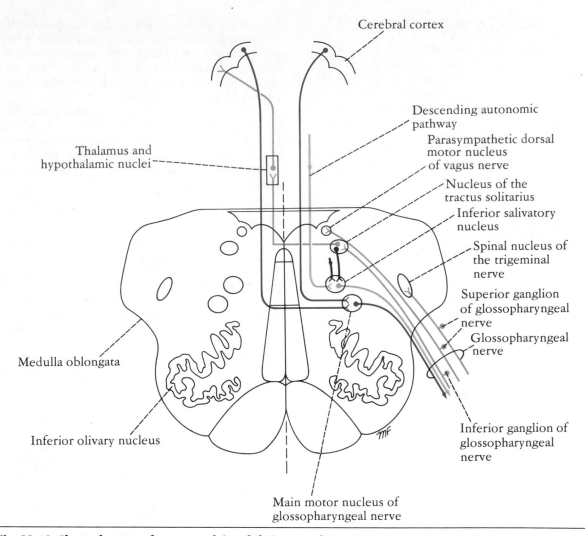

Fig. 23-16. Glossopharyngeal nerve nuclei and their central connections.

ramen. The superior and inferior glossopharyngeal sensory ganglia are situated on the nerve here. The nerve then descends through the upper part of the neck in company with the internal jugular vein and the internal carotid artery to reach the posterior border of the stylopharyngeus muscle, which it supplies. The nerve then passes forward between the superior and middle constrictor muscles of the pharynx to give sensory branches to the mucous membrane of the pharynx and the posterior third of the tongue (Fig. 23-17).

VAGUS NERVE (CRANIAL NERVE X)

The vagus nerve is a motor and a sensory nerve.

Vagus Nerve Nuclei

The vagus nerve has three nuclei: (1) the main motor nucleus, (2) the parasympathetic nucleus, and (3) the sensory nucleus.

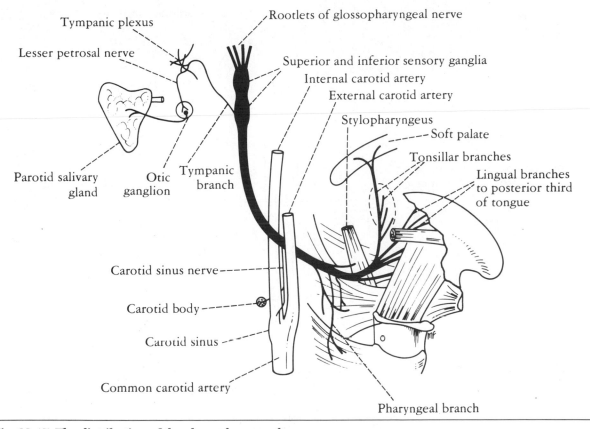

Fig. 23-17. The distribution of the glossopharyngeal nerve.

Main Motor Nucleus

This nucleus lies deep in the reticular formation of the medulla oblongata and is formed by the nucleus ambiguus (Fig. 23-18). It receives corticonuclear fibers from both cerebral hemispheres. The efferent fibers supply the constrictor muscles of the pharynx and the intrinsic muscles of the larynx (Fig. 23-19).

Parasympathetic Nucleus

This nucleus forms the dorsal nucleus of the vagus and lies beneath the floor of the lower part of the fourth ventricle posterolateral to the hypoglossal nucleus (Fig. 23-18). It receives afferent fibers from the hypothalamus through the descending autonomic pathways. It also receives other afferents, including those from the glossopharyngeal nerve (carotid sinus reflex). The efferent fibers are distributed to the involuntary muscle of the bronchi, heart, esophagus, stomach, small intestine, and large intestine as far as the distal one-third of the transverse colon (Fig. 23-19).

Sensory Nucleus

This nucleus is the lower part of the **nucleus of the tractus solitarius**. Sensations of taste travel through the peripheral axons of nerve cells situated in the **inferior ganglion on the vagus nerve**. The central processes of those cells synapse on nerve cells in the nucleus (Fig. 23-18). Efferent fibers

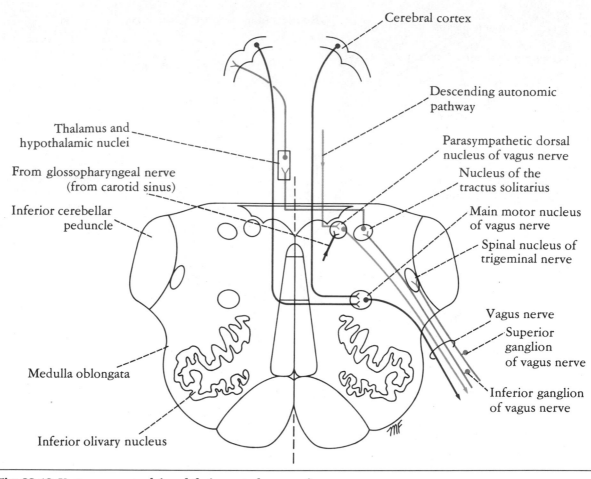

Fig. 23-18. Vagus nerve nuclei and their central connections.

cross the median plane and ascend to the ventral group of nuclei of the opposite thalamus as well as to a number of hypothalamic nuclei. From the thalamus, the axons of the thalamic cells pass through the internal capsule and corona radiata to end in the postcentral gyrus.

It is interesting to note that afferent information concerning common sensation enters the brainstem through the superior ganglion of the vagus nerve but ends in the **spinal nucleus of the trigeminal nerve.**

Course of the Vagus Nerve

The vagus nerve leaves the anterolateral surface of the upper part of the medulla oblongata as a series

of rootlets in a groove between the olive and the inferior cerebellar peduncle (Fig. 23-18). The nerve passes laterally through the posterior cranial fossa and leaves the skull through the jugular foramen. The vagus nerve possesses two sensory ganglia, a rounded **superior ganglion**, situated on the nerve within the jugular foramen, and a cylindrical **inferior ganglion**, which lies on the nerve just below the foramen. Below the inferior ganglion the cranial root of the accessory nerve joins the vagus nerve and is distributed mainly in its pharyngeal and recurrent laryngeal branches.

The vagus nerve descends vertically in the neck within the carotid sheath with the internal jugular vein and the internal and common carotid arteries.

The **right vagus nerve** enters the thorax and

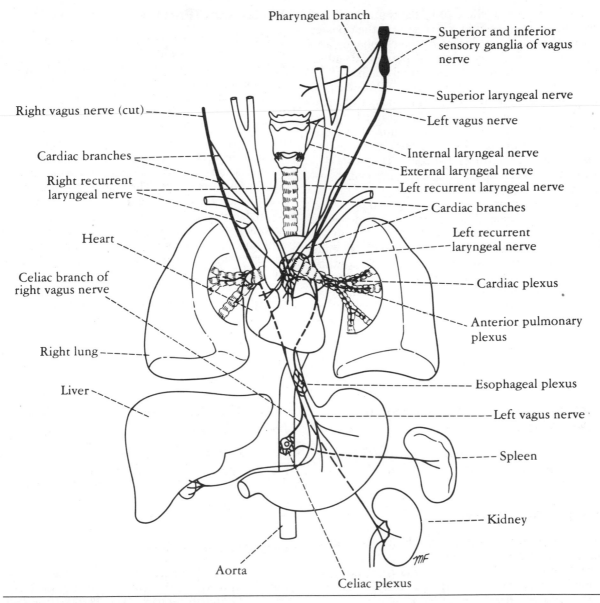

Pharyngeal branch

Superior and inferior sensory ganglia of vagus nerve

Superior laryngeal nerve

Right vagus nerve (cut)

Left vagus nerve

Internal laryngeal nerve

Cardiac branches

External laryngeal nerve

Right recurrent laryngeal nerve

Left recurrent laryngeal nerve

Cardiac branches

Heart

Left recurrent laryngeal nerve

Celiac branch of right vagus nerve

Cardiac plexus

Anterior pulmonary plexus

Right lung

Esophageal plexus

Liver

Left vagus nerve

Spleen

Kidney

Aorta

Celiac plexus

Fig. 23-19. Distribution of the vagus nerve.

passes posterior to the root of the right lung contributing to the pulmonary plexus. It then passes on to the posterior surface of the esophagus and contributes to the **esophageal plexus**. It enters the abdomen through the esophageal opening of the diaphragm. The posterior vagal trunk (which is the name now given to the right vagus) is distributed to the posterior surface of the stomach and by a large celiac branch to the duodenum, liver, kidneys, and small and large intestines as far as the distal third of the transverse colon. This wide distribution is accomplished through the celiac, superior mesenteric, and renal plexuses.

The **left vagus nerve** enters the thorax and crosses the left side of the aortic arch and descends behind the root of the left lung contributing to the **pulmonary plexus**. The left vagus then descends on the anterior surface of the esophagus contributing to the **esophageal plexus**. It enters the abdomen through the esophageal opening of the diaphragm. The anterior vagal trunk (which is the name now given to the left vagus) divides into several branches, which are distributed to the stomach, liver, upper part of the duodenum, and head of the pancreas.

ACCESSORY NERVE (CRANIAL NERVE XI)

The accessory nerve is a motor nerve that is formed by the union of a cranial and a spinal root.

Cranial Root (Part)

The cranial root is formed from the axons of nerve cells of the nucleus ambiguus (Fig. 23-20). The nucleus receives corticonuclear fibers from both cerebral hemispheres. The efferent fibers of the nucleus emerge from the anterior surface of the medulla oblongata between the olive and the inferior cerebellar peduncle. The nerve runs laterally in the posterior cranial fossa and joins the spinal root. The two roots unite and leave the skull through the jugular foramen. The roots then separate and the cranial root joins the vagus nerve and is distributed in its pharyngeal and recurrent laryngeal branches to the muscles of the soft palate, pharynx, and larynx.

Spinal Root (Part)

The spinal root is formed from axons of nerve cells in the **spinal nucleus**, which is situated in the anterior gray column of the spinal cord in the upper five cervical segments (Fig. 23-20). The spinal nucleus is thought to receive corticospinal fibers from both cerebral hemispheres.

The nerve fibers emerge from the spinal cord midway between the anterior and posterior nerve roots of the cervical spinal nerves. The fibers form a nerve trunk that ascends into the skull through the foramen magnum. The spinal root passes laterally and joins the cranial root as they pass through the jugular foramen. After a short distance, the spinal root separates from the cranial root and runs downward and laterally and enters the deep surface of the sternocleidomastoid muscle, which it supplies (Fig. 23-21). The nerve then crosses the posterior triangle of the neck and passes beneath the trapezius muscle, which it supplies.

The accessory nerve thus brings about movements of the soft palate, pharynx, and larynx and controls the movement of two large muscles in the neck.

HYPOGLOSSAL NERVE (CRANIAL NERVE XII)

The hypoglossal nerve is a motor nerve and supplies all the intrinsic muscles of the tongue and, in addition, the styloglossus, the hyoglossus, and the genioglossus muscles.

Hypoglossal Nucleus

The hypoglossal nucleus is situated close to the midline immediately beneath the floor of the lower part of the fourth ventricle (Fig. 23-22). It receives corticonuclear fibers from both cerebral hemispheres. However, the cells responsible for supplying the genioglossus muscle (Fig. 23-23) only receive corticonuclear fibers from the opposite cerebral hemisphere.

The hypoglossal nerve fibers pass anteriorly through the medulla oblongata and emerge as a series of roots in the groove between the pyramid and the olive (Fig. 23-22).

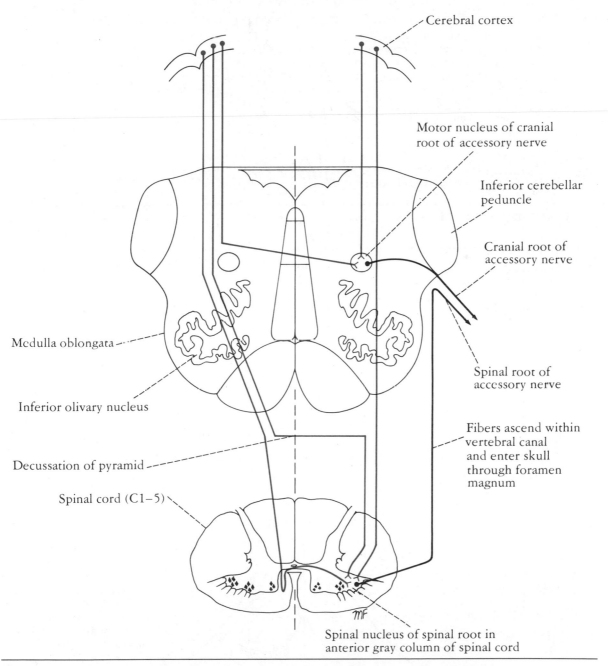

Cerebral cortex

Motor nucleus of cranial
root of accessory nerve

Inferior cerebellar
peduncle

Cranial root of
accessory nerve

Spinal root of
accessory nerve

Fibers ascend within
vertebral canal
and enter skull
through foramen
magnum

Medulla oblongata

Inferior olivary nucleus

Decussation of pyramid

Spinal cord (C1–5)

Spinal nucleus of spinal root in
anterior gray column of spinal cord

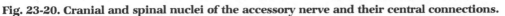

Fig. 23-20. Cranial and spinal nuclei of the accessory nerve and their central connections.

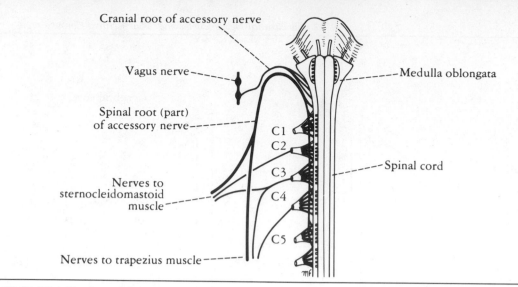

Fig. 23-21. Distribution of the accessory nerve.

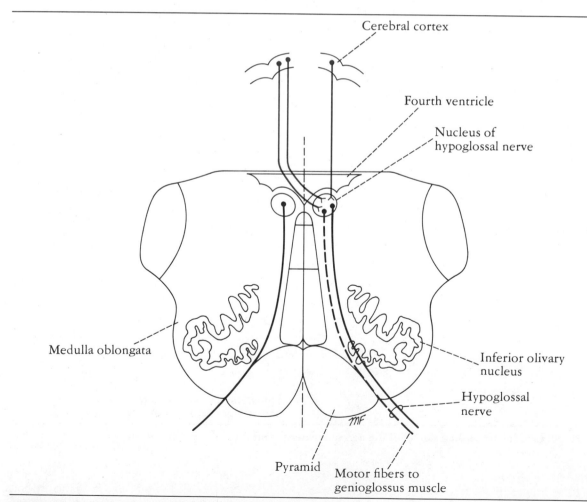

Fig. 23-22. Hypoglossal nucleus and its central connections.

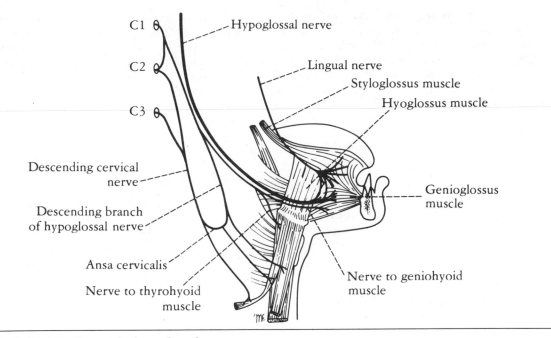

Fig. 23-23. Distribution of the hypoglossal nerve.

Course of the Hypoglossal Nerve

The hypoglossal nerve fibers emerge on the anterior surface of the medulla oblongata between the pyramid and the olive (Fig. 23-22). It crosses the posterior cranial fossa and leaves the skull through the hypoglossal canal. The nerve passes downward and forward in the neck between the internal carotid artery and the internal jugular vein until it reaches the lower border of the posterior belly of the digastric muscle. Here, it turns forward and crosses the internal and external carotid arteries and the loop of the lingual artery. It passes deep to the posterior margin of the mylohyoid muscle lying on the lateral surface of the hyoglossus muscle. The nerve then sends branches to the muscles of the tongue (Fig. 23-23).

In the upper part of its course, the hypoglossal nerve is joined by C1 fibers from the cervical plexus.

The hypoglossal nerve thus controls the movements and shape of the tongue.

CLINICAL NOTES

GENERAL CONSIDERATIONS

The 12 pairs of cranial nerves supply information to the brain from outlying receptor organs and bring about changes in peripheral effector organs by means of appropriate motor nerves. Unfortunately for the student, the nerve cells are not arranged simply, as in the spinal cord, but are grouped together to form **nuclei** that are found in different situations at different levels of the brain-stem. Moreover, whereas spinal nerves possess afferent somatic fibers, afferent visceral fibers, efferent somatic fibers, and efferent visceral fibers, cranial nerves, in addition, possess special afferent fibers (e.g., visual and auditory) and special visceral afferent fibers (e.g., taste).

When the central connections of the different cranial nerve nuclei were discussed in the previous section a simplified practical version was given, since many of the precise connections of the cranial nerve nuclei are still not known. Because the delicate movements of the eyes, the larynx, and the face require carefully integrated muscle action and the fine control of muscle tone, it must be assumed that the motor nuclei of the various cranial nerves receive input from the cerebellum, the red nucleus, the reticular formation, and the corpus striatum in the same manner as the lower motor neurons of the spinal cord.

Three points of clinical value should be remembered:

1. Bilateral corticonuclear connections are present for all the cranial motor nuclei **except** that part of the facial nucleus that supplies the muscles of the lower part of the face and that part of the hypoglossal nucleus that supplies the genioglossus muscle.
2. The cranial nerves that possess afferent sensory fibers have cell bodies that are found in ganglia along the course of the nerves; these are equivalent to the posterior root ganglia. In the case of the olfactory nerves, the cells are the olfactory receptors.
3. In situations where the cranial nerve nuclei are close together, it is very rare for a disease process to affect one nucleus only. For example, the cell groups of the nucleus ambiguus serve the glossopharyngeal, the vagus, and the cranial root of the accessory nerve, and functional loss involving all three nerves is a common finding.

CLINICAL EXAMINATION OF CRANIAL NERVES

The systematic examination of the 12 cranial nerves is an important part of the examination of every neurological patient. It may reveal a lesion of a cranial nerve nucleus, or its central connections, or it may show an interruption of the lower motor neurons.

The Olfactory Nerve

First determine that the nasal passages are clear. Then apply some easily recognizable aromatic substance, such as oil of peppermint, oil of cloves, or tobacco, to each nostril in turn. Ask the patient whether he can smell anything; then ask him to identify the smell. It should be remembered that food flavors depend on the sense of smell and not on the sense of taste. Fractures of the anterior cranial fossa or cerebral tumors of the frontal lobes may produce lesions of the olfactory nerves, with consequent loss of the sense of smell (**anosmia**).

A lesion of the olfactory cortex on one side is unlikely to produce complete anosmia because fibers from each olfactory tract travel to both cerebral hemispheres.

Optic Nerve

First ask the patient whether he has noted any change in his eyesight. **Visual acuity** should be tested for near and distant vision. Near vision is tested by asking the patient to read a card with a standard size of type. Each eye is tested in turn, with or without spectacles. Distant vision is tested by asking the patient to read Snellen's type at a distance of 20 feet.

The **visual fields** should then be tested. The patient and the examiner sit facing each other at a distance of 2 feet. The patient is asked to cover his right eye and the examiner covers his own left eye. The patient is asked to look into the pupil of the examiner's right eye. A small object is then moved in an arc around the periphery of the field of vision, and the patient is asked whether he can see the object. The extent of his field of vision is compared with the normal examiner's field. The other eye then is tested. It is important not to miss loss or impairment of vision in the central area of the field (**central scotoma**).

Lesions of the Visual Pathway

Lesions of the optic pathway may have many pathologic causes. Expanding tumors of the brain and neighboring structures, such as the pituitary gland and the meninges, and cerebrovascular accidents are commonly responsible. The most widespread effects on vision occur where the nerve fibers of the visual pathway are tightly packed together, such as in the optic nerve or the optic tract.

Circumferential Blindness. This may be caused by hysteria or optic neuritis (Fig. 23-24 [1]). Optic neuritis may occur following spread of infection from the sphenoid and ethmoid sinuses; the

Fig. 23-24. Visual field defects associated with lesions of the optic pathways.
1. **Right-sided circumferential blindness due to retrobulbar neuritis.**
2. **Total blindness of right eye due to division of right optic nerve.**
3. **Right nasal hemianopia due to partial lesion of right side of optic chiasma.**
4. **Bitemporal hemianopia due to complete lesion of optic chiasma.**
5. **Left temporal hemianopia and right nasal hemianopia due to lesion of right optic tract.**
6. **Left temporal and right nasal hemianopia due to lesion of right optic radiation.**
7. **Left temporal and right nasal hemianopia due to lesion of right visual cortex.**

nerve is infected as it passes through the optic canal to enter the orbital cavity.

Total Blindness of One Eye. This would follow complete section of one optic nerve (Fig. 23-24 [2]).

Nasal Hemianopia. This would follow a partial lesion of the optic chiasma on its lateral side (Fig. 23-24 [3]).

Bitemporal Hemianopia. This would follow a sagittal section of the optic chiasma (Fig. 23-24 [4]). This condition is most commonly produced by a tumor of the pituitary gland exerting pressure on the optic chiasma.

Contralateral Homonymous Hemianopia. This would follow division of the optic tract or optic radiation or destruction of the visual cortex on one side; the lesion would produce the same hemianopia for both eyes, i.e., homonymous hemianopia (Fig. 23-24 [5, 6, and 7]). If the right optic tract is divided, for example, a left temporal hemianopia and a right nasal hemianopia will occur.

Examination of the Fundi

The ocular fundus should be examined with an ophthalmoscope. The patient is asked to look at a distant object. When the right eye is examined, the physician should use his right eye and hold the ophthalmoscope in his right hand. He should systematically examine the fundus, looking first at the optic disc, then at the retina, then at the blood vessels, and finally at the macula.

The **optic disc** is creamy pink in color and the lateral margin is seen clearly. The center of the disc is paler in color and hollowed out.

The retina is pinkish red in color and there should be no hemorrhages or exudates.

The **blood vessels** should consist of four main arteries with their accompanying veins. Carefully examine the arteriovenous crossings. The veins should not be indented by the arteries.

The **macula** is examined by asking the patient to look directly at the light of the ophthalmoscope. It should look slightly darker than the surrounding retina.

Oculomotor, Trochlear, and Abducent Nerves

The oculomotor, trochlear, and abducent nerves innervate the muscles that move the eyeball; they are usually examined at the same time.

To examine the extraocular muscles, the patient's head is fixed, and he is asked to move the eyes, in turn, to the left, to the right, upward, and downward, as far as possible in each direction. He should then be asked to look upward and laterally, upward and medially, downward and medially, and downward and laterally.

The pupillary reactions to convergence associated with accommodation and the direct and consensual pupillary reactions to light are tested. The nervous pathways involved in the pupillary reflexes are described on page 425.

Oculomotor Nerve

The oculomotor nerve supplies all the extraocular muscles except the superior oblique and the lateral rectus. It also supplies the striated muscle of the levator palpebrae superioris and the smooth muscle concerned with accommodation, namely, the sphincter pupillae and the ciliary muscle.

In a complete lesion of the oculomotor nerve, the eye cannot be moved upward, downward, or inward. At rest, the eye looks laterally (external strabismus) owing to the activity of the lateral rectus and downward owing to the activity of the superior oblique. The patient sees double (diplopia). There is drooping of the upper eyelid (ptosis) due to paralysis of the levator palpebrae superioris. The pupil is widely dilated and nonreactive to light owing to paralysis of the sphincter pupillae and unopposed action of the dilator (supplied by the sympathetic). Accommodation of the eye is paralyzed.

Incomplete lesions of the oculomotor nerve are common and may spare the extraocular muscles or the intraocular muscles. The condition in which the innervation of the extraocular muscles is spared with selective loss of the autonomic innervation of the sphincter pupillae and ciliary muscle is called **internal ophthalmoplegia**. The condition in which the sphincter pupillae and the ciliary muscle are spared with paralysis of the extraocular muscles is called **external ophthalmoplegia**.

The possible explanation for the involvement of the autonomic nerves and the sparing of the remaining fibers is that the parasympathetic autonomic fibers are superficially placed within the oculomotor nerve and are likely to be first affected by compression. The nature of the disease also plays a role. For example, in cases of diabetes with impaired nerve conduction (diabetic neuropathy), the autonomic fibers are unaffected whereas the nerves to the extraocular muscles are paralyzed.

The conditions most commonly affecting the oculomotor nerve are diabetes, aneurysm, tumor, trauma, inflammation, and vascular disease. See lesions of the oculomotor nerve in the midbrain (Benedikt's syndrome) on page 243.

Trochlear Nerve

The trochlear nerve supplies the superior oblique muscle, which rotates the eye downward and laterally.

In lesions of the trochlear nerve the patient complains of double vision on looking straight downward, because the images of the two eyes are tilted relative to each other. This is because the superior oblique is paralyzed, and the eye turns medially as well as downward. In fact the patient has great difficulty in turning the eye downward and laterally.

Abducent Nerve

The abducent nerve supplies the lateral rectus muscle, which rotates the eye laterally.

In a lesion of the abducent nerve the patient cannot turn the eye laterally. When the patient is looking straight ahead, the lateral rectus is paralyzed, and the unopposed medial rectus pulls the eyeball medially, causing **internal strabismus**.

Trigeminal Nerve

The trigeminal nerve has sensory and motor roots. The sensory root passes to the trigeminal ganglion, from which emerge the ophthalmic (V1), maxillary (V2), and mandibular (V3) divisions. The motor root joins the mandibular division.

The sensory function may be tested by using cotton and a pin over each area of the face supplied by the divisions of the trigeminal nerve (Fig. 23-9). Note that there is very little overlap of the dermatomes and that the skin covering the angle of the jaw is innervated by branches from the cervical plexus (C2 and C3). In lesions of the ophthalmic division, the cornea and conjunctiva will be insensitive to touch.

The motor function may be tested by asking the patient to clench his teeth. The masseter and the temporalis muscles can be palpated and felt to contract.

Facial Nerve

The facial nerve supplies the muscles of facial expression, supplies the anterior two-thirds of the tongue with taste fibers, and is secretomotor to the lacrimal, submandibular, and sublingual glands.

To test the facial nerve, the patient is asked to show the teeth by separating the lips with the teeth clenched. Normally, equal areas of the upper and lower teeth are revealed on both sides. Should a lesion of the facial nerve be present on one side the mouth is distorted. A greater area of teeth is revealed on the side of the intact nerve, since the mouth is pulled up on that side. Another useful test is to ask the patient to close both eyes firmly. The examiner then attempts to open the eyes by gently raising the patient's upper lids. On the side of the lesion the orbicularis oculi is paralyzed so that the eyelid on that side is easily raised.

The sensation of taste on each half of the anterior two-thirds of the tongue can be tested by placing on the tongue small amounts of sugar, salt, vinegar, and quinine for the sweet, salt, sour, and bitter sensations.

Facial Nerve Lesions

The facial nerve may be injured or may become dysfunctional anywhere along its long course from the brainstem to the face. Its anatomical relationship to other structures greatly assists in the localization of the lesion. If the abducent nerve (supplies the lateral rectus muscle) and the facial nerve are not functioning, this would suggest a lesion in the pons of the brain. If the vestibulocochlear nerve (balance and hearing) and the facial nerve are not functioning, this would suggest a lesion in the internal acoustic meatus. If the patient is excessively sensitive to sound in one ear, the lesion probably involves the nerve to the stapedius muscle, which arises from the facial nerve in the facial canal.

Loss of taste over the anterior two-thirds of the tongue implies that the facial nerve is damaged proximal to the point where it gives off the chorda tympani branch.

A firm swelling of the parotid salivary gland associated with impaired function of the facial nerve is strongly indicative of a cancer of the parotid gland with involvement of the nerve within the gland.

Deep lacerations of the face may involve branches of the facial nerve.

It should be remembered that the part of the facial nucleus that controls the muscles of the upper part of the face receives corticonuclear fibers from both cerebral hemispheres. Therefore it follows that with a lesion involving the upper motor neurons only the muscles of the lower part of the face will be paralyzed (Fig. 23-25). However, in patients with a lesion of the facial nerve motor nucleus or the facial nerve itself, that is, a lower motor neuron lesion, all the muscles on the affected side of the face will be paralyzed (Fig. 23-25). The lower eyelid will droop, and the angle of the mouth will sag. Tears will flow over the lower eyelid, and saliva will dribble from the corner of the mouth. The patient will be unable to close the eye and will be unable to expose the teeth fully on the affected side.

In patients with hemiplegia, the emotional movements of the face are usually preserved. This indicates that the upper motor neurons controlling these **mimetic movements** have a course separate

Fig. 23-25. Facial expression defects associated with lesions of:
1. Upper motor neurons.
2. Lower motor neurons.

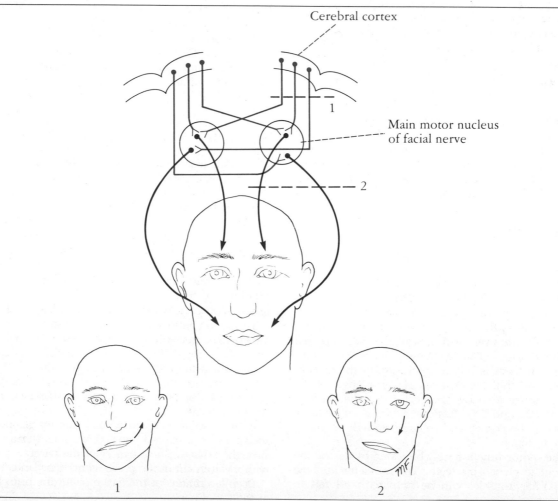

from that of the main corticobulbar fibers. A lesion involving this separate pathway alone results in a loss of emotional movements, but voluntary movements are preserved. A more extensive lesion will produce both mimetic and voluntary facial paralysis.

Bell's Palsy

Bell's palsy is a dysfunction of the facial nerve, as it lies within the facial canal; it is usually unilateral. The site of the dysfunction will determine which aspects of facial nerve function do not work.

The swelling of the nerve within the bony canal causes pressure on the nerve fibers; this results in a temporary loss of function of the nerve producing a lower motor neuron type of facial paralysis. The cause of Bell's palsy is not known; it sometimes follows exposure of the face to a cold draft.

Vestibulocochlear Nerve

The vestibulocochlear nerve innervates the utricle and saccule, which are sensitive to static changes in equilibrium; the semicircular canals, which are sensitive to changes in dynamic equilibrium; and the cochlea, which is sensitive to sound.

Vestibular function may be investigated with **caloric tests**. These involve the raising and lowering of the temperature in the external auditory meatus, which induces convection currents in the semicircular canals and stimulates the vestibular nerve endings.

Disturbances of vestibular function include giddiness (**vertigo**) and **nystagmus**. Vestibular nystagmus is an uncontrollable rhythmical oscillation of the eyes and the fast phase is away from the side of the lesion. Nystagmus is essentially a disturbance in the reflex control of the extraocular muscles, which is mainly a function of the semicircular canals.

Disturbances of cochlear function are manifested clinically as deafness and tinnitus. The patient's ability to hear a voice or a vibrating tuning fork should be tested; each ear should be tested separately.

Glossopharyngeal Nerve

The glossopharyngeal nerve supplies the stylopharyngeus muscle and sends secretomotor fibers to the parotid gland. Sensory fibers innervate the posterior one-third of the tongue for general sensation and taste.

The integrity of this nerve may be evaluated by testing the patient's general sensation or taste on the posterior third of the tongue.

Isolated lesions of the glossopharyngeal nerve are rare and usually also involve the vagus nerve.

Vagus Nerve

The vagus nerve innervates many important organs, but the examination of this nerve depends upon testing the function of the branches to the pharynx, soft palate, and larynx. The **pharyngeal** or **gag reflex** may be tested by touching the lateral wall of the pharynx with a spatula. This should immediately cause the patient to gag; that is, the pharyngeal muscles will contract. The afferent neuron of the pharyngeal reflex runs in the glossopharyngeal nerve, and the efferent neurons run in the glossopharyngeal (to the stylopharyngeus muscle) and vagus nerves (pharyngeal constrictor muscles). Unilateral lesions of the vagus will show little or no gag reflex on that side.

The innervation of the soft palate may be tested by asking the patient to say "ah." Normally, the soft palate rises and the uvula moves backward in the midline.

All the muscles of the larynx are supplied by the recurrent laryngeal branch of the vagus, except the cricothyroid muscle, which is supplied by the external laryngeal branch of the superior laryngeal branch of the vagus. Hoarseness or absence of the voice may occur as a symptom of vagal nerve palsy. The movements of the vocal cords may be tested by means of a laryngoscopic examination. Lesions involving the vagus nerve in the posterior cranial fossa commonly involve the glossopharyngeal, accessory, and hypoglossal nerves also.

Accessory Nerve

The accessory nerve supplies the sternocleidomastoid and the trapezius muscles by means of its spinal root. The patient should be asked to rotate his head to one side against resistance, when the sternocleidomastoid of the opposite side will be brought into action. Then he should be asked to shrug his shoulders, when the trapezius muscles come into action.

Lesions of the spinal part of the accessory nerve will result in paralysis of the sternocleidomastoid and trapezius muscles. The sternocleidomastoid muscle will atrophy and there will be weakness in turning the head to the opposite side. The trapezius muscle will also atrophy and the shoulder will droop on that side; there will also be weakness and difficulty in raising the arm above the horizontal.

Lesions of the spinal part of the accessory nerve may occur anywhere along its course and may result from tumors or trauma from stab or gunshot wounds in the neck.

Hypoglossal Nerve

The hypoglossal nerve supplies the intrinsic muscles of the tongue and the styloglossus, hyoglossus, and genioglossus muscles. To test the integrity of the nerve the patient is asked to put out his tongue; if there is a lower motor neuron lesion, the tongue will be observed to deviate toward the paralyzed side. The tongue will be smaller on the side of the lesion, owing to muscle atrophy, and fasciculation may accompany or precede the atrophy. Remember that the greater part of the hypoglossal nucleus receives corticonuclear fibers from both cerebral hemispheres. However, the part of the nucleus that supplies the genioglossus receives corticonuclear fibers only from the opposite cerebral hemisphere. If a patient has a lesion of the corticonuclear fibers, there will be no atrophy or fibrillation of the tongue and on protrusion the tongue will deviate to the side opposite the lesion. (Note that the genioglossus is the muscle that pulls the tongue forward.)

Lesions of the hypoglossal nerve may occur anywhere along its course and may result from tumor, demyelinating diseases, syringomyelia, and vascular accidents. Injury of the nerve in the neck may also follow stab and gunshot wounds.

CLINICAL PROBLEMS

Answers on Page 609

1. A 60-year-old woman was seen as an outpatient because she had suddenly developed double vision. She was watching her favorite television program the day before when it suddenly occurred. She had no other symptoms. After a complete physical examination it was found that her right eye, when at rest, was turned medially and she was unable to turn it laterally. A moderate amount of glucose was found in her urine and she had an abnormally elevated blood glucose level. When closely questioned, she admitted that recently she had noticed having to pass water more frequently, especially at night. She also said she often felt thirsty. She had lost 28 pounds during the past two years. Using your knowledge of neuroanatomy, can you explain the problem in her right eye? Do you think there is any connection between her glucosuria, high blood glucose, polyuria, polydipsia, and weight loss and her eye condition?

2. An 18-year-old man was admitted to the hospital unconscious after a serious motorcycle accident. After a complete physical examination and lateral and anteroposterior radiographs of the skull, it was found that the patient had a fracture involving the anterior cranial fossa. It also was noted that he had a slight but continuous blood-stained watery discharge from his left nostril. Three days later, he recovered consciousness and a further physical examination revealed that he could no longer smell. This was tested by asking him to recognize the smell of coffee, oil of cloves, and oil of peppermint. Using your knowledge of neuroanatomy, can you diagnose what is wrong with this patient? Is it possible for normal individuals with an acute sense of smell to be unable to recognize common scents? Could a tumor that had destroyed the olfactory cortex of one cerebral hemisphere be responsible for the anosmia in this patient?

3. A 72-year-old man with a known history of cerebrovascular problems visited his physician because three days previously he had begun to have trouble reading the paper. He complained that the print started to tilt and that he was beginning to see double. He also said that he found it difficult to see the steps when he descended the staircase to the physician's office. On physical examination, the patient had

weakness of movement of the right eye both downward and laterally. Using your knowledge of neuroanatomy, explain this patient's signs and symptoms. If we assume that a cranial nerve nucleus is the site of the lesion, is it the right one or the left one that is involved?

4. A 73-year-old man consulted his physician because he was becoming deaf. His only other complaints were that he didn't think he was as tall as he used to be and he was annoyed to find that each year he had to buy a size larger hat. The physician diagnosed osteitis deformans (Paget's disease) and explained to the medical students that this is a disease of bones involving bone absorption and new bone formation. These bony changes lead to enlargement of the skull, deformities of the vertebral column, and bowing of the long bones of the legs. The physician asked the students whether there was any connection between the bone disease and the patient's deafness and which other cranial nerve they would be particularly interested in testing. How would you have answered these questions?

5. A neurologist was visited by a 25-year-old man who complained of a feeling of heaviness in both legs and giddiness on walking. On examination, it was found that the patient had widely disseminated lesions involving the corticospinal tracts, the posterior white column, and the optic nerves. A diagnosis of multiple sclerosis (M.S.) was made. This disease of unknown origin primarily involves the white matter of the brain and spinal cord. Do you think this patient's symptoms of vertigo could be accounted for by this disease?

6. A 54-year-old woman with left-sided hemiplegia was examined by a fourth-year medical student. He very carefully tested each cranial nerve and noted any defects. During the examination, he stood behind the patient and gently grasped the trapezius muscles between his fingers and thumbs and asked the patient to shrug her shoulders against resistance. He was surprised to find that there was no evidence of weakness in either trapezius muscle and there was no muscle wasting. Would you expect to find evidence of weakness or wasting in the trapezius muscles of a patient with hemiplegia?

7. A 35-year-old man was admitted to the hospital with a complaint of severe pain of the right forehead and right eye. The pain had started three weeks previously and had progressively increased since then. One week ago he started to see double and this morning his wife had noticed that his right eye was turning out laterally. The physician in charge made a careful neurological workup on this patient and found a lateral deviation of the right eye, dilatation of the right pupil with loss of direct and consensual light reflexes, paralysis of accommodation on the right, and paralysis of all right-sided ocular movement except laterally. He initially advised the patient to have CT and MRI scans of the skull and later ordered a right-sided carotid arteriogram. The film showed an aneurysm of the internal carotid artery on the right side. Can you explain the signs and symptoms of this patient? Can you relate the signs and symptoms to the aneurysm?

8. During ward rounds, the neurologist demonstrated the signs and symptoms of neurosyphilis to a group of students. The patient was a 62-year-old man. The physician asked the students to note that both the patient's pupils were small and fixed and were not altered by shining a light in the eyes or shading the eyes. It was noted, however, that the pupils narrowed when the patient was asked to look from a distant object to the tip of his nose. Moreover, the pupils dilated again when he looked in the distance. "This is a good example of the Argyll Robertson pupil," said the physician. Using your knowledge of neuroanatomy, can you explain this curious pupillary reaction?

9. Describe the effects of a lesion at the following points along the visual pathway of the right eye:
   (a) Section of the right optic nerve
   (b) Midline section of the optic chiasma
   (c) Section of the right optic tract
   (d) Section of the right optic radiation
   (e) Destruction of the cortex of the right occipital pole

10. A 58-year-old woman was diagnosed as having an advanced carcinoma of the nasopharynx with neoplastic infiltration of the posterior cranial fossa. How would you test for the integrity of the ninth, tenth, and eleventh cranial nerves?

11. A 32-year-old woman with syringomyelia was found on physical examination to have impair-

ment of appreciation of pain and temperature of the face but preservation of light touch. Using your knowledge of neuroanatomy, can you explain this dissociated sensory loss in the face?

12. A 64-year-old man was seen as an outpatient. When he was asked to protrude his tongue, it turned to the right. The right half of the tongue was wrinkled and wasted. He attended his physician because he had a chronic cough and was rapidly losing weight. A diagnosis of right-sided bronchogenic carcinoma was made. How can you explain the tongue findings? Is there a possible connection between the paralysis of the tongue and the bronchogenic carcinoma?

13. A 55-year-old man woke up one morning to find the right side of his face paralyzed. When examined by his physician, he was found to have complete paralysis of the entire right side of the face. He was also found to have severe hypertension. The patient talked with a slightly slurred speech. The physician told the patient that he thought he had suffered a mild stroke and that he should be treated in bed. Do you think the physician's diagnosis was correct?

14. A physician turned to a group of students and said, "I think this patient has an advanced neoplasm in the posterior cranial fossa with involvement of the medulla oblongata and in particular the nuclei of the vagus nerve." What are the nuclei of the vagus nerve? Is it possible to have abnormal movements of the vocal cords in a patient with hemiplegia? Is it possible to have a solitary lesion of the vagal nuclei without involvement of other cranial nerve nuclei?

NATIONAL BOARD TYPE QUESTIONS

Answers on Page 621

IN THE FOLLOWING QUESTIONS, ANSWER:
   (a) IF (1), (2), AND (3) ONLY ARE CORRECT
   (b) IF (1) AND (3) ONLY ARE CORRECT
   (c) IF (2) AND (4) ONLY ARE CORRECT
   (d) IF (4) ONLY IS CORRECT, OR
   (e) IF ALL ARE CORRECT

1. The nuclei associated with the facial nerve include the following:
   (1) Nucleus of tractus solitarius
   (2) Superior salivatory nucleus
   (3) Lacrimal nucleus
   (4) Nucleus ambiguus

2. A patient with a unilateral upper motor neuron paralysis of the facial muscles can smile in response to a joke with both sides of his face, but not voluntarily. This can be explained as follows:
   (1) The corticobulbar fibers controlling voluntary movement of the facial muscles have been destroyed by a lesion.
   (2) A second separate pathway, possibly originating in the hypothalamus and descending to the motor nucleus of the facial nerve, is intact.
   (3) The facial nerve is intact.
   (4) There is a lesion involving the lower motor neuron.

3. Which of the following structure(s) participate(s) in the reception of sound?
   (1) Lateral lemniscus
   (2) Trigeminal nerve
   (3) Facial nerve
   (4) Medial lemniscus

4. The cerebral cortex plays an essential role in the following reflexes:
   (1) Corneal reflex
   (2) Consensual light reflex
   (3) Pupillary light reflex
   (4) Accommodation reflex

5. The nasal visual field of the right eye is projected to:
   (1) Nasal retina of the right eye
   (2) Right lateral geniculate body
   (3) Left lateral geniculate body
   (4) Both banks of the right calcarine fissure

6. Right pupillary constriction associated with light directed at the left eye requires the:
   (1) Left pretectal nucleus
   (2) Left optic radiation
   (3) Right Edinger-Westphal nucleus
   (4) Optic chiasma

Match the cranial nerve nuclei listed below on the left with the appropriate descending tracts

terminating on them listed on the right. An answer may be used more than once.

7. Inferior salivatory nucleus of the glossopharyngeal nerve
8. Nucleus of abducent nerve
9. Nucleus of facial nerve supplying muscles of lower part of face
10. Trigeminal motor nucleus
11. Nucleus of trochlear nerve

(a) Crossed corticobulbar tracts
(b) Uncrossed corticobulbar tracts
(c) Crossed and uncrossed corticobulbar tracts
(d) None of the above

Select the best response:

12. (a) A lesion involving the hypoglossal nerve will result in deviation of the tongue toward the same side as the lesion, when the tongue is protruded.
   (b) The hypoglossal nerve conducts taste impulses from the posterior third of the tongue.
   (c) The hypoglossal nerve emerges from the brainstem between the olive and the inferior cerebellar peduncle.
   (d) The hypoglossal nerve carries with it fibers from the third and fourth cervical nerves.
   (e) The fibers of the accessory nerve wind round the motor nucleus of the hypoglossal nerve beneath the floor of the fourth ventricle.
13. Which of the following statements concerning the trigeminal nuclei is (are) correct?
   (a) The main sensory nucleus lies within the medulla oblongata.
   (b) The spinal nucleus extends inferiorly as far as the fifth cervical segment.
   (c) Proprioceptive impulses from the muscles of mastication reach the mesencephalic nucleus along fibers that are part of the unipolar neurons of the nucleus.
   (d) The sensations of pain and temperature terminate in the main sensory nucleus.
   (e) The trigeminal lemniscus contains only efferent fibers from the ipsilateral sensory nuclei of the trigeminal nerve.

Match the cranial nerves listed below on the left with the appropriate function or structure supplied on the right.

14. Spinal part of accessory nerve
15. Oculomotor nerve
16. Trigeminal nerve
17. Facial nerve
18. Trochlear nerve
19. Glossopharyngeal nerve
20. Vagus nerve

(a) Muscles of mastication
(b) Opens the eye
(c) Sternocleidomastoid muscle
(d) Taste anterior two-thirds of the tongue
(e) None of the above

IN EACH OF THE FOLLOWING QUESTIONS, ANSWER:
   (a) IF (1) ONLY IS CORRECT
   (b) IF (2) ONLY IS CORRECT
   (c) IF BOTH (1) AND (2) ARE CORRECT, AND
   (d) IF NEITHER (1) NOR (2) IS CORRECT

21. Which of the following statements is (are) correct concerning the olfactory pathways?
   (1) The olfactory receptor cells are located in the mucous membrane of the nasal cavity above the level of the superior concha.
   (2) The olfactory nerve fibers are unmyelinated.
22. Which of the following statements is (are) correct concerning the optic nerve?
   (1) The nerve fibers of the optic nerve are surrounded by Schwann cells.
   (2) The optic nerve is surrounded by an extension of the subarachnoid space.
23. Which of the following statements is (are) correct?
   (1) Internal ophthalmoplegia is a condition in which the nerve supply to the sphincter pupillae and the ciliary muscle is lost.
   (2) External ophthalmoplegia is a condition in which the nerve supply to the superior oblique muscle is lost.
24. Which of the following statements is (are) correct concerning the nuclei of the trigeminal nerve?
   (1) The main sensory nucleus lies in the brainstem medial to the motor nucleus.
   (2) Proprioceptive impulses from the sternocleidomastoid and trapezius muscles end in the mesencephalic nucleus.
25. Which of the following statements is (are) correct concerning the facial nerve?

(1) The facial nerve leaves the posterior cranial fossa with the vestibulocochlear nerve and enters the internal acoustic meatus.

(2) The superior salivatory nucleus of the facial nerve innervates the parotid salivary gland.

ADDITIONAL READING

Altner, H. Physiology of taste. In R. R. Schmidt (ed.), *Fundamentals of Sensory Physiology* (2nd ed.). New York: Heidelberg and Berlin: Springer-Verlag, 1981. P. 218.

Ashworth, B., and Isherwood, I. *Clinical Neuro-Ophthalmology* (2nd ed.). Oxford: Blackwell, 1981.

Baker, R., Evinger, C., and McCrea, R. A. Some thoughts about the three neurons in the vestibular ocular reflex. *Ann. NY Acad. Sci.* 374:171, 1981.

Bender, M. B., and Bodis-Wollner, I. Visual dysfunction in optic tract lesions. *Ann. Neurol.* 3:187, 1978.

Brazis, P. W., Masden, J. C., and Biller, J. *Localization in Clinical Neurology* (2nd ed.). Boston: Little, Brown, 1990.

Büttner, V., and Dichgans, J. The vestibulo-ocular reflex and related functions. In S. Lessell and J. T. W. Van Dalen (eds.), *Neuro-Ophthalmology*. Amsterdam: Elsevier, and New York: Oxford University Press, 1984. Vol. 3, P. 205.

Crosby, E. C., Humphrey, T., and Lauer, E. W. *Correlative Anatomy of the Nervous System*. New York: Macmillan, 1962.

Dubner, R., Sessle, B. J., and Storey, A. T. Jaw, facial, and tongue reflexes. In R. Dubner, B. J. Sessle, and A. T. Storey (eds.), *The Neural Basis of Oral and Facial Function*. Amsterdam: Elsevier, 1978. P. 246.

Fitzgerald, M. J. T., Comerford, P. T., and Tuffery, A. Sources of innervation of the neuromuscular spindles in sternomastoid and trapezius. *J. Anat.* 134:471, 1982.

Frisen, L. The neurology of visual activity. *Brain* 103:639, 1980.

Hussein, M., Wilson, L. A., and Illingworth, R. Patterns of sensory loss following fractional posterior fossa Vth nerve section for trigeminal neuralgia. *J. Neurol. Neurosurg. Psychiatry* 45:786, 1982.

Judge, R. D., and Zuidema, G. D. *Physical Diagnosis: A Physiologic Approach to Clinical Examination* (2nd ed.). Boston: Little, Brown, 1968.

Masterson, R. B. Neural mechanisms for sound localization. *Annu. Rev. Physiol.* 46:275, 1984.

Merritt, H. H. *A Textbook of Neurology* (5th ed.). Philadelphia: Lea & Febiger, 1973.

Moran, D. T., Rowley, J. C., Jafek, B. W., and Lovell, M. A. The fine structure of the olfactory mucosa in man. *J. Neurocytol.* 11:721, 1982.

Ongeboer de Visser, B. W. The corneal reflex: Electrophysiological and anatomical data in man. *Prog. Neurobiol.* 15:71, 1980.

Parker, D. E. The vestibular apparatus. *Sci. Am.* 243:98, 1980.

Rinn, W. E. The neuropsychology of facial expression: A review of the neurological and psychological mechanisms for producing facial expressions. *Psychol. Bull.* 95:52, 1984.

Rudge, P. *Clinical Neurology*. Edinburgh: Churchill Livingstone, 1983.

Sawchenko, P. E. Central connections of the sensory and motor nuclei of the vagus nerve. *J. Auton. Nerv. Syst.* 9:13, 1983.

Sears, E. S., and Franklin, G. M. *Diseases of the Cranial Nerves in Neurology*. New York: Grune & Stratton, 1980. P. 471.

Snell, R. S. *Clinical Anatomy for Medical Students* (4th ed.). Boston: Little, Brown, 1992.

Snell, R. S., and Lemp, M. A. *Clinical Anatomy of the Eye*. Boston: Blackwell, 1989.

Spillane, J. D. *An Atlas of Clinical Neurology* (2nd ed.). New York and London: Oxford University Press, 1975.

Walton, J. N. *Brain's Diseases of the Nervous System*. New York and London: Oxford University Press, 1977.

Warr, W. B. Parallel ascending pathways from the cochlear nucleus. In William D. Neff (ed.), *Contributions to Sensory Physiology*. New York: Academic Press, 1982. Vol. 7, P. 1.

Williams, P. L., Warwick, R., Dyson, M., and Bannister, L. H. (eds.). *Gray's Anatomy* (37th Brit. ed.). Philadelphia: Saunders, 1990.

Wilson, V. J., and Peterson, B. W. Central pathways for vestibular reflexes. In B. V. Brooks (ed.) *Handbook of Physiology*, Section 1: *The Nervous System*. Bethesda, Maryland: American Physiological Society, 1981. Vol. 2, Part 1, P. 671.

Chapter 24
The Thalamus and
Its Connections

The thalamus is a large, egg-shaped mass of gray matter that forms the major part of the diencephalon. There are two thalami and one is situated on each side of the third ventricle (Figs. 24-1 and 13-3). The anterior end of the thalamus is narrow and rounded and forms the posterior boundary of the interventricular foramen. The posterior end is expanded to form the **pulvinar**, which overhangs the superior colliculus (Fig. 24-2). The inferior surface is continuous with the tegmentum of the midbrain. The medial surface of the thalamus forms part of the lateral wall of the third ventricle and is usually connected to the opposite thalamus by a band of gray matter (Fig. 24-2), the **interthalamic connection** (interthalamic adhesion).

SUBDIVISIONS OF THE THALAMUS

The thalamus is covered on its superior surface by a thin layer of white matter, called the **stratum zonale** (Fig. 24-1), and on its lateral surface by another layer, the **external medullary lamina** (Fig.

24-1). The gray matter of the thalamus is divided by a vertical sheet of white matter, the **internal medullary lamina**, into medial and lateral halves (Figs. 24-1 and 24-3). The internal medullary lamina consists of nerve fibers that pass from one thalamic nucleus to another. Anterosuperiorly, the internal medullary lamina splits so that it is Y-shaped. The thalamus thus is subdivided into three main parts; the **anterior part** lies between the limbs of the Y, and the **medial and lateral parts** lie on the sides of the stem of the Y (Fig. 24-3).

Each of the three parts of the thalamus contains a group of thalamic nuclei (Fig. 24-3). Moreover, smaller nuclear groups are situated within the internal medullary lamina, and some are located on the medial and lateral surfaces of the thalamus.

ANTERIOR PART OF THE THALAMUS

This part of the thalamus contains the **anterior thalamic nuclei** (Fig. 24-3). They receive the mammillothalamic tract from the mammillary

Fig. 24-1. Coronal section of the cerebral hemispheres, showing the position and relations of the thalamus.

nuclei. These anterior thalamic nuclei also receive reciprocal connections with the cingulate gyrus and hypothalamus. The function of the anterior thalamic nuclei is closely associated with that of the limbic system and is concerned with emotional tone and the mechanisms of recent memory.

MEDIAL PART OF THE THALAMUS

This part of the thalamus contains the large **dorsomedial nucleus** and several smaller nuclei (Fig. 24-3). The dorsomedial nucleus has two-way connections with the whole prefrontal cortex of the frontal lobe of the cerebral hemisphere. It also has similar connections with the hypothalamic nuclei. It is interconnected with all other groups of thalamic nuclei. The medial part of the thalamus is responsible for the integration of a large variety of sensory information, including somatic, visceral,

and olfactory information, and the relation of this information to one's emotional feelings and subjective states.

LATERAL PART OF THE THALAMUS

The nuclei are subdivided into a dorsal tier and a ventral tier (Fig. 24-3).

DORSAL TIER OF THE NUCLEI

This tier includes the **lateral dorsal nucleus**, the **lateral posterior nucleus**, and the **pulvinar**. The details of the connections of these nuclei are not clear. They are known, however, to have interconnections with other thalamic nuclei, and with the parietal lobe, cingulate gyrus, and occipital and temporal lobes.

Fig. 24-2. Posterior view of the brainstem, showing the thalamus and the tectum of the midbrain.

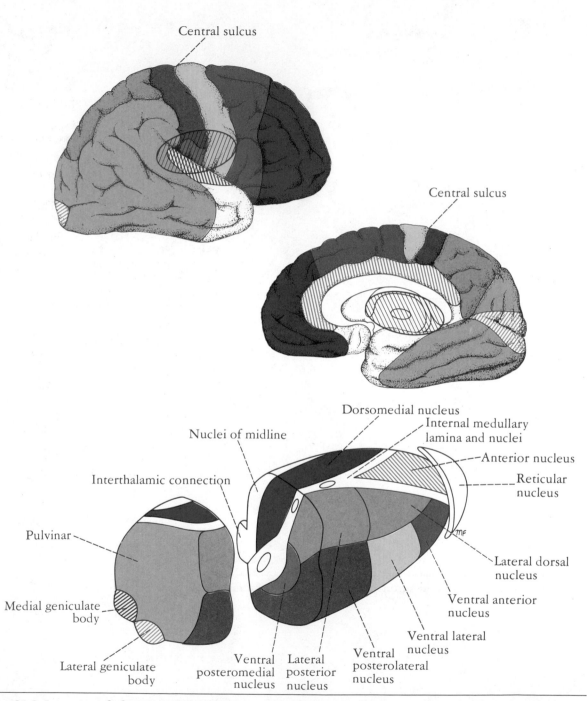

Fig. 24-3. Important thalamocortical projections. Adapted from an original painting by Frank H. Netter, M.D., from *The CIBA Collection of Medical Illustrations*, copyright by CIBA Pharmaceutical Company, Division of CIBA-GEIGY Corporation.

VENTRAL TIER OF THE NUCLEI

This tier consists of the following in a craniocaudal sequence:

1. **Ventral anterior nucleus** (Fig. 24-3). This nucleus is connected to the reticular formation, the substantia nigra, the corpus striatum, and the premotor cortex as well as to many of the other thalamic nuclei. Since this nucleus lies on the pathway between the corpus striatum and the motor areas of the frontal cortex, it probably influences the activities of the motor cortex.

2. **Ventral lateral nucleus** (Fig. 24-3). This nucleus has connections similar to those of the ventral anterior nucleus but, in addition, has a major input from the cerebellum and a minor input from the red nucleus. Its main projections pass to the motor and premotor regions of the cerebral cortex. Here again this thalamic nucleus probably influences motor activity.

3. **Ventral posterior nucleus.** This nucleus is subdivided into the **ventral posteromedial nucleus** and the **ventral posterolateral nucleus** (Fig. 24-3). The ventral posteromedial nucleus receives the ascending trigeminal and gustatory pathways, while the ventral posterolateral nucleus receives the important ascending sensory tracts, the medial and spinal lemnisci. The thalamocortical projections from these important nuclei pass through the posterior limb of the internal capsule and corona radiata to the primary somatic sensory areas of the cerebral cortex in the postcentral gyrus (areas 3, 1, and 2).

Other Nuclei of the Thalamus

These nuclei include the intralaminar nuclei, the midline nuclei, the reticular nucleus, and the medial and lateral geniculate bodies.

The **intralaminar nuclei** are small collections of nerve cells within the internal medullary lamina (Fig. 24-3). They receive afferent fibers from the reticular formation as well as fibers from the spinothalamic and trigeminothalamic tracts; they send efferent fibers to other thalamic nuclei, which in turn project to the cerebral cortex, and fibers to the corpus striatum.

The **midline nuclei** consist of groups of nerve cells adjacent to the third ventricle and in the interthalamic connection (Fig. 24-3). They receive afferent fibers from the reticular formation. Their precise functions are unknown.

The **reticular nucleus** is a thin layer of nerve cells sandwiched between the external medullary lamina and the posterior limb of the internal capsule (Fig. 24-3). Afferent fibers converge on this nucleus from the cerebral cortex and the reticular formation and its output is mainly to other thalamic nuclei. The function of this nucleus is not fully understood, but it may be concerned with a mechanism by which the cerebral cortex regulates thalamic activity.

The **medial geniculate body** forms part of the auditory pathway and is a swelling on the posterior surface of the thalamus beneath the pulvinar (Fig. 24-3). Afferent fibers to the medial geniculate body form the **inferior brachium** and come from the inferior colliculus. It will be remembered that the inferior colliculus receives the termination of the fibers of the lateral lemniscus. The medial geniculate body receives auditory information from both ears but predominantly from the opposite ear.

The efferent fibers leave the medial geniculate body to form the auditory radiation, which passes to the auditory cortex of the superior temporal gyrus. The **lateral geniculate body** forms part of the visual pathway and is a swelling on the undersurface of the pulvinar of the thalamus (Fig. 24-3). The nucleus consists of six layers of nerve cells and is the terminus of all but a few fibers of the optic tract (except the fibers passing to the pretectal nucleus). The fibers are the axons of the ganglion cell layer of the retina and come from the temporal half of the ipsilateral eye and from the nasal half of the contralateral eye, the latter fibers crossing the midline in the optic chiasma. Each lateral geniculate body, therefore, receives visual information from the opposite field of vision.

The efferent fibers leave the lateral geniculate body to form the visual radiation, which passes to the visual cortex of the occipital lobe.

Connections of the Thalamus

The following important neuronal loops exist between the thalamic nuclei and other areas of the central nervous system:

1. Every thalamic nucleus (except the reticular nucleus) sends axons to different parts of the cere-

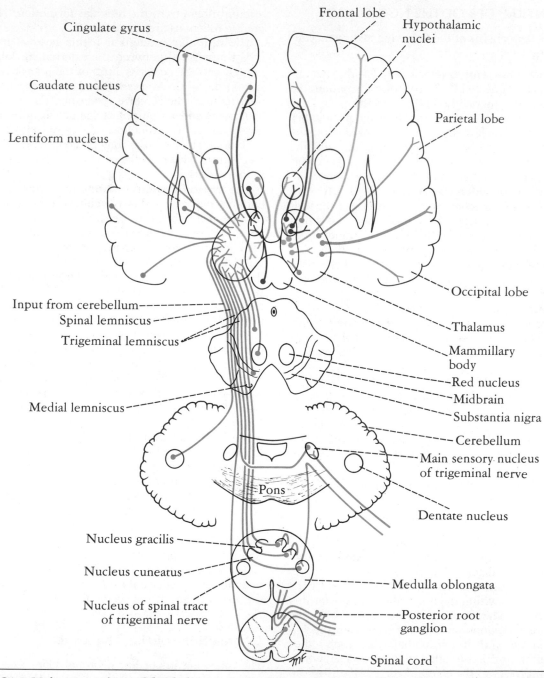

Fig. 24-4. Main connections of the thalamus. On the left are shown the afferent fibers and on the right the efferent fibers.

bral cortex (Fig. 24-3) and every part of the cerebral cortex sends reciprocal fibers back to the thalamic nuclei. This would indicate that information received by the thalamus is always shared with the cerebral cortex and that the cortex and thalamus can modify each other's activities.

2. The thalamus is an important relay station for two sensory-motor axonal loops involving the cerebellum and the basal nuclei: (a) the cerebellar-rubro-thalamic-cortical-ponto-cerebellar loop and (b) the cortical-striatal-pallidal-thalamic-cortical loop, both of which are necessary for normal voluntary movement.

The main connections of the various thalamic nuclei are summarized in Figure 24-4.

Function of the Thalamus

It is not considered essential for a practicing physician to have a detailed knowledge of all the thalamic nuclei and their connections. Although an enormous amount of research has been devoted to this area, we still know very little about the functional significance of many of the nuclei.

The following basic principles should be committed to memory:

1. The thalamus is made up of complicated collections of nerve cells that are centrally placed in the brain and are interconnected.
2. A vast amount of sensory information of all types (except smell) converges on the thalamus and presumably is integrated through the interconnections between the nuclei. The resulting information pattern is distributed to other parts of the central nervous system. It is probable that olfactory information is first integrated at a lower level with taste and other sensations and is relayed to the thalamus from the amygdaloid complex and hippocampus through the mammillothalamic tract.

3. Anatomically and functionally, the thalamus and the cerebral cortex are closely linked. The fiber connections have been established, and it is known that following removal of the cortex the thalamus can appreciate crude sensations. However, the cerebral cortex is required for the interpretation of sensations based on past experiences.

4. The thalamus possesses certain very important nuclei whose connections have been clearly established. These include the ventral posteromedial nucleus, the ventral posterolateral nucleus, the medial geniculate body, and the lateral geniculate body. Their positions and connections should be learned.

5. The large dorsomedial nucleus has extensive connections with the frontal lobe cortex and hypothalamus. There is considerable evidence that this nucleus lies on the pathway that is concerned with subjective feeling states and the personality of the individual.

6. The intralaminar nuclei are closely connected with the activities of the reticular formation and they receive much of their information from this source. Their strategic position enables them to control the level of overall activity of the cerebral cortex. The intralaminar nuclei are thus able to influence the levels of consciousness and alertness in an individual.

CLINICAL NOTES

Since the thalamus is such an important relay and integrative center, it follows that disease of this area of the central nervous system will have profound effects. The thalamus may be invaded by neoplasm, undergo degeneration following disease of its arterial supply, or be damaged by hemorrhage.

LESIONS OF THE THALAMUS

Sensory Loss

These lesions usually result from thrombosis or hemorrhage of one of the arteries supplying the thalamus. Damage to the ventral posteromedial nucleus and the ventral posterolateral nucleus will result in the loss of all forms of sensation, including light touch, tactile localization and discrimination, and muscle joint sense from the opposite side of the body.

Thalamic Syndrome

This syndrome may occur as the patient is recovering from a thalamic infarct. Spontaneous pain, which is often excessive and unpleasant, occurs on the opposite side of the body. The painful sensation may be aroused by light touch or cold and may fail to respond to powerful analgesic drugs.

Abnormal involuntary movements and the **thalamic hand** are described on page 257.

CLINICAL PROBLEMS

For clinical problems concerning the thalamus, see page 257.

NATIONAL BOARD TYPE QUESTIONS

Answers on Page 621

In each of the following questions, answer:
- (a) If (1) only is correct
- (b) If (2) only is correct
- (c) If both (1) and (2) are correct, and
- (d) If neither (1) nor (2) is correct

1. Which of the following statements is (are) correct?
   (1) All types of sensory information, with the exception of smell, reach the thalamic nuclei via afferent fibers.
   (2) Very few afferent fibers reach the thalamic nuclei from the cerebral cortex.

2. Which of the following statements is (are) correct?
   (1) The intralaminar nuclei of the thalamus are closely connected with the reticular formation.
   (2) The intralaminar nuclei can influence the levels of consciousness and alertness.

3. Which of the following statements is (are) correct?
   (1) The thalamus is covered on its superior surface by the external medullary lamina.
   (2) The stratum zonale is an area of gray matter lying on the lateral surface of the thalamus.

4. Which of the following statements is (are) correct?
   (1) The Y-shaped internal medullary lamina subdivides the thalamus into three main parts.
   (2) The ventral posteromedial nucleus receives the ascending trigeminal and gustatory pathways.

5. Which of the following axonal loops is (are) correct concerning the thalamus and voluntary movement?
   (1) The cerebellar-rubro-thalamic-cortical-ponto-cerebellar loop.
   (2) The mammillary body–thalamus–amygdaloid nucleus–dentate gyrus loop.

In the following questions, answer:
- (a) If (1), (2), and (3) only are correct
- (b) If (1) and (3) only are correct
- (c) If (2) and (4) only are correct
- (d) If (4) only is correct, or
- (e) If all are correct

6. Which of the following statements is (are) correct concerning the thalamic nuclei?
   (1) The reticular nucleus is part of the reticular formation.
   (2) The ventral posterolateral nucleus receives the ascending sensory tracts of the medial and spinal lemnisci.
   (3) The intralaminar nuclei lie within the external medullary lamina.
   (4) The projections from the ventral posterolateral nucleus ascend to the postcentral gyrus through the posterior limb of the internal capsule.

7. Which of the following statements is (are) correct concerning the medial geniculate body?
   (1) The medial geniculate body receives auditory information from the inferior colliculus and from the lateral lemniscus.
   (2) The medial geniculate body receives auditory information from both ears but predominantly from the opposite ear.
   (3) The medial geniculate body projects to the auditory cortex of the superior temporal gyrus.
   (4) The medial geniculate body projects from the posterior surface of the thalamus.

8. Which of the following statements is (are) correct concerning the lateral geniculate body?
   (1) The lateral geniculate body receives most of the fibers of the optic tract.
   (2) Each lateral geniculate body receives visual information from the opposite field of vision.
   (3) The lateral geniculate body has a nucleus made up of six layers of nerve cells.
   (4) The lateral geniculate body is part of the midbrain at the level of the red nucleus.

ADDITIONAL READING

Ajmone Marsan, C. The thalamus: Data on its functional anatomy and on some aspects of thalamocortical integration. *Arch. Ital. Biol.* 103:847, 1965.

Angevine, J. B., Jr., Locke, S., and Yakovlev, P. Limbic nuclei of thalamus and connections of limbic cortex; thalamocortical projections of the magnocellular medial dorsal nucleus in man. *Arch. Neurol.* 10:165, 1964.

Bertrand, G., Jasper, H. H., and Wong, A. Microelectrode study of the human thalamus, functional organization in the ventrobasal complex. *Confin. Neurol.* 29:81, 1967.

Carpenter, M. B. Ventral tier thalamic nuclei. In D. Williams (ed.), *Modern Trends in Neurology.* London and Washington, D.C.:Butterworth, 1967. P. 1.

Guyton, A. C. *Textbook of Medical Physiology* (7th ed.). Philadelphia and London: Saunders, 1986.

Houser, C. R., Vaughn, J. E., Barber, R. P., and Roberts, E. GABA neurons are the major cell type of the nucleus reticularis thalami. *Brain Res.* 200:341, 1980.

Jones, E. G. *The Thalamus.* New York: Plenum, 1985.

Markowitsch, H. J. Thalamic mediodorsal nucleus and memory: A critical evaluation of studies in animals and man. *Neurosci. Behav. Rev.* 6:351, 1982.

Purpura, D., and Yahr, M. D. *The Thalamus.* New York: Columbia University Press, 1966.

Scheibel, M. A., and Scheibel, A. B. The organization of the nucleus reticularis thalami; a Golgi study. *Brain Res.* 1:43, 1966.

Steriade, M. Mechanisms underlying cortical activation: Neuronal organization and properties of the midbrain reticular core and intralaminar thalamic nuclei. In O. Pompeiano and C. A. Marsan (eds.), *Awareness.* New York: Raven, 1981. P. 327.

Van Buren, J. M., and Borke, R. C. *Variations and Connections of the Human Thalamus.* Berlin and Vienna: Springer, 1972.

Chapter 25
The Hypothalamus and Its Connections

The hypothalamus, although small in size, is a very important part of the central nervous system. It controls the autonomic nervous system and the endocrine system and thus indirectly controls body homeostasis. The hypothalamus is well placed for this purpose, lying in the center of the limbic system. It is the site of numerous converging and diverging neuronal pathways and through its adequate blood supply it is able to sample the blood chemistry. The hypothalamus makes appropriate controlling responses following the integration of its nervous and chemical inputs.

The hypothalamus is that part of the diencephalon that extends from the region of the optic chiasma to the caudal border of the mammillary bodies. It lies below the thalamus and forms the floor and the inferior part of the lateral walls of the third ventricle (Fig. 25-1). Anterior to the hypothalamus is an area that for functional reasons is often included in the hypothalamus. Because it extends forward from the optic chiasma to the lamina terminalis and the anterior commissure, it is referred to as the preoptic area. Caudally, the hy-

pothalamus merges into the tegmentum of the midbrain. The lateral boundary of the hypothalamus is formed by the internal capsule.

When observed from below (Fig. 25-2), the hypothalamus is seen to be related to the following structures, from anterior to posterior: (1) the optic chiasma, (2) the tuber cinereum and the infundibulum, and (3) the mammillary bodies.

HYPOTHALAMIC NUCLEI

The following principal groups of nuclei are present. For purposes of description, the nuclei are divided by an imaginary parasagittal plane into medial and lateral zones. Lying within the plane are the columns of the fornix and the mammillothalamic tract, which serve as markers (Figs. 25-3 and 25-4).

Medial Zone

In the medial zone, the following hypothalamic nuclei may be recognized, from anterior to poste-

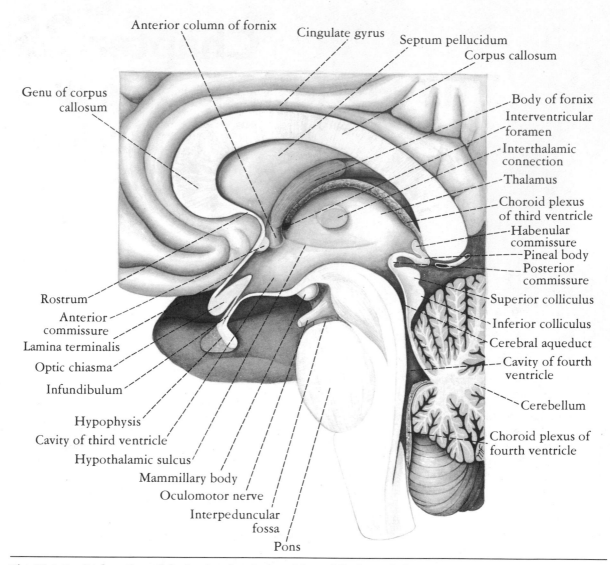

Fig. 25-1. Sagittal section of the brain, showing position of the hypothalamus.

rior: (1) the **preoptic nucleus**, (2) the **paraventricular nucleus**, (3) the **dorsomedial nucleus**, (4) the **ventromedial nucleus**, (5) the **infundibular nucleus**, and (6) the **posterior nucleus**.

Lateral Zone

In the lateral zone, the following hypothalamic nuclei may be recognized, from anterior to posterior: (1) the **supraoptic nucleus**, (2) the **large lateral** nucleus, (3) the **tuberomammillary nucleus**, and (4) the **lateral tuberal nuclei**.

Some of the nuclei, for example, the preoptic nucleus, extend into both the medial and lateral zones. The mammillary body with its medial and lateral mammillary nuclei overlaps both zones. The **suprachiasmatic nucleus** also overlaps both zones and consists of a small group of neurons lying just above the optic chiasma; it receives nerve fibers from the retina. It should be emphasized

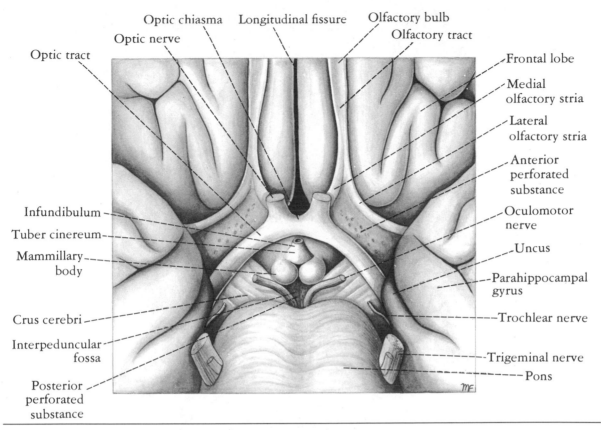

Fig. 25-2. Inferior surface of the brain, showing parts of the hypothalamus.

that most of the hypothalamic nuclei have ill-defined boundaries.

AFFERENT CONNECTIONS OF THE HYPOTHALAMUS

The hypothalamus, which lies in the center of the limbic system, receives many afferent fibers from the viscera, the olfactory mucous membrane, the cerebral cortex, and the limbic system.

The afferent connections are numerous and complex; only the main pathways (Fig. 25-5) are described here:

1. **Visceral and somatic afferents** reach the hypothalamus through collateral branches of the lemniscal afferent fibers and through the reticular formation.

2. **Olfaction** travels through the medial forebrain bundle.

3. **Corticohypothalamic fibers** arise from the frontal lobe of the cerebral cortex and pass directly to the hypothalamus.

4. **Hippocampohypothalamic fibers** pass from the hippocampus through the fornix to the mammillary body. Many neurophysiologists regard the hypothalamus as the main output pathway of the limbic system.

5. **Amygdalohypothalamic fibers** pass from the amygdaloid complex to the hypothalamus through the stria terminalis and by a route that passes inferior to the lentiform nucleus.

6. **Thalamohypothalamic fibers** arise from the dorsomedial and midline thalamic nuclei.

7. **Tegmental fibers** arise from the midbrain.

Fig. 25-3. Sagittal section of the brain, showing the hypothalamic nuclei.
A. Medial zone nuclei lying medial to the plane of the fornix and the mammillothalamic tract.
B. Lateral zone nuclei lying lateral to the plane of the fornix and the mammillothalamic tract.

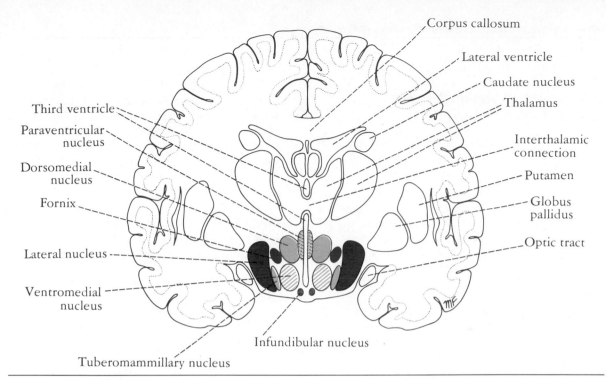

Fig. 25-4. Coronal section of cerebral hemispheres, showing position of hypothalamic nuclei.

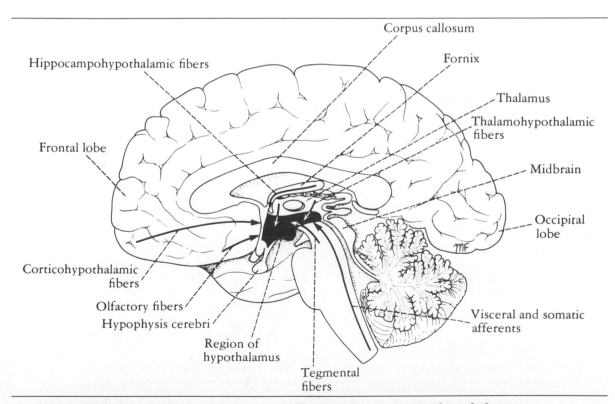

Fig. 25-5. Sagittal section of brain, showing main afferent pathways entering hypothalamus.

EFFERENT CONNECTIONS OF THE HYPOTHALAMUS

The efferent connections of the hypothalamus are also numerous and complex, and only the main pathways (Fig. 25-6) are described here:

1. The **mammillothalamic tract** arises in the mammillary body and terminates in the anterior nucleus of the thalamus. Here the pathway is relayed to the cingulate gyrus.
2. The **mammillotegmental tract** arises from the mammillary body and terminates in the cells of the reticular formation in the tegmentum of the midbrain.
3. **Descending fibers to the brainstem and spinal cord** influence the peripheral neurons of the autonomic nervous system. It is believed that, through a series of neurons in the reticular formation, the hypothalamus is connected to the parasympathetic nuclei of the oculomotor, facial, glossopharyngeal, and vagus nerves in the brainstem. In a similar manner, the reticulo-

spinal fibers probably connect the hypothalamus with sympathetic cells of origin in the lateral gray horns of the first thoracic segment to the second lumbar segment of the spinal cord and the sacral parasympathetic outflow at the level of the second, third, and fourth sacral segments of the spinal cord.

CONNECTIONS OF THE HYPOTHALAMUS WITH THE HYPOPHYSIS CEREBRI

The hypothalamus is connected to the hypophysis cerebri (pituitary gland) by two pathways: (1) nerve fibers that travel from the supraoptic and paraventricular nuclei to the posterior lobe of the hypophysis, and (2) long and short portal blood vessels that connect sinusoids in the median eminence and infundibulum with capillary plexuses in the anterior lobe of the hypophysis (Fig. 25-7). These pathways enable the hypothalamus to influence the activities of the endocrine glands.

Fig. 25-6. Sagittal section of brain, showing main efferent pathways leaving hypothalamus.

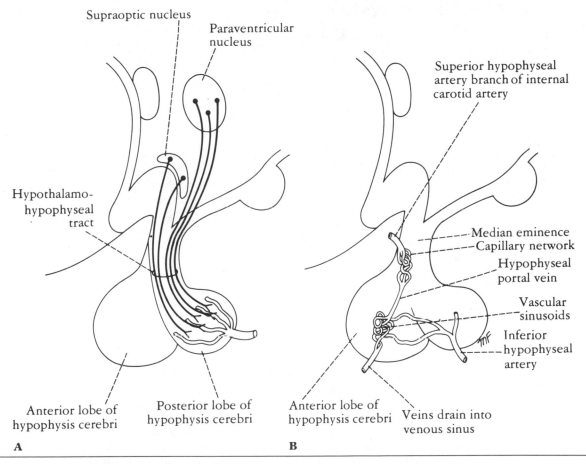

Supraoptic nucleus

Paraventricular nucleus

Hypothalamo-hypophyseal tract

Superior hypophyseal artery branch of internal carotid artery

Median eminence
Capillary network
Hypophyseal portal vein
Vascular sinusoids
Inferior hypophyseal artery

Anterior lobe of hypophysis cerebri

Posterior lobe of hypophysis cerebri

Anterior lobe of hypophysis cerebri

Veins drain into venous sinus

A   B

**Fig. 25-7. A. Hyothalamohypophyseal tract.
B. Hypophyseal portal system.**

HYPOTHALAMOHYPOPHYSEAL TRACT

The hormones **vasopressin** and **oxytocin** are synthesized in the nerve cells of the supraoptic and paraventricular nuclei. The hormones are passed along the axons together with carrier proteins called **neurophysins** and are released at the axon terminals (Fig. 25-7). Here the hormones are absorbed into the bloodstream in the capillaries of the posterior lobe of the hypophysis. The hormone vasopressin (antidiuretic hormone) is produced mainly in the nerve cells of the supraoptic nucleus. Its function is to cause **vasoconstriction.** It also has an important **antidiuretic function**, causing an increased absorption of water in the distal convoluted tubules and collecting tubules of the kidney. The other hormone is oxytocin, which is produced mainly in the paraventricular nucleus. Oxytocin stimulates the contraction of the smooth muscle of the uterus and causes contraction of the myoepithelial cells that surround the alveoli of the mammary gland.

The supraoptic nucleus, which produces vasopressin, acts as an **osmoreceptor**. Should the osmotic pressure of the blood circulating through the nucleus be too high, the nerve cells increase their production of vasopressin and the antidiuretic effect of this hormone will increase the reabsorption of water from the kidney. By this means, the osmotic pressure of the blood will return to normal limits.

HYPOPHYSEAL PORTAL SYSTEM

The hypophyseal portal system is formed on each side from the superior hypophyseal artery, which is a branch of the internal carotid artery (Fig. 25-7). The artery enters the median eminence and divides into tufts of capillaries. These capillaries drain into long and short descending vessels that end in the anterior lobe of the hypophysis by dividing into vascular sinusoids that pass between the secretory cells of the anterior lobe.

The portal system carries **releasing hormones** and **release-inhibiting hormones**, which are produced in the neurons of the hypothalamus, to the secretory cells of the anterior lobe of the hypophysis. The releasing hormones stimulate the production and release of **adrenocorticotropic hormone** (ACTH), **follicle-stimulating hormone** (FSH), **luteinizing hormone** (LH), **thyrotropic hormone** or **thyroid-stimulating hormone** (TSH) and **growth hormone** (GH). The release of inhibiting hormones inhibits the release of the **melanocyte-stimulating hormone** (MSH) and **luteotropic hormone** (LTH). LTH (also known as the **lactogenic hormone** or **prolactin**) stimulates the corpus luteum to secrete progesterone and the mammary gland to produce milk. The growth hormone inhibitory hormone (somatostatin) inhibits the release of growth hormone.

The neurons of the hypothalamus that are responsible for the production of the releasing hormones and the release-inhibiting hormones are influenced by the afferent fibers passing to the hypothalamus. They also are influenced by the level of the hormone produced by the target organ controlled by the hypophysis. Should the level of thyroxine in the blood, for example, fall, then the releasing factor for the thyrotropic hormone would be produced in increased quantities.

FUNCTIONS OF THE HYPOTHALAMUS

AUTONOMIC CONTROL

The hypothalamus has a controlling influence on the autonomic nervous system and appears to integrate the autonomic and neuroendocrine systems, thus preserving body homeostasis. Essentially, the hypothalamus should be regarded as a higher nervous center for the control of lower autonomic centers in the brainstem and spinal cord (Fig. 25-8).

Electrical stimulation of the hypothalamus in animal experiments shows that the anterior hypothalamic area and the preoptic area influence parasympathetic responses; these include lowering of the blood pressure, slowing of the heart rate, contraction of the bladder, increased motility of the gastrointestinal tract, increased acidity of the gastric juice, salivation, and pupillary constriction.

Stimulation of the posterior and lateral nuclei causes sympathetic responses, which include elevation of blood pressure, acceleration of the heart rate, cessation of peristalsis in the gastrointestinal tract, pupillary dilation, and hyperglycemia. These responses would lead one to believe that there exist in the hypothalamus areas that might be termed "parasympathetic and sympathetic centers." However, it has been shown that considerable overlap of function occurs in these areas.

Fig. 25-8. Diagram depicting the hypothalamus as the chief center of the brain for controlling the internal milieu of the body.

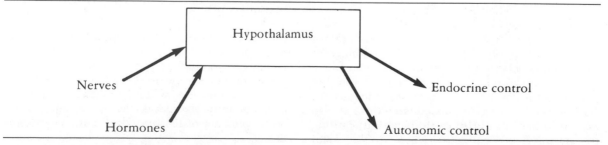

ENDOCRINE CONTROL

The nerve cells of the hypothalamus, by producing the **releasing factors** or **release-inhibiting factors**, control the production of **ACTH, FSH, LH, TSH, GH, MSH,** and **LTH.** Some of these hormones act directly on body tissues, while others, such as **ACTH,** act through an endocrine organ, which in turn produces additional hormones that influence the activities of general body tissues. It should be pointed out that each stage is controlled by negative or positive feedback mechanisms.

NEUROSECRETION

The secretion of vasopressin and oxytocin by the supraoptic and paraventricular nuclei is discussed on page 477.

TEMPERATURE REGULATION

The anterior portion of the hypothalamus controls those mechanisms that dissipate heat loss. Experimental stimulation of this area causes dilatation of skin blood vessels and sweating, which lower the body temperature. Stimulation of the posterior portion of the hypothalamus results in vasoconstriction of the skin blood vessels and inhibition of sweating; there also may be shivering, in which the skeletal muscles produce heat.

REGULATION OF FOOD AND WATER INTAKE

Stimulation of the lateral region of the hypothalamus initiates eating and increases food intake. This lateral region sometimes is referred to as the **hunger center.** Stimulation of the medial region of the hypothalamus inhibits eating and reduces food intake. This area is referred to as the **satiety center.**

Experimental stimulation of other areas in the lateral region of the hypothalamus causes an immediate increase in water intake; this area is referred to as the **thirst center.** In addition, the hypothalamus exerts a careful control on the osmolarity of the blood through the secretion of vasopressin by the posterior lobe of the hypophysis and its influence on the distal convoluted tubules and collecting tubules of the kidneys.

EMOTION AND BEHAVIOR

Emotion and behavior are a function of the hypothalamus, the limbic system, and the prefrontal cortex. Some authorities believe that the hypothalamus is the integrator of afferent information received from other areas of the nervous system, and brings about the physical expression of emotion; it can produce an increase in the heart rate, elevate the blood pressure, cause dryness of the mouth, flushing or pallor of the skin, and sweating, and can often produce a massive peristaltic activity of the gastrointestinal tract.

CONTROL OF CIRCADIAN RHYTHMS

The hypothalamus controls many circadian rhythms, including body temperature, adrenocortical activity, eosinophil count, and renal secretion. Sleeping and wakefulness, although dependent on the activities of the thalamus, the limbic system, and the reticular activating system, are also controlled by the hypothalamus. Lesions of the anterior part of the hypothalamus seriously interfere with the rhythm of sleeping and waking. The suprachiasmatic nucleus, which receives afferent fibers from the retina, appears to play an important role in controlling the biological rhythms. Nerve impulses generated in response to variations in the intensity of light are transmitted via this nucleus to influence the activities of many of the hypothalamic nuclei.

CLINICAL NOTES

It is clear that the hypothalamus consists of a number of complex, ill-defined nuclei situated in the floor and lower lateral walls of the third ventricle. The activities of the hypothalamus are modified by information received along numerous afferent pathways from different parts of the central nervous system (especially from the limbic system and the prefrontal cortex) and by the plasma levels of circulating hormones. It exerts its influence on bodily functions through the autonomic nervous system and the endocrine system.

Although small in size, the hypothalamus should not be interpreted as a structure of little importance. It is the chief center of the brain for maintaining the internal milieu of the body (Fig. 25-8). There is hardly a tissue in the body that escapes its influence.

The connections of the hypothalamus are extremely complicated and only the major pathways should be committed to memory for use in clinical work.

CLINICAL DISORDERS ASSOCIATED WITH HYPOTHALAMIC LESIONS

The hypothalamus may be the site of inflammation, neoplasm, or vascular disorder. Because of its deep-seated central position, it can be pressed upon by tumors of the surrounding brain tissue or may be compressed as the result of the development of internal hydrocephalus. Its widespread influence on many homeostatic and behavioral functions means that a lesion of the hypothalamus will produce a large number of different syndromes. Thus, it is important to remember that an acute lesion is more likely to produce signs and symptoms than a slowly growing tumor.

Obesity and Wasting

Severe obesity can occur as the result of hypothalamic lesions. It is generally associated with genital hypoplasia or atrophy.

Wasting is less common than obesity in hypothalamic disease. Severe cachexia is suggestive of damage to the hypophysis (pituitary gland).

Sexual Disorders

In children there may be sexual retardation and, rarely, sexual precocity with hypothalamic lesions. After puberty, the patient with hypothalamic disease may have impotence or amenorrhea.

Hyperthermia and Hypothermia

Hyperthermia can follow lesions of the hypothalamus caused by head injury or following surgical operations in the region of the hypothalamus. The patient with hyperthermia is otherwise normal and has no signs of malaise, which occurs with pyrexia secondary to infections.

Hypothermia also can follow a lesion of the hypothalamus.

Diabetes Insipidus

This disease results from a lesion of the supraoptic nucleus or from the interruption of the nervous pathway to the posterior lobe of the hypophysis. Characteristically, the patient passes large volumes of urine of low specific gravity. As a result, the patient is extremely thirsty and drinks large quantities of fluids. The condition must be distinguished from diabetes mellitus, in which there is glucosuria.

Disturbances of Sleep

The occurrence of either frequent short periods of sleep during the waking hours or insomnia has been observed in patients with hypothalamic lesions.

Emotional Disorders

Attacks of unexplained weeping or laughter, uncontrollable rage, depressive reactions, or even maniacal outbursts all have been observed in patients with hypothalamic lesions.

CLINICAL PROBLEMS

Answers on Page 610

1. A 17-year-old boy was admitted into the medical ward for observation. The tentative diagnosis was *Fröhlich's syndrome.* He had a three-month history of severe headaches. More recently, he had had attacks of vomiting, and one week ago he had noticed problems with his eyesight. The

patient said that he had difficulty seeing objects on the lateral side of both eyes. His parents were concerned that he was putting on weight, because he was especially fat over the lower part of the trunk. On physical examination, the boy was found to be 6 feet 3 inches tall; he had excessive trunk obesity. The testes and penis were small, and the pubic and axillary hair was absent. A lateral radiograph of the skull showed enlargement of the sella turcica with erosion of the dorsum sellae. An examination of the eye fields confirmed that the patient had partial bitemporal hemianopia. Using your knowledge of neuroanatomy, explain the symptoms and signs of this patient.

2. A 40-year-old woman was involved in an automobile accident in which she sustained severe head injuries. Following a slow but uneventful recovery, she was released from the hospital without any residual signs or symptoms. Six months later, the patient started to complain of frequency of micturition and was passing very large quantities of pale urine. She also said that she always seemed thirsty and would often drink 10 glasses of water in one morning. Using your knowledge of neuroanatomy and neurophysiology, do you think there is any connection between the urinary symptoms and her automobile accident?

3. Do you think it is possible that a patient with hydrocephalus could have a malfunctioning hypothalamus? If so, can you explain the connection?

4. Sherrington once stated in a scientific publication in 1947 that the hypothalamus should be regarded as the "head ganglion" of the autonomic nervous system. What is the relationship that exists between the hypothalamus and the autonomic nervous system?

5. Explain what is meant by the terms the *hypothalamohypophyseal tract* and the *hypophyseal portal system*.

NATIONAL BOARD TYPE QUESTIONS

Answers on Page 621

IN EACH OF THE FOLLOWING QUESTIONS, ANSWER:

(a) IF (1) ONLY IS CORRECT
(b) IF (2) ONLY IS CORRECT
(c) IF BOTH (1) AND (2) ARE CORRECT, AND
(d) IF NEITHER (1) NOR (2) IS CORRECT

1. Which of the following statements is (are) correct?
   (1) The hypothalamus lies below the thalamus in the tectum of the midbrain.
   (2) The hypothalamus lies in the center of the limbic system.

2. Which of the following statements is (are) correct?
   (1) The nuclei of the hypothalamus are divided by an imaginary plane formed by the columns of the fornix and the mammillothalamic tract into medial and lateral groups.
   (2) The suprachiasmatic nucleus overlaps both medial and lateral groups of nuclei and receives nerve fibers from the retina.

3. Which of the following statements is (are) correct?
   (1) When seen from the inferior aspect, the hypothalamus is related to the following structures from anterior to posterior: (a) the tuber cinereum (b) the optic chiasma, and (c) the mammillary bodies.
   (2) The lateral boundary of the hypothalamus is formed by the internal capsule.

4. Which of the following statements concerning the nuclei of the hypothalamus is (are) correct?
   (1) The margins of the different nuclei can be clearly seen with the naked eye.
   (2) The mamillary body overlaps both the medial and lateral groups of nuclei.

5. Which of the following statements is (are) correct?
   (1) The preoptic area of the hypothalamus is located between the lamina terminalis and the optic chiasma.
   (2) The blood-brain barrier is absent in the median eminence of the hypothalamus, thus permitting the neurons to sample the chemical content of the plasma directly.

In the following questions, answer:

    (a) If (1), (2), AND (3) ONLY ARE CORRECT
    (b) If (1) AND (3) ONLY ARE CORRECT
    (c) If (2) AND (4) ONLY ARE CORRECT
    (d) If (4) ONLY IS CORRECT, OR
    (e) If ALL ARE CORRECT

6. Which of the following statements concerning the afferent fibers passing to the hypothalamus is (are) correct?
   (1) Fibers pass from the hippocampus to the mammillary bodies, bringing information from the limbic system.
   (2) Fibers ascend to the dorsomedial nucleus from the posterior lobe of the hypophysis cerebri.
   (3) Olfactory impulses reach the hypothalamus through the median forebrain bundle.
   (4) The pineal gland sends fibers via the habenular commissure to the hypothalamus.

7. Which of the following statements concerning the hypothalamus is (are) correct?
   (1) Visceral and somatic afferents reach the hypothalamic nuclei via the medial and lateral lemnisci.
   (2) The hypothalamus appears to integrate the autonomic and neuroendocrine systems, thus preserving homeostasis.
   (3) The nerve cells of the hypothalamus produce releasing and release-inhibiting factors that control the production of various hormones.
   (4) The anterior portion of the hypothalamus controls those mechanisms that dissipate heat loss.

8. Which of the following statements concerning the functional activities of the hypothalamus is (are) true?
   (1) The lateral region of the hypothalamus is concerned with the initiation of eating and increasing food intake.
   (2) It is probable that the hypothalamus brings about the physical changes associated with emotion, such as increased heart rate and flushing or pallor of the skin.
   (3) The suprachiasmatic nucleus plays an important role in controlling circadian rhythm.
   (4) The hypothalamus controls the lower autonomic centers by means of pathways through the reticular formation.

9. Which of the following statements concerning the hypothalamohypophyseal tract is (are) correct?
   (1) The nerve cells of the supraoptic and paraventricular nuclei produce the hormones vasopressin and oxytocin.
   (2) The hormones travel in the axons of the tract with protein carriers called neurophysins.
   (3) Vasopressin stimulates the distal convoluted tubules and collecting tubules of the kidney, causing increased absorption of water from the urine.
   (4) Oxytocin inhibits the contraction of the smooth muscle of the uterus.

10. Which of the following statements concerning the hypophyseal portal system is (are) correct?
    (1) The blood vessels commence superiorly in the mammillary bodies and end inferiorly in the vascular sinusoids of the anterior lobe of the hypophysis cerebri.
    (2) The portal system carries releasing hormones and release-inhibiting hormones to the secretory cells of the anterior lobe of the hypophysis.
    (3) Afferent nerve fibers entering the hypothalamus have no influence on the production of the releasing hormones by the nerve cells.
    (4) The production of the releasing hormones and the release-inhibiting hormones can be influenced by the level of the hormone produced by the target organ controlled by the hypophysis.

ADDITIONAL READING

Adams, J. H., Daniel, P. M., and Prichard, M. Observations on the portal circulation of the pituitary gland. *Neuroendocrinology* 1:193, 1966.

Anderson, G. H., Li, E. T. S., and Glanville, N. T. Brain mechanisms and the quantitative and qualitative aspects of food intake. *Brain Res. Bull.* 12:167, 1984.

Bauer, H. G. Endocrine and other clinical manifestations of hypothalamic disease. *J. Clin. Endocrinol. Metab.* 14:13, 1954.

Bisset, G. W., Hilton, S. M., and Poisner, A. M. Hypothalamic pathways for the independent release of vasopressin and oxytocin. *Proc. R. Soc. Lond. [Biol.]* 166:422, 1966.

Braak, H., and Braak, E. The hypothalamus of the human adult: Chiasmatic region. *Anat. Embryol.* 176: 315, 1987.

Buijs, R. M. Vasopressin and oxytocin—their role in neurotransmission. *Pharmacol. Ther.* 22:127, 1983.

Burgus, R., and Guillemin, R. Hypothalamic releasing factors. *Annu. Rev. Biochem.* 39:499, 1970.

Emmers, R. Interaction of neural systems which control body water. *Brain Res.* 49:323, 1973.

Ganong, W. F. Neural centers regulating visceral function. In W. F. Ganong (ed.), *The Nervous System.* Los Altos, California: Lange, 1979. P. 163.

Ganten, D., and Pfaff, D. *Morphology of Hypothalamus and Its Connections.* Berlin: Springer-Verlag, 1986.

Grossman, S. P. A reassessment of the brain mechanisms that control thirst. *Neurosci. Behav. Rev.* 8:95, 1984.

Guyton, A. C. *Textbook of Medical Physiology* (7th ed.). Philadelphia: Saunders, 1986.

Haymaker, W., Anderson, E., and Nauta, W. J. H. *The Hypothalamus.* Springfield, Illinois: Thomas, 1969.

Knigge, K. M., and Silverman, A. J. Anatomy of the endocrine hypothalamus. In R. O. Greep and E. B. Astwood (eds.), *Handbook of Physiology*, Section 7: *Endocrinology.* Washington, D.C.: American Physiological Society, 1974. Vol. 4, P. 1.

Langevin, H., and Iversen, L. L. A new method for the microdissection of the human hypothalamus, with mapping of cholinergic, GABA, and catecholamine systems in twelve nuclei and areas. *Brain* 103:623, 1980.

McCann, S. M., and Porter, J. C. Hypothalamic pituitary stimulating and inhibiting hormones. *Physiol. Rev.* 49:240, 1969.

Morton, R. A quantitative analysis of the normal neuron population of the hypothalamic magnocellular nuclei in man and of their projections to the neurohypophysis. *J. Comp. Neurol.* 136:143, 1969.

Nilaver, G. Chemical anatomy of the hypothalamus. *Neurol. Clin.* 4:701, 1986.

Raisman, G. W., and Field, P. M. Anatomical considerations relevant to the interpretation of neuroendocrine experiments. In L. Martini and W. F. Ganong (eds.), *Frontiers in Neuroendocrinology.* London: Oxford University Press, 1971. P. 3.

Reichlin, S., Baldessarini, R. J., and Martin, J. B. (eds.). *The Hypothalamus.* New York: Raven, 1980.

Saper, C. B., Loewy, A. D., Swanson, L. W., Cowan, W. M., et al. Direct hypothalamo-autonomic connections. *Brain Res.* 117:305, 1976.

Swaab, D. F., and Schade, J. P. Integrative hypothalamic activity. In *Progress in Brain Research.* New York: American Elsevier, 1974. Vol. 41.

Swanson, L. W., and Sawchenko, P. E. Hypothalamic integration: Organization of the paraventricular and supraoptic nuclei. *Annu. Rev. Neurosci.* 6:269, 1983.

Chapter 26
The Autonomic Nervous System

The autonomic nervous system exerts control over the functions of many organs and tissues in the body. Along with the endocrine system, it brings about fine internal adjustments necessary for the optimal internal environment of the body.

The autonomic nervous system, like the somatic nervous system, has afferent, connector, and efferent neurons. The afferent impulses originate in visceral receptors and travel via afferent pathways to the central nervous system, where they are integrated through connector neurons at different levels and then leave via efferent pathways to visceral effector organs.

The efferent pathways of the autonomic system are made up of preganglionic and postganglionic neurons. The cell bodies of the preganglionic neurons are situated in the lateral gray column of the spinal cord and in the motor nuclei of the third, seventh, ninth, and tenth cranial nerves. The axons of these cell bodies synapse on the cell bodies of the postganglionic neurons that are collected together to form **ganglia** outside the central nervous system.

The control exerted by the autonomic system is widespread, since one preganglionic axon may synapse with several postganglionic neurons. Large collections of afferent and efferent nerve fibers and their associated ganglia form **autonomic plexuses** in the thorax, abdomen, and pelvis.

The visceral receptors include chemoreceptors, baroreceptors, and osmoreceptors. Pain receptors are present in viscera and certain types of stimuli, such as oxygen lack or stretch, may cause extreme pain.

ORGANIZATION OF THE AUTONOMIC NERVOUS SYSTEM

The autonomic nervous system innervates involuntary structures such as the heart, the smooth muscles, and the glands. The system is distributed throughout the central and peripheral nervous systems; is divided into two parts, the **sympathetic** and the **parasympathetic**; and, as emphasized above, consists of both afferent and efferent nerve fibers. This division between sympathetic and parasympathetic is made on the basis of anatomical differences, differences in the neurotransmitters, and differences in the physiological effects.

SYMPATHETIC PART OF THE AUTONOMIC NERVOUS SYSTEM

The sympathetic system is the larger of the two parts of the autonomic system and is widely distributed throughout the body, innervating the heart and lungs, the muscle in the walls of many blood vessels, the hair follicles and the sweat glands, and many abdominopelvic viscera.

The function of the sympathetic system is to prepare the body for an emergency. The heart rate is increased, arterioles of the skin and intestine are constricted, those of skeletal muscle are dilated, and the blood pressure is raised. There is a redistribution of blood so that it leaves the skin and gastrointestinal tract and passes to the brain, heart, and skeletal muscle. In addition the sympathetic nerves dilate the pupils, inhibit smooth muscle of the bronchi, intestine, and bladder wall, and close

the sphincters. The hair is made to stand on end and sweating occurs.

The sympathetic system consists of the efferent outflow from the spinal cord, two ganglionated sympathetic trunks, important branches, plexuses, and regional ganglia.

Efferent Nerve Fibers (Sympathetic Outflow)

The lateral gray columns (horns) of the spinal cord from the first thoracic segment to the second lumbar segment (sometimes third lumbar segment) possess the cell bodies of the sympathetic connector neurons (Fig. 26-1). The myelinated axons of these cells leave the cord in the anterior nerve roots and pass via the **white rami communicantes** to the **paravertebral ganglia** of the **sympathetic trunk**. Once these fibers (preganglionic) reach the ganglia in the sympathetic trunk, they are distributed as follows:

1. They synapse with an excitor neuron in the ganglion (Fig. 26-1 and 26-2). The gap between the

Fig. 26-1. General arrangement of somatic part of nervous system (*on left*) compared with autonomic part of nervous system (*on right*).

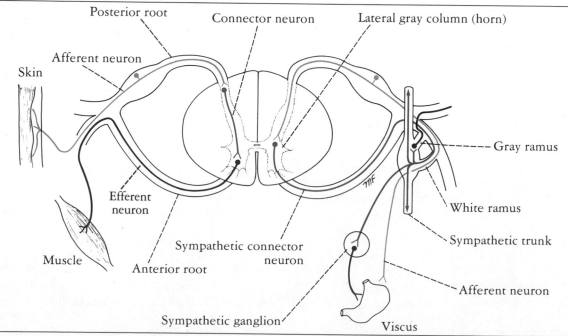

two neurons is bridged by the neurotransmitter **acetylcholine**. The postganglionic nonmyelinated axons leave the ganglion and pass to the thoracic spinal nerves as **gray rami communicantes** (the gray rami are gray colored because the nerve fibers are devoid of myelin). They are distributed in branches of the spinal nerves to smooth muscle in the blood vessel walls, sweat glands, and arrector pili muscles of the skin.

2. They travel cephalad in the sympathetic trunk to synapse in ganglia in the cervical region (Fig. 26-2). The postganglionic nerve fibers pass via gray rami communicantes to join the cervical spinal nerves. Many of the preganglionic fibers entering the lower part of the sympathetic trunk from the lower thoracic and upper two lumbar segments of the spinal cord travel caudal to synapse in ganglia in the lower lumbar and sacral regions. Here again, the postganglionic nerve fibers pass via gray rami communicantes to join the lumbar, sacral, and coccygeal spinal nerves (Fig. 26-2).

3. They may pass through the ganglia of the sympathetic trunk without synapsing. These myelinated fibers leave the sympathetic trunk as the **greater splanchnic**, **lesser splanchnic**, and **lowest** or **least splanchnic nerves**. The greater splanchnic nerve is formed from branches from the fifth to the ninth thoracic ganglia. It descends obliquely on the sides of the bodies of the thoracic vertebrae and pierces the crus of the diaphragm to synapse with excitor cells in the ganglia of the **celiac plexus**, the **renal plexus**, and the suprarenal medulla. The lesser splanchnic nerve is formed from branches of the tenth and eleventh thoracic ganglia. It descends with the greater splanchnic nerve and pierces the diaphragm to join excitor cells in ganglia in the lower part of the **celiac plexus**. The lowest splanchnic nerve (when present) arises from the twelfth thoracic ganglion, pierces the diaphragm and synapses with excitor neurons in the ganglia of the **renal plexus**. The splanchnic nerves, therefore, are formed of preganglionic fibers. The postganglionic fibers arise from the excitor cells in the peripheral plexuses and are distributed to the smooth muscle and glands of the viscera. A few preganglionic fibers, travelling in the greater splanchnic nerve, end directly on the cells of the **suprarenal medulla**. These medullary cells, which may be regarded as modified sympathetic excitor neurons, are responsible for the secretion of epinephrine and norepinephrine.

Afferent Nerve Fibers

The afferent myelinated nerve fibers travel from the viscera through the sympathetic ganglia without synapsing. They pass to the spinal nerve via white rami communicantes and reach their cell bodies in the posterior root ganglion of the corresponding spinal nerve (Fig. 26-1). The central axons then enter the spinal cord and may form the afferent component of a local reflex arc or ascend to higher centers, such as the hypothalamus.

Sympathetic Trunks

The sympathetic trunks are two ganglionated nerve trunks that extend the whole length of the vertebral column (Fig. 26-2). In the neck, each trunk has three ganglia; in the thorax, eleven or twelve; in the lumbar region, four or five; and in the pelvis, four or five. In the neck, the trunks lie anterior to the transverse processes of the cervical vertebrae; in the thorax, they are anterior to the heads of the ribs or lie on the sides of the vertebral bodies; in the abdomen, they are anterolateral to the sides of the bodies of the lumbar vertebrae; and in the pelvis, they are anterior to the sacrum. Below, the two trunks end by joining together to form a single ganglion, the **ganglion impar**.

PARASYMPATHETIC PART OF THE AUTONOMIC NERVOUS SYSTEM

The activities of the parasympathetic part of the autonomic system are directed toward conserving and restoring energy. The heart rate is slowed, pupils are constricted, peristalsis and glandular activity is increased, sphincters are opened, and the bladder wall is contracted.

Efferent Nerve Fibers (Craniosacral Outflow)

The connector nerve cells of the parasympathetic part of the autonomic nervous system are located in the brainstem and the sacral segments of the spinal cord (Fig. 26-2).

Fig. 26-2. Efferent part of autonomic nervous system. Preganglionic parasympathetic fibers are shown in solid blue, postganglionic parasympathetic fibers in interrupted blue. Preganglionic sympathetic fibers are shown in solid red, postganglionic sympathetic fibers in interrupted red.

Those nerve cells located in the brainstem form nuclei in the following cranial nerves: the **oculomotor** (parasympathetic or Edinger-Westphal nucleus), the **facial** (superior salivatory nucleus and lacrimatory nucleus), the **glossopharyngeal** (inferior salivatory nucleus), and the **vagus** nerves (dorsal nucleus of the vagus). The axons of these connector nerve cells are myelinated and emerge from the brain within the cranial nerves.

The sacral connector nerve cells are found in the gray matter of the **second, third, and fourth sacral segments of the spinal cord**. These cells are not sufficiently numerous to form a lateral gray horn, as do the sympathetic connector neurons in the thoracolumbar region. The myelinated axons leave the spinal cord in the anterior nerve roots of the corresponding spinal nerves. They then leave the sacral nerves and form the **pelvic splanchnic nerves** (Fig. 26-2).

The efferent fibers of the craniosacral outflow are pregangionic and synapse in peripheral ganglia located close to the viscera they innervate. Here, again, acetylcholine is the neurotransmitter. The cranial parasympathetic ganglia are the **ciliary, pterygopalatine, submandibular, and otic** (Fig. 26-2). In certain locations the ganglion cells are placed in nerve plexuses, such as the **cardiac plexus, pulmonary plexus, myenteric plexus (Auerbach's plexus)**, and **mucosal plexus (Meissner's plexus)**; the last two plexuses are associated with the gastrointestinal tract. The pelvic splanchnic nerves synapse in ganglia in the **hypogastric plexuses**. Characteristically, the postganglionic parasympathetic fibers are nonmyelinated and of relatively short length as compared with sympathetic postganglionic fibers.

AFFERENT NERVE FIBERS

The afferent myelinated fibers travel from the viscera to their cell bodies, located either in the sensory ganglia of the cranial nerves or in the posterior root ganglia of the sacrospinal nerves. The central axons then enter the central nervous system and take part in the formation of local reflex arcs, or pass to higher centers of the autonomic nervous system, such as the hypothalamus.

It is important to realize that the afferent component of the autonomic system is identical to the afferent component of somatic nerves and that it forms part of the general afferent segment of the entire nervous system. The nerve endings in the autonomic afferent component may not be activated by such sensations as heat or touch but rather by stretch or lack of oxygen. Once the afferent fibers gain entrance to the spinal cord or brain, they are thought to travel alongside, or mixed with, the somatic afferent fibers.

The Large Autonomic Plexuses

Large collections of sympathetic and parasympathetic efferent nerve fibers and their associated ganglia, together with visceral afferent fibers, form autonomic nerve plexuses in the thorax, abdomen, and pelvis. Branches from these plexuses innervate the viscera. In the thorax there are the cardiac, pulmonary, and esophageal plexuses. In the abdomen the plexuses are associated with the aorta and its branches, and subdivisions of these autonomic plexuses are named according to the branch of the aorta along which they are lying: celiac, superior mesenteric, inferior mesenteric, and aortic plexuses. In the pelvis there are the superior and inferior hypogastric plexuses.

Autonomic Ganglia

The autonomic ganglion is the site where preganglionic nerve fibers synapse on postganglionic neurons (Fig. 26-3). Ganglia are situated along the course of efferent nerve fibers of the autonomic nervous system. Sympathetic ganglia form part of the sympathetic trunk or are prevertebral in position. Parasympathetic ganglia, on the other hand, are situated close to or within the walls of the viscera.

An autonomic ganglion consists of a collection of multipolar neurons together with capsular or satellite cells and a connective tissue capsule. Nerve bundles are attached to each ganglion and consist of preganglionic nerve fibers that enter the ganglion, postganglionic nerve fibers that have arisen from neurons within the ganglion and are leaving the ganglion, and afferent and efferent nerve fibers that pass through the ganglion without synapsing. The preganglionic fibers are myelinated, small, and relatively slow-conducting B fibers. The postganglionic fibers are unmyelinated, smaller, and slower-conducting C fibers.

Fig. 26-3. A. An autonomic ganglion as an integrator.
B. The liberation of acetylcholine at an autonomic synapse.

While an autonomic ganglion is the site where preganglionic fibers synapse on postganglionic neurons, the presence of small interneurons and collateral branches suggests that a ganglion may play a greater role than simply relaying information; it probably serves some integrative function (Fig. 26-3).

Preganglionic Transmitters

As the preganglionic nerve fibers approach their termination they wind around and between the dendritic processes of the postganglionic neuron, making multiple synaptic contacts. When the wave of excitation reaches the synaptic contacts the synaptic transmitter is liberated, crosses the synaptic cleft, and excites the postganglionic neuron (Fig. 26-3 B and 26-4).

The synaptic transmitter that excites the postganglionic neurons in both sympathetic and parasympathetic ganglia is **acetylcholine**. The action of acetylcholine in autonomic ganglia is quickly terminated by hydrolysis by **acetylcholinesterase**. The small ganglionic interneurons contain **dopamine**, which is thought to act as a transmitter.

The structure of synapses in autonomic ganglia shows the characteristic membrane thickening and small clear vesicles. In addition, there are some

Fig. 26-4. The efferent parts of the autonomic nervous system and the chemical transmitter substances released at the nerve endings.

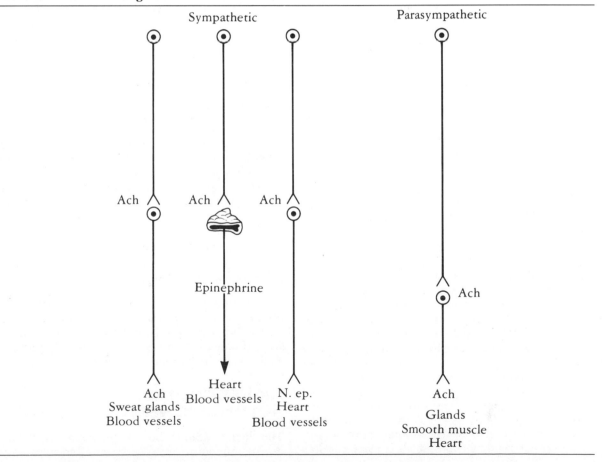

Sympathetic   Parasympathetic

Ach   Ach   Ach

Epinephrine   Ach

Ach   Heart   N. ep.   Ach
Sweat glands   Blood vessels   Heart   Glands
Blood vessels   Blood vessels   Smooth muscle
                                        Heart

larger granular vesicles. The smaller vesicles contain acetylcholine; the content of the granular vesicles is unknown.

Ganglion Blocking Agents

There are two types of ganglion blocking agents. **Nicotine** acts as a blocking agent in high concentrations, first by stimulating the postganglionic neuron by causing depolarization, and then by maintaining depolarization of the excitable membrane. **Hexamethonium** and **tetraethylammonium** block ganglia by competing with acetylcholine at the receptor sites.

Postganglionic Nerve Endings

The postganglionic fibers terminate on the effector cells without special discrete endings. The axons run between the gland cells and the smooth and cardiac muscle fibers and lose their covering of Schwann cells. At sites where transmission occurs, clusters of vesicles are present within the axoplasm (see Fig. 5-18). The site on the axon may lie at some distance from the effector cell so that the transmission time may be slow at these endings. The diffusion of the transmitter through the large extracellular distance also permits a given nerve to have an action on a large number of effector cells.

Postganglionic Transmitters

Parasympathetic postganglionic nerve endings liberate **acetylcholine** as their transmitter substance (Fig. 26-4). The acetylcholine traverses the synaptic cleft and binds reversibly with the cholinergic receptor on the postsynaptic membrane. Within 2 to 3 msec it is hydrolyzed into acetic acid and choline by the enzyme **acetylcholinesterase**, which is located on the surface of the nerve and receptor membranes. The choline is reabsorbed into the nerve ending and used again for synthesis of acetylcholine.

Most sympathetic postganglionic nerve endings liberate **norepinephrine** as their transmitter substance. In addition, some sympathetic postganglionic nerve endings, particularly those that end on cells of sweat glands, release **acetylcholine**.

Sympathetic endings that use norepinephrine are called **adrenergic endings**. There are two major kinds of receptors in the effector organs, called **alpha** and **beta receptors**.

Two subgroups of alpha receptors (alpha-1 and alpha-2 receptors) and two subgroups of beta receptors (beta-1 and beta-2 receptors) have been described. Norepinephrine has a greater effect on alpha receptors than on beta receptors. On the other hand, beta receptors are more strongly stimulated by other adrenergic drugs such as **isoproterenol**. As a general rule alpha receptor sites are associated with most of the excitatory functions of the sympathetic system (e.g., smooth muscle contraction, vasoconstriction, diaphoresis), whereas the beta receptor sites are associated with most of the inhibitory functions (e.g., smooth muscle relaxation). Beta-2 receptors are predominant in the lung and stimulation results in bronchodilation. The myocardium, where beta receptors are associated with excitation, is an exception.

The action of norepinephrine on the receptor site of the effector cell is terminated by reuptake into the nerve terminal where it is stored in presynaptic vesicles; it is protected from inactivation by the enzyme **monoamine oxidase**.

Blocking of Cholinergic Receptors

In the case of the parasympathetic and the sympathetic postganglionic nerve endings that liberate acetylcholine as the transmitter substance, the receptors on the effector cells are **muscarinic**. This means that the action can be blocked by **atropine**. Atropine is a competitive antagonist to the muscarinic actions and it occupies the cholinergic receptor sites on the effector cells.

Blocking of Adrenergic Receptors

The alpha-adrenergic receptor can be blocked by **phenoxybenzamine** and the beta-adrenergic receptor can be blocked by **propranolol**. The synthesis and storage of norepinephrine at sympathetic endings can be inhibited by **reserpine**.

HIGHER CONTROL OF THE AUTONOMIC NERVOUS SYSTEM

The hypothalamus has a controlling influence on the autonomic nervous system and appears to

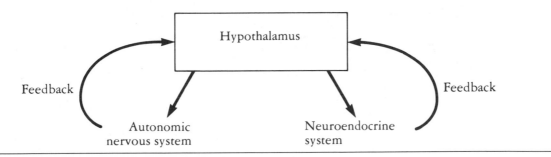

Fig. 26-5. The hypothalamus as the control center for the autonomic nervous system and the neuroendocrine system.

integrate the autonomic and neuroendocrine systems, thus preserving body homeostasis (Fig. 26-5). Essentially, the hypothalamus should be regarded as a higher nervous center for the control of lower autonomic centers in the brainstem and spinal cord.

Stimulation of the anterior region of the hypothalamus can influence parasympathetic responses, whereas stimulation of the posterior part of the hypothalamus gives rise to sympathetic responses. In addition, lower brainstem centers such as **vasopressor**, **vasodilator**, **cardioaccelerator**, **cardiodecelerator**, and **respiratory centers** have been found in the reticular formation as the result of experimental stimulation in lower animals. It is believed that the various levels of control are exerted as the result of interconnections of the different regions by ascending and descending pathways. The neurons of the thoracolumbar outflow of the sympathetic part of the system and the neurons of the craniosacral outflow of the parasympathetic part of the system receive their control through the descending tracts of the reticular formation.

It has long been known that stimulation of different parts of the cerebral cortex and the limbic system can produce autonomic effects and it is assumed that this is brought about through the hypothalamus. In this connection, the work of Miller et al. in 1970 is of interest. They suggest that the autonomic nervous system can be brought under voluntary control to some extent and that patients with hypertension, for example, possibly can be trained to reduce their blood pressure.

THE "ENTERIC NERVOUS SYSTEM"

The so-called enteric nervous system, consisting of the myenteric and mucosal plexuses of the gastrointestinal tract, has recently received considerable attention by researchers. No longer can these plexuses be regarded as simply parasympathetic plexuses containing preganglionic and postganglionic nerve fibers and nerve cells. It has been shown that contractions of the smooth muscle in the gut wall can occur in the absence of the myenteric plexus, but the coordinated purposeful contractions, as seen with peristalsis and segmental movements, require the presence of a nerve plexus, even though this may be isolated from the central nervous system.

Different types of neurons have been recognized in the plexuses. Some neurons are bipolar or unipolar and are thought to be sensory and involved in local reflex activity; other neurons send axons to the celiac and mesenteric plexuses. Preganglionic parasympathetic fibers synapse on nerve cells that give rise to postganglionic fibers that innervate the smooth muscle and glands. Postganglionic sympathetic fibers have been seen to terminate on parasympathetic nerve cells and probably exert an inhibitory role in parasympathetic activity. Internuncial neurons are also present. It is interesting to note that the nerve cells and their processes are surrounded by neuroglia-like cells that closely resemble astrocytes in the central nervous system. It has been suggested that while the enteric plexuses can coordinate the activities of the gut wall, the

Fig. 26-6. This man is making good use of the sympathetic part of his autonomic nervous system.

parasympathetic and sympathetic inputs modulate these activities.

FUNCTIONS OF THE AUTONOMIC NERVOUS SYSTEM

The autonomic nervous system, along with the endocrine system, maintains the stability of the internal environment of the body. By means of its fine control it brings about the internal adjustments that are necessary for the optimal internal environment of the body. The endocrine control is slower and exerts its influence by means of hormones, which are transported in the bloodstream.

The autonomic nervous system functions for the most part at the subconscious level. We are not aware, for example, that our pupils are dilating or that our arteries are constricting. The system should not be regarded as an isolated portion of the nervous system, for we know that it can play a role with somatic activity in expressing emotion and that certain autonomic activities, such as micturition, can be brought under voluntary control. The various activities of the autonomic and endocrine systems are integrated within the hypothalamus.

The sympathetic and parasympathetic components of the autonomic system cooperate in maintaining the stability of the internal environment. The sympathetic part prepares and mobilizes the body in an emergency (Fig. 26-6), when there is sudden severe exercise, fear, or rage. The parasympathetic part aims at conserving and storing energy, for example, in the promotion of digestion

Fig. 26-7. There is nothing like a good, large meal and a comfortable armchair to facilitate the activities of the parasympathetic part of the autonomic nervous system.

and the absorption of food by increasing the secretions of the glands of the gastrointestinal tract and stimulating peristalsis (Fig. 26-7).

The sympathetic and parasympathetic parts of the autonomic system usually have antagonistic control over a viscus. For example, the sympathetic activity will increase the heart rate, whereas the parasympathetic will cause slowing of the heart rate. The sympathetic activity will make the bronchial smooth muscle relax but it is contracted by the parasympathetic.

It should be pointed out, however, that many viscera do not possess this fine dual control from the autonomic system. The smooth muscle of the hair follicles (the arrector pili muscle) is made to contract by the sympathetic activity, and there is no parasympathetic control.

The activities of some viscera are kept under a constant state of inhibition by one or the other components of the autonomic nervous system. The heart in a trained athlete is maintained at a slow rate by the activities of the parasympathetic system. This is of considerable importance, because the heart is a more efficient pump when contracting slowly than when contracting very quickly. To put it another way, if the heart is contracting excessively fast, the duration of diastole may be so reduced between contractions that the ventricles do not have time to fill.

IMPORTANT ANATOMICAL, PHYSIOLOGICAL, AND PHARMACOLOGICAL DIFFERENCES BETWEEN THE SYMPATHETIC AND PARASYMPATHETIC PARTS OF THE AUTONOMIC SYSTEM (TABLE 26-1)

1. The sympathetic efferent nerve fibers originate (Fig. 26-2) from nerve cells in the lateral gray column of the spinal cord between the first thoracic and second lumbar segments (the **thoracic outflow**). The parasympathetic efferent nerve fibers originate from nerve cells in the third, seventh, ninth, and tenth cranial nerves and in the gray matter of the second, third, and fourth sacral segments of the cord (the **craniosacral outflow**).
2. The sympathetic ganglia are located either in the paravertebral sympathetic trunks or in the prevertebral ganglia, such as the celiac ganglion (Fig. 26-2). The parasympathetic ganglion cells are located as small ganglia close to the viscera or within plexuses within the viscera.
3. The sympathetic part of the autonomic system has long postganglionic fibers, whereas the parasympathetic system has short fibers (Fig. 26-5).
4. The sympathetic part of the system has a wide-

spread action on the body as the result of the preganglionic fibers synapsing on many postganglionic neurons and the suprarenal medulla releasing the sympathetic transmitters epinephrine and norepinephrine, which are distributed throughout the body through the bloodstream (Fig. 26-4). The parasympathetic part of the autonomic system has a more discrete control, since the preganglionic fibers synapse on only a few postganglionic neurons and there is no comparable organ to the suprarenal medulla.
5. The sympathetic postganglionic endings liberate norepinephrine at most endings and acetylcholine at a few endings (e.g., sweat glands). The parasympathetic postganglionic endings liberate acetylcholine (Fig. 26-4).
6. The sympathetic part of the autonomic system prepares the body for emergencies and severe muscular activity, whereas the parasympathetic part conserves and stores energy.

To assist with the learning of the different actions of these two components of the autonomic system it might be helpful to imagine the sympathetic activity to be maximal in a man who finds himself suddenly alone in a field with a bull who is about to charge (Fig. 26-6). His hair will stand on end with fear; his skin will be pale as the result of vasoconstriction, which causes a redistribution of blood away from the skin and viscera to the heart muscle and skeletal muscle. His upper eyelids will be raised and his pupils widely dilated so that he can see where to run. His heart rate will rise and the peripheral resistance of the arterioles will be increased, causing a rise in blood pressure. His bronchi will dilate to permit maximum respiratory flow of air. His peristaltic activity will be inhibited and his gut sphincters will be contracted. His vesical sphincter will also be contracted (this is certainly not the time to be thinking of defecation or micturition). Glycogen will be converted into glucose for energy and he will sweat to lose body heat.

On the other hand, the parasympathetic activity will be great in a man who has fallen asleep in an armchair after a satisfying meal (Fig. 26-7). His heart rate will be slow and his blood pressure will not be high. His upper eyelids will droop or be closed and his pupils will be constricted. His breathing will be noisy owing to bronchial constriction. His abdomen may rumble owing to ex-

Table 26-1. Comparison of Anatomical, Physiological, and Pharmacological Characteristics of the Sympathetic and Parasympathetic Parts of the Autonomic Nervous System

	Sympathetic	Parasympathetic
Action	Prepares body for emergency	Conserves and restores energy
Outflow	T1–L2 (3)	CN 3, 7, 9, and 10; S2, 3, and 4
Preganglionic fibers	Myelinated	Myelinated
Ganglia	Paravertebral (sympathetic trunks); prevertebral (e.g., celiac, superior mesenteric, inferior mesenteric)	Small ganglia close to viscera (e.g., otic, ciliary) or ganglion cells in plexuses (e.g., cardiac, pulmonary)
Neurotransmitter within ganglia	Acetylcholine	Acetylcholine
Ganglion-blocking agents	Hexamethonium and tetraethylammonium by competing with acetylcholine	Hexamethonium and tetraethylammonium by competing with acetylcholine
Postganglionic fibers	Long, nonmyelinated	Short, nonmyelinated
Characteristic activity	Widespread due to many postganglionic fibers and liberation of epinephrine and norepinephrine from suprarenal medulla	Discrete action with few postganglionic fibers
Neurotransmitter at postganglionic endings	Norepinephrine at most endings and acetylcholine at few endings (sweat glands)	Acetylcholine at all endings
Blocking agents on receptors of effector cells	Alpha-adrenergic receptors—phenoxybenzamine, beta-adrenergic receptors—propranolol	Atropine, scopolamine
Agents inhibiting synthesis and storage of neurotransmitter at postganglionic endings	Reserpine	
Agents inhibiting hydrolysis of neurotransmitter at site of effector cells		Acetylcholinesterase blockers (e.g., neostigmine)

Drugs mimicking autonomic activity	Sympathomimetic drugs
	    Phenylephrine: alpha receptors
	    Isoproterenol: beta receptors
		Parasympathomimetic drugs
		    Pilocarpine
		    Methacholine

Higher control	Hypothalamus	Hypothalamus

cessive peristaltic activity. He may feel the inclination to defecate or micturate.

SOME IMPORTANT AUTONOMIC INNERVATIONS (TABLE 26-2)

Eye

UPPER LID

The upper lid is raised by the levator palpebrae superioris muscle. The major part of this muscle is formed by skeletal muscle and this receives its innervation from the oculomotor nerve. A small part of the muscle is composed of smooth muscle fibers that are innervated by sympathetic postganglionic fibers from the superior cervical sympathetic ganglion (Fig. 26-8). Division of the cervical sympathetic nerve fibers paralyzes the smooth muscle and causes drooping of the upper lid (ptosis).

IRIS

The smooth muscle fibers of the iris consist of circular and radiating fibers. The circular fibers form the sphincter pupillae and the radial fibers form the dilator pupillae.

The sphincter pupillae is supplied by parasympathetic fibers from the parasympathetic nucleus (Edinger-Westphal nucleus) of the oculomotor nerve (Fig. 26-8). After synapsing in the **ciliary ganglion**, the postganglionic fibers pass forward to the eyeball in the **short ciliary nerves**. (The ciliary muscle of the eye is also supplied by the short ciliary nerves; see page 425.)

The dilator pupillae is supplied by postganglionic fibers from the superior cervical sympathetic ganglion (Fig. 26-8). The postganglionic fibers reach the orbit along the internal carotid and ophthalmic arteries. They pass uninterrupted through the ciliary ganglion and reach the eyeball in the **short ciliary nerves**. Other sympathetic fibers reach the eyeball in the long ciliary nerves.

Salivary Glands

SUBMANDIBULAR AND SUBLINGUAL GLANDS

Parasympathetic secretomotor supply originates in the **superior salivatory nucleus** of the facial nerve (Fig. 26-8). The preganglionic fibers pass to the **submandibular ganglion** and other small ganglia close to the duct through the **chorda tympani nerve** and the **lingual nerve**. Postganglionic fibers reach the submandibular gland either directly or along the duct. Postganglionic fibers to the sublingual gland travel through the lingual nerve.

Sympathetic postganglionic fibers arise from the superior cervical sympathetic ganglion and reach the glands as a plexus of nerves around the external carotid, facial, and lingual arteries. They function as vasoconstrictor fibers.

PAROTID GLAND

Parasympathetic secretomotor fibers from the **inferior salivatory nucleus** of the glossopharyngeal nerve supply the gland (Fig. 26-9). The preganglionic nerve fibers pass to the otic ganglion through the **tympanic branch of the glossopharyngeal nerve** and the **lesser petrosal nerve**. Postganglionic fibers reach the gland through the auriculotemporal nerve.

Sympathetic postganglionic fibers arise from the superior cervical sympathetic ganglion and reach the gland as a plexus of nerves around the external carotid artery.

Lacrimal Gland

The parasympathetic secretomotor nerve supply to the lacrimal gland originates in the **lacrimatory nucleus** of the facial nerve (Fig. 26-9). The preganglionic fibers reach the **pterygopalatine ganglion** through the **nervus intermedius** and its **great petrosal branch** and through the **nerve of the pterygoid canal**. The postganglionic fibers leave the ganglion and join the maxillary nerve. They then pass into its **zygomatic branch** and the **zygomaticotemporal nerve**. They reach the lacrimal gland within the **lacrimal nerve**.

The sympathetic postganglionic fibers arise from the superior cervical sympathetic ganglion and travel in the plexus of nerves around the internal carotid artery. They join the **deep petrosal nerve**, the **nerve of the pterygoid canal**, the **maxillary nerve**, the **zygomatic nerve**, and **zygomaticotemporal nerve**, and, finally, the lacrimal nerve.

Table 26-2. Effects of Autonomic Nervous System on Organs of the Body

Organ		Sympathetic action	Parasympathetic action
Eye	Pupil	Dilates	Constricts
	Ciliary muscle	Relaxes	Contracts
Glands	Lacrimal, parotid, submandibular, sublingual, nasal	Reduces secretion by causing vasoconstriction of blood vessels	Increases secretion
	Sweat	Increases secretion	
Heart	Cardiac muscle	Increases force of contraction	Decreases force of contraction
	Coronary arteries (mainly controlled by local metabolic factors)	Dilates (beta receptors), constricts (alpha receptors)	
Lung	Bronchial muscle	Relaxes (dilates bronchi)	Contracts (constricts bronchi), increases secretion
	Bronchial secretion		
	Bronchial arteries	Constricts	Dilates
Gastrointestinal tract	Muscle in walls	Decreases peristalsis	Increases peristalsis
	Muscle in sphincters	Contracts	Relaxes
	Glands	Reduces secretion by vasoconstriction of blood vessels	Increases secretion
Liver		Breaks down glycogen into glucose	
Gallbladder		Relaxes	Contracts
Kidney		Decreases output due to constriction of arteries	
Urinary bladder	Bladder wall (detrusor)	Relaxes	Contracts
	Sphincter vesicae	Contracts	Relaxes
Erectile tissue of penis and clitoris			Relaxes, causes erection
Ejaculation		Contracts smooth muscle of vas deferens, seminal vesicles, and prostate	
Systemic arteries			
Skin		Constricts	
Abdominal		Constricts	
Muscle		Constricts (alpha receptors), dilates (beta receptors), dilates (cholinergic)	
Erector pili muscles		Contracts	
Suprarenal			
Cortex		Stimulates	
Medulla		Liberates epinephrine and norepinephrine	

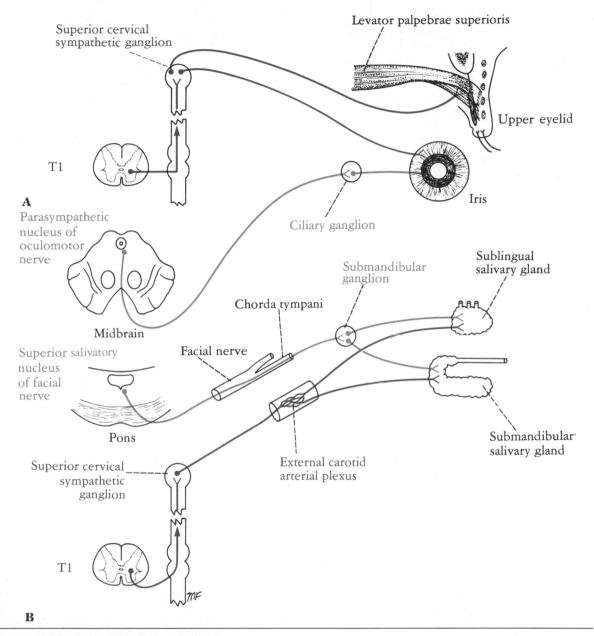

Fig. 26-8. The autonomic innervation of:
A. The upper eyelid and iris.
B. The sublingual and submandibular salivary glands.

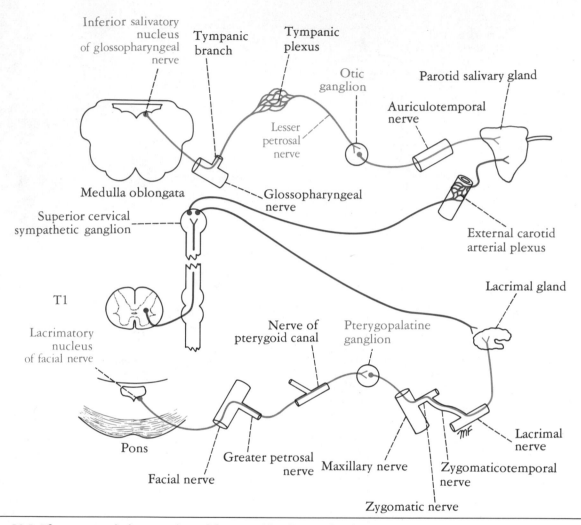

Fig. 26-9. The autonomic innervation of the parotid salivary gland and the lacrimal gland.

Heart

The sympathetic postganglionic fibers arise from the cervical and upper thoracic portions of the sympathetic trunks (Fig. 26-10). Postganglionic fibers reach the heart by way of the **superior, middle,** and **inferior cardiac branches** of the cervical portion of the sympathetic trunk and a number of **cardiac branches** from the thoracic portion of the sympathetic trunk. The fibers pass through the **cardiac plexuses** and terminate on the **sinoatrial** and **atrioventricular nodes,** on cardiac muscle fibers, and on coronary arteries. Activation of these

nerves results in cardiac acceleration, increased force of contraction of the cardiac muscle, and dilatation of the coronary arteries. The coronary dilatation is mainly produced in response to local metabolic needs rather than by direct nerve stimulation of the coronary arteries.

The parasympathetic preganglionic fibers originate in the **dorsal nucleus of the vagus nerve** and descend into the thorax in the vagus nerves. The fibers terminate by synapsing with postganglionic neurons in the **cardiac plexuses**. Postganglionic fibers terminate on the **sinoatrial** and

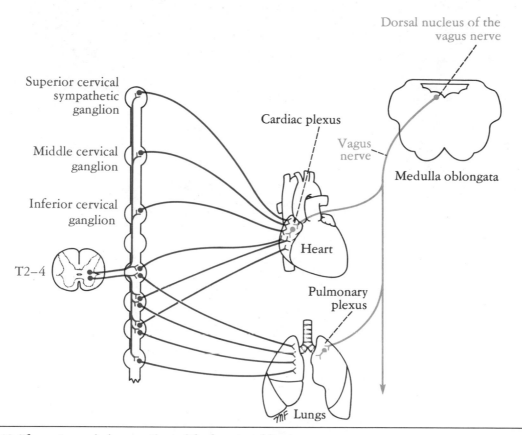

Fig. 26-10. The autonomic innervation of the heart and lungs.

atrioventricular nodes and on the coronary arteries. Activation of these nerves results in a reduction in the rate and force of contraction of the heart and a constriction of the coronary arteries. Here again, the coronary constriction is mainly produced by the reduction in local metabolic needs rather than by direct stimulation of the coronary arteries.

Lungs

The sympathetic postganglionic fibers arise from the second to the fifth thoracic ganglia of the sympathetic trunk (Fig. 26-10). The fibers pass through the pulmonary plexuses and enter the lung, where they form networks around the bronchi and blood vessels. The sympathetic fibers produce bronchodilatation and are vasoconstrictor.

The parasympathetic preganglionic fibers arise from the dorsal nucleus of the vagus and descend

to the thorax within the vagus nerves. The fibers terminate by synapsing with postganglionic neurons in the pulmonary plexuses. The postganglionic fibers enter the lung, where they form networks around the bronchi and blood vessels. The parasympathetic fibers produce bronchoconstriction and vasodilatation and increase glandular secretion.

Gastrointestinal Tract

STOMACH AND INTESTINE AS FAR AS THE SPLENIC FLEXURE

Preganglionic parasympathetic fibers enter the abdomen in the **anterior (left)** and **posterior (right) vagal trunks** (Fig. 26-11). The fibers are distributed to many abdominal viscera and to the gastrointestinal tract from the stomach to the splenic

Fig. 26-11. The autonomic innervation of the gastrointestinal tract.

flexure of the colon. The fibers that pass to the gastrointestinal tract terminate on postganglionic neurons in the **myenteric (Auerbach's)** and **submucosal (Meissner's) plexuses**. The postganglionic fibers supply the smooth muscle and glands. The parasympathetic nerves stimulate peristalsis and relax the sphincters; they also stimulate secretion.

Sympathetic preganglionic nerve fibers pass through the thoracic part of the sympathetic trunk and enter the **greater** and **lesser splanchnic nerves**. These descend into the abdomen and synapse with postganglionic neurons in the **celiac** and **superior mesenteric ganglia**. The postganglionic nerve fibers are distributed to the stomach and intestine as nerve plexuses around the branches of the celiac and superior mesenteric arteries. The sympathetic nerves inhibit peristalsis and cause contraction of the sphincters; they also inhibit secretion (see the enteric nervous system, p. 493).

Descending Colon, Pelvic Colon, and Rectum

The preganglionic parasympathetic fibers originate in the gray matter of the spinal cord from the second to the fourth sacral segments (Fig. 26-11). The fibers pass through the **pelvic splanchnic nerves** and the nerve plexuses around the branches of the inferior mesenteric artery. They terminate on postganglionic neurons in the myenteric (Auerbach's) and submucosal (Meissner's) plexuses. The postganglionic fibers supply the smooth muscle and glands. The parasympathetic nerves stimulate peristalsis and secretion.

The sympathetic preganglionic nerve fibers pass through the lumbar part of the sympathetic trunk and synapse with postganglionic neurons in the **inferior mesenteric plexus**. Postganglionic fibers are distributed to the bowel as nerve plexuses around the branches of the inferior mesenteric arteries. The sympathetic nerves inhibit peristalsis and secretion.

Kidney

Preganglionic sympathetic fibers pass through the lower thoracic part of the sympathetic trunk and the lowest thoracic splanchnic nerve to join the **renal plexus** around the renal artery (Fig. 26-12). The preganglionic fibers synapse with postganglionic neurons in the renal plexus. The postganglionic fibers are distributed to the branches of the renal artery. The sympathetic nerves are vasoconstrictor to the renal arteries within the kidney.

Preganglionic parasympathetic fibers enter the renal plexus from the vagus. Here they synapse with postganglionic neurons whose fibers are distributed to the kidney along the branches of the renal artery. The parasympathetic nerves are thought to be vasodilator in action.

Medulla of Suprarenal Gland

Preganglionic sympathetic fibers descend to the gland in the **greater splanchnic nerve**, a branch

Fig. 26-12. The autonomic innervation of the kidney and suprarenal gland.

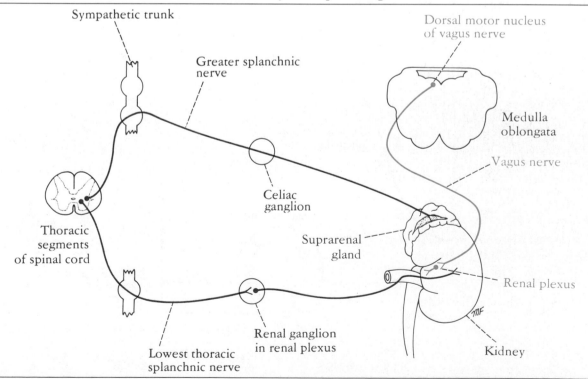

of the thoracic part of the sympathetic trunk (Fig. 26-12). The nerve fibers terminate on the secretory cells of the medulla, which are comparable to postganglionic neurons. Acetylcholine is the transmitter substance between the nerve endings and the secretory cells, as at any other preganglionic endings. The sympathetic nerves stimulate the secretory cells of the medulla to increase the output of epinephrine and norepinephrine. There is no parasympathetic innervation of the medulla of the suprarenal gland.

Involuntary Internal Sphincter of the Anal Canal

The circular smooth muscle coat is thickened at the upper end of the anal canal to form the involuntary internal sphincter. The sphincter is innervated by

postganglionic sympathetic fibers from the **hypogastric plexuses** (Fig. 26-13). Each hypogastric plexus receives sympathetic fibers from the **aortic plexus** and from the lumbar and pelvic parts of the sympathetic trunks. The sympathetic nerves cause the internal anal sphincter to contract.

Urinary Bladder

The muscular coat of the bladder is composed of smooth muscle, which at the bladder neck is thickened to form the **sphincter vesicae**. The nerve supply of the smooth muscle is from the hypogastric plexuses (Fig. 26-13). The sympathetic postganglionic fibers originate in the first and second lumbar ganglia of the sympathetic trunk and travel to the hypogastric plexuses. The parasympathetic preganglionic fibers arise as the pelvic splanchnic

Fig. 26-13. The autonomic innervation of the sphincters of the anal canal and urinary bladder.

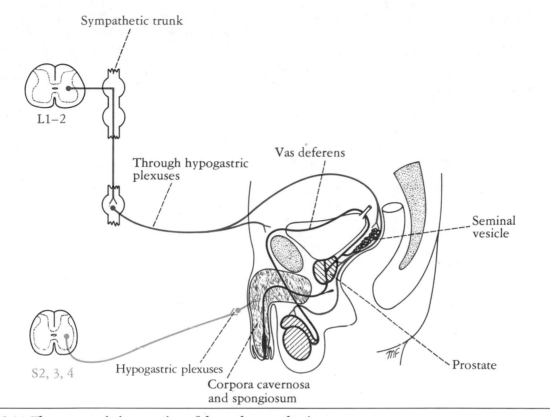

Fig. 26-14. **The autonomic innervation of the male reproductive tract.**

nerves from the second, third, and fourth sacral nerves; they pass through the hypogastric plexuses to reach the bladder wall, where they synapse with postganglionic neurons.

The sympathetic nerves* inhibit contraction of the smooth muscle of the bladder wall (detrusor) and stimulate the contraction of the sphincter vesicae. The parasympathetic nerves stimulate the contraction of the smooth muscle of the bladder

---

*The sympathetic nerves to the detrusor muscle are now thought to have little or no action on the smooth muscle of the bladder wall and are distributed mainly to the blood vessels. The sympathetic nerves to the sphincter vesicae are thought to play only a minor role in causing contraction of the sphincter in maintaining urinary continence. However, in the male, the sympathetic innervation of the sphincter causes active contraction of the bladder neck during ejaculation (brought about by sympathetic action), thus preventing seminal fluid from entering the bladder.

wall and in some way inhibit the contraction of the sphincter vesicae.

Erection of the Penis and Clitoris

In erection, the genital **erectile tissue** becomes engorged with blood. The initial vascular engorgement is controlled by the parasympathetic part of the autonomic nervous system. The parasympathetic preganglionic fibers originate in the gray matter of the second, third, and fourth sacral segments of the spinal cord (Fig. 26-14). The fibers enter the hypogastric plexuses and synapse on the postganglionic neurons. The postganglionic fibers join the internal pudendal arteries and are distributed along their branches, which enter the erectile tissue. The parasympathetic nerves cause vasodilatation of the arteries and greatly increase the blood flow to the erectile tissue.

Ejaculation

The nervous impulses that pass to the genital organs are thought to leave the spinal cord at the first and second lumbar segments in the preganglionic sympathetic fibers (Fig. 26-14). Many of these fibers synapse with postganglionic neurons in the first and second lumbar ganglia. Other fibers may synapse in ganglia in the lower lumbar or pelvic parts of the sympathetic trunks. The postganglionic fibers are then distributed to the **vas deferens**, the **seminal vesicles**, and the **prostate** through the **hypogastric plexuses**. The sympathetic nerves stimulate the contractions of the smooth muscle in the walls of these structures and cause the spermatozoa, together with the secretions of the seminal vesicles and prostate, to be discharged into the urethra.

Uterus

Preganglionic sympathetic nerve fibers leave the spinal cord at segmental levels T12 and L1 and are believed to synapse with ganglion cells in the sympathetic trunk or possibly in the inferior hypogastric plexuses (Fig. 26-15). The postganglionic fibers supply the smooth muscle of the uterus. Parasympathetic preganglionic fibers leave the spinal cord at levels S2, S3, and S4 and synapse with ganglion cells in the inferior hypogastric plexuses (Fig. 26-15). Although it is recognized that the uterine muscle is largely under hormonal control, sympathetic innervation may cause uterine contraction and vasoconstriction, whereas parasympathetic fibers have the opposite effect.

Afferent pain fibers from the fundus and the body of the uterus ascend to the spinal cord through the hypogastric plexuses, entering it through the posterior roots of the tenth, eleventh, and twelfth thoracic spinal nerves (Fig. 26-15). Fibers from the cervix run in the pelvic splanchnic nerves, and enter the spinal cord through the posterior roots of the second, third, and fourth sacral nerves.

Arteries of the Upper Limb

The arteries of the upper limb are innervated by sympathetic nerves. The preganglionic fibers orig-inate from cell bodies in the second to the eighth thoracic segments of the spinal cord (Fig. 26-16). They pass to the sympathetic trunk through white rami and ascend in the trunk to synapse in the middle cervical, inferior cervical, first thoracic, or stellate ganglia. The postganglionic fibers join the nerves that form the brachial plexus and are distributed to the arteries within the branches of the plexus. The sympathetic nerves cause vasoconstriction of cutaneous arteries and vasodilatation of arteries that supply skeletal muscle.

Arteries of the Lower Limb

The arteries of the lower limb are also innervated by sympathetic nerves (Fig. 26-16). The preganglionic fibers originate from cell bodies in the lower three thoracic and upper two or three lumbar segments of the spinal cord. The preganglionic fibers pass to the lower thoracic and upper lumbar ganglia of the sympathetic trunk through white rami. The fibers synapse in the lumbar and sacral ganglia, and the postganglionic fibers reach the arteries through branches of the lumbar and sacral plexuses.

SOME IMPORTANT PHYSIOLOGICAL REFLEXES INVOLVING THE AUTONOMIC NERVOUS SYSTEM

Visual Reflexes

Direct and Consensual Light Reflexes

Afferent nervous impulses travel from the retina through the optic nerve, optic chiasma, and optic tract (see Fig. 23-3). A small number of fibers leave the optic tract and synapse on nerve cells in the **pretectal nucleus**, which lies close to the superior colliculus. The impulses are passed by axons of the pretectal nerve cells to the parasympathetic nuclei (Edinger-Westphal nuclei) of the oculomotor nerve on both sides. Here the fibers synapse and the parasympathetic nerves travel through the oculomotor nerve to the **ciliary ganglion** in the orbit. Finally, postganglionic parasympathetic fibers pass through the **short ciliary nerves** to the eyeball and the constrictor pupillae muscle of the iris. Both

T10–T12

Afferent pain fibers

Sympathetic trunk

T12–L1

Uterus

Through
hypogastric
plexuses

Through
hypogastric plexuses

S2, S3, S4

Fig. 26-15. The autonomic innervation of the uterus; the pathway taken by the afferent sensory fibers is also shown.

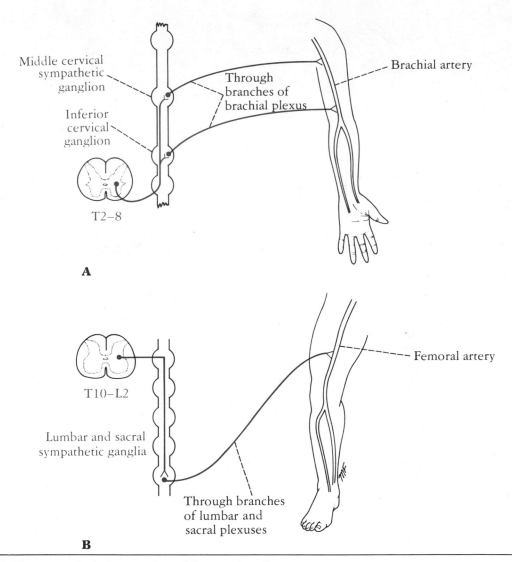

Fig. 26-16. The sympathetic innervation of the arteries of:
A. The upper limb.
B. The lower limb.

pupils constrict in the consensual light reflex, since the pretectal nucleus sends fibers to the parasympathetic nuclei on both sides of the midbrain.

Accommodation Reflex

When the eyes are directed from a distant to a near object, contraction of the medial recti brings about convergence of the ocular axes, the lens thickens to increase its refractive power by contraction of the ciliary muscle, and the pupils constrict to restrict the light waves to the thickest central part of the lens. The afferent impulses travel through the optic nerve, the optic chiasma, the optic tract, the lateral geniculate body, and the optic radiation to the visual cortex (see Fig. 23-3). The latter is connected to the eyefield of the frontal cortex. From here, cortical fibers descend through the internal capsule to the oculomotor nuclei in the midbrain. The oculomotor nerve travels to the medial recti muscles. Some of the descending cortical fibers synapse with the parasympathetic nuclei (Edinger-Westphal nuclei) of the oculomotor nerve on both sides. Here the fibers synapse and the parasympathetic preganglionic fibers travel through the oculomotor nerve to the **ciliary ganglion** in the orbit. Finally, postganglionic parasympathetic fibers pass through the **short ciliary nerves** to the ciliary muscle and the constrictor pupillae muscle of the iris.

Cardiovascular Reflexes

The **carotid sinus** and the **aortic arch** serve as baroreceptors. As the blood pressure rises, nerve endings situated in the walls of these vessels are stimulated. The afferent fibers from the carotid sinus ascend in the glossopharyngeal nerve and terminate in the **nucleus solitarius** (see Figs. 23-16 and 23-17). The afferent fibers from the aortic arch ascend in the vagus nerve. Connector neurons in the medulla oblongata activate the parasympathetic nucleus (dorsal nucleus) of the vagus, which slows the heart rate. At the same time, reticulospinal fibers descend to the spinal cord and inhibit the preganglionic sympathetic outflow to the heart and cutaneous arterioles. The combined effect of stimulation of the parasympathetic action on the heart and inhibition of the sympathetic action on the heart and peripheral blood vessels reduces the rate and force of contraction of the heart and reduces the peripheral resistance of the blood vessels. As a consequence of this effect, the blood pressure falls. The blood pressure of the individual is thus established by the afferent information received from the baroreceptors and the modulator of the autonomic nervous system, namely, the hypothalamus; the latter, in turn, can be influenced by other, higher centers in the central nervous system.

The **Bainbridge right atrial reflex** is another example of a cardiovascular reflex. The nerve endings are situated in the wall of the right atrium and in the walls of the venae cavae. These endings are stimulated by a rise of venous pressure. The afferent fibers ascend in the vagus to the medulla oblongata and terminate on the **nucleus of the tractus solitarius** (see Fig. 23-18). Connector neurons inhibit the parasympathetic nucleus (dorsal) of the vagus, and reticulospinal fibers stimulate the thoracic sympathetic outflow to the heart, resulting in cardiac acceleration.

CLINICAL NOTES

From the foregoing description, it must now be clear to the reader that the autonomic nervous system is not an isolated part of the nervous system. It should be regarded as the part of the nervous system that, with the endocrine system, is particularly involved in maintaining the stability of the internal environment of the body. Its activities are modified by the hypothalamus, whose function is to integrate vast amounts of afferent information received from other areas of the nervous system, and to translate changing hormonal levels of the bloodstream into appropriate nervous and hormonal activities.

DEGENERATION AND REGENERATION OF AUTONOMIC NERVES

The structural changes are identical to those found in other areas of the peripheral and central parts of the nervous system. Functional recoveries following sympathectomy operations can be explained only by the assumption either that the operative procedure was inadequate and nerve fibers were left intact or regenerated or that alternative nervous pathways existed and were left undisturbed.

The denervation of viscera supplied by autonomic nerves is followed by their increased sensitivity to the agent that was previously the transmitter substance. One explanation is that following nerve section there may be an increase in the number of receptor sites on the postsynaptic membrane. Another possibility, which applies to endings where norepinephrine is the transmitter, is that the reuptake of the transmitter by the nerve terminal is interfered with in some way.

DISEASES INVOLVING THE AUTONOMIC NERVOUS SYSTEM

Horner's Syndrome

This syndrome comprises (1) constriction of the pupil, (2) drooping of the upper lid, (3) enophthalmos, (4) vasodilation of skin arterioles, and (5) anhydrosis. It is caused by an interruption of the sympathetic nerve supply to the orbit, the skin arterioles, and sweat glands. The lesions responsible may occur in the brainstem or cervical part of the spinal cord, and interrupt the reticulospinal tracts descending from the hypothalamus to the sympathetic outflow in the lateral gray column of the first thoracic segment of the spinal cord. Such lesions include **multiple sclerosis** and **syringomyelia**. Traction on the stellate ganglion from a **cervical rib,** or involvement of the ganglion in a metastatic lesion, may interrupt the peripheral part of the sympathetic pathway.

Argyll Robertson Pupil

This condition is characterized by a small pupil, which is of fixed size and does not react to light, but contracts with accommodation. It is usually due to a syphilitic lesion interrupting the fibers that run from the pretectal nucleus to the parasympathetic nuclei (Edinger-Westphal nuclei)

of the oculomotor nerve on both sides. The fact that the pupil constricts with accommodation implies that the connections between the parasympathetic nuclei and the constrictor pupillae muscle of the iris are intact.

Frey's Syndrome

Frey's syndrome is an interesting complication that sometimes follows penetrating wounds of the parotid gland. During the process of healing, the postganglionic parasympathetic secretomotor fibers traveling in the auriculotemporal nerve grow out and join the distal end of the great auricular nerve, which supplies the sweat glands of the overlying facial skin. By this means, a stimulus intended for saliva production instead produces sweat secretion.

Hirschsprung's Disease (Megacolon)

Hirschsprung's disease is a congenital condition in which there is a failure of development of the myenteric plexus (Auerbach's plexus) in the distal part of the colon. The involved part of the colon possesses no parasympathetic ganglion cells and peristalsis is absent. This effectively blocks the passage of feces and the proximal part of the colon becomes enormously distended.

Urinary Bladder Following Spinal Cord Injuries

Injuries to the spinal cord are followed by disruption of the nervous control of micturition. The normal bladder is innervated as follows:

Sympathetic innervation is from the first and second lumbar segments of the spinal cord.
Parasympathetic innervation is from the second, third, and fourth sacral segments of the spinal cord.
Sensory nerve fibers enter the spinal cord at the above segments.

The **atonic bladder** occurs during the phase of spinal shock immediately following the injury and may last from a few days to several weeks. The bladder wall muscle is relaxed, the sphincter vesicae tightly contracted (loss of inhibition from higher levels), and the sphincter urethrae relaxed.

The bladder becomes greatly distended and finally overflows. Depending on the level of the cord injury, the patient either will or will not be aware that the bladder is full.

The **automatic reflex bladder** occurs after the patient has recovered from spinal shock, provided that the cord lesion lies above the level of the parasympathetic outflow (S2, 3, and 4). This is the type of bladder normally found in infancy. The bladder fills and empties reflexly. Stretch receptors in the bladder wall are stimulated as the bladder fills, and the afferent impulses pass to the spinal cord (S2, 3, and 4). Efferent impulses pass down to the bladder muscle, which contracts; the sphincter vesicae and the urethral sphincter both relax. This simple reflex occurs every 1 to 4 hours.

The **autonomous bladder** is the condition that occurs if the sacral segment of the spinal cord is destroyed. The bladder is without any external reflex control. The bladder wall is flaccid, and the capacity of the bladder is greatly increased. It merely fills to capacity and overflows; continual dribbling is the result. The bladder may be partially emptied by manual compression of the lower part of the anterior abdominal wall, but infection of the urine and back pressure effects on the ureters and kidneys are inevitable.

ACT OF DEFECATION FOLLOWING SPINAL CORD INJURIES

The act of defecation involves a coordinated reflex that results in the emptying of the descending colon, pelvic colon, rectum, and anal canal. It is assisted by a rise in the intraabdominal pressure brought about by contraction of the muscles of the anterior abdominal wall. The involuntary internal sphincter of the anal canal normally is innervated by postganglionic sympathetic fibers from the hypogastric plexuses and the voluntary external sphincter of the anal canal is innervated by the inferior rectal nerve. The desire to defecate is initiated by stimulation of the stretch receptors in the wall of the rectum.

Following severe spinal cord injuries, the patient is not aware of rectal distention. Moreover, the parasympathetic influence on the peristaltic activity of the descending colon, sigmoid colon, and rectum is lost. In addition, control over the abdominal musculature and sphincters of the anal canal may be severely impaired. The rectum, now an isolated structure, responds by contracting when the pressure within its lumen rises. This local reflex response is much more efficient if the sacral segments of the spinal cord are intact. At best, however, the force of the contractions of the rectal wall is small and constipation and impaction are the usual outcome. The treatment of patients with spinal cord injuries is to empty the rectum with biweekly enemas; the use of suppositories also may be helpful.

ERECTION AND EJACULATION FOLLOWING SPINAL CORD INJURIES

As described previously, erection of the penis or clitoris is controlled by the parasympathetic nerves that originate from the second, third, and fourth sacral segments of the spinal cord. Bilateral damage to the reticulospinal tracts in the spinal cord above the second sacral segment of the spinal cord will result in loss of erection. Later, when the effects of spinal shock have disappeared, spontaneous or reflex erection may occur if the sacral segments of the spinal cord are intact.

Ejaculation is controlled by sympathetic nerves that originate in the first and second lumbar segments of the spinal cord. Ejaculation brings about a flow of seminal fluid into the prostatic urethra. The final ejection of the fluid from the penis is the result of the rhythmic contractions of the bulbospongiosus muscles, which compress the urethra. The bulbospongiosus muscles are innervated by the pudendal nerve (S2, 3, and 4). Discharge of the seminal fluid into the bladder is prevented by the contraction of the sphincter vesicae, which is innervated by the sympathetic nerves (L1 and 2). As in the case of erection, severe bilateral damage to the spinal cord results in loss of ejaculation. Later, reflex ejaculation may be possible in patients with spinal cord transections in the thoracic or cervical regions. Some individuals have a normal ejaculation without external emission and the seminal fluid passes into the bladder, owing to paralysis of the sphincter vesicae.

SYMPATHECTOMY AS A METHOD OF TREATING ARTERIAL DISEASE

RAYNAUD'S DISEASE

This is a vasospastic disorder involving the digital arteries of the upper limb. The disorder is usually bilateral and an attack is provoked by exposure to cold. There is pallor or cyanosis of the fingers as well as severe pain. Gangrene of the tips of the fingers may occur.

In mild cases of Raynaud's disease, the treatment is the avoidance of cold and no smoking (smoking causes vasoconstriction). In more severe cases, drugs that inhibit sympathetic activity, such as reserpine, bring about arterial vasodilatation with consequent increase in blood flow to the fingers. Cervicothoracic preganglionic sympathectomy has been used but the long-term results are disappointing.

INTERMITTENT CLAUDICATION

This condition, which is common in men, is due to arterial occlusive disease of the leg. Ischemia of the muscles produces a cramplike pain on exercise. Lumbar preganglionic sympathectomy may be advocated as a form of treatment, in order to bring about vasodilatation and an increase in blood flow through the collateral circulation. Preganglionic sympathectomy is performed by removing the upper three lumbar ganglia and the intervening parts of the sympathetic trunk.

HYPERTENSION

In the past severe essential hypertension was treated by bilateral thoracolumbar sympathectomy to reduce the vasomotor control over the peripheral resistance and thus lower the blood pressure. Today, chemical blocking agents of the sympathetic system are widely used with great success and the resulting reduction in the force of myocardial contraction reduces the arterial blood pressure.

REFERRED PAIN

Most viscera are innervated only by autonomic nerves. It therefore follows that visceral pain is conducted along afferent autonomic nerves. Visceral pain is diffuse and poorly localized, whereas somatic pain is intense and discretely localized. Visceral pain frequently is referred to skin areas that are innervated by the same segments of the spinal cord as the painful viscus (Fig. 26-17). The explanation for referred pain is unknown. One theory is that the nerve fibers from the viscus and the dermatome ascend in the central nervous system along a common pathway and the cerebral cortex is incapable of distinguishing between the sites of origin. Another theory is that under normal conditions the viscus does not give rise to painful stimuli, whereas the skin area repeatedly receives noxious stimuli. Since both afferent fibers enter the spinal cord at the same segment, the brain interprets the information as coming from the skin rather than from the viscus.

Inadequate blood supply to the myocardium (myocardial ischemia) results in the patient's experiencing severe pain over the middle of the sternum, often spreading to one or both arms, the root of the neck, and even the jaw. The pain is assumed to be caused by the accumulation of metabolites and by oxygen deficiency, which stimulate the sensory nerve endings in the myocardium. The afferent nerve fibers ascend to the central nervous system through the cardiac branches of the sympathetic trunk and enter the spinal cord through the posterior roots of the upper four thoracic nerves. Note that the cardiac pain is not felt in the heart; rather, it is referred to the skin areas supplied by the corresponding spinal nerves. The skin areas supplied by the upper four intercostal nerves and by the intercostobrachial nerve (T2) are therefore affected. A certain amount of spread of nervous information must occur within the central nervous system, for the pain is sometimes felt in the neck and jaw.

Another common example of referred pain occurs during the early stages of an acute appendicitis. Initially, visceral pain in the appendix is produced by distention of its lumen or spasm of its muscle. The afferent pain fibers enter the spinal cord at the level of the tenth thoracic segment, having ascended through the superior mesenteric plexus and the lesser splanchnic nerve. A vague referred pain is felt in the region of the umbilicus, which is innervated by the tenth intercostal nerve. Later, the pain shifts to the right iliac fossa, where the inflamed appendix irritates the parietal peri-

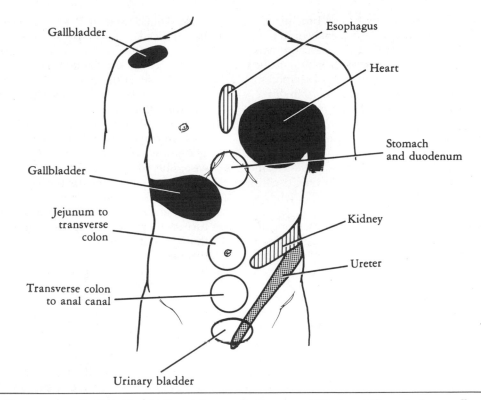

Gallbladder

Esophagus

Heart

Gallbladder

Stomach
and duodenum

Jejunum to
transverse
colon

Kidney

Transverse colon
to anal canal

Ureter

Urinary bladder

Fig. 26-17. Some areas of referred pain from viscera. In the case of the heart the pain is usually referred to the left side of the thorax; occasionally it is referred to both sides.

toneum, which is innervated by the twelfth thoracic and first lumbar spinal nerves. Here, the pain is precise, severe, and localized.

CAUSALGIA

Causalgia is a painful condition of the arm or leg accompanied by trophic changes in the affected skin and nails. It commonly follows crushing or partial division of the median nerve in the arm or the tibial nerve in the leg. It is thought that the descending impulses in the sympathetic postganglionic fibers in some way evoke ascending impulses in the afferent pain fibers at the site of injury. In many instances sympathectomy has relieved the pain of causalgia.

CLINICAL PROBLEMS

Answers on Page 611

1. A 35-year-old man was getting off the back of a truck when it started to move. Having placed his feet on the ground, he grabbed a rail on the truck with his right hand and held on. The truck continued along the road for one block before it stopped. In the meantime, the man had been dragged along the road as he held onto the truck. He was seen in the emergency room in a state of shock, with cuts and abrasions to his legs. On careful examination of his right arm, the following muscles were found to be paralyzed: the flexor carpi ulnaris, the flexor digitorum profundus, the palmar and dorsal interossei, and the thenar and hypothenar muscles. There was also loss of sensation on the medial side of the arm, forearm, and hand. The

deep tendon reflex for the biceps brachii was present but the triceps reflex was absent. It also was noted that the pupil of the right eye was constricted and that there was drooping of the right upper eyelid. The right eyeball seemed to be less prominent than the left. The skin of the right cheek felt warmer and drier and was redder in color than the left cheek. Using your knowledge of neuroanatomy, can you explain the clinical findings?

2. A 3-year-old boy was taken to a pediatrician with a history since infancy of chronic constipation and abdominal distention. The child's mother said that the constipation was getting progressively worse. It was not responding to laxatives, and she was finding it necessary to give her son an enema once a week to relieve his abdominal distention. On physical examination, the child's abdomen was obviously distended and a doughlike mass could be palpated along the course of the descending colon in the left iliac fossa. Examination of the rectum showed it to be empty and not dilated. Following an enema and repeated colonic irrigation with saline solution, the patient was given a barium enema followed by a radiographic examination. The radiograph showed a grossly distended descending colon and an abrupt change in lumen diameter where the descending colon joined the sigmoid colon. It was interesting to note that the child failed to empty the colon of the barium enema. Using your knowledge of the autonomic nerve supply to the colon, what is the diagnosis? How would you treat this patient?

3. A nervous 25-year-old woman attended her physician because she was experiencing attacks of painful discoloration of the fourth and fifth fingers of both hands. She said that her symptoms had started two years previously, during the winter, and affected first her right hand and in subsequent attacks, her left hand as well. Initially, her fingers turned white on exposure to cold and then became deep blue in color. The color change was confined to the distal half of each finger and was accompanied by an aching pain. Holding her hands over a hot stove or going into a hot room was the only treatment that relieved the pain. As the pain disappeared, she said, her fingers became red

and swollen. She told her physician that she had noticed that her fingers were moist with sweat during some of the attacks. Using your knowledge of neuroanatomy, make the diagnosis. What is the autonomic nerve supply to the blood vessels of the upper limb? How would you treat this patient?

4. An obese 45-year-old mother of six children was examined by her physician because her symptoms were suggestive of gallbladder disease. She complained of having severe attacks of colicky pain beneath the right costal margin, which often radiated through to the back beneath the right scapula. The physician turned to a medical student and said, "Note that the patient complains of referred pain to the back." What did he mean by that statement? Explain the phenomenon of referred pain to the back and sometimes the right shoulder in gallbladder disease.

5. Examination of a patient with neurosyphilis indicated that the pupil of her left eye was small and fixed and did not react to light, but contracted when the patient was asked to look at a near object. What is the innervation of the iris? Using your knowledge of neuroanatomy, state where you believe the neurological lesion to be situated to account for these defects.

6. A 36-year-old man was admitted to the emergency room following a gunshot wound to the lower back. Radiographic examination revealed that the bullet was lodged in the vertebral canal at the level of the third lumbar vertebra. A complete neurological examination revealed the symptoms and signs that indicate a complete lesion of the cauda equina. What is the autonomic nerve supply to the bladder? Is this patient going to have any interference with bladder function?

7. A professor of physiology, during the course of his lecture, repeatedly referred to the *sympathetic outflow* and the *parasympathetic outflow*. What is meant by these terms?

8. A 40-year-old black man was found, on routine medical examination, to have essential hypertension. His blood pressure readings were 180 systolic and 100 diastolic (mm Hg). How would you treat this patient medically? What is the action of the various types of drugs that are commonly used in the treatment of hypertension?

9. What transmitter substances are liberated at the following nerve endings: (a) preganglionic sympathetic, (b) preganglionic parasympathetic, (c) postganglionic parasympathetic, (d) postganglionic sympathetic fibers to the heart muscle, and (e) postganglionic sympathetic fibers to the sweat glands of the hand?

10. What is meant by the terms *alpha* and *beta receptors* at sympathetic postganglionic nerve endings?

NATIONAL BOARD TYPE QUESTIONS

Answers on Page 621

IN EACH OF THE FOLLOWING QUESTIONS, ANSWER:
 (a) IF (1) ONLY IS CORRECT
 (b) IF (2) ONLY IS CORRECT
 (c) IF BOTH (1) AND (2) ARE CORRECT, AND
 (d) IF NEITHER (1) NOR (2) IS CORRECT

1. Which of the following statements is (are) correct?
 (1) The enteric nervous system is made up of the submucous plexus of Meissner and the myenteric plexus of Auerbach.
 (2) The nerve fibers of the enteric nervous system are ensheathed by neuroglia-like cells.

2. Which of the following statements is (are) correct?
 (1) The activities of the parasympathetic part of the autonomic nervous system aim at conserving and restoring energy.
 (2) The parasympathetic part of the autonomic system contains both afferent and efferent nerve fibers.

3. Which of the following statements is (are) correct?
 (1) The pretectal nucleus is concerned with the light reflex.
 (2) An Argyll Robertson pupil indicates that the accommodation reflex for near vision is normal but that the light reflex is lost.

4. Which of the following statements is (are) correct?
 (1) White rami communicantes are limited to the thoracic part of the sympathetic trunk.
 (2) Gray rami communicantes contain postganglionic sympathetic fibers.

5. Which of the following statements is (are) correct?
 (1) The greater splanchnic nerves are formed of myelinated axons.
 (2) The lesser splanchnic nerves arise from the tenth and eleventh ganglia of the thoracic part of the sympathetic trunks.

6. Which of the following statements is (are) correct?
 (1) The hypothalamus has very little control of the autonomic nervous system.
 (2) The cerebral cortex has no control over the autonomic nervous system.

Select the best response:

7. The following statements concerning the Horner's syndrome are correct **except**:
 (a) The pupil is constricted.
 (b) There is ptosis of the upper eyelid.
 (c) The patient has vasoconstriction of the facial skin arterioles.
 (d) There is an absence of facial sweating.
 (e) There is enophthalmos.

8. The following statements concerning the sympathetic outflow are incorrect **except**:
 (a) The nerve cells are situated in the posterior gray column (horn) of the spinal cord.
 (b) The preganglionic fibers leave the spinal cord in the posterior roots of the spinal nerves.
 (c) The outflow is restricted to T1–L2 segments of the spinal cord.
 (d) The descending fibers from supraspinal levels pass down the spinal cord to the sympathetic outflow in the posterior white column.
 (e) Many preganglionic nerve fibers synapse in the posterior root ganglia of the spinal nerves.

9. Norepinephrine is secreted by:
 (a) Preganglionic sympathethic fibers
 (b) Preganglionic parasympathetic fibers
 (c) Postganglionic parasympathetic fibers
 (d) Postganglionic sympathetic fibers
 (e) Preganglionic fibers to the suprarenal medulla

10. The parasympathetic innervation controlling the parotid salivary gland arises from which of the following cranial nerves?
    (a) Facial nerve
    (b) Oculomotor nerve
    (c) Vagus nerve
    (d) Carotid plexus
    (e) Glossopharyngeal nerve

11. Which of the following statements best describes the parasympathetic part of the autonomic nervous system?
    (a) It is associated with the thoracolumbar part of the spinal cord.
    (b) Effects are local and discrete due to preganglionic neurons synapsing with few postganglionic neurons.
    (c) It has short preganglionic axons.
    (d) It is active during an emotional crisis.
    (e) Its activity mobilizes glucose from glycogen.

12. Anticholinesterase drugs act at synapses by:
    (a) Mimicking the action of acetylcholine at its receptor sites
    (b) Preventing the release of acetylcholine
    (c) Increasing the secretion of acetylcholine
    (d) Blocking the breakdown of acetylcholine
    (e) Preventing the uptake of acetylcholine by the nerve ending

13. Atropine has the following effect on the autonomic nervous system:
    (a) It is an anticholinesterase drug.
    (b) It increases the activity of norepinephrine.
    (c) It blocks the action of acetylcholine on effector sites in the parasympathetic system.
    (d) It blocks norepinephrine reuptake by presynaptic terminals in the sympathetic system.
    (e) It blocks norepinephrine receptor sites.

Match the glands listed on the left with the most appropriate autonomic ganglion listed on the right. Answers may be used more than once.

14. Submandibular gland
15. Lacrimal gland
16. Nasal glands
17. Parotid gland
18. Sublingual gland

(a) Otic ganglion
(b) Submandibular ganglion
(c) Pterygopalatine ganglion
(d) Ciliary ganglion
(e) None of the above

Match the autonomic ganglia listed on the left with the most appropriate viscus or muscle listed on the right. Answers may be used more than once.

19. Superior cervical ganglion
20. Ciliary ganglion
21. Celiac ganglion
22. Inferior mesenteric ganglion
23. Superior mesenteric ganglion

(a) Levator palpebrae superioris (smooth muscle only)
(b) Vermiform appendix
(c) Constrictor pupillae
(d) Descending colon
(e) None of the above

Match the cranial nerves listed on the left with the appropriate nuclei listed below on the right. Answers may be used more than once.

24. Facial nerve
25. Oculomotor nerve
26. Glossopharyngeal nerve
27. Hypoglossal nerve

(a) Inferior salivatory nucleus
(b) Edinger-Westphal nucleus
(c) Lacrimatory nucleus
(d) None of the above

In the following questions, answer:
    (a) IF (1), (2), AND (3) ONLY ARE CORRECT
    (b) IF (1) AND (3) ONLY ARE CORRECT
    (c) IF (2) AND (4) ONLY ARE CORRECT
    (d) IF (4) ONLY IS CORRECT, OR
    (e) IF ALL ARE CORRECT

28. Which of the following statements is (are) correct, concerning the spinal cord level of the parasympathetic outflow?
    (1) S1, and 2
    (2) S3, 4, and 5
    (3) S1, 2, and 3
    (4) S2, 3, and 4

29. Which of the following statements is (are) correct concerning the autonomic innervation of the urinary bladder?
    (1) The parasympathetic brings about contraction of the bladder wall muscle and relaxation of the sphincter vesicae.
    (2) The sympathetic causes inhibition of the bladder wall muscle and contraction of the sphincter vesicae.

(3) The afferent fibers from the bladder reach the spinal cord at the first and second lumbar segments and the second, third, and fourth sacral segments.

(4) The sympathetic causes contraction of the sphincter urethrae.

30. Which of the following statements is (are) correct concerning the autonomic innervation of the heart?

(1) The parasympathetic nerves cause dilatation of the coronary arteries.

(2) The postganglionic fibers terminate on the sinoatrial and atrioventricular nodes.

(3) The sympathetic postganglionic fibers liberate acetylcholine at their nerve endings.

(4) The sympathetic nerves cause cardiac acceleration and increased force of contraction of the heart.

In Figure 26-18, match the numbered areas of referred pain listed on the left with the appropriate viscus originating the pain listed on the right. Answers may be used more than once.

31. Number 1
32. Number 2
33. Number 3
34. Number 4

(a) Heart
(b) Appendix
(c) Gallbladder
(d) Stomach
(e) None of the above

Fig. 26-18. Areas of referred pain.

ADDITIONAL READING

Appenzeller, D. *The Autonomic Nervous System. An Introduction to Basic and Clinical Concepts* (3rd ed.). Amsterdam: Elsevier Biomedical Press, 1982.

Axelrod, J. The metabolism of catecholamines in vivo and in vitro. *Pharmacol. Rev.* 11:402, 1959.

Bannister, R. (ed.). *Autonomic Failure.* London and Toronto: Oxford University Press, 1983.

Bors, E., and Porter, R. W. Neurosurgical considerations in bladder dysfunction. *Urol. Int.* 25:114, 1970.

Bulygin, I. A. A consideration of the general principles of organization of sympathetic ganglia. *J. Auton. Nerv. Syst.* 8:303, 1983.

de Dombal, F. T. *Diagnosis of Acute Abdominal Pain.* Edinburgh: Churchill Livingstone, 1980.

Eccles, J. C. *The Physiology of Synapses.* Berlin and Vienna: Springer, 1964.

Fitzgerald, G. A. Peripheral presynaptic adrenoreceptor regulation of norepinephrine release in humans. *Fed. Proc.* 43:1379, 1984.

Gershon, M. D. The enteric nervous system. *Annu. Rev. Neurosci.* 4:227, 1981.

Goodman, L. S., and Gilman, A. *The Pharmacological Basis of Therapeutics* (3rd ed.). New York and London: Macmillan, 1965.

Grundy, D. *Gastrointestinal Motility.* Lancaster and Boston: MTP Press, 1985.

Hirsch, E. F., and Borghard-Erdle, A. M. The innervation of the human heart. *Arch. Pathol. Lab. Med.* 71:384, 1961.

Kalsner, S. Limitations of presynaptic theory: No support for feedback control of autonomic effects. *Fed. Proc.* 43:1358, 1984.

Karczmar, A. G., Koketsu, K., and Nishi, S. (eds.). *Autonomic and Enteric Ganglia.* New York: Plenum, 1986.

Kuntz, A. *The Autonomic Nervous System.* Philadelphia: Lea & Febiger, 1953.

Kuru, M. Nervous control of micturition. *Physiol. Rev.* 45:425, 1965.

Lepor, H., Gregerman, M., Crosby, R., Mostofi, F. K., and Walsh, P. C. Precise localization of the autonomic nerves from the pelvic plexus to the corpora cavernosa: A detailed anatomical study of the adult male pelvis. *J. Urol.* 133:207, 1985.

Mei, N. Recent studies on intestinal vagal afferent innervation. Functional implications. *J. Auton. Nerv. Syst.* 9:199, 1983.

Merritt, H., and Moore, M. The Argyll Robertson pupil. *Arch. Neurol. Psychiatry* 30:357, 1933.

Miller, N. E., DiCara, L. V., Solomon, H., et al. Learned modifications of autonomic functions: A review and some new data. *Circ. Res.* (Suppl. 1, Psychological Aspects of Hypertension) 27:3, 1970.

Mitchell, G. A. G. *Anatomy of the Autonomic Nervous System.* Edinburgh: Livingstone, 1953.

Mitchell, G. A. G. *Cardiovascular Innervation.* Edinburgh: Livingstone, 1956.

Nathan, P. W., and Smith, M. C. The location of descending fibers to sympathetic neurons supplying the eye and sudomotor neurons supplying the head and neck. *J. Neurol. Neurosurg. Psychiatry* 49: 187, 1986.

Pick, J. *The Autonomic Nervous System: Morphological, Comparative, Clinical and Surgical Aspects.* Philadelphia: Lippinott, 1970.

Procacci, P., and Zoppi, M. Pathophysiology and clinical aspects of visceral and referred pain. In J. J. Bonica, D. Lindblom, A. Iggo, L. E. Jones, and C. Benedetti (eds.), *Advances in Pain Research and Therapy.* New York: Raven, 1983. Vol. 5. P. 643.

Snell, R. S. *Clinical Anatomy for Medical Students* (4th ed.). Boston: Little, Brown, 1992.

Snell, R. S. The histochemical appearances of cholinesterase in the parasympathetic nerves supplying the submandibular and sublingual salivary glands of the rat. *J. Anat. (Lond.)* 92:534, 1958.

Snell, R. S. The histochemical appearances of cholinesterase in the superior cervical sympathetic ganglion and the changes which occur after preganglionic nerve section. *J. Anat. (Lond.)* 92:408, 1958.

Snider, S. R., and Kuchel, O. Dopamine: An important hormone of the sympathoadrenal system. *Endocr. Rev.* 4:291, 1983.

Swanson, L. W., and Mogenson, G. J. Neural mechanisms for the functional coupling of autonomic, endocrine and somatomotor responses in adaptive behavior. *Brain Res. Rev.* 3:1, 1981.

Westfall, T. C. Evidence that noradrenergic transmitter release is regulated by presynaptic receptors. *Fed. Proc.* 43:1352, 1984.

White, J. C., Smithwick, R. H., and Simeone, F. A. *The Autonomic Nervous System: Anatomy, Physiology and Surgical Applications.* New York and London: Macmillan, 1952.

Chapter 27
The Meninges of the Brain

The brain and spinal cord are surrounded by three membranes, or meninges: the dura mater, the arachnoid mater, and the pia mater.

DURA MATER OF THE BRAIN

The dura mater is conventionally described as two layers, the endosteal layer and the meningeal layer (Fig. 27-1). These are closely united except along certain lines, where they separate to form **venous sinuses**.

The **endosteal layer** is nothing more than the periosteum covering the inner surface of the skull bones. At the foramen magnum it does **not** become continuous with the dura mater of the spinal cord. Around the margins of all the foramina in the skull it becomes continuous with the **periosteum** on the outside of the skull bones. At the sutures, it is continuous with the **sutural ligaments** (Fig. 27-1). It is most strongly adherent to the bones over the base of the skull.

The **meningeal layer** is the dura mater proper. It is a dense, strong fibrous membrane covering the brain (Figs. 27-2 and 27-3) and is continuous through the foramen magnum with the dura mater of the spinal cord. It provides tubular sheaths for the cranial nerves as the latter pass through the foramina in the skull. Outside the skull, the sheaths fuse with the epineurium of the nerves (Fig. 27-2).

The meningeal layer sends inward four septa, which divide the cranial cavity into freely communicating spaces that lodge the subdivisions of the brain (Figs. 27-1 and 27-3). The function of these septa is to restrict the displacement of the brain associated with acceleration and deceleration, when the head is moved.

The **falx cerebri** is a sickle-shaped fold of dura mater that lies in the midline between the two cerebral hemispheres (Figs. 27-1 and 27-3). Its narrow anterior end is attached to the internal frontal crest and the crista galli. Its broad posterior part blends in the midline with the upper surface of the **tentorium cerebelli**. The **superior sagittal sinus** runs in its upper fixed margin; the **inferior sagittal sinus** runs in its lower concave free margin; and the **straight sinus** runs along its attachment to the tentorium cerebelli.

The **tentorium cerebelli** is a crescent-shaped

Skin
Superficial fascia
Epicranial aponeurosis
Loose connective tissue
Pericranium (periosteum)
Outer table of parietal bone
Diploë
Inner table of parietal bone
Cerebral vein in subarachnoid space
Inferior sagittal sinus

Superficial nerves of scalp
Superficial vein of scalp
Skin
Emissary vein
Diploic vein
Superior sagittal sinus
Arachnoid granulation
Endosteal layer of dura
Meningeal layer of dura
Arachnoid
Cerebral artery in subarachnoid space
Pia mater
Cerebral cortex
Falx cerebri

A

Facial and vestibulocochlear nerves
Great cerebral vein
Straight sinus
Tentorium cerebelli
Glossopharyngeal, vagus, and accessory nerves
Hypoglossal nerve
Abducent nerve

Diploic vein
Superior sagittal sinus
Inferior sagittal sinus
Falx cerebri
Trochlear nerve
Oculomotor nerve
Trigeminal nerve
Optic nerve
Olfactory bulb
Sphenoparietal sinus
Superior petrosal sinus

B

Fig. 27-1. A. Coronal section of upper part of head showing: layers of scalp, sagittal suture of skull, falx cerebri, venous sinuses, arachnoid granulations, emissary veins, and relation of cerebral blood vessels to subarachnoid space.
B. Interior of skull, showing dura mater and its contained venous sinuses.

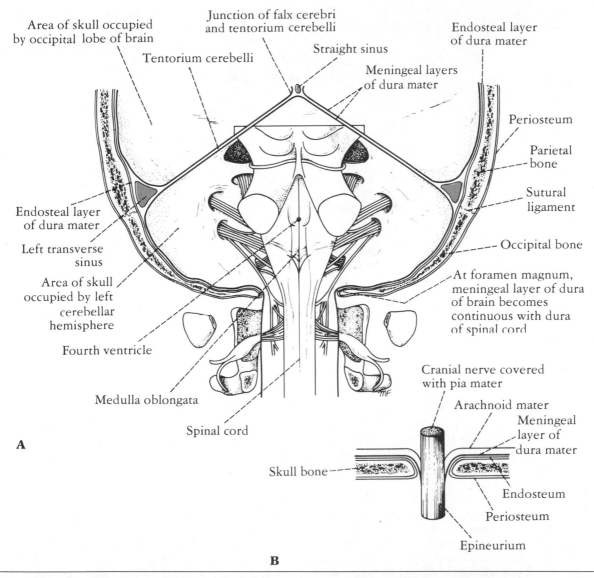

Area of skull occupied
by occipital lobe of brain

Junction of falx cerebri
and tentorium cerebelli

Tentorium cerebelli

Straight sinus

Endosteal layer
of dura mater

Meningeal layers
of dura mater

Periosteum

Parietal
bone

Sutural
ligament

Occipital bone

At foramen magnum,
meningeal layer of dura
of brain becomes
continuous with dura
of spinal cord

Endosteal layer
of dura mater

Left transverse
sinus

Area of skull
occupied by left
cerebellar
hemisphere

Fourth ventricle

Medulla oblongata

Spinal cord

A

Cranial nerve covered
with pia mater

Arachnoid mater

Meningeal
layer of
dura mater

Endosteum

Periosteum

Epineurium

Skull bone

B

Fig. 27-2. A. Posterior view of interior of skull after removal of the occipital and parietal bones. Shows the
arrangement of the endosteal and meningeal layers of the dura mater. The brainstem has been left in situ.
B. The arrangement of the meninges as a cranial nerve passes through a foramen in the skull.

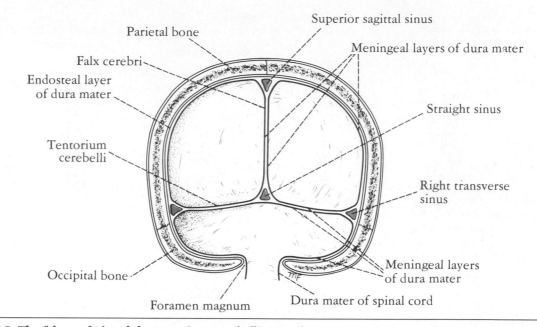

Fig. 27-3. The falx cerebri and the tentorium cerebelli. Note the continuity between the meningeal layer of dura mater within the skull and the dura mater of the spinal cord at the foramen magnum.

fold of dura mater that roofs over the posterior cranial fossa (Figs. 27-1 and 27-4). It covers the upper surface of the cerebellum and supports the occipital lobes of the cerebral hemispheres. In the anterior edge there is a gap, the **tentorial notch**, for the passage of the midbrain (Fig. 27-4), which produces an inner free border and an outer attached or fixed border. The fixed border is attached to the posterior clinoid processes, the superior borders of the petrous bones, and the margins of the grooves for the transverse sinuses on the occipital bone. The free border runs forward at its two ends, crosses the attached border, and is affixed to the anterior clinoid process on each side. At the point where the two borders cross, the third and fourth cranial nerves pass forward to enter the lateral wall of the cavernous sinus (Fig. 27-4).

Close to the apex of the petrous part of the temporal bone, the lower layer of the tentorium is pouched forward beneath the superior petrosal sinus, to form a recess for the trigeminal nerve and the trigeminal ganglion.

The falx cerebri and the falx cerebelli are attached to the upper and lower surfaces of the tentorium, respectively. The straight sinus runs along its attachment to the falx cerebri; the superior petrosal sinus, along its attachment to the petrous bone; and the **transverse sinus**, along its attachment to the occipital bone (Figs. 27-1 and 27-4).

The **falx cerebelli**, a small, sickle-shaped fold of dura mater attached to the internal occipital crest, projects forward between the two cerebellar hemispheres. Its posterior fixed margin contains the **occipital sinus**.

The **diaphragma sellae** is a small, circular fold of dura mater that forms the roof for the sella turcica (Figs. 27-4 and 27-6). A small opening in its center allows passage of the stalk of the **hypophysis cerebri** (Fig. 27-6).

DURAL NERVE SUPPLY

This nerve supply is mainly derived from branches of the **trigeminal nerve**, the **upper three cervical nerves**, the **cervical part of the sympathetic trunk**, and the **vagus nerve**.

Pain receptors in the dura above the tentorium send their impulses via the trigeminal nerve, and a

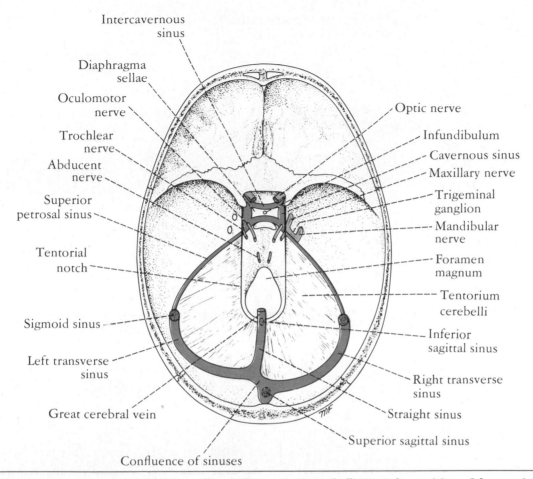

Intercavernous sinus

Diaphragma sellae

Oculomotor nerve

Trochlear nerve

Abducent nerve

Superior petrosal sinus

Tentorial notch

Sigmoid sinus

Left transverse sinus

Great cerebral vein

Confluence of sinuses

Optic nerve

Infundibulum

Cavernous sinus

Maxillary nerve

Trigeminal ganglion

Mandibular nerve

Foramen magnum

Tentorium cerebelli

Inferior sagittal sinus

Right transverse sinus

Straight sinus

Superior sagittal sinus

Fig. 27-4. Superior view of diaphragma sellae and tentorium cerebelli. Note the position of the cranial nerves and venous sinuses.

headache is referred to the skin of the forehead and face. Pain impulses arising from below the tentorium in the posterior cranial fossa travel via the upper three cervical nerves, and the headache is referred to the back of the head and neck.

DURAL ARTERIAL SUPPLY

Numerous arteries supply the dura mater from the **internal carotid, maxillary, ascending pharyngeal, occipital** and **vertebral arteries**. From the clinical standpoint, the most important is the **middle meningeal artery**, which is commonly damaged in head injuries (Fig. 27-5).

The **middle meningeal artery** arises from the maxillary artery in the infratemporal fossa. It enters the cranial cavity through the **foramen spinosum** and then lies between the meningeal and endosteal layers of dura. The artery then runs forward and laterally in a groove on the upper surface of the squamous part of the temporal bone. The anterior (frontal) branch deeply grooves or tunnels the anterior-inferior angle of the parietal bone (Fig. 27-5), and its course corresponds roughly to the line of the underlying precentral gyrus of the brain. The posterior (parietal) branch curves backward and supplies the posterior part of the dura mater (Fig. 27-7).

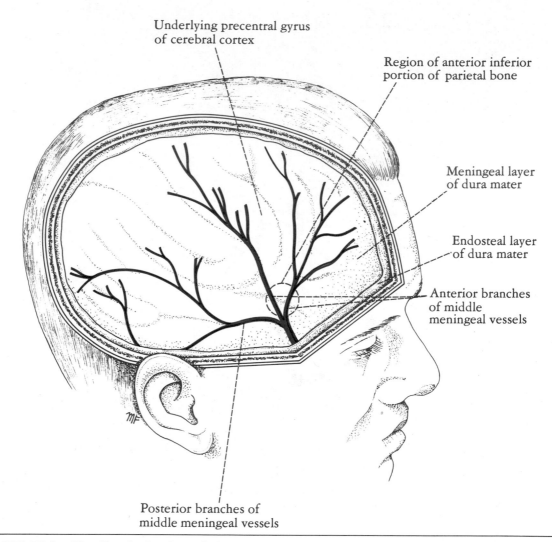

Underlying precentral gyrus of cerebral cortex

Region of anterior inferior portion of parietal bone

Meningeal layer of dura mater

Endosteal layer of dura mater

Anterior branches of middle meningeal vessels

Posterior branches of middle meningeal vessels

Fig. 27-5. Right side of head, showing relations of middle meningeal vessels to layers of dura mater and skull.

The **meningeal veins** lie in the endosteal layer of dura (Fig. 27-5). The middle meningeal vein follows the branches of the middle meningeal artery and drains into the pterygoid venous plexus or the sphenoparietal sinus. The veins lie lateral to the arteries.

DURAL VENOUS SINUSES

The venous sinuses of the cranial cavity are situated between the layers of the dura mater (Figs. 27-1,

27-3, 27-4, 27-6, and 27-7). Their main function is to receive blood from the brain through the cerebral veins and the cerebrospinal fluid from the subarachnoid space through the **arachnoid villi** (see Figs. 18-1 and 18-10). The blood in the dural sinuses ultimately drains into the internal jugular veins in the neck. The dural sinuses are lined by endothelium, and their walls are devoid of muscular tissue. They contain no valves. **Emissary veins,** which are also valveless, connect the dural venous sinuses with the **diploic veins** of the skull and with the veins of the scalp (Fig. 27-1).

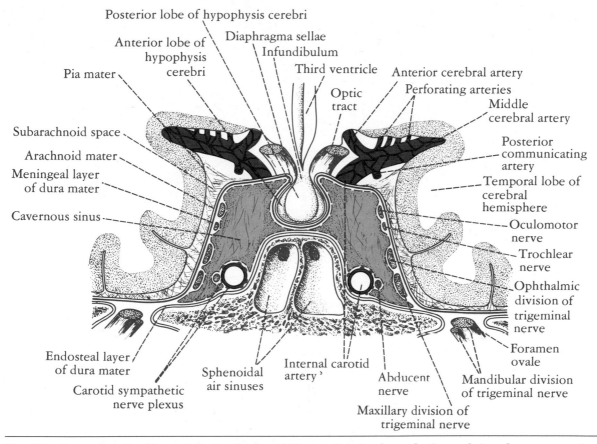

Fig. 27-6. Coronal section through body of sphenoid bone, showing hypophysis cerebri and cavernous sinuses. Note the position of the internal carotid artery and the cranial nerves.

The **superior sagittal sinus** occupies the upper fixed border of the falx cerebri (Figs. 27-1 and 27-4). It begins anteriorly at the foramen cecum, where it occasionally receives a vein from the nasal cavity. It runs posteriorly, grooving the vault of the skull, and at the internal occipital protuberance it deviates to one or the other side (usually the right) and becomes continuous with the corresponding **transverse sinus**. The sinus communicates through small openings with two or three irregularly shaped **venous lacunae** on each side (Fig. 27-7). Numerous arachnoid villi and granulations project into the lacunae, which also receive the diploic and meningeal veins (Fig. 27-1).

The superior sagittal sinus receives in its course the **superior cerebral veins** (Figs. 27-1 and 28-5). At the internal occipital protuberance it is dilated to form the **confluence of the sinuses** (Fig. 27-4).

Here, the superior sagittal sinus usually becomes continuous with the right transverse sinus; it is connected to the opposite transverse sinus and receives the **occipital sinus**.

The **inferior sagittal sinus** occupies the free lower margin of the falx cerebri (Fig. 27-1). It runs backward and joins the **great cerebral vein** at the free margin of the tentorium cerebelli, to form the straight sinus (Figs. 27-1 and 27-4). It receives a few cerebral veins from the medial surface of the cerebral hemispheres.

The **straight sinus** occupies the line of junction of the falx cerebri with the tentorium cerebelli (Figs. 27-1 and 27-4). It is formed by the union of the **inferior sagittal sinus** with the **great cerebral vein**. It ends by turning to the left (sometimes to the right) to form the **transverse sinus**.

The **transverse sinuses** are paired structures

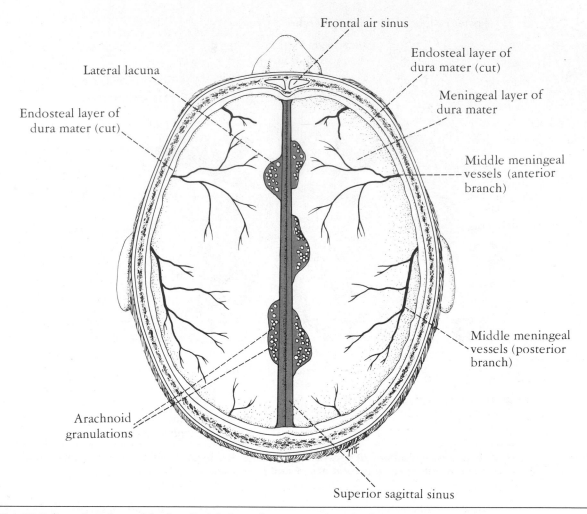

Frontal air sinus

Endosteal layer of
dura mater (cut)

Meningeal layer of
dura mater

Lateral lacuna

Endosteal layer of
dura mater (cut)

Middle meningeal
vessels (anterior
branch)

Middle meningeal
vessels (posterior
branch)

Arachnoid
granulations

Superior sagittal sinus

Fig. 27-7. Superior view of the head with the calvarium removed. The greater part of the endosteal layer of dura mater has been removed, exposing the underlying meningeal layer of dura and the interior of the superior sagittal venous sinus.

and they begin at the internal occipital protuberance (Figs. 27-3 and 27-4). The right sinus is usually continuous with the superior sagittal sinus, and the left is continuous with the straight sinus. Each sinus occupies the attached margin of the tentorium cerebelli, grooving the occipital bone and the posteroinferior angle of the parietal bone. They receive the **superior petrosal sinuses**, the **inferior cerebral** and **cerebellar veins**, and the **diploic veins**. They end by turning downward as the **sigmoid sinuses** (Fig. 27-4).

The **sigmoid sinuses** are a direct continuation of the transverse sinuses. Each sinus turns downward and medially and grooves the mastoid part of the temporal bone (Fig. 27-4). It is here that the sinus lies posterior to the mastoid antrum. The sinus then turns forward and then inferiorly through the posterior part of the jugular foramen, to become continuous with the **superior bulb** of the **internal jugular vein**.

The **occipital sinus** is a small sinus occupying the attached margin of the falx cerebelli. It commences near the foramen magnum, where it communicates with the **vertebral veins** and drains into the **confluence of sinuses**.

The **cavernous sinuses** are situated in the middle cranial fossa on each side of the body of the sphenoid bone (Fig. 27-6). Numerous trabeculae cross their interior, giving them a spongy appearance; hence the name. Each sinus extends from the superior orbital fissure in front to the apex of the petrous part of the temporal bone behind.

The **internal carotid artery**, surrounded by its **sympathetic nerve plexus**, runs forward through the sinus (Fig. 27-6). The **abducent nerve** also passes through the sinus. The internal carotid artery and the nerves are separated from the blood by an endothelial covering.

The **third and fourth cranial nerves**, and the **ophthalmic and maxillary divisions of the trigeminal nerve**, run forward in the lateral wall of the sinus (Fig. 27-6). They lie between the endothelial lining and the dura mater. The tributaries are the **superior and inferior ophthalmic veins**, the **inferior cerebral veins**, the **sphenoparietal sinus**, and the **central vein of the retina**.

The sinus drains posteriorly into the **superior and inferior petrosal sinuses**, and inferiorly into the **pterygoid venous plexus**.

The two sinuses communicate with each other by means of the **anterior and posterior intercavernous sinuses**, which run in the diaphragma sellae anterior and posterior to the stalk of the hypophysis cerebri (Fig. 27-4). Each sinus has an important communication with the facial vein through the superior ophthalmic vein. (This is a route by which infection can travel from the facial skin to the cavernous sinus.)

The **superior and inferior petrosal sinuses** are small sinuses situated on the superior and inferior borders of the petrous part of the temporal bone on each side of the skull (Fig. 27-4). Each superior sinus drains the cavernous sinus into the transverse sinus, and each inferior sinus drains the cavernous sinus into the internal jugular vein.

ARACHNOID MATER OF THE BRAIN

The arachnoid mater is a delicate, impermeable membrane covering the brain and lying between the pia mater internally and the dura mater externally (Fig. 27-1). It is separated from the dura by a potential space, the **subdural space**, filled by a film of fluid; it is separated from the pia by the **subarachnoid space**, which is filled with **cerebrospinal fluid**. The outer and inner surfaces of the arachnoid are covered with flattened mesothelial cells.

The arachnoid bridges over the sulci on the surface of the brain, and in certain situations the arachnoid and pia are widely separated to form the **subarachnoid cisternae**. The **cisterna cerebellomedullaris** lies between the inferior surface of the cerebellum and the roof of the fourth ventricle. The **cisterna interpeduncularis** lies between the two cerebral peduncles. All the cisternae are in free communication with one another and with the remainder of the subarachnoid space.

In certain areas, the arachnoid projects into the venous sinuses to form **arachnoid villi**. The arachnoid villi are most numerous along the superior sagittal sinus. Aggregations of arachnoid villi are referred to as **arachnoid granulations** (Fig. 27-7). Arachnoid villi serve as sites where the cerebrospinal fluid diffuses into the bloodstream (see p. 346).

The arachnoid is connected to the pia mater across the fluid-filled subarachnoid space by delicate strands of fibrous tissue.

It is important to remember that structures passing to and from the brain to the skull or its foramina must pass through the subarachnoid space. All the cerebral arteries and veins lie in the space, as do the cranial nerves (Figs. 27-1 and 27-6). The arachnoid fuses with the epineurium of the nerves at their point of exit from the skull (Fig. 27-2B). In the case of the **optic nerve**, the arachnoid forms a sheath for the nerve, which extends into the orbital cavity through the optic canal and fuses with the sclera of the eyeball (Fig. 27-8). Thus, the subarachnoid space extends around the optic nerve as far as the eyeball.

The **cerebrospinal fluid** is produced by the **choroid plexuses** within the lateral, third, and fourth ventricles of the brain. It escapes from the ventricular system of the brain through the three foramina in the roof of the fourth ventricle and so enters the subarachnoid space. It now circulates both upward over the surfaces of the cerebral hemispheres and downward around the spinal cord. The spinal subarachnoid space extends down

Eyeball
Sclera
Meningeal layer
of dura mater
Arachnoid mater
Pia mater
Optic nerve
Subarachnoid space filled
with cerebrospinal fluid

Fig. 27-8. Sagittal section of the eyeball, showing the attachment of the meninges to the sclera. Note the extension of the subarachnoid space around the optic nerve to the eyeball.

as far as the **second sacral vertebra** (see p. 344). Eventually, the fluid enters the bloodstream by passing into the arachnoid villi and diffusing through their walls.

In addition to removing waste products associated with neuronal activity, the cerebrospinal fluid provides a fluid medium in which the brain floats. This mechanism effectively protects the brain from trauma. In addition, the fluid is now believed to play a role in hormonal transport (see p. 345).

PIA MATER OF THE BRAIN

The pia mater is a vascular membrane covered by flattened mesothelial cells. It closely invests the brain, covering the gyri and descending into the deepest sulci (Fig. 27-1). It extends out over the cranial nerves and fuses with their epineurium. The cerebral arteries entering the substance of the brain carry a sheath of pia with them.

The pia mater forms the **tela choroidea** of the roof of the third and fourth ventricles of the brain, and it fuses with the ependyma to form the choroid plexuses in the lateral, third, and fourth ventricles of the brain.

CLINICAL NOTES

FUNCTIONAL SIGNIFICANCE OF THE MENINGES

The brain and spinal cord have been shown to be enclosed within three concentric membranous sheaths. The outermost is thick, tough, and fibrous and is called the **dura mater**; the middle membrane is thin and delicate and is known as the

arachnoid mater; and the innermost is delicate and vascular and closely applied to the surfaces of the brain and spinal cord and is known as the **pia mater**.

The dura mater of the brain has an outer **endosteal layer**, which serves as the periosteum of the bones of the skull, and an inner **meningeal**

layer, which by virtue of its toughness serves to protect the underlying nervous tissue. The meningeal layer also protects the cranial nerves by forming a sheath that covers each cranial nerve for a short distance as it passes through foramina in the skull. It is in the dura that the large venous sinuses are located. These convey venous blood from the brain and meninges to the internal jugular vein in the neck.

The sickle-shaped partition of dura called the **falx cerebri**, which is positioned vertically between the cerebral hemispheres, and the horizontal sheet, the **tentorium cerebelli**, which projects forward between the cerebrum and cerebellum, serve to limit excessive movements of the brain within the skull. The small vertical sheet, the falx cerebelli, extends forward in the cleft between the cerebellar hemispheres and performs a similar function.

The arachnoid mater is a much thinner membrane than the dura and forms a loose covering for the brain. It bridges over the sulci and dips down into the deep fissure between the cerebral hemispheres. The interval between the arachnoid and pia mater is known as the **subarachnoid space** and is filled with **cerebrospinal fluid**. The cerebrospinal fluid gives buoyancy to the brain and protects the nervous tissue from mechanical forces applied to the skull. The **arachnoid granulations** are essentially small diverticula of the subarachnoid space; they have a covering of arachnoid and an outer covering of endothelium and project into the venous sinuses. They serve as sites where the cerebrospinal fluid diffuses into the bloodstream.

The pia mater is a vascular membrane that closely invests and supports the brain. A sheath of pia accompanies the branches of the cerebral arteries as they enter the substance of the brain.

Clinically, the dura mater is commonly called the **pachymeninx** and the arachnoid and pia mater, the **leptomeninges**.

Movements of the Brain in Relationship to the Meninges in Head Injuries

When a moving patient's head is suddenly halted, the momentum of the brain causes it to travel onward until its movement is resisted by the skull or the strong septa of dura mater. In lateral movements, the lateral surface of one hemisphere hits the side of the skull and the medial surface of the opposite hemisphere hits the side of the falx cerebri. In superior movements, the superior surfaces of the cerebral hemispheres hit the vault of the skull and the superior surface of the corpus callosum hits the sharp free edge of the falx cerebri; the superior surface of the cerebellum presses against the inferior surface of the tentorium cerebelli.

Movements of the brain relative to the skull and dural septa may seriously injure the cranial nerves that are tethered as they pass through the various foramina. Furthermore, the fragile cortical veins that drain into the dural sinuses may be torn, resulting in severe **subdural or subarachnoid hemorrhage**. The tortuous arteries, with their strong walls, are rarely damaged.

Intracranial Hemorrhage and the Meninges

EXTRADURAL HEMORRHAGE

Extradural hemorrhage results from injuries to the meningeal arteries or veins. The most common artery to be damaged is the **anterior division of the middle meningeal artery**. A comparatively minor blow to the side of the head, resulting in fracture of the skull in the region of the anterior-inferior portion of the parietal bone, may sever the artery. Arterial or venous injury is especially liable to occur if the vessels enter a bony canal in this region. Bleeding occurs and strips up the meningeal layer of dura from the internal surface of the skull. The intracranial pressure rises, and the enlarging blood clot exerts local pressure on the underlying motor area in the precentral gyrus. Blood also passes laterally through the fracture line, to form a soft swelling under the temporalis muscle.

In order to stop the hemorrhage, the torn artery or vein must be ligated or plugged. The burr hole through the skull wall should be placed about 1½ inches (4 cm) above the midpoint of the zygomatic arch.

SUBDURAL HEMORRHAGE

Subdural hemorrhage results from tearing of the **superior cerebral veins** at their point of entrance into the superior sagittal sinus. The cause is usually a blow on the front or the back of the head, causing excessive anteroposterior displacement of the brain within the skull.

This condition, which is much more common than middle meningeal hemorrhage, can be produced by a sudden minor blow. Once the vein is torn, blood under low pressure begins to accumulate in the potential space between the dura and the arachnoid. In about half the cases the condition is bilateral.

Acute and chronic forms of the clinical condition occur, depending on the speed of accumulation of fluid in the subdural space. For example, if the patient starts to vomit, the venous pressure will rise as the result of a rise in the intrathoracic pressure. Under these circumstances, the extradural blood clot will rapidly increase in size and produce acute symptoms. In the chronic form, over a course of several months, the small blood clot will attract fluid by osmosis, so that a hemorrhagic cyst is formed, which gradually expands and produces pressure symptoms. In both forms, the blood clot must be removed through burr holes in the skull.

SUBARACHNOID AND CEREBRAL HEMORRHAGES

Subarachnoid and cerebral hemorrhages are described on page 545.

Intracranial Hemorrhage in the Infant

Intracranial hemorrhage may occur during birth and may result from excessive molding of the head. Bleeding may occur from the cerebral veins or the venous sinuses. Excessive anteroposterior compression of the head often tears the anterior attachment of the falx cerebri from the tentorium cerebelli. Bleeding then takes place from the great cerebral veins, the straight sinus, or the inferior sagittal sinus.

Headache

The brain itself is insensitive to pain. It follows that headaches are due to the stimulation of receptors outside the brain.

MENINGEAL HEADACHES

The dura mater receives its sensory nerve supply from the trigeminal and the first three cervical nerves. The dura above the tentorium is innervated by the trigeminal nerve, and the headache is referred to the forehead and face. The dura below the tentorium is innervated by the cervical nerves, and the headache is referred to the back of the head and neck. **Meningitis**, or inflammation of the meninges, causes severe headache over the entire head and back of the neck.

HEADACHES CAUSED BY CEREBRAL TUMORS

An expanding tumor with its associated raised intracranial pressure produces severe, continuous, and progressive headache, caused by the irritation and stretching of the dura. A tumor above the tentorium tends to produce a headache referred to the front of the head, while a tumor below the tentorium produces a headache referred to the back of the head.

MIGRAINE HEADACHE

This is a common form of headache, which may be unilateral or bilateral, recurring at intervals, and associated with prodromal visual disturbances. The prodromal visual disturbances are thought to be due to sympathetic vasoconstriction of the cerebral arteries supplying the visual cortex. The headache is due chiefly to the dilatation and stretching of the external carotid artery and its branches. The disease thus affects both intracranial and extracranial arteries and its cause is unknown, although genetic, hormonal, and biochemical factors may initiate an attack.

ALCOHOLIC HEADACHE

This type of headache is due to the direct toxic affect of alcohol on the meninges.

HEADACHES DUE TO DISEASES OF THE TEETH, PARANASAL SINUSES, AND EYES

Dental infection and sinusitis are common causes of headache. The pain is referred to the skin of the face and the forehead along the branches of the trigeminal nerve. Tonic spasm of the ciliary muscle of the eye, when attempting to focus on an object for prolonged periods (e.g., reading small print), may cause severe orbital headache. This commonly occurs in individuals who need lenses for the correction of presbyopia.

CLINICAL PROBLEMS

Answers on Page 613

1. A visiting neurologist concluded his lecture on the "late effects of head injuries" by saying that the disabilities experienced by a patient are likely to be greater following damage to the dominant hemisphere than to the opposite hemisphere, and that the effect would be much greater in adults than in children. There is no question that this statement is true, but have you thought of the structures that exist within the skull that are clearly there to limit damage to the cerebral hemispheres and other parts of the brain? Which blood vessels are damaged more commonly, the cerebral arteries or the cerebral veins? Are cranial nerves likely to be damaged in head injuries? If so, which ones are damaged most commonly and what is the reason for their increased susceptibility?

2. While performing an autopsy on a patient who had died of a meningioma, the pathologist explained to a group of students that these tumors arise from the arachnoid mater. He explained that they occur in those areas in which the arachnoid pierces the dura to form the arachnoid villi that project into the dural venous sinuses. He then asked the students where they would expect to find meningiomas? Could you answer that question?

3. A 10-year-old girl was admitted to hospital for surgical correction of medial strabismus of the right eye. Twenty-four hours after the successful completion of the operation it was noted that her right eyeball was projecting forward excessively (proptosis) and the conjunctiva of the right eye was inflamed. A watery, purulent discharge could be expressed from beneath the eyelids. The ophthalmologist was greatly concerned because he did not want the complication of cavernous sinus thrombosis to occur. What is the connection between infection of the eye and cavernous sinus thrombosis? Do you think that cavernous sinus thrombosis is a serious condition?

4. A 41-year-old man was found, on examination, to have paralysis of the lateral rectus muscle of his left eye; the left pupil was dilated but reacted slowly to light, and there was some anesthesia of the skin over the left forehead. A carotid arteriogram revealed the presence of an aneurysm of the right internal carotid artery situated in the cavernous sinus. Using your knowledge of anatomy, can you explain the clinical findings on physical examination?

5. A 45-year-old woman was found on ophthalmoscopic examination to have edema of both optic discs (*bilateral papilledema*) and congestion of the retinal veins. The cause of the condition was found to be a rapidly growing intracranial tumor. Using your knowledge of anatomy, explain the papilledema. Why does the patient exhibit bilateral papilledema?

6. A pediatrician was observing a 6-year-old boy playing with his toys. He noted that the child had perfectly normal use of his arms but that his legs were stiff and, when he walked, he tended to cross his legs and had a scissorlike gait. A diagnosis of cerebral diplegia* secondary to birth injuries was made. Apparently the child was born prematurely and he was a breech presentation. Using your knowledge of anatomy, explain what happens to the fetal skull bones during delivery. Why are the dural venous sinuses likely to be damaged at birth? Why is cerebral hemorrhage more likely to occur in a premature baby with a malpresentation?

7. A 25-year-old woman was admitted to the emergency room unconscious. She had apparently been hit on the side of the head by a car while crossing the road. Within an hour, her state of unconsciousness deepened. On examination, she was found to have a large, doughlike swelling over the right temporalis muscle. She also had

---

*Congenital cerebral diplegia is believed by some authorities to occur early in fetal life and to be caused by a viral infection that arrests cerebral development.

the signs of right-sided hemiplegia. Later, a right-sided, fixed, dilated pupil developed. A lateral radiograph of the skull showed a fracture line across the groove for the anterior division of the right middle meningeal artery. Her coma deepened, and she died 4 hours after the accident. Using your knowledge of neuroanatomy, make a diagnosis in this case. Explain the clinical findings. How could you account for the homolateral hemiplegia?

8. A 50-year-old woman visited her physician complaining of a severe headache of 3 days' duration. She said that the headache had started getting very severe about 1 hour after she had hit her head on the mantelpiece after bending down to poke the fire. She was admitted to the hospital for observation. Three hours later it was noticed that she was becoming mentally confused and also that she was developing a right-sided hemiplegia on the side of the body opposite the head injury. She had exaggeration of the deep reflexes and a positive Babinski response on the right side. Examination of the cerebrospinal fluid with a lumbar puncture showed a raised pressure with the presence of blood in the fluid. Radiographic examination showed no fracture of the skull. A diagnosis of subdural hematoma was made. What exactly is a subdural hematoma?

NATIONAL BOARD TYPE QUESTIONS

Answers on Page 621

IN EACH OF THE FOLLOWING QUESTIONS, ANSWER:
- (a) IF (1) ONLY IS CORRECT
- (b) IF (2) ONLY IS CORRECT
- (c) IF BOTH (1) AND (2) ARE CORRECT, AND
- (d) IF NEITHER (1) NOR (2) IS CORRECT

1. Which of the following statements is (are) correct?
   (1) Both layers of the dura mater covering the brain are continuous through the foramen magnum with the dura covering the spinal cord.
   (2) The meningeal layer of dura mater is continuous with the sutural ligaments of the skull.

2. Which of the following statements is (are) correct?
   (1) As each cranial nerve passes through a foramen in the skull, it is surrounded by a tubular sheath of pia, arachnoid, and dura mater.
   (2) The cranial venous sinuses run between the meningeal and endosteal layers of dura mater.

3. Which of the following statements is (are) correct?
   (1) The meninges extend anteriorly through the optic canal and fuse with the sclera of the eyeball.
   (2) The cisterna cerebellomedularis is filled with blood and lies between the inferior surface of the cerebellum and the roof of the fourth ventricle.

4. Which of the following statements is (are) correct?
   (1) The arachnoid mater is permeable to cerebrospinal fluid.
   (2) The cerebrospinal fluid in the arachnoid villi is able to drain into the venous sinuses through small tubules lined with endothelial cells.

Select the best response:

5. The following statements concerning the tentorium cerebelli are correct **except**:
   (a) The free border is attached anteriorly to the anterior clinoid processes.
   (b) It is formed from the meningeal layer of the dura mater.
   (c) It separates the cerebellum from the occipital lobes of the brain.
   (d) The sigmoid sinus lies within its attached border to the occipital bone.
   (e) In the anterior edge there is the tentorial notch.

6. The following statements concerning headache are correct **except**:
   (a) Brain tissue is insensitive to pain.
   (b) Intracranial pain arises from receptors situated in the dura mater.
   (c) An expanding cerebral tumor located in the posterior cranial fossa would produce pain referred to the face.
   (d) Migraine headache is due to dilatation of the external carotid artery and its branches.

(e) Headaches associated with presbyopia are due to tonic spasm of the ciliary muscles of the eyes.

7. The following statements concerning the subarachnoid space are true **except**:
   (a) It is filled with cerebrospinal fluid.
   (b) It extends inferiorly as far as the second sacral vertebra.
   (c) It contains the cerebral arteries and veins.
   (d) The cranial nerves lie outside the subarachnoid space in sheaths derived from the dura mater.
   (e) The arachnoid villi project into the venous sinuses as minute out-pouchings of the subarachnoid space.

In the following questions, answer:
   (a) IF (1), (2), AND (3) ONLY ARE CORRECT
   (b) IF (1) AND (3) ONLY ARE CORRECT
   (c) IF (2) AND (4) ONLY ARE CORRECT
   (d) IF (4) ONLY IS CORRECT, OR
   (e) IF ALL ARE CORRECT

8. Which of the following statements is (are) correct concerning the cavernous sinus?
   (1) It has passing through it the internal carotid artery and the abducent nerve.
   (2) It has the oculomotor, trochlear, and ophthalmic divisions of the trigeminal nerve in its lateral wall.
   (3) It is related medially to the pituitary gland and the sphenoid air sinus.
   (4) It communicates anteriorly via the superior ophthalmic vein with the facial vein.

9. Which of the following structures limit(s) rotatory movements of the brain within the skull?
   (1) The falx cerebri
   (2) The falx cerebelli
   (3) The body of the sphenoid bone
   (4) The diaphragma sellae

10. Which of the following nerves serve(s) as sensory nerves to the dura mater?
   (1) Glossopharyngeal nerve
   (2) Trigeminal nerve
   (3) Hypoglossal nerve
   (4) Upper three cervical nerves

ADDITIONAL READING

Bannister, R. *Brain's Clinical Neurology* (6th ed.). London and New York: Oxford University Press, 1985.

Bruyn, G. W. Biochemistry of Migraine. *Headache* 20:235, 1980.

Doogan, D. P. Prophylaxis of migraine with beta-blockers. *Practitioner* 227:441, 1983.

Snell, R. S. *Clinical Anatomy for Medical Students* (4th ed.). Boston: Little, Brown, 1992.

Williams, P. L., Warwick, R., Dyson, M., and Bannister, L. H. (eds.). *Gray's Anatomy* (37th Brit. ed.). Philadelphia: Saunders, 1989.

Chapter 28
The Blood Supply of the Brain

ARTERIES OF THE BRAIN

The brain is supplied by the two internal carotid and the two vertebral arteries. The four arteries lie within the subarachnoid space, and their branches anastomose on the inferior surface of the brain to form the **circulus arteriosus** (circle of Willis).

Internal Carotid Artery

The internal carotid artery begins at the bifurcation of the common carotid artery (Fig. 28-1), where it usually possesses a localized dilatation, called the **carotid sinus**. It ascends the neck and perforates the base of the skull by passing through the carotid canal of the temporal bone. The artery then runs horizontally forward through the cavernous sinus and emerges on the medial side of the anterior clinoid process by perforating the dura mater. It now enters the subarachnoid space by piercing the arachnoid mater and turns posteriorly to the region of the anterior perforated substance of the brain at the medial end of the lateral cerebral sulcus. Here, it divides into the **anterior** and **middle cerebral arteries** (Figs. 28-1 and 28-2).

Branches of the Cerebral Portion of the Internal Carotid Artery

1. The **ophthalmic artery** arises as the internal carotid artery emerges from the cavernous sinus (Fig. 28-1). It enters the orbit through the optic canal below and lateral to the optic nerve. It supplies the eye and other orbital structures and its terminal branches supply the frontal area of the scalp, the ethmoid and frontal sinuses, and the dorsum of the nose.
2. The **posterior communicating artery** is a small vessel that originates from the internal carotid artery close to its terminal bifurcation (Figs. 28-1 and 28-2). The posterior communicating artery runs posteriorly above the oculomotor nerve to join the posterior cerebral artery, thus forming part of the **circulus arteriosus**.
3. The **choroidal artery**, a small branch, also originates from the internal carotid artery close to its terminal bifurcation. The choroidal artery

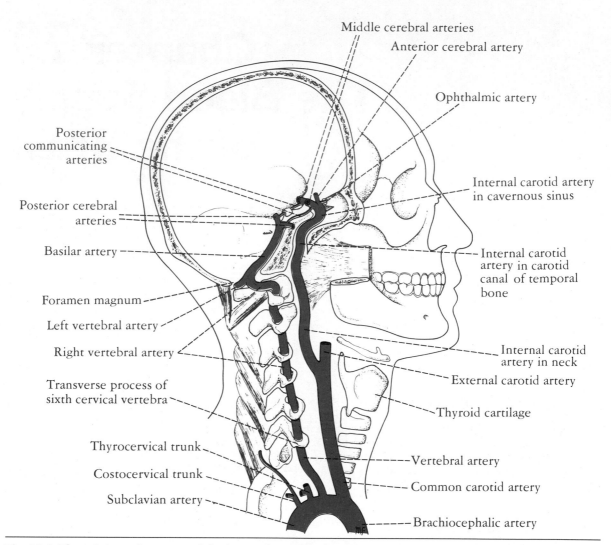

Middle cerebral arteries

Anterior cerebral artery

Ophthalmic artery

Posterior communicating arteries

Internal carotid artery in cavernous sinus

Posterior cerebral arteries

Basilar artery

Internal carotid artery in carotid canal of temporal bone

Foramen magnum

Left vertebral artery

Right vertebral artery

Transverse process of sixth cervical vertebra

Internal carotid artery in neck

External carotid artery

Thyroid cartilage

Thyrocervical trunk

Costocervical trunk

Subclavian artery

Vertebral artery

Common carotid artery

Brachiocephalic artery

Fig. 28-1. The origin and courses of the internal carotid and vertebral arteries as they ascend the neck to enter the skull.

passes posteriorly close to the optic tract, enters the inferior horn of the lateral ventricle, and ends in the choroid plexus. It gives off numerous small branches to surrounding structures, including the crus cerebri, the lateral geniculate body, the optic tract, and the internal capsule.

4. The **anterior cerebral artery** is the smaller terminal branch of the internal carotid artery (Fig. 28-2). It runs forward and medially superior to the optic nerve and enters the longitudinal fissure of the cerebrum. Here, it is joined to the

anterior cerebral artery of the opposite side by the **anterior communicating artery**. It curves backward over the corpus callosum, and, finally, anastomoses with the posterior cerebral artery (Figs. 28-3 and 28-7). The **cortical branches** supply all the medial surface of the cerebral cortex as far back as the parieto-occipital sulcus (Fig. 28-3). They also supply a strip of cortex about 1 inch (2.5 cm) wide on the adjoining lateral surface. The anterior cerebral artery thus supplies the "leg area" of the precentral gyrus. A

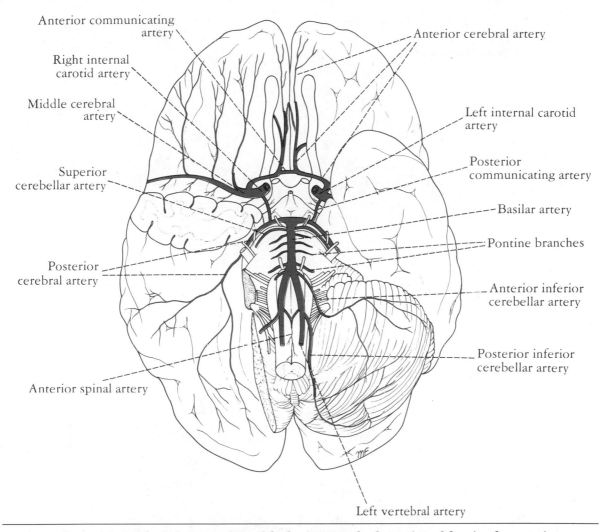

Anterior communicating artery

Right internal carotid artery

Middle cerebral artery

Superior cerebellar artery

Posterior cerebral artery

Anterior spinal artery

Anterior cerebral artery

Left internal carotid artery

Posterior communicating artery

Basilar artery

Pontine branches

Anterior inferior cerebellar artery

Posterior inferior cerebellar artery

Left vertebral artery

Fig. 28-2. The arteries of the inferior surface of the brain. Note the formation of the circulus arteriosus. Part of the right terminal lobe has been removed to show the course of the middle cerebral artery.

group of **central branches** pierces the anterior perforated substance and helps to supply parts of the lentiform and caudate nuclei and the internal capsule.

5. The **middle cerebral artery**, the largest branch of the internal carotid, runs laterally in the lateral cerebral sulcus (Fig. 28-2). **Cortical branches** supply the entire lateral surface of the hemisphere, except for the narrow strip supplied by the anterior cerebral artery, the occipital pole, and the inferolateral surface of the hemisphere, which are supplied by the posterior cerebral

artery (Fig. 28-3). This artery thus supplies all the motor area except the "leg area." **Central branches** enter the anterior perforated substance and supply the lentiform and caudate nuclei and the internal capsule (Fig. 28-4).

Vertebral Artery

The vertebral artery, a branch of the first part of the subclavian artery, ascends the neck by passing through the foramina in the transverse processes of the upper six cervical vertebrae (Fig. 28-1). It en-

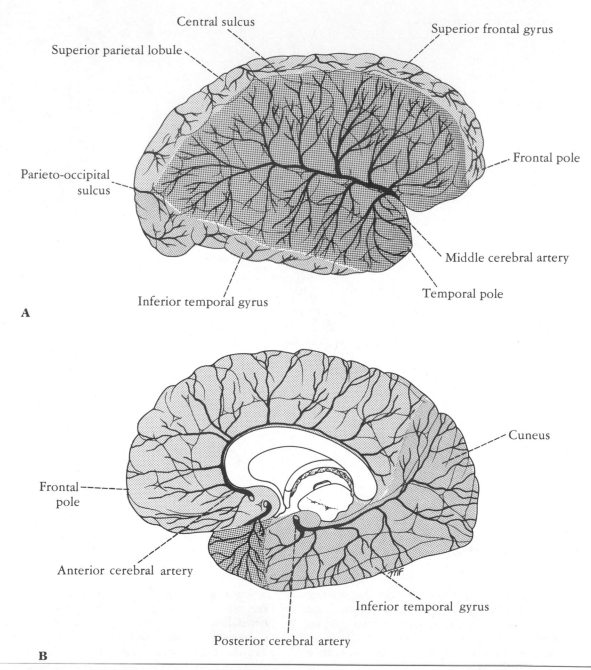

Fig. 28-3. Areas supplied by the cerebral arteries.
A. The lateral surface of the right cerebral hemisphere.
B. The medial surface of the right cerebral hemisphere. The area supplied by the anterior cerebral artery is colored blue, that supplied by the middle cerebral artery is red, and that supplied by the posterior cerebral artery is brown.

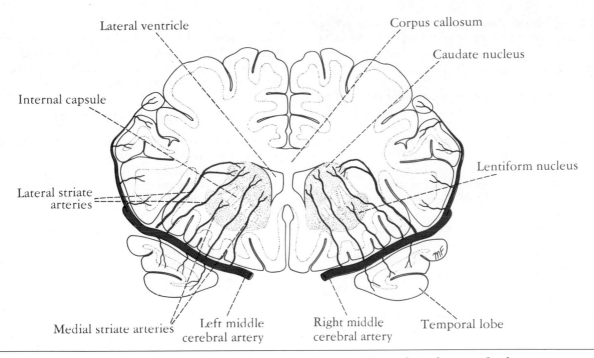

Fig. 28-4. Coronal section of cerebral hemispheres, showing arterial supply to deep cerebral structures from the middle cerebral artery.

ters the skull through the foramen magnum and pierces the dura mater and arachnoid to enter the subarachnoid space. It then passes upward, forward, and medially on the medulla oblongata (Fig. 28-2). At the lower border of the pons, it joins the vessel of the opposite side to form the **basilar artery**.

Branches of the Cranial Portion of the Vertebral Artery

1. The **meningeal branches** are small and supply the bone and dura in the posterior cranial fossa.
2. The **posterior spinal artery** may arise from the vertebral artery or the posterior inferior cerebellar artery. It descends on the posterior surface of the spinal cord close to the posterior roots of the spinal nerves. The branches are reinforced by radicular arteries that enter the vertebral canal through the intervertebral foramina. For the detailed distribution of this artery, see page 173.
3. The **anterior spinal artery** is formed from a contributory branch from each vertebral artery near its termination (Fig. 28-2). The single ar-

tery descends on the anterior surface of the medulla oblongata and spinal cord and is embedded in the pia mater along the anterior median fissure. The artery is reinforced by radicular arteries that enter the vertebral canal through the intervertebral foramina. For the detailed distribution of this artery, see page 173.
4. The **posterior inferior cerebellar artery**, the largest branch of the vertebral artery, passes on an irregular course between the medulla and the cerebellum (Figs. 28-2, 28-11, and 28-13). It supplies the inferior surface of the vermis, the central nuclei of the cerebellum, and the undersurface of the cerebellar hemisphere; it also supplies the medulla oblongata and the choroid plexus of the fourth ventricle.
5. The **medullary arteries** are very small branches that are distributed to the medulla oblongata.

Basilar Artery

The basilar artery, formed by the union of the two vertebral arteries (Fig. 28-1), ascends in a groove on the anterior surface of the pons (Figs. 28-2, 28-

12, and 28-13). At the upper border of the pons, it divides into the two posterior cerebral arteries.

Branches of the Basilar Artery

1. The **pontine arteries** are numerous small vessels that enter the substance of the pons (Figs. 28-2, 28-12, and 28-13).
2. The **labyrinthine artery** is a long, narrow artery that accompanies the facial and the vestibulocochlear nerves into the internal acoustic meatus and supplies the internal ear. It often arises as a branch of the anterior inferior cerebellar artery.
3. The **anterior inferior cerebellar artery** passes posteriorly and laterally and supplies the anterior and inferior parts of the cerebellum (Figs. 28-2, 28-12, and 28-13). A few branches pass to the pons and the upper part of the medulla oblongata.
4. The **superior cerebellar artery** arises close to the termination of the basilar artery (Figs. 28-2 and 28-10 through 28-13). It winds around the cerebral peduncle and supplies the superior surface of the cerebellum. It also supplies the pons, the pineal gland, and the superior medullary velum.
5. The **posterior cerebral artery** curves laterally and backward around the midbrain and is joined by the posterior communicating branch of the internal carotid artery (Figs. 28-1, 28-2, and 28-10 through 28-13). **Cortical branches** supply the inferolateral and medial surfaces of the temporal lobe and the lateral and medial surfaces of the occipital lobe (Fig. 28-3). Thus the posterior cerebral artery supplies the visual cortex. **Central branches** pierce the brain substance and supply parts of the thalamus and the lentiform nucleus, and the midbrain, the pineal, and the medial geniculate bodies. A **choroidal branch** enters the inferior horn of the lateral ventricle and supplies the choroid plexus; it also supplies the choroid plexus of the third ventricle.

The **circulus arteriosus** lies in the interpeduncular fossa at the base of the brain. It is formed by the anastomosis between the two internal carotid arteries and the two vertebral arteries (Fig. 28-2). The anterior communicating, anterior cerebral, internal carotid, posterior communicating, posterior cerebral, and basilar arteries all contribute to the circle. The circulus arteriosus allows blood that enters by either internal carotid or vertebral arteries to be distributed to any part of both cerebral hemispheres. Cortical and central branches arise from the circle and supply the brain substance.

Arteries to Specific Brain Areas

The **corpus striatum** and the **internal capsule** are supplied mainly by the medial and lateral striate central branches of the middle cerebral artery (Fig. 28-4); the central branches of the anterior cerebral artery supply the remainder of these structures.

The **thalamus** is supplied mainly by branches of the posterior communicating, basilar, and posterior cerebral arteries.
The **midbrain** is supplied by the posterior cerebral, superior cerebellar, and basilar arteries.
The **pons** is supplied by the basilar and the anterior, inferior, and superior cerebellar arteries.
The **medulla oblongata** is supplied by the vertebral, anterior and posterior spinal, posterior inferior cerebellar, and basilar arteries.
The **cerebellum** is supplied by the superior cerebellar, anterior inferior cerebellar, and posterior inferior cerebellar arteries.

Nerve Supply of Cerebral Arteries

The cerebral arteries receive a rich supply of sympathetic postganglionic nerve fibers. These fibers are derived from the superior cervical sympathetic ganglion. Stimulation of these nerves causes vasoconstriction of the cerebral arteries. However, under normal conditions, the local blood flow is mainly controlled by the concentrations of carbon dioxide, hydrogen ions, and oxygen present in the nervous tissue; a rise in the carbon dioxide and hydrogen ion concentrations and a lowering of the oxygen tension bring about a vasodilatation.

VEINS OF THE BRAIN

The veins of the brain have no muscular tissue in their very thin walls, and they possess no valves. They emerge from the brain and lie in the subarachnoid space. They pierce the arachnoid mater and the meningeal layer of the dura and drain into the cranial venous sinuses (Fig. 28-5).

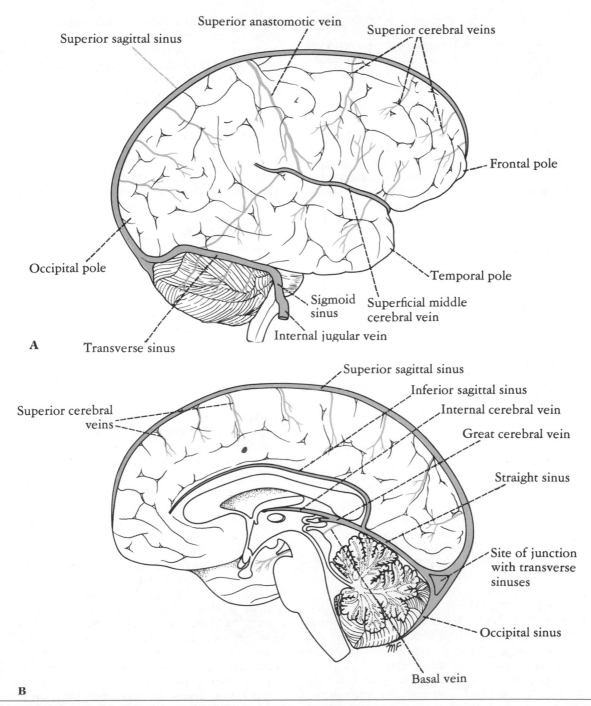

Fig. 28-5. The venous drainage of the right cerebral hemisphere.
A. Lateral surface.
B. Medial surface.

External Cerebral Veins

The **superior cerebral veins** pass upward over the lateral surface of the cerebral hemisphere and empty into the superior sagittal sinus (Fig. 28-5).

The **superficial middle cerebral vein** drains the lateral surface of the cerebral hemisphere. It runs inferiorly in the lateral sulcus and empties into the cavernous sinus (Fig. 28-5).

The **deep middle cerebral vein** drains the insula and is joined by the **anterior cerebral** and **striate veins** to form the **basal vein**. The basal vein ultimately joins the great cerebral vein, which in turn drains into the straight sinus (Fig. 28-5).

Internal Cerebral Veins

There are two internal cerebral veins and they are formed by the union of the **thalamostriate vein** and the **choroid vein** at the interventricular foramen. The two veins run posteriorly in the tela choroidea of the third ventricle and unite beneath the splenium of the corpus callosum to form the great cerebral vein, which empties into the straight sinus.

Veins of Specific Brain Areas

The **midbrain** is drained by veins that open into the basal or great cerebral veins.

The **pons** is drained by veins that open into the basal vein, cerebellar veins, or neighboring venous sinuses.

The **medulla oblongata** is drained by veins that open into the spinal veins and neighboring venous sinuses.

The **cerebellum** is drained by veins that empty into the great cerebral vein or adjacent venous sinuses.

CLINICAL NOTES

In spite of the recent decrease in cerebrovascular disease, it has been estimated that it is responsible for about 50 percent of all adult neurological hospital admissions.

CEREBRAL CIRCULATION

The brain has been shown to be supplied with arterial blood from the two internal carotid arteries and the two vertebral arteries, which unite anteriorly to form the basilar artery. The circulus arteriosus (**circle of Willis**), which lies in the interpeduncular fossa at the base of the brain, is formed by anastomoses between the internal carotid arteries, the basilar artery, and their branches.

In 1951, McDonald and Potter showed that the blood supply to half of the brain is provided by the internal carotid and vertebral arteries on that side, and that their respective streams come together in the posterior communicating artery at a point where the pressure of the two is equal and they do not mix (Fig. 28-14). If, however, the internal carotid or vertebral artery is occluded, the blood passes forward or backward across that point to compensate for the reduction in blood flow. The circulus arteriosus also permits the blood to flow across the midline, as shown when the internal carotid or vertebral artery on one side is occluded. It also has been shown that the two streams of blood from the vertebral arteries remain separate and on the same side of the lumen of the basilar artery and do not mix.

Although the cerebral arteries anastomose with one another at the circulus arteriosus and by means of branches on the surface of the cerebral hemispheres, once they enter the brain substance no further anastomoses occur.

The most important factor in forcing the blood through the brain is the arterial blood pressure. This is opposed by such factors as a raised intracranial pressure, increased blood viscosity, and narrowing of the vascular diameter. Cerebral blood flow remains remarkably constant in spite of changes in the general blood pressure. This autoregulation of the circulation (Best and Taylor, 1973) is accomplished by a compensatory lowering of the cerebral vascular resistance when the arterial pressure is lowered and a raising of the vascular resistance when the arterial pressure is raised. Needless to say, this autoregulation fails to maintain an adequate blood flow, should the arterial blood pressure fall to a very low level.

The diameter of the cerebral blood vessels is the main factor contributing to the cerebrovascular resistance. While it is known that they are innervated by sympathetic postganglionic nerve fibers and that they respond to norepinephrine, they apparently play little or no part in the control of cerebrovascular resistance in normal human beings. The most powerful vasodilator substances for cerebral blood vessels are an increase in carbon dioxide or hydrogen ion concentration; a reduction in oxygen concentration also causes vasodilatation. It has recently been shown that an increase in neuronal activity in different parts of the brain causes a local increase in blood flow.

The cerebral blood flow in patients can be measured by the intracarotid injection or inhalation of radioactive krypton or xenon. A cerebral blood flow of 50 to 60 ml/100 g of brain per minute is considered normal.

CEREBRAL ISCHEMIA

Vascular lesions of the brain are extremely common and the resulting neurological defect will depend on the size of the artery occluded, the state of the collateral circulation, and the area of the brain involved. Clinical studies and the examination of postmortem material have focused attention on the high frequency of lesions in the common carotid, internal carotid, and vertebral arteries in the neck.

Impairment of cerebral blood flow may be caused by a large number of conditions, and the more important may be considered under the following headings: (1) diseases that produce alteration in blood pressure, (2) diseases of arterial walls, and (3) diseases that result in blockage of the arterial lumen.

DISEASES THAT PRODUCE ALTERATION IN BLOOD PRESSURE

Interruption of Cerebral Circulation

Irreversible brain damage with death of nervous tissue rapidly follows complete arrest of cerebral blood flow. It has been estimated that neuronal function ceases after about one minute and that irreversible changes start to occur after about 4 minutes, although this time may be longer if the patient's body has been cooled.* Cardiac arrest due to coronary thrombosis is the most common cause of this condition.

Postural Hypotension

Patients who get up after being confined to bed for several days, soldiers who stand at attention for long periods on a hot day, and worshipers kneeling in church—all may experience the accumulation of venous blood in the limbs or impaired venous return to the heart, with a consequent fall in the cardiac output and a lowered arterial blood pressure. The general arterial pressure has to be lowered considerably before the cerebral blood flow is diminished.

Physical and Psychological Shock

The profound and prolonged fall in blood pressure that may follow physical trauma such as an automobile accident or extensive surgery, especially in the elderly, in whom the cerebral arteries are already narrowed by disease, may cause the patient to lose consciousness. Hyperventilation in anxiety states may reduce the cerebral blood flow by lowering the carbon dioxide content of the blood.

Change in Blood Viscosity

In polycythemia vera, the cerebral blood flow is considerably reduced as the result of an increase in the viscosity of the blood (Brain and Walton, 1969).

Carotid Sinus Syndrome

The carotid sinus, situated at the proximal end of the internal carotid artery, is extremely sensitive to changes in arterial blood pressure. Distention of the arterial wall causes a reflex slowing of the heart rate and a fall in blood pressure. This occurs as the result of an increased number of nervous impulses passing up the sinus nerve, a branch of the glossopharyngeal nerve, which connects with the car-

---

*It must be emphasized that brain damage may be reversed, if the blood flow can be restored even after 5 minutes.

dioinhibitory and vasomotor centers. Hypersensitivity of the reflex or external pressure may cause the blood pressure to fall suddenly and produce cerebral ischemia and loss of consciousness.

Diseases of the Heart

Any severe cardiac disease, such as coronary thrombosis, auricular fibrillation, or heart block, that results in a marked fall in cardiac output will result in a severe fall in general arterial blood pressure and reduction in cerebral blood flow.

Diseases of the Arterial Walls

The most common cause of narrowing of the lumen of the arteries that supply the brain is atheroma. This disease may affect the main arteries supplying the brain in their course through the neck as well as their course within the skull. Moreover, the impairment of the cerebral circulation may be worsened by an attack of coronary thrombosis, with its associated hypotension, shock due to surgical procedures, severe anemia, or even rotation of the head with external pressure on the carotid arteries.

Atheromatous degeneration of the cerebral arteries occurs most commonly in middle or old age and often complicates diabetes and hypertension. When actual blockage of an artery occurs, the effect will depend on the size and location of the vessel. The nerve cells and their fibers will degenerate in the avascular area and the surrounding neuroglia will proliferate and invade the area. In patients with generalized narrowing of the cerebral arteries without blockage of a single artery, the brain will undergo a diffuse atrophy. It should be remembered that a very narrow atheromatous artery may be blocked by a thrombus, thus totally closing the lumen.

DISEASES THAT RESULT IN BLOCKAGE OF THE ARTERIAL LUMEN

Embolism of a cerebral artery may occur in two forms: (1) by far the most common, a thrombus, and (2) fat globules. The thrombus may develop anywhere on the endothelial lining from the left side of the heart to the parent vessels of the cerebral arteries. A common site of origin is an atheromatous plaque on the internal carotid, common carotid, or vertebral artery. Another area is the site of endocarditis on the mitral or aortic valve or the endocardial lining of a myocardial infarction following a coronary thrombosis. In women, cerebral thrombosis is more common among those taking oral contraceptives, especially those taking a high-dose estrogen-progesterone combination.

Fat embolism usually follows severe fractures of one of the long bones. Fat globules from the macerated yellow marrow enter the nutrient veins, pass through the pulmonary circulation, and end up blocking multiple small cerebral end arteries.

CEREBRAL ANEURYSMS

Congenital Aneurysms

Congenital aneurysms occur most commonly at the site where two arteries join in the formation of the circulus arteriosus. At this point, there is a deficiency in the tunica media and this is complicated by the development of atheroma, which so weakens the arterial wall that a local dilatation occurs. The aneurysm may press on neighboring structures, such as the optic nerve or the third, fourth, or sixth cranial nerve, and produce signs or symptoms, or may suddenly rupture into the subarachnoid space. In the latter case, a severe pain in the head suddenly develops, followed by mental confusion. Death may quickly occur, or the patient may survive the first bleeding only to die a few days or weeks later. Clipping or ligating the neck of the aneurysm offers the best chance of recovery.

Other types of aneurysms are rare and include those due to softening of the arterial wall following the lodging of an infected embolus, those due to damage of the internal carotid artery as it lies within the cavernous sinus following a fracture of the skull, and those that are associated with disease of the arterial wall such as atheroma.

INTRACRANIAL HEMORRHAGE

Intracranial hemorrhage may result from trauma or cerebral vascular lesions. Four varieties will be considered: (1) extradural, (2) subdural, (3) subarachnoid, and (4) cerebral. Extradural and subdural hemorrhage are described on page 37.

Subarachnoid Hemorrhage

Subarachnoid hemorrhage usually results from leakage or rupture of a congenital aneurysm on the cerebral arterial circle or, less commonly, from an angioma or contusion and laceration of the brain and meninges. The symptoms, which are sudden in onset, will include severe headache, stiffness of the neck, and loss of consciousness. The diagnosis is established by the use of computed tomography (CT scanning). The dense areas of the blood in the subarachnoid space can be identified. The withdrawal of heavily blood-stained cerebrospinal fluid through a lumbar puncture is also diagnostic, but this method has been replaced by the use of CT scans.

Cerebral Hemorrhage

Cerebral hemorrhage generally is due to rupture of an atheromatous artery and is most common in patients with hypertension. It usually occurs in individuals of middle age and often involves a rupture of the thin-walled lenticulostriate artery, a branch of the middle cerebral artery. The important corticonuclear and corticospinal fibers in the internal capsule are damaged, producing hemiplegia on the opposite side of the body. The patient immediately loses consciousness, and the paralysis is evident when consciousness is regained. In some cases, the hemorrhage bursts into the lateral ventricle, resulting in deeper unconsciousness and corticospinal lesions on both sides of the body. Hemorrhage may also occur into the pons and cerebellum.

CT AND MR SCANNING

Computerized tomography (CT) and magnetic resonance (MR) are techniques that are indispensable in making the diagnosis in different forms of cerebrovascular disease. The diagnosis can usually be made with speed, accuracy, and safety. An intracranial blood clot can be recognized by its density. These techniques have largely replaced cerebral angiography (see pp. 38 and 39).

CEREBRAL ANGIOGRAPHY

The technique of cerebral angiography is used for the detection of abnormalities of the blood vessels, the detection and localization of space-occupying lesions such as tumors, hematomas, or abscesses, or the determination of the vascular pattern of tumors to aid in the diagnosis of their pathology. Under general anesthesia, with the patient in the supine position, the head is centered on a radiographic apparatus that will take repeated radiographs at 2-second intervals. Both anteroposterior and lateral projections are obtained. A radiopaque medium is injected rapidly into the lumen of the common carotid or vertebral artery or is indirectly introduced into one of these arteries through a catheter inserted into the radial or femoral artery. As the radiopaque material is rapidly introduced, a series of films are exposed. By this means, the cerebral arteries, the capillary flush, and the veins may be demonstrated. Examples of normal carotid and vertebral angiograms are shown in Figures 28-6 through 28-13.

Cerebral angiography is an invasive technique that unfortunately has a morbidity of 0.5 to 2.5 percent. CT and MR scans should therefore be used whenever possible. Positive emission tomography (PET) scans will probably be used extensively in the future.

Fig. 28-6. Lateral internal carotid arteriogram. Male aged 20 years.

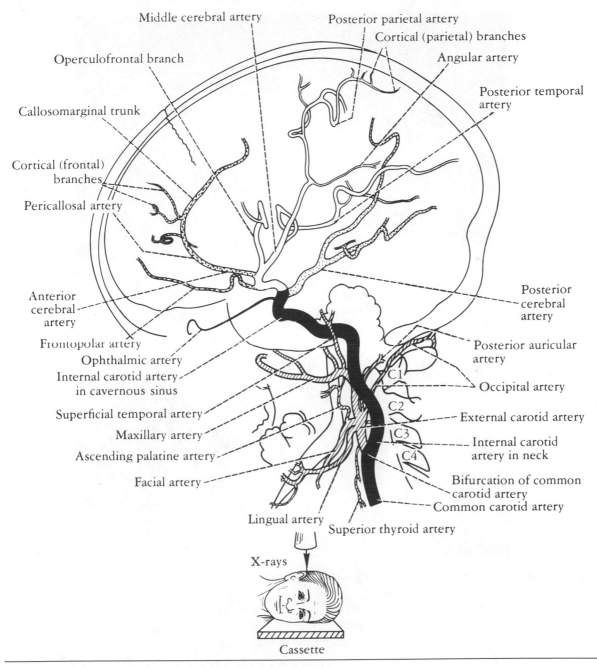

Fig. 28-7. Main features seen in radiograph in Figure 28-6.

Fig. 28-8. Anteroposterior internal carotid arteriogram. Male aged 20 years.

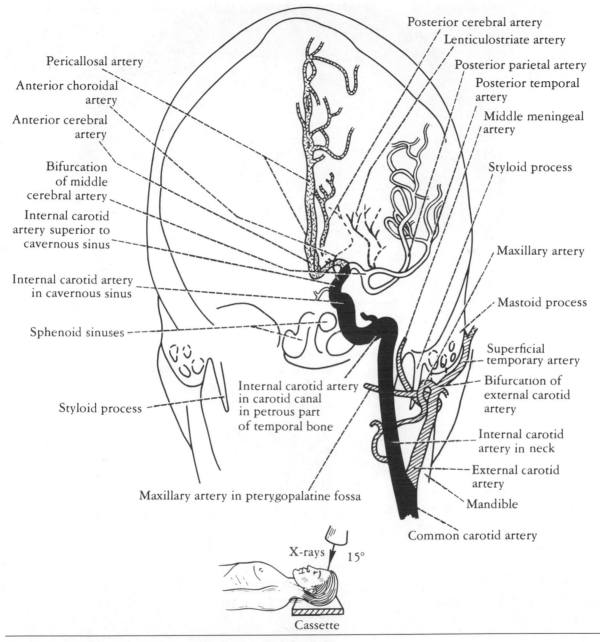

Pericallosal artery

Anterior choroidal artery

Anterior cerebral artery

Bifurcation of middle cerebral artery

Internal carotid artery superior to cavernous sinus

Internal carotid artery in cavernous sinus

Sphenoid sinuses

Styloid process

Internal carotid artery in carotid canal in petrous part of temporal bone

Maxillary artery in pterygopalatine fossa

Posterior cerebral artery

Lenticulostriate artery

Posterior parietal artery

Posterior temporal artery

Middle meningeal artery

Styloid process

Maxillary artery

Mastoid process

Superficial temporary artery

Bifurcation of external carotid artery

Internal carotid artery in neck

External carotid artery

Mandible

Common carotid artery

X-rays 15°

Cassette

Fig. 28-9. Main features seen in radiograph in Figure 28-8.

Fig. 28-10. Lateral vertebral arteriogram. Male aged 20 years.

Fig. 28-11. Main features shown in radiograph in Figure 28-10.

Fig. 28-12. Anteroposterior (angled) vertebral arteriogram. Woman aged 35 years.

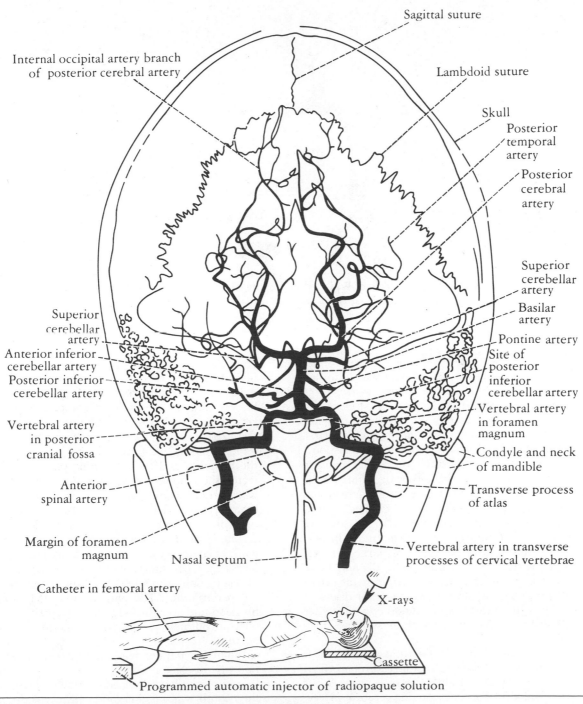

Fig. 28-13. Main features shown in radiograph in Figure 28-12.

	Right internal carotid
	Left internal carotid
	Right vertebral
	Left vertebral

Fig. 28-14. The circus arteriosus (circle of Willis) showing the distribution of blood from the four main arteries.

CLINICAL PROBLEMS

Answers on Page 614

1. While examining a patient who was admitted to the emergency room following a stroke, the neurologist turned to the medical student and asked him what the circulus arteriosus of Willis is, and what functions it normally performs. How would you have answered that question?

2. A distinguished neurosurgeon, while giving a lecture on cerebrovascular accidents, made the following statement: "It is generally agreed that there are no anastomoses of clinical importance between the terminal end arteries within the brain substance, but there are many important anastomoses between the large arteries, both within and outside the skull, and these may play a major role in determining the extent of brain damage in cerebral vascular disease." Comment on this statement and name the sites at which important arterial anastomoses take place.

3. During examination of a carotid angiogram, it was noted that the contrast medium had filled the anterior and middle cerebral arteries but had failed to fill the posterior cerebral artery. On careful following of the contrast medium, it was seen to enter the posterior communicating artery but to extend no farther. Can you explain this phenomenon in a normal person?

4. A 58-year-old man, while sitting quietly eating his evening meal, suddenly complained of a very severe headache. A few moments later, he slumped forward over the table and lost consciousness. He was immediately admitted to the hospital, and the examining physician detected the following physical signs. The patient was in deep coma, his face was flushed, his breathing was deep and slow (14 respirations per minute), and the right cheek blew out during expiration. Periodically, the breathing would become rapid and deep (hyperpnea), alternating with intervals of complete cessation of respiration (apnea). The pulse rate was slow (50 per minute). The patient lay quietly with his head and eyes turned to the left, he had urinary incontinence, and his temperature was normal.

When the patient was examined for alteration of muscle tone, the right side of the face looked somewhat flattened, the right corner of the mouth was sagging, and saliva was drooling out of that side of the mouth. The muscle tone of the limbs appeared to be less on the right side than on the left, and the tone on the left appeared to be within normal limits; the change in muscle tone was greater in the right arm than in the right leg. The right abdominal reflexes were absent and there was also a positive Babinski response on the right side.

Three days later, the patient slowly regained consciousness; the right arm and, to a lesser extent, the right leg were paralyzed, but movements on the left side were normal. As the days passed, it was clear that the lower part of the right side of the face was paralyzed, the patient had some difficulty in swallowing, and he was unable to speak. During the next two weeks, the muscles of the limbs on the right side became hypertonic and the tendon reflexes were hyperactive. It was observed that the patient had some sensory loss on the right side. What is your diagnosis?

5. A 65-year-old woman collapsed in the street and was admitted to the emergency room in a coma. Twenty-four hours later she recovered consciousness and was found to have paralysis on the left side of the body, mainly involving the lower limb. There was also some sensory loss on the left side of the body. She was able to swallow normally and did not appear to have difficulty with her speech. What is your diagnosis?

6. A 45-year-old man was admitted to the hospital after collapsing in his home three days previously. He was found by a friend on the floor of his sitting room in a partial state of unconsciousness. On physical examination, he was found to have right-sided homonymous hemianopia, although careful examination of the fields of vision showed that the macular regions were normal. Right-sided hemianesthesia and hemianalgesia also were present, although the patient complained of severe burning pain in the right leg. During the first 24 hours in the hospital, the patient demonstrated mild right-sided hemiparesis of the flaccid type, which disappeared within two days. What is your diagnosis? Be specific in describing the branches of the artery that are involved.

7. During the course of an autopsy on a patient who had recently died of cerebrovascular disease, the pathologist made the comment that in atherosclerosis of the cerebral arteries, the atheromatous plaques tend to occur where the main arteries divide or where the arteries suddenly curve. It is thought that at these sites the pressure flow changes may be a factor in the causation of the disease process. Using your knowledge of anatomy, name as many sites as you can where the main cerebral arteries divide or undergo abrupt change in their course.

8. Having carefully examined a male patient with cerebrovascular disease, the physician met with the family to discuss the nature of the illness, the course of treatment, and the prognosis. The daughter asked the physician what was meant by the term *stroke* and what the common causes are. He was also asked why the clinical findings vary so much from patient to patient. Using your knowledge of the anatomy and physiology of cerebral blood flow, can you explain why patients with cerebrovascular disease present such a variety of syndromes?

9. The classic sign of cerebrovascular disease is hemiplegia, yet we know that most patients also exhibit sensory deficits of different types. Using your knowledge of the anatomical distribution of the cerebral arteries, discuss the main types of sensory loss that you may find in such patients.

10. During the discussion of the symptoms and signs of a 70-year-old woman who had been admitted to the hospital for the treatment of cerebrovascular disease, a fourth-year medical student made the comment that he was surprised to find that many of the signs and symptoms were bilateral in this patient. He said that the three previous patients he had examined had displayed only unilateral signs and symptoms. Using your knowledge of neuroanatomy, explain why some patients exhibit bilateral signs and symptoms while in others the syndrome is clearly unilateral.

11. Neurologists speak frequently of the dominant hemisphere, and if cerebrovascular disease should involve that hemisphere one would expect the patient possibly to have global or total sensorimotor aphasia. Can you explain this phenomenon?

12. Can you explain why patients with a thrombosis of the middle cerebral artery often present with homonymous hemianopia as well as hemiplegia and hemianesthesia?

13. During the neurobiology course, the professor of neuroanatomy emphasized the importance of knowing the structure and blood supply of

the internal capsule. He explained the arrangement of the ascending and descending tracts within the capsule and showed how they were concentrated into a small area between the thalamus and caudate nucleus medially and the lentiform nucleus laterally. Clearly, an interruption of the blood supply to this vital area would produce widespread neurological defects. What is the blood supply to the internal capsule?

14. A 36-year-old man visited his physician with a complaint that on three occasions during the past six months he had fainted at work. During careful questioning, the patient stated that on each occasion he had fainted while sitting at his desk and while interviewing office personnel; he added that the person being interviewed sat in a chair immediately to the right of the desk. He said that before each fainting attack he felt dizzy; then he lost consciousness, only to recover within a few moments. The previous evening, he had a similar dizzy spell when he turned his head quickly to the right to talk to a friend in the street. The physician noted that the patient wore a stiff collar that was rather close-fitting. When the physician commented on this, the patient stated that he always wore this type of collar to work. No abnormal physical signs were found. Using your knowledge of anatomy and physiology, you would make what diagnosis?

15. A 45-year-old man, a company director, rose to give his annual after-dinner speech to the board when he suddenly experienced an "agonizing, crushing" pain over the sternum. Feeling giddy and weak, he fell back in his chair. A few moments later, he lapsed into unconsciousness. An attendant at the dinner, who had received some training in cardiopulmonary resuscitation while a member of the armed forces, ran forward and noted that the patient had stopped breathing. He quickly started mouth-to-mouth resuscitation and cardiac compression and kept going until ambulance personnel arrived to take the patient to the hospital. The physician in the intensive care unit at the hospital later told the patient that his life had been saved by the alertness and competence of the attendant at the dinner. Using your knowledge of neurophysiology, state how long brain tissue can survive when there is complete cardiac arrest and breathing has ceased.

16. A 62-year-old man with a history of hypertension visited his physician because the day before he had temporarily lost the sight of his right eye. He explained that the sight loss was partial and lasted about half an hour. On close questioning, the patient admitted that he had had similar episodes of blindness in the same eye during the previous six months, but they had lasted only a few minutes. The patient also mentioned that there were days when he could not remember the names of people and things. He also had recently experienced severe right-sided headaches. When asked about his activities, he said that he could not walk as well as he used to and his left leg sometimes felt weak and numb. While performing a careful physical examination, the physician heard with his stethoscope a distinct systolic bruit over the right side of the neck. Given that the patient has vascular disease of the brain, which artery is likely to be involved in the disease process? What special clinical investigations could you perform in order to confirm the diagnosis?

17. A 39-year-old man was admitted to the hospital with a history of a sudden excruciating, generalized headache while gardening. This was followed, 10 minutes later, by the patient's collapsing to the ground in a state of unconsciousness. After being carried indoors and placed on a settee, the patient regained consciousness but appeared confused. He complained of a severe headache and a stiff neck. Physical examination revealed some rigidity of the neck but nothing further. A careful neurological examination three days later revealed some loss of tone in the muscles of the left leg. Using your knowledge of anatomy, make the diagnosis. What is the reason for the neck rigidity?

18. A 26-year-old man, on leaving a bar after a few drinks, stepped into the road at 1:00 A.M. and was struck by a passing car. Fortunately, the car was traveling slowly and struck the patient's head a glancing blow. One hour later, the patient was found by a policeman, unconscious on the sidewalk. Physical examination at the local hospital found that the patient had recovered consciousness for a few minutes, but

then he had quickly relapsed into an unconscious state. The right pupil was dilated and the muscle tone of the left leg was found to be less than normal. A positive Babinski sign was obtained on the left side. Examination of the scalp showed a severe bruise over the right temple and a lateral radiograph of the skull showed a fracture of the anterior inferior angle of the parietal bone. A CT scan showed a dense area extending from anterior to posterior along the inner table of the right parietal bone. What is the diagnosis? Let us suppose that the equipment for performing a CT scan was unavailable and that it was decided to perform a lumbar puncture; this test revealed a raised cerebrospinal fluid pressure and the fluid was very slightly bloodstained. Can you explain these additional findings?

19. A 50-year-old woman visited her physician complaining of headaches, drowsiness, and mental confusion. On close questioning, the patient distinctly remembered striking her head against a closet door when bending down three weeks previously. A CT scan revealed the presence of a large space-occupying lesion over the right frontal lobe of the brain. What is the possible diagnosis in this case?

20. A 55-year-old man with a history of hypertension collapsed in the street while walking to work. He complained of a sudden severe headache. After 5 minutes, his face began to sag on the right side and his speech became slurred. On admission to the hospital, his right arm and leg were found to be weaker than the left, and the muscles were hypotonic. The eyes were deviated to the left. Later, the right arm and leg showed complete paralysis and were insensitive to pinprick. A positive Babinski sign was present on the right side. Two hours later, the patient relapsed into a deep coma with bilateral dilated fixed pupils. Later, the respirations became deep and irregular, and the patient died six hours later. Using your knowledge of neuroanatomy, make the diagnosis.

NATIONAL BOARD TYPE QUESTIONS

Answers on Page 621

IN EACH OF THE FOLLOWING QUESTIONS, ANSWER:

(a) IF (1) ONLY IS CORRECT
(b) IF (2) ONLY IS CORRECT
(c) IF BOTH (1) AND (2) ARE CORRECT, AND
(d) IF NEITHER (1) NOR (2) IS CORRECT

1. Which of the following statements is (are) correct?
   (1) The brain receives its blood supply directly and indirectly from the two internal carotid and the two vertebral arteries that lie within the subarachnoid space.
   (2) The circulus arteriosus is formed by the anterior cerebral, the internal carotid, the posterior cerebral, the basilar, and the anterior and posterior communicating arteries.

2. Which of the following statements is (are) correct concerning the arteries supplying the brain?
   (1) The cerebral arteries anastomose on the surface of the brain.
   (2) There are no anastomoses between the branches of the cerebral arteries once they have entered the substance of the brain.

3. Which of the following statements concerning the blood supply of the internal capsule is (are) correct?
   (1) It is supplied by the central branches of the middle cerebral artery.
   (2) It is supplied by the central branches of the anterior cerebral artery.

Match the areas of the cerebral cortex listed on the left with the most likely cerebral arterial supply listed on the right. Answers may be used more than once.

4. Precentral gyrus (face area)
5. Postcentral gyrus (foot area)
6. Cuneus
7. Inferior temporal gyrus
8. Wernicke's area

(a) Middle cerebral
(b) Anterior cerebral
(c) Posterior cerebral
(d) None of the above

Match the arteries listed on the left with the most likely main stem arteries from which they arose, listed on the right. Answers may be used more than once.

9. Ophthalmic artery
10. Pontine arteries
11. Posterior communicating artery
12. Posterior spinal artery
13. Posterior inferior cerebellar artery

(a) Basilar artery
(b) Internal carotid artery
(c) Vertebral artery
(d) External carotid artery
(e) None of the above

Match the veins listed on the left with the most likely cranial venous sinuses listed on the right into which they drain. Answers may be used more than once.

14. Superior cerebral veins
15. Great cerebral vein
16. Superior cerebellar veins

(a) Inferior sagittal sinus
(b) Transverse sinus
(c) Straight sinus
(d) Superior sagittal sinus
(e) None of the above

In the following questions, answer:

(a) If (1), (2), AND (3) ONLY ARE CORRECT
(b) If (1) AND (3) ONLY ARE CORRECT
(c) If (2) AND (4) ONLY ARE CORRECT
(d) If (4) ONLY IS CORRECT, OR
(e) If ALL ARE CORRECT

17. Which of the following statements is (are) correct concerning cerebral blood flow?

Fig. 28-15. The arteries of the inferior surface of the brain.

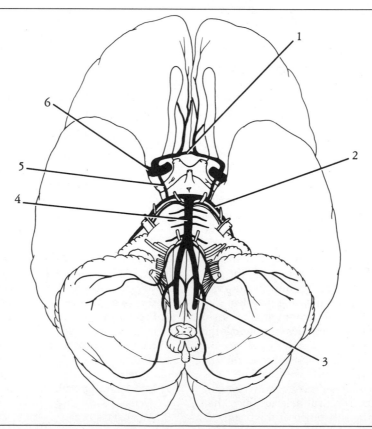

(1) Cerebral blood flow varies widely with changes in the general blood pressure.

(2) The sympathetic postganglionic fibers exert very little control over the diameter of the cerebral blood vessels.

(3) A high oxygen tension in the cerebral blood causes vasodilation of the cerebral blood vessels.

(4) One of the most powerful vasodilators of cerebral blood vessels is carbon dioxide.

18. Which of the following statements is (are) correct concerning cerebral ischemia?

(1) Atheromatous degeneration of a cerebral artery may cause degeneration of the nerve cells in the avascular area and proliferation of the microglial cells in the surrounding area.

(2) Neuronal function ceases after the blood flow has stopped for about 1 minute.

(3) Irreversible cerebral damage starts to occur after the blood flow has ceased for about 4 minutes.

(4) Cooling of the patient's body following a cerebrovascular accident speeds up cerebral degeneration.

In Figure 28-15, match the numbered arteries listed on the left with the appropriate arteries listed on the right. Any answer may be used more than once.

19. Number 1
20. Number 2
21. Number 3
22. Number 4
23. Number 5
24. Number 6

(a) Middle cerebral artery
(b) Anterior communicating artery
(c) Posterior cerebral artery
(d) Basilar artery
(e) None of the above

ADDITIONAL READING

Ascher, G. F., Ganti, S. R., and Hilal, S. K. Cerebral Angiography. In R. N. Rosenberg (ed.), *The Science and Practice of Clinical Medicine.* Vol. 5, Neurology. New York: Grune & Stratton, 1980.

Bannister, R. *Brain's Clinical Neurology* (6th ed.). London and New York: Oxford University Press, 1985.

Bes, A. (ed.). *Proceedings of the Eleventh International Symposium on Cerebral Blood Flow and Metabolism.* New York: Raven, 1983.

Best, C. H., and Taylor, N. B. *Physiological Basis of Medical Practice* (9th ed.). Baltimore: Williams & Wilkins, 1973.

Brain, W. R., and Walton, J. N. *Brain's Diseases of the Nervous System* (7th ed.). New York and London: Oxford University Press, 1969.

Brazis, P. W., Masden, J. C., and Biller, J. *Localization in Clinical Neurology* (2nd ed.). Boston: Little, Brown, 1990.

Capra, N. F. Anatomy of the Cerebral Venous System. In J. P. Kapp and H. H. Schmidek (eds.), *Cerebral Venous System and Its Disorders.* New York: Grune & Stratton, 1984. P. 1.

Denny-Brown, D. Recurrent cerebro-vascular episodes. *Arch. Neurol. (Chicago)* 2:194, 1960.

Duvernoy, H. M. *The Superficial Veins of the Human Brain.* Berlin: Springer-Verlag, 1975.

Duvernoy, H. M., Delon, S., and Vanson, J. L. Cortical blood vessels of the human brain. *Brain Res. Bull.* 7:519, 1981.

Duvernoy, H. M., Delon, S., and Vanson, J. L. The vascularization of the human cerebellar cortex. *Brain Res. Bull.* 11:419, 1983.

Krayenbühl, H. A., and Yasargil, M. G. *Cerebral Angiography.* Philadelphia: Lippincott, 1968.

McDonald, D. A., and Potter, J. M. The distribution of blood to the brain. *J. Physiol. (Lond.)* 114:356, 1951.

Reed, G., and Devous, M. Cerebral blood flow autoregulation and hypertension. *Am. J. Med. Sci.* 289:37, 1985.

Rowland, L. P. (ed.). *Merritt's Textbook of Neurology* (7th ed.). Philadelphia: Lea & Febiger, 1984.

Snell, R. S. *Clinical Anatomy for Medical Students* (4th ed.). Boston: Little, Brown, 1992.

Snell, R. S., and Wyman, A. C. *An Atlas of Normal Radiographic Anatomy.* Boston: Little, Brown, 1976.

Warwick, R., Williams, P. L., Dyson, M., and Bannister, L. H. (eds.). *Gray's Anatomy* (37th Brit. ed.). Philadelphia: Saunders, 1990.

Weisberg, L. A., Strub, R. L., and Garcia, C. A. Stroke. In *Essentials of Clinical Neurology*, Baltimore: University Park Press, 1983. P. 147.

Chapter 29
The Development of the Central Nervous System

This chapter is a brief overview of the development of the central nervous system. It has been included to assist the students who have difficulty in visualizing the relationship of different parts of the central nervous system to one another; it also serves to explain in many instances how the different nerve tracts insinuate themselves between the central masses of gray matter.

EARLY DEVELOPMENT

During the third week of development, the ectoderm on the dorsal surface of the embryo between the primitive knot and the buccopharyngeal membrane becomes thickened to form the **neural plate**. The plate, which is pear-shaped and wider cranially, develops a longitudinal **neural groove**. The groove now deepens so that it is bounded on either side by **neural folds** (Fig. 29-1). With further development, the neural folds fuse, converting the neural groove into a **neural tube**. Fusion starts at about the midpoint along the groove and extends cranially and caudally so that in the earliest stage the cavity of the tube remains in communication

with the amniotic cavity through the **anterior and posterior neuropores** (Fig. 29-1). The anterior neuropore closes first, and 2 days later the posterior neuropore closes. Meanwhile, the neural tube has sunk beneath the surface ectoderm.

During the invagination of the neural plate to form the neural groove, the cells forming the lateral margin of the plate do not become incorporated in the neural tube but form a strip of ectodermal cells that lie between the neural tube and the covering ectoderm. This strip of ectoderm is called the **neural crest** (Fig. 29-1), and subsequently this group of cells will migrate ventrolaterally on each side around the neural tube. Ultimately the neural crest cells will differentiate into the cells of the **posterior root ganglia**, the **sensory ganglia of the cranial nerves, autonomic ganglia, the cells of the suprarenal medulla**, and the **melanocytes**. It also believed that these cells give rise to mesenchymal cells in the head and neck.

Meanwhile, the cephalic end of the neural tube dilates to form **three primary brain vesicles**: the **forebrain vesicle**, the **midbrain vesicle**, and the

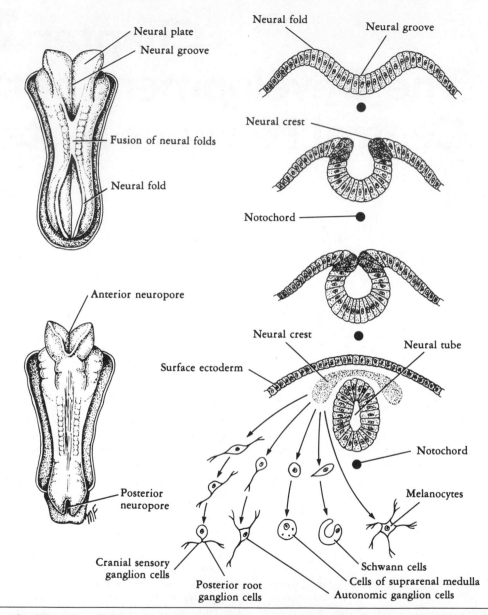

Fig. 29-1. The formation of the neural plate, neural groove, and neural tube. The cells of the neural crest differentiate into the cells of the posterior root ganglia, the sensory ganglia of cranial nerves, autonomic ganglia, neurilemmal cells (Schwann cells), the cells of the suprarenal medulla, and melanocytes.

hindbrain vesicle (Fig. 29-2). The rest of the tube elongates and remains smaller in diameter; it will form the **spinal cord**.

SPINAL CORD

The wall of the neural tube consists of a thick layer of pseudostratified epithelium, the **neuroepithelium** (Fig. 29-2). Repeated division of the neuroepithelial cells results in an increase in length and diameter of the tube. Eventually the **primitive neurocytes** are formed that are incapable of further division. These cells migrate peripherally to

form the **mantle layer** (Fig. 29-2). The mantle layer will form the **gray matter** of the spinal cord. The primitive neurocytes now give rise to nerve fibers that grow peripherally and form a layer external to the mantle layer called the **marginal layer**. The nerve fibers in the marginal layer become myelinated and form the **white matter** of the spinal cord.

While the primitive neurocytes are being formed, the neuroepithelial cells also give rise to the **astrocytes** and the **oligodendrocytes** of the neuroglia. Later the **microglial cells**, which are derived from the surrounding mesenchyme, migrate into the de-

Fig. 29-2. A. Expansion of the cephalic end of the neural tube to form the forebrain, midbrain, and hindbrain vesicles. B and C. Cross section of the developing neural tube in the region of the spinal cord. The cells of the neuroepithelial layer have been widely separated for clarity.

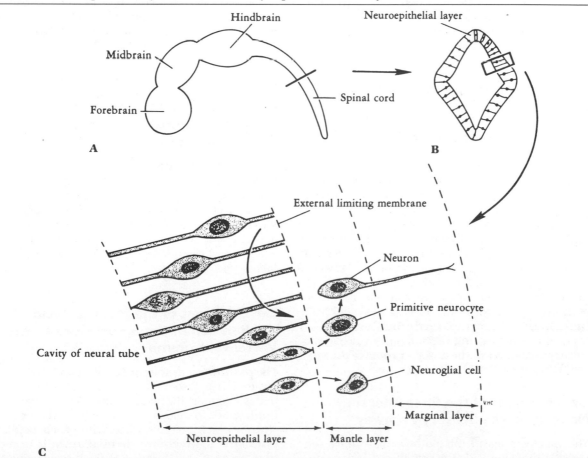

veloping spinal cord along with blood vessels. The **ependymal cells** are formed from the neuroepithelial cells that line the neural tube.

The cavity of the neural tube now becomes narrowed to form a dorsoventral cleft with thick lateral walls and thin floor and roof plates (Fig. 29-3). The mantle layer of the lateral wall of the tube forms a large anterior thickening known as the **basal plate** and a smaller posterior thickening known as the **alar plate** (Fig. 29-3). The neurocytes in the basal plate will form the motor anterior column (horn) cells, while the neurocytes in the alar plate will become the sensory cells of the posterior column. The motor basal plate and the sensory alar plate are separated on each side by the **sulcus limitans**.

Continued forward growth of the basal plates on each side of the midline forms a deep longitudinal groove called the **anterior median fissure** (Fig. 29-3). The alar plates also increase in size and extend medially, compressing the posterior part of the lumen of the neural tube. Ultimately the walls of the posterior portion of the tube fuse, forming the **posterior median septum**. The remainder of the neural tube becomes the **central canal** (Fig. 29-3).

Further Development of the Motor Neurons

The medial group of motor neurons form large multipolar cells whose axons will leave the anterior surface of the spinal cord to supply the musculature of the body.

The lateral group of neurons gives rise to axons that will leave the anterior surface of the spinal cord as autonomic preganglionic fibers. Between the first thoracic and second or third lumbar segments of the mature spinal cord, the lateral group of neurons will form the **lateral gray column (horn)**, i.e., the **sympathetic outflow**. Collectively, the axons leaving the anterior surface of the spinal cord will form the **anterior roots of the spinal nerves** (Fig. 29-3).

Development of the First Afferent Neurons in the Sensory Pathway

The first neurons in this pathway have their cell bodies situated outside the spinal cord and are derived from the neural crest (Figs. 29-1 and 29-3). The neural crest cells migrate to a posterolateral position on either side of the developing spinal cord and become segmented into cell clusters. Some of the cells in each cluster now differentiate into primitive neurocytes. Each primitive neurocyte develops two processes, a peripheral process and a central process. The peripheral processes grow out laterally to become typical axons of sensory nerve fibers. The central processes, also axons, grow into the posterior part of the developing spinal cord and either end in the posterior gray column or ascend through the marginal layer (white matter) to one of the higher brain centers. These central processes are referred to collectively as the **posterior root of the spinal nerve** (Fig. 29-3). The peripheral processes join the anterior root to form the **spinal nerve**.

Some of the neural crest cells form the **capsular** or **satellite cells**, which surround the unipolar nerve cell bodies in a ganglion. Each **posterior root ganglion** is thus formed of the unipolar neurons and the capsular cells.

Further Development of the Sensory Neurons in the Posterior Gray Column

The primitive neurocytes that have entered the alar plates now develop processes that enter the marginal layer (white matter) of the cord on the same side and either ascend or descend to a higher or lower level. Other nerve cells send processes to the opposite side of the cord through the floor plate, where they ascend or descend for variable distances (Fig. 29-3).

Development of the Meninges and the Relation of the Spinal Cord to the Vertebral Column

The **pia mater**, **arachnoid mater**, and **dura mater** are formed from the mesenchyme (sclerotome) that surrounds the neural tube. The **subarachnoid space** develops as a cavity in the mesenchyme, which becomes filled with **cerebrospinal fluid**. The **ligamentum denticulatum** is formed from areas of condensation of the mesenchyme.

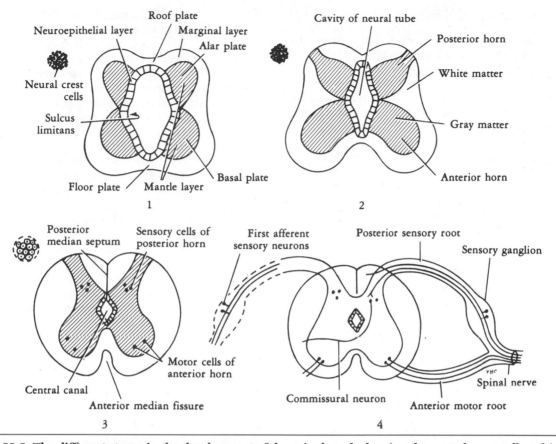

Fig. 29-3. The different stages in the development of the spinal cord, showing the neural crest cells, which will form the first afferent neurons in the sensory pathway.

During the first two months of intrauterine life, the spinal cord is the same length as the vertebral column. Thereafter the developing vertebral column grows more rapidly than the spinal cord, so that at birth the coccygeal end of the cord lies at the level of the third lumbar vertebra. In the adult, the lower end of the spinal cord lies at the level of the lower border of the body of the first lumbar vertebra. As a result of this disproportion in the rate of growth of the vertebral column and spinal cord, the anterior and posterior roots of the spinal nerves below the first lumbar segment of the spinal cord descend within the vertebral canal until they reach their appropriate exits through the intervertebral foramina. Moreover the pia mater, which attached the coccygeal end of the spinal cord to the coccyx, now extends down as a slender fibrous strand from the lower end of the cord to the coccyx and forms the **filum terminale**. The obliquely coursing anterior and posterior roots of the spinal nerves and the filum terminale, which now occupy the lower end of the vertebral canal, form collectively the **cauda equina**.

It is now understood how the cauda equina is enclosed within the subarachnoid space down as far as the level of the second sacral vertebra. It is in this region, below the level of the lower end of the spinal cord, that a **lumbar puncture** can be performed (see p. 32).

As the result of the development of the limb buds during the fourth month and the additional sensory and motor neurons, the spinal cord becomes swollen in the cervical and lumbar regions to form the **cervical** and **lumbar enlargements**.

BRAIN

Once the neural tube has closed, the **three primary vesicles**—the **forebrain vesicle**, the **midbrain vesicle**, and the **hindbrain vesicle**—complete their development (Fig. 29-4). The forebrain vesicle will form the forebrain **(prosencephalon)**, the midbrain vesicle will form the midbrain **(mesencephalon)**, and the hindbrain vesicle will form the hindbrain **(rhombencephalon)**.

By the fifth week the forebrain and hindbrain vesicles divide into two secondary vesicles (Fig. 29-4). The forebrain vesicle forms (1) the **telencephalon**, with its primitive cerebral hemispheres, and (2) the **diencephalon**, which develops optic vesicles. The hindbrain vesicle forms (1) the **metencephalon**, the future pons and cerebellum, and (2) the **myelencephalon**, or medulla oblongata.

The basic pattern of the ventricular system now is established. The cavity in each cerebral hemisphere is known as the **lateral ventricle**. The cavity of the diencephalon is known as the **third ventricle**. With continued growth, the cavity of the midbrain vesicle becomes small and forms the **cerebral aqueduct** or **aqueduct of Sylvius**. The cavity of the hindbrain vesicle forms the **fourth ventricle**, which is continuous with the central canal of the spinal cord. The lateral ventricles communicate with the third ventricle through the **interventricular foramina (foramina of Monro)**. The ventricular system and the central canal of the spinal cord are lined with ependyma and are filled with cerebrospinal fluid. In the earliest stages, the cerebrospinal fluid within the ventricular system is not continuous with that of the subarachnoid space.

Early in development, the embryo is a flat disc and the neural tube is straight. Later, with the development of the head fold and tail fold, the neural tube becomes curved.

Medulla Oblongata (Myelencephalon)

The walls of the hindbrain vesicle initially show the typical organization seen in the neural tube, with the anterior thickenings, the **basal plates**, and the posterior thickenings, the **alar plates**, the two being separated by the **sulcus limitans** (Fig. 29-5). As development proceeds, the lateral walls are moved laterally (like an opening clamshell) at higher levels by the expanding fourth ventricle. As a result, the alar plates come to lie lateral to the basal plates. The neurons of the basal plate form the motor nuclei of cranial nerves IX, X, XI, and XII and are situated in the floor of the fourth ventricle medial to the sulcus limitans. The neurons of the alar plate form the sensory nuclei of cranial nerves V, VIII, IX, and X and the **gracile and cuneate nuclei**. Other cells of the alar plate migrate ventrolaterally and form the **olivary nuclei**.

The roof plate becomes stretched into a thin layer of ependymal tissue. The vascular mesenchyme lying in contact with the outer surface of the roof plate forms the pia mater, and the two layers together form the **tela choroidea**. Vascular tufts of tela choroidea project into the cavity of the fourth ventricle to form the **choroid plexus** (Fig. 29-5). Between the fourth and fifth months, local resorptions of the roof plate occur, forming paired lateral foramina, the **foramina of Luschka**, and a median foramen, the **foramen of Magendie**. These important foramina allow the escape of the cerebrospinal fluid, which is produced in the ventricles, into the subarachnoid space (see p. 343).

The floor plate remains narrow and forms the region of the median sulcus. In the marginal layer on the anterior aspect of the medulla, descending axons from the neurons in the motor areas of the cerebral cortex (precentral gyrus) produce prominent swellings called the **pyramids**.

Pons (Ventral Part of the Metencephalon)

The pons arises from the anterior part of the metencephalon (Fig. 29-6), but it also receives a cellular contribution from the alar part of the myelencephalon.

The neurons of the basal plates form the motor nuclei of cranial nerves V, VI, and VII. The neurons of the ventromedial part of each alar plate form the main sensory nucleus of cranial nerve V, a sensory nucleus of cranial nerve VII, and the vestibular and cochlear nuclei of cranial nerve VIII; they also form the **pontine nuclei**. The axons of the pontine nuclei grow transversely to enter the developing cerebellum of the opposite side, thus forming the **transverse pontine fibers** and the **middle cerebellar peduncle**.

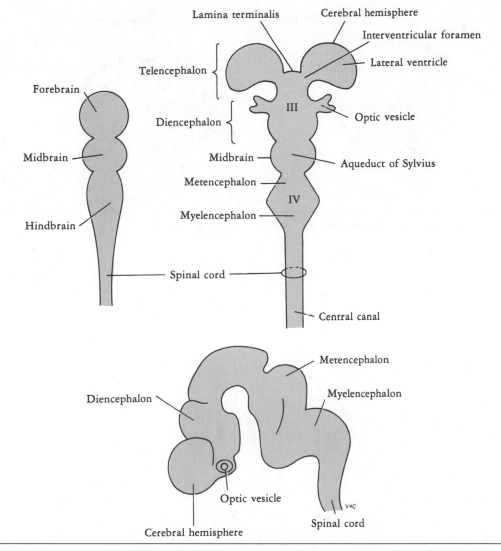

Fig. 29-4. The division of the forebrain vesicle into the telencephalon and the diencephalon, and the hindbrain vesicle into the metencephalon and myelencephalon. Also shown is the way in which the cerebral hemisphere on each side develops as a diverticulum from the telencephalon.

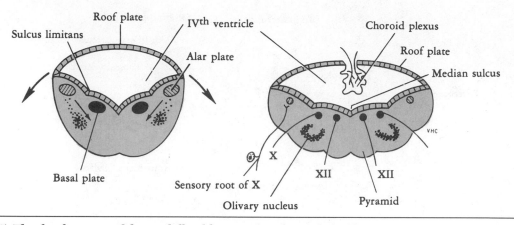

Fig. 29-5. The development of the medulla oblongata (myelencephalon).

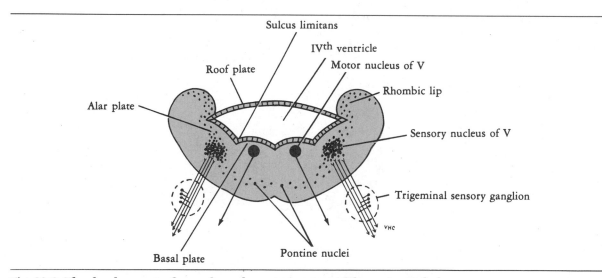

Fig. 29-6. The development of pons from the anterior part of the metencephalon.

Cerebellum (Posterior Part of the Metencephalon)

The cerebellum is formed from the posterior part of the alar plates of the metencephalon. On each side, the alar plates bend medially to form the **rhombic lips** (Fig. 29-7). As they enlarge, the lips project caudally over the roof plate of the fourth ventricle and unite with each other in the midline to form the cerebellum (Figs. 29-7 and 29-8). At the twelfth week, a small midline portion, the **ver-** mis, and two lateral portions, the **cerebellar hemispheres**, may be recognized. At about the end of the fourth month, fissures develop on the surface of the cerebellum and the characteristic folia of the adult cerebellum gradually develop.

The primitive neurocytes derived from the neuroepithelium migrate toward the surface of the cerebellum and eventually give rise to the neurons forming the **cerebellar cortex**. Other neurocytes remain close to the ventricular surface and differentiate into the **dentate** and other deep cerebellar

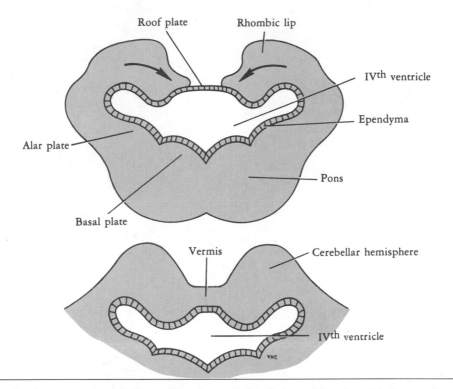

Fig. 29-7. The development of cerebellum. Also shown is the fusion of the rhombic lips in the midline to form the dumbell-shaped cerebellum.

nuclei. With further development, the axons of neurons forming these nuclei grow out into the mesencephalon (midbrain) to reach the forebrain and these fibers will form the greater part of the **superior cerebellar peduncle**. Later, the growth of the axons of the **pontocerebellar fibers** and the **corticopontine fibers** will connect the cerebral cortex with the cerebellum, and so the **middle cerebellar peduncles** will be formed. The **inferior cerebellar peduncle** will be formed largely by the growth of sensory axons from the spinal cord, the vestibular nuclei, and olivary nuclei.

Midbrain (Mesencephalon)

The midbrain develops from the midbrain vesicle, the cavity of which becomes much reduced to form the **cerebral aqueduct or aqueduct of Sylvius** (Fig. 29-9). The sulcus limitans separates the alar plate from the basal plate on each side, as seen in the developing spinal cord. The primitive neuro-

cytes in the basal plates will differentiate into the neurons forming the nuclei of the **third** and **fourth cranial nerves** and possibly the **red nuclei**, the **substantia nigra**, and the **reticular formation**. The marginal layer of each basal plate enlarges considerably, thus forming the **basis pedunculi** by the descent of nerve fibers from the cerebral cortex to the lower motor centers in the pons and spinal cord, i.e., the **corticopontine, corticobulbar**, and **corticospinal tracts**.

The two alar plates and the original roof plate form the **tectum**. The primitive neurocytes in the alar plates differentiate into the sensory neurons of the **superior** and **inferior colliculi** (Fig. 29-9). Four swellings representing the four colliculi appear on the posterior surface of the midbrain. The superior colliculi are associated with visual reflexes and the inferior colliculi are associated with auditory reflexes.

With further development, the fibers of the fourth cranial nerve emerge on the posterior sur-

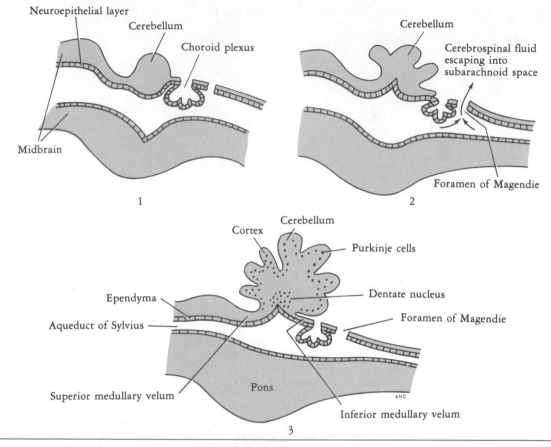

Fig. 29-8. Sagittal sections of the developing cerebellum.

face of the midbrain and decussate completely in the superior medullary velum. The fibers of the third cranial nerve emerge on the anterior surface between the cerebral peduncles.

Forebrain (Prosencephalon)

The forebrain develops from the forebrain vesicle. The roof and floor plates remain thin, whereas the lateral walls become thick, as in the developing spinal cord. At an early stage, a lateral diverticulum called the **optic vesicle** appears on each side of the forebrain. That part of the forebrain that lies rostral to the optic vesicle is the telencephalon, and the remainder is the diencephalon (Fig. 29-10). The optic vesicle and stalk ultimately will form the retina and optic nerve.

The telencephalon now develops a lateral diverticulum on each side of the cerebral hemisphere, and its cavity is known as the **lateral ventricle**. The anterior part of the third ventricle therefore is formed by the medial part of the telencephalon and ends at the **lamina terminalis**, which represents the rostral end of the neural tube. The opening into each lateral ventricle is the future **interventricular foramen**.

Fate of the Diencephalon

The cavity of the diencephalon forms the greater part of the third ventricle (Fig. 29-10). Its roof shows a small diverticulum immediately anterior to the midbrain, which will form the **pineal body**. The remainder of the roof forms the **choroid**

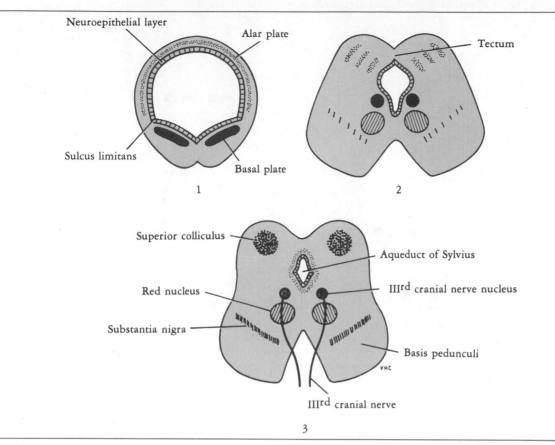

Fig. 29-9. The successive stages in the development of the midbrain.

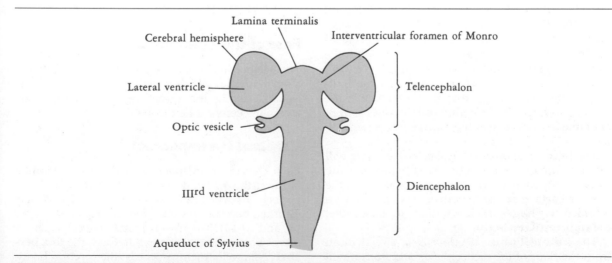

Fig. 29-10. The division of the forebrain vesicle into the telencephalon and the diencephalon.

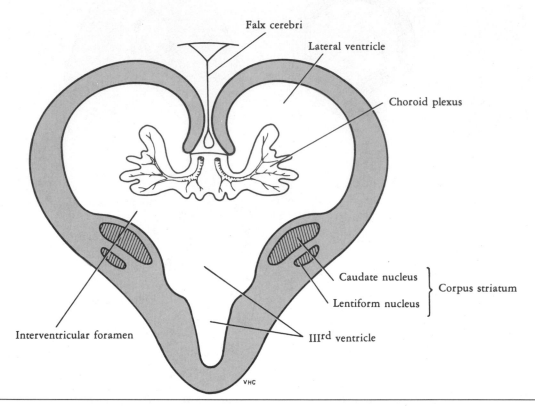

Falx cerebri

Lateral ventricle

Choroid plexus

Caudate nucleus

Lentiform nucleus

Corpus striatum

Interventricular foramen

IIIrd ventricle

VHC

Fig. 29-11. Coronal section of the cerebral hemispheres showing the developing choroid plexuses in the third and lateral ventricles.

plexus of the third ventricle (Fig. 29-11). In the lateral wall of the third ventricle the **thalamus** arises as a thickening of the alar plate on each side. Posterior to the thalamus, the **medial** and **lateral geniculate bodies** develop as solid buds. With the continued growth of the two thalami, the ventricular cavity becomes narrowed, and in some individuals the two thalami may meet and fuse in the midline to form the **interthalamic connection** of gray matter that crosses the third ventricle (Fig. 29-12).

The lower part of the alar plate on each side will differentiate into a large number of **hypothalamic nuclei**. One of these becomes conspicuous on the inferior surface of the hypothalamus and forms a rounded swelling on each side of the midline called the **mammillary body**.

The **infundibulum** develops as a diverticulum from the floor of the diencephalon and from it will

originate the **stalk** and **pars nervosa of the hypophysis**.

Fate of the Telencephalon

The telencephalon forms the anterior end of the third ventricle, which is closed by the lamina terminalis, while the diverticulum on either side forms the cerebral hemisphere.

Cerebral Hemispheres

Each cerebral hemisphere arises at the beginning of the fifth week of development. As it expands superiorly, its walls thicken and the interventricular foramen becomes reduced in size (Figs. 29-10, 29-11, and 29-12). The mesenchyme between each cerebral hemisphere condenses to form the **falx cerebri**. As development proceeds, the cerebral hemi-

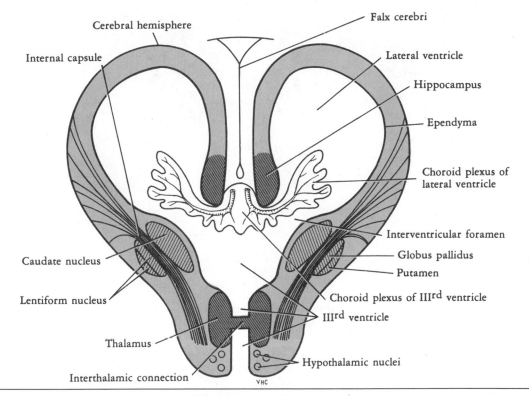

Fig. 29-12. Coronal section of the cerebral hemispheres showing the choroid plexuses in the third and lateral ventricles. Also shown are the caudate and lentiform nuclei and the thalami. The ascending and descending nerve tracts can be seen passing between the masses of gray matter to form the internal capsule.

spheres grow and expand rapidly, first anteriorly to form the **frontal lobes**, then laterally and superiorly to form the **parietal lobes**, and finally posteriorly and inferiorly to produce the **occipital** and **temporal lobes.** As the result of this great expansion, the hemispheres cover the midbrain and hindbrain (Fig. 29-13).

The medial wall of the cerebral hemisphere remains thin and is formed by the ependymal cells. This area becomes invaginated by vascular mesoderm, which forms the **choroid plexus of the lateral ventricle** (Fig. 29-12). The occipital lobe of the cerebral hemisphere is separated from the cerebellum by mesenchyme, which condenses to form the **tentorium cerebelli**.

Meanwhile, the neuroepithelium lining the floor of the forebrain vesicle proliferates, producing large numbers of primitive neurocytes. These col-

lectively form a projection that encroaches on the cavity of the lateral ventricle and is known as the **corpus striatum** (Fig. 29-11). Later this differentiates into two parts: the dorsomedial portion, the **caudate nucleus**, and a ventrolateral part, the **lentiform nucleus.** The latter becomes subdivided into a lateral part, the **putamen**, and a medial part, the **globus pallidus** (Fig. 29-12). As each hemisphere expands, its medial surface approaches the lateral surface of the diencephalon so that the caudate nucleus and thalamus come in close contact.

A further longitudinal thickening occurs in the wall of the forebrain vesicle that protrudes into the lateral ventricle and forms the **hippocampus** (Fig. 29-12).

While these various masses of gray matter are developing within each cerebral hemisphere, ma-

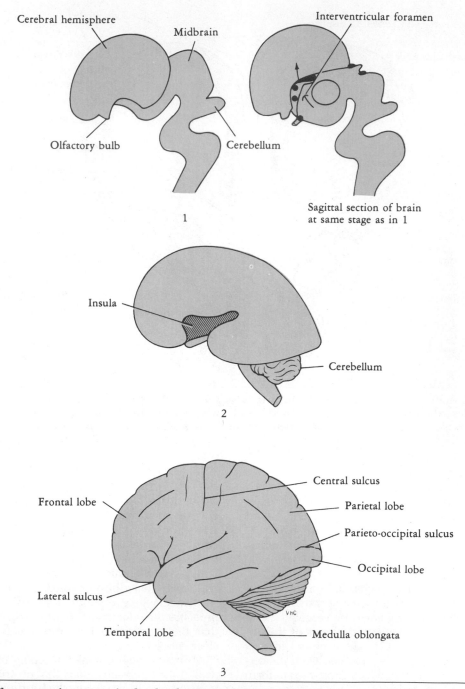

Fig. 29-13. The successive stages in the development of the cerebral cortex.

turing neurons in different parts of the nervous system are sending axons either to or from the differentiating cortex. These axons form the large **ascending and descending tracts**, which, as they develop, are forced to pass between the thalamus and caudate nucleus medially and the lentiform nucleus laterally. The compact bundle of ascending and descending tracts is known as the **internal capsule** (Fig. 29-12). The **external capsule** consists of a few cortical projection fibers that pass lateral to the lentiform nucleus.

Cerebral Cortex

As each cerebral hemisphere rapidly expands, the **convolutions** or **gyri** separated by **fissures** or **sulci** become evident on its surface. The cortex covering the lentiform nucleus remains as a fixed area called the **insula** (Fig. 29-13). Later this region becomes buried in the **lateral sulcus** as the result of overgrowth of the adjacent temporal, parietal, and frontal lobes.

The neuroepithelial cells lining the cavity of the cerebral hemisphere produce large numbers of primitive neurocytes and **neuroglial cells** that migrate out into the marginal layer. The remaining neuroepithelial cells ultimately will form the **ependyma**, which lines the lateral ventricle. In the twelfth week, the cortex becomes very cellular because of the migration of large numbers of primitive neurocytes. At term, the neurocytes have become differentiated and have assumed a stratified appearance as the result of the presence of incoming and outgoing fibers. Different areas of the cortex soon show specific cell types; thus the motor cortex contains a large number of **pyramidal cells**, whereas the sensory areas are characterized mainly by **granular cells**.

Commissures

The **lamina terminalis**, which is the cephalic end of the neural tube, forms a bridge between the two cerebral hemispheres and enables nerve fibers to pass from one cerebral hemisphere to the other (Fig. 29-10).

The **anterior commissure** is the first commissure to develop. It runs in the lamina terminalis and connects the olfactory bulb and the temporal lobe of the cortex on one side with the same structures of the opposite hemisphere.

The **fornix** is the second commissure to develop and connects the cortex of the hippocampus in each hemisphere.

The **corpus callosum**, the largest and most important commissure, is the third commissure to develop. Its first fibers connect the frontal lobes of both sides and later the parietal lobes. As the corpus callosum increases in size because of increased numbers of fibers, it arches back over the roof of the developing third ventricle. The remains of the lamina terminalis, which lie between the corpus callosum and the fornix, become stretched out to form a thin septum, the **septum pellucidum**. The **optic chiasma** is formed in the inferior part of the lamina terminalis; it contains fibers from the medial halves of the retinae, which cross the midline to join the optic tract of the opposite side and so pass to the **lateral geniculate body** and the **superior colliculus**.

MYELINATION IN THE CENTRAL NERVOUS SYSTEM

The myelin sheath in the central nervous system is formed and maintained by the oligodendrocytes of the neuroglia (see p. 96).

Myelination in the spinal cord begins first in the cervical region, and from here the process extends caudally. The fibers of the anterior nerve roots are myelinated before those of the posterior nerve roots. The process of myelination begins within the cord at about the fourth month, and the sensory fibers are affected first. The last affected are the descending motor fibers.

Myelination in the brain begins at about the sixth month of fetal life but is restricted to the fibers of the basal ganglia. Later the sensory fibers passing up from the spinal cord myelinate, but the progress is slow so that at birth the brain still is largely unmyelinated. In the newborn there is very little cerebral function; motor reactions such as respiration, sucking, and swallowing are essentially reflex. After birth, the corticobulbar, corticospinal, tectospinal, and corticopontocerebellar fibers begin to myelinate. This process of myelination is not haphazard but systematic, occurring in different nerve fibers at specific times. The corticospinal fibers, for example, start to myelinate at about 6 months after birth, and the process is largely complete by the end of the second year. It is believed that some nerve fibers in the brain and spinal cord do not complete myelination until puberty.

CLINICAL NOTES

CONGENITAL ANOMALIES

Practically any part of the nervous system may show defects of development, and these produce a wide variety of clinical signs and symptoms. Only the common defects of the central nervous system will be considered here. Spina bifida, hydrocephalus, and anencephaly each occur about 6 times per 1,000 births and are therefore the more common congenital anomalies.

Spina Bifida

In spina bifida, the spines and arches of one or more adjacent vertebrae fail to develop. The condition occurs most frequently in the lower thoracic, lumbar, and sacral regions. Beneath this defect the meninges and spinal cord may or may not be involved to varying degrees. The condition is a result of failure of the mesenchyme, which grows in between the neural tube and the surface ectoderm, to form the vertebral arches in the affected region. The types of spina bifida are as follows:

1. **Spina bifida occulta.** The spines and arches of one or more vertebrae, usually in the lumbar region, are absent, and the vertebral canal remains open posteriorly (Fig. 29-14). The spinal cord and nerve roots usually are normal. The defect is covered by the postvertebral muscles and cannot be seen from the surface. A small tuft of hair or a fatty tumor may be present over the defect. Most cases are symptomless and are diagnosed by chance when the vertebral column is x-rayed.
2. **Meningocele.** The meninges project through the defect in the vertebral arches, forming a cystic swelling beneath the skin and containing cerebrospinal fluid, which communicates with the subarachnoid space (Fig. 29-14). The spinal cord and nerves usually are normal.
3. **Meningomyelocele.** The normal spinal cord, or cauda equina, lies within the meningeal sac, which projects through the vertebral arch defect (Fig. 29-14). The spinal cord or nerve roots are adherent to the inner wall of the sac.
4. **Myelocele.** The neural tube fails to close in the region of the defect (Fig. 29-14). An oval raw area is found on the surface; this represents the neural groove whose lips are noted fused. The central canal discharges clear cerebrospinal fluid onto the surface.
5. **Syringomyelocele.** This condition is rare. A mengomyelocele is present, and in addition the central canal of the spinal cord at the level of the bony defect is grossly dilated (Fig. 29-14).

Spina bifida occulta is the commonest defect. The next most common defect is myelocele, and many afflicted infants are born dead. If the child is born alive, death from infection of the spinal cord occurs within a few days.

Most cases of spina bifida occulta require no treatment. A meningocele should be removed surgically within a few days of birth. Infants with meningomyelocele should also be treated surgically. The sac is opened and the spinal cord or nerves are freed and carefully replaced in the vertebral canal. The meninges are sutured over the cord and the postvertebral muscles are approximated.

Hydrocephalus

Hydrocephalus is an abnormal increase in the volume of cerebrospinal fluid within the skull. The condition may be associated with spina bifida and meningocele. Hydrocephalus alone may be caused by stenosis of the cerebral aqueduct or, more commonly, by the normal single channel being represented by many inadequate minute tubules. Another cause, which is progressive, is the overgrowth of neuroglia around the aqueduct. Inadequate development or failure of development of the interventricular foramen, or the foramina of Magendie and Luschka, may also be responsible.

In cases of hydrocephalus with spina bifida, the **Arnold-Chiari phenomenon** may occur. During

Spina bifida occulta

Meningocele

Meningomyelocele

Myelocele

Syringomyelocele

Fig. 29-14. The different types of spina bifida.

development, the cephalic end of the spinal cord is fixed by virtue of the brain's residing in the skull, and in the presence of spina bifida the caudal end of the cord may also be fixed. The longitudinal growth of the vertebral column is more rapid and greater than that of the spinal cord, and this results in traction pulling the medulla and part of the cerebellum through the foramen magnum. This displacement of the hindbrain downward obstructs the flow of cerebrospinal fluid through the foramina in the roof of the fourth ventricle.

Hydrocephalus may occur before birth, and if it is advanced, it could obstruct labor. It usually is noticed during the first few months of life because of the enlarging head, which may attain a huge size, sometimes measuring more than 30 inches in diameter (Fig. 29-15). The cranial sutures are widely separated and the anterior fontanelle is much enlarged. The veins of the scalp are distended and the eyes look downward. Cranial nerve paralyses are common. The ventricles of the brain become markedly dilated. This ventricular expansion occurs largely at the expense of the white matter, and the neurons of the cerebral cortex are mostly spared. This results in the preservation of cerebral function, but the destruction of the tracts, especially the corticobulbar and corticospinal tracts, produces a progressive loss of motor function.

If the condition is diagnosed by sonography while the fetus is in utero, it is now possible to perform prenatal surgery with the introduction of a catheter into the ventricles of the brain and the drainage of the cerebrospinal fluid into the amniotic cavity. Should the diagnosis be delayed until after birth, a drainage tube fitted with a nonreturn valve can connect the ventricles to the internal jugular vein in the neck.

Anencephaly

In anencephaly the greater part of the brain and the vault of the skull are absent (Fig. 29-16). The anomaly is caused by the failure of the rostral end of the neural tube to develop and as a consequence its cavity remains open. In place of the normal neural tissue are thin-walled vascular channels resembling the choroid plexus and masses of neural

Fig. 29-15. Hydrocephalus. Note the large size of the head. (Courtesy of Dr. G. Avery.)

Fig. 29-16. An example of anencephaly. Note that the greater part of the brain and the vault of the skull are absent. In the posterior view, the remainder of the brain is exposed. (Courtesy of Dr. M. Platt.)

tissue. Although the eyes are present, the optic nerves are absent. The condition commonly involves the spinal cord, and the neural tube remains open in the cervical region. The condition is commonly diagnosed before birth with sonography or x-ray studies. Most anencephalic infants are stillborn or die shortly after birth.

CLINICAL PROBLEMS

Answers on Page 617

1. A 10-year-old boy fell off his bicycle and hurt his back. Following a complete physical examination in the Emergency Department, nothing abnormal was found. An x-ray examination, however, revealed the complete absence of the spine and laminae of the fifth lumbar vertebra. How would you explain the presence of the bony defect?

2. A male child was delivered normally to a 20-year-old woman. A pediatrician examined the infant and found a large swelling in the lower part of his back over the fourth and fifth lumbar vertebrae. On closer examination, the summit of the swelling had an oval raw area from which a clear fluid was discharging. The legs showed hyperextension of the knees, and the feet were held in the position of talipes calcaneus. What is the diagnosis? How would you explain the congenital defect on the back?

3. A 2-month-old girl was taken to a pediatrician because her mother was concerned about the size of her head. "She looks top-heavy," she said. Examination showed the head to be large and globular in shape. The anterior fontanelle was greatly enlarged and extended posteriorly to the enlarged posterior fontanelle. The enlarged head contrasted markedly with the small face. Neurological examination revealed some evidence of optic atrophy on both sides and there was increased tone in the muscles of both lower limbs. What is the diagnosis? How can you explain this congenital anomaly? What is the prognosis if the patient is left untreated?

NATIONAL BOARD TYPE QUESTIONS

Answers on Page 621

IN EACH OF THE FOLLOWING QUESTIONS, ANSWER:
- (a) IF (1) ONLY IS CORRECT
- (b) IF (2) ONLY IS CORRECT
- (c) IF BOTH (1) AND (2) ARE CORRECT, AND
- (d) IF NEITHER (1) NOR (2) IS CORRECT

1. Which of the following statements concerning the neural tube is (are) correct?
   (1) It is lined by pseudostratified epithelium, the neuroepithelium.
   (2) The primitive neurocytes migrate peripherally to form the mantle layer, which later forms the gray matter.

2. Which of the following statements concerning the neural crest cells is (are) correct?
   (1) They are formed from the central portion of the neural plate.
   (2) They give rise to the posterior root ganglia, the autonomic ganglia, the Schwann cells, and the cells of the suprarenal medulla.

3. Which of the following statements concerning the developing spinal cord is (are) correct?
   (1) The alar plates form the neurons in the posterior gray columns.
   (2) The nerve cells of the sympathetic outflow are formed from the basal plates.

4. Which of the following statements concerning the vertebral levels of the developing spinal cord is (are) correct?
   (1) In the adult the lower end of the spinal cord lies at the level of the lower border of the first lumbar vertebra.
   (2) At birth the lower end of the spinal cord lies at the level of the third sacral vertebra.

5. Which of the following statements concerning the development of the cerebellum is (are) correct?
   (1) It is formed from the dorsal part of the alar plates of the metencephalon.
   (2) The neurons of the deep cerebellar nuclei are derived from the neuroepithelium lining the cavity of the hindbrain vesicle.

6. Which of the following statements concerning the development of the midbrain is (are) true?
   (1) The neurocytes in the basal plates will form the nuclei of the trochlear and oculomotor nerves.
   (2) The neurocytes of the superior and inferior colliculi are also formed from the neurocytes in the basal plates.

Select the best response:

7. The following statements concerning the fate of the forebrain vesicle are correct except:
   (a) The optic vesicle divides up the forebrain vesicle into the telencephalon and the diencephalon.
   (b) The thalamus is formed from the alar plates in the lateral walls of the diencephalon.
   (c) The lamina terminalis is formed from the rostral end of the telencephalon.
   (d) The pars nervosa of the hypophysis is formed from the floor of the diencephalon.
   (e) The hypothalamic nuclei are formed from the basal plates of the diencephalon.

8. The following statements concerning the development of the cerebral hemispheres are correct except:
   (a) The corpus striatum is formed from the proliferation of the neuroepithelium lining the floor of the forebrain vesicle.
   (b) The interventricular foramen is formed by the cavity of the telencephalon.
   (c) The choroid plexus of the lateral ventricle is formed by vascular mesenchyme covered by ependymal cells.
   (d) The internal capsule is formed by the developing ascending and descending tracts growing between the developing thalamus and caudate nucleus medially and the lentiform nucleus laterally.
   (e) The cortical neurons develop in situ and do not migrate out laterally from the neuroepithelial cells lining the cavity of the cerebral hemisphere.

9. The following statements concerning the development of myelination in the brain are correct except:
   (a) Myelination begins at birth.
   (b) The sensory fibers are myelinated first.
   (c) The process of myelination is not haphazard.
   (d) Myelination of the nerve tracts is largely complete by the second year of life.

(e) Myelination is carried out by oligodendrocytes and not by neurons.
10. The following statements concerning the condition of spina bifida are correct **except**:
    (a) It is one of the more common congenital anomalies of the central nervous system.
    (b) The commonest form of spina bifida is syringomyelocele.

(c) The condition occurs most often in the lower thoracic, lumbar, and sacral regions.
(d) In a myelocele, the neural tube fails to close in the region of the defect.
(e) Most cases of spina bifida occulta require no treatment.

ADDITIONAL READING

Adams, R. D., Schatzki, R., and Scoville, W. B. The Arnold-Chiari malformation. *N. Engl. J. Med.* 225:135, 1941.

Angevine, J. B., and Sidman, R. L. Autoradiographic study of cell migration during histogenesis of cerebral cortex in the mouse. *Nature* 192:766, 1961.

Bering, E. A. Pathophysiology of Hydrocephalus. In K. Shulman (ed.), *Workshop in Hydrocephalus.* Philadelphia: Children's Hospital, 1965.

Dennison, W. M. Spina Bifida. In J. C. Mustarde (ed.), *Plastic Surgery in Infancy and in Childhood.* Edinburgh: Livingstone, 1971. Pp. 381–385.

Eckstein, H. B. Management of Hydrocephalus. In *Proceedings of a Symposium on Spina Bifida.* London: National Foundation for Research into Poliomyelitis and Other Crippling Diseases, 1965.

Forrest, D. M., Hole, R., and Wynne, J. M. Treatment of infantile hydrocephalus using the Holter valve. *Dev. Med. Child. Neurol. [Suppl.]* 11:27, 1966.

Hewitt, W. The development of the human internal capsule and lentiform nucleus. *J. Anat.* 95:191, 1961.

Holmes, R. L., and Sharp, J. A. *The Human Nervous System: A Developmental Approach.* London: Churchill Livingstone, 1969.

Hoytema, G. J., and Van Den Berg, R. Embryological studies of the posterior fossa in connection with Arnold-Chiari malformation. *Dev. Med. Child. Neurol. [Suppl.]* 11:61, 1966.

Laurence, K. M., and Weeks, R. Abnormalities in the Central Nervous System. In A. P. Norman (ed.), *Congenital Abnormalities in Infancy.* Oxford, Engl.: Blackwell, 1971.

Leikola, A. The neural crest: Migrating cells in embryonic development. *Folia Morphol.* 24:155, 1976.

Ostertag, C. B., and Mundinger, R. Diagnosis of normal pressure hydrocephalus using CT with CSF enhancement. *Neuroradiology* 16:216, 1978.

Answers to Clinical Problems

CHAPTER I

1. Very often a physician thinks he knows what these terms mean but to his embarassment he finds out that he has forgotten. (a)*Neuron* is the name given to a nerve cell and all its processes. (b) *Neuroglia* is the term used to describe the specialized supporting tissue found within the central nervous system. (For details, see p. 77.) (c) Gray matter consists of nerve cells and the proximal portions of their processes embedded in neuroglia. (d) White matter consists of nerve fibers embedded in neuroglia. It is white in color because of the presence of myelin around the nerve fibers. (For details, see p. 91.) (e) Cerebrospinal fluid is the fluid found within the ventricular system of the brain and spinal cord and within the subarachnoid space.

2. The white matter of the spinal cord is divided, for purposes of description, into anterior, lateral, and posterior white columns. The posterior column lies between the entry of the posterior nerve roots and the midline posteriorly; the lateral column lies between the emergence of the anterior nerve roots and the entry of the posterior nerve roots. In the spinal cord there is an inner core of gray matter that is surrounded by an outer covering of white matter.

3. The autonomic nervous system is distributed throughout the central and peripheral nervous systems. Historically, the tendency has been to regard it as a special part of the nervous system because, anatomically, physiologically, and pharmacologically, it has been shown to be concerned with the control of involuntary structures. The autonomic system possesses both afferent and efferent nervous pathways.

4. Although the spinal cord is roughly cylindrical throughout its length, in the cervical region, where it gives origin to the brachial plexus, and in the lower thoracic and lumbar regions, where it gives origin to the lumbosacral plexus, there are fusiform enlargements, called the cervical and lumbar enlargements. The spinal cord tapers off inferiorly into the conus medullaris. At this particular operation the cervical enlargement of the cord had been exposed.

5. Carcinoma of the thyroid, breast, kidney, lung, and prostate commonly gives rise to metastases in bone. (a) The pain in the back was caused by the carcinoma invading and destroying the tenth thoracic vertebral body. (b) Compression of the posterior nerve root of the tenth thoracic spinal nerve by the carcinoma of the vertebral column produced the hyperesthesia and hyperalgesia over the right tenth intercostal space. (c) Muscular weakness of the legs was caused by pressure on the descending motor nerve fibers in the spinal cord by the carcinoma's invasion of the vertebral canal. (d) Although there is disproportionate growth in length of the vertebral column during development compared with that of the spinal cord, the upper cervical segments of the spinal cord still lie posterior to the vertebral bodies of the same number; however, the spinal cord in the adult terminates inferiorly at the level of the lower border of the first lumbar vertebra and, therefore, the first and second lumbar segments of the spinal cord lie at the level of the tenth thoracic vertebral body.

6. This patient had a severe fracture dislocation between the seventh and eighth thoracic vertebrae. The vertical arrangement of the articular processes and the low mobility of this region because of the thoracic cage mean that a dislocation can occur in this region only if the articular processes are fractured by a great force. The small circular vertebral canal leaves little space around the spinal cord, so that severe cord injuries are certain.

7. Each spinal nerve is formed by the union of a posterior sensory root and an anterior motor root and leaves the vertebral canal by traveling through an intervertebral foramen. Each foramen is bounded superiorly and inferiorly by the pedicles of adjacent vertebrae, anteriorly by the lower part of the vertebral body and by the intervertebral disc, and posteriorly by the articular processes and the joint between them. In this patient the fifth thoracic vertebral body had collapsed and the intervertebral foramina on both sides had been considerably reduced in size, causing compression of the posterior sensory roots and the spinal nerves. The consequent irritation of the sensory fibers was responsible for the pain.

8. This patient had symptoms suggestive of irritation of the left sixth cervical posterior nerve root. The radiograph revealed narrowing of the space between the fifth and sixth cervical vertebral bodies, suggesting a herniation of the nucleus pulposus of the intervertebral disc at this level. The MRI showed the nucleus pulposus extending posteriorly beyond the annulus fibrosus, thus confirming the diagnosis.

9. The herniation occurred on the right side and was relatively small. The pain occurred in the distribution of the fifth lumbar and first sacral segments of the spinal cord, and the posterior sensory roots of these segments of the cord were pressed upon on the right side.

10. In a 5-year-old child, the spinal cord terminates inferiorly at about the level of the second lumbar vertebra (certainly no lower than the third lumbar vertebra). With the child lying on his side and comforted by a nurse, and with the operator using an aseptic technique, the skin is anesthetized in the midline just below the fourth lumbar spine. The fourth lumbar spine lies on an imaginary line joining the highest points on the iliac crests. The lumbar puncture needle, fitted with a stylet, is then passed carefully into the vertebral canal. The needle will pass through the following anatomical structures before it enters the subarachnoid space: (a) skin, (b) superficial fascia, (c) supraspinous ligament, (d) interspinous ligament, (e) ligamentum flavum, (f) areolar tissue containing the internal vertebral venous plexus, (g) dura mater, and (h) arachnoid mater.

11. Caudal analgesia (anesthesia) is very effective in producing a painless labor if it is performed skillfully. The anesthetic solutions are introduced into the sacral canal through the sacral hiatus. Sufficient solution is given so that the nerve roots up as far as T11 and 12 and L1 are blocked. This will make the uterine contractions painless during the first stage of labor. If the nerve fibers of S2, 3, and 4 are also blocked, the perineum will be anesthetized.

12. A blow on the side of the head may easily fracture the thin anterior part of the parietal bone. The anterior branch of the middle meningeal artery commonly enters a bony canal in this region and is sectioned at the time of the fracture. The resulting hemorrhage causes gradual ac-

cumulation of blood under high pressure outside the meningeal layer of the dura mater. The pressure is exerted on the underlying brain as the blood clot enlarges, and the symptoms of confusion and irritability become apparent. This is followed later by drowsiness. Pressure on the lower end of the motor area of the cerebral cortex (the right precentral gyrus) causes twitching of the facial muscles and, later, twitching of the left arm muscles. As the blood clot progressively enlarges, the intracranial pressure rises and the patient's condition deteriorates.

13. The cerebral aqueduct is the narrow channel in the midbrain that connects the third ventricle to the fourth ventricle; it is filled with cerebrospinal fluid. The cerebrospinal fluid produced in the lateral ventricles and the third ventricle is unable to escape into the fourth ventricle if the cerebral aqueduct is blocked. The increased volume of cerebrospinal fluid accumulated in the third and lateral ventricles produces the clinical condition of hydrocephalus, which is accompanied by enlargement of the head.

14. A detailed account of the various changes that occur in the skull in patients with an intracranial tumor is given on page 38. A patient suspected of having an intracranial tumor should **not** undergo a lumbar puncture. The withdrawal of cerebrospinal fluid may lead to a sudden displacement of the cerebral hemisphere through the opening in the tentorium cerebelli into the posterior cranial fossa, or herniation of the medulla oblongata and cerebellum through the foramen magnum. CT scans or MRIs are now used in making the diagnosis.

15. The brain is floating in the cerebrospinal fluid within the skull, so that blows to the head or sudden deceleration leads to displacement of the brain. This may produce severe cerebral damage, stretching or distortion of the brainstem, avulsion of cranial nerves, and, commonly, rupture of tethering cerebral veins. (For further details, see p. 37.) A crash helmet helps to protect the brain by cushioning the blow and thus slowing up the brain's rate of deceleration.

16. (a) Contrecoup injury to the brain is an injury to the pole of the brain opposite the site of impact, where the brain is thrown against the skull wall. (b) Subarachnoid hemorrhage—a hemorrhage into the subarachnoid space—results from leakage or rupture of a congenital aneurysm on the cerebral arterial circle, or, less commonly, a tumor of an artery (angioma). (c) Subdural hemorrhage is a hemorrhage into the space between the meningeal layer of dura and the arachnoid mater. It results from tearing of the superior cerebral veins at their point of entrance into the superior sagittal sinus. (d) Cerebral hemorrhage is a hemorrhage into the substance of the brain.

17. The brain and spinal cord are enclosed by the skull and vertebrae. The meninges, the cerebrospinal fluid in the subarachnoid space, and a large number of blood vessels and venous sinuses are also contained within these bony structures. Expanding intracranial lesions, because of their bulk, increase the intracranial pressure and compress the ventricular system. The ventricular circulation of cerebrospinal fluid will or will not be interfered with, depending on the site of the lesion. The raised intracranial pressure is initially compensated for by a reduction in cerebrospinal fluid volume, as the result of an increased rate of absorption. A continued rise in intracranial pressure ultimately compresses the cerebral veins and venous sinuses, causing an accumulation of tissue fluid in the brain (cerebral edema) and reduced absorption of cerebrospinal fluid (see p. 38). At this point, a vicious circle has been established and the intracranial pressure continues to rise. Arterial blood is continually being pumped into the rigid bony case from the outside, but the veins and sinuses, which drain the cerebrospinal fluid and blood from the case, are being pressed upon.

18. In the newborn the bones of the vault of the skull are not closely knit at sutures, as in the adult, but are separated by unossified membranous intervals called *fontanelles*. The anterior and posterior fontanelles are clinically the most important. The anterior fontanelle is bounded by the two halves of the frontal bone anteriorly and the two parietal bones posteriorly. By the age of 18 months, it is very small and no longer clinically palpable. The posterior fontanelle is bounded by the two parietal bones anteriorly and the occipital bone posteriorly. By the end of the first year it can no longer be palpated. Pal-

pation of the fontanelles enables the physician to determine the state of intracranial pressure. For example, a bulging fontanelle indicates raised intracranial pressure.

The adult skull may be likened to an eggshell because it possesses a certain limited resilience, beyond which it splinters. A young child's skull, on the other hand, may be likened to a table tennis ball because a localized blow produces a depression without splintering. (For further details see p. 33).

19. The cerebellum is part of the hindbrain and is situated posterior to the fourth ventricle (the cavity of the hindbrain) and posterior to the pons and medulla oblongata. A medulloblastoma is a common tumor found in children, especially in the cerebellum. It is a rapidly growing malignant tumor. The cerebellum is situated in the posterior cranial fossa of the skull.

20. The surface layer of each cerebral hemisphere is called the cortex. The cerebral cortex is thrown into folds or gyri, separated by fissures or sulci. The larger sulci are used arbitrarily to subdivide the surface of each hemisphere into lobes. The lobes are named from the bones of the cranium under which they lie. The frontal lobe lies beneath the frontal bone of the skull and is situated anterior to the central sulcus and superior to the lateral sulcus.

CHAPTER 2

1. The following are some of the pathogenic mechanisms that may influence the neuron and thus initiate mental deficiency:

(a) Abnormal chromatin. Down's syndrome or mongolism is one of the most common examples of mental retardation. Nearly all who have Down's syndrome have an extra chromosome of number 21, making a total of 47 chromosomes. A few have a translocation of one of the parts of a 21 chromosome.

A single genetic defect may result in errors of metabolism. A failure of development of the enzyme required to form the hormone thyroxin will result in lack of normal brain development. The enzymatic defect resulting in the failure of hydroxylation of phenylalanine to tyrosine produces phenylketonuria. The accumulation of phenylalanine in the body fluids causes mental retardation. Galactosemia is a further example of an inborn error in metabolism.

(b) Maternal and fetal infection with the rubella virus, fetal cytomegalovirus, and *Toxoplasma gondii*, a protozoan infection, can all produce mental deficiency.

(c) Atomic radiations and x-ray therapy of the gravid uterus can inhibit the normal development of the nervous system.

(d) Maternal ingestion of drugs such as thalidomide can cause fetal brain defects.

(e) Autoimmune diseases. In Hashimoto's disease, for example, the thyroid gland fails to develop adequately owing to the formation of autoantibodies to thyroid tissue. Athyrotic cretins result, with accompanying mental deficiency.

(f) Excessive amounts of bilirubin in the blood (hyperbilirubinemia), associated with hemolytic disease of the newborn, can produce severe cerebral injury (kernicterus). The mental deficiency is usually associated with other neurological defects, including cranial nerve palsies, convulsive disorders, and aphasias.

It is clear from the above list that the pediatrician can treat and prevent the maldevelopment of neurons, and thus reduce the incidence of mental deficiency, by knowing what drugs the mother is taking, by knowing the genetic history of the family, by making an early diagnosis of cretinism, and by recognizing phenylketonuria and galactosemia.

2. The radial nerve is made up of nerve fibers derived from motor, sensory, and autonomic neurons. By definition the nerve fibers, or nerve cell processes, are referred to as neurites. The short neurites are called dendrites and the long neurites are called axons. It is customary to refer to those neurites that conduct the nervous impulse toward the cell body as the dendrites and to those that conduct the impulses away from the cell body as the axons. However, in the case of the unipolar sensory neurons found in the posterior root ganglia, the neurite carrying nervous information toward the cell body has all the structural characteristics of an axon and

is referred to as an axon. Thus the radial nerve, which is composed of sensory and motor fibers, is made up of axons.

3. The nucleolus in any cell is concerned with the synthesis of ribonucleic acid (RNA). The large size is probably related to the very large volume of cytoplasm possessed by certain neurons. For example, the axons of the motor nerve cells that supply the muscles of the sole of the foot are situated in the lumbar and sacral regions of the spinal cord; thus the axons may measure as much as 4 feet long.

4. (a) It is a general rule that all reparative phenomena throughout the body occur more readily in the young than in the old. (b) As the distal end of a peripheral nerve is approached, fewer branches remain and thus there are fewer structures yet to innervate; consequently, there are fewer possibilities of nerve fibers innervating the wrong structure during the process of regeneration. Moreover, the more distal the injury the less the metabolism of the proximal nerve cell body is affected by the injury. (c) This is a physiological fact. A very severe nerve injury close to its nerve cell body may result in the death of the entire neuron. (d) The physiology of sensory neurons is more susceptible to change by retrograde phenomena than that of motor neurons.

5. If the wound is not infected, the best time to perform a nerve suture is about 3 weeks after the injury. Satisfactory results have been obtained after a delay of as much as 14 months, provided that paralyzed muscles have not been overstretched and joint adhesions have been avoided by passive movements of the joints. In other words, the neuron still retains the ability to regenerate its processes even after 14 months, but the degree of recovery of function will depend a great deal on the care that the denervated structures have received in the intervening time.

6. Golgi type I neurons have long axons that form the long fiber tracts of the brain and spinal cord and form the nerve fibers of peripheral nerves. Golgi type II neurons have short axons that terminate in the neighborhood of the cell body or are entirely absent. There are many more type II neurons in the nervous system than type I.

7. (a) Nissl substance is composed of vesicles, tubules, or stacks of flat cisternae. Associated with the vesicles are dense granules measuring 10 to 30 nm in diameter and containing ribonucleoprotein. The Nissl substance is responsible for synthesizing protein. (b) Golgi apparatus is composed of clusters of flattened cisternae and vesicles made up of smooth-surfaced endoplasmic reticulum. It is thought to serve as an intracellular storage area, and to be active in lysosome production. It may also be involved in the synthesis of cell membranes. (c) Lysosomes are membrane-bound vesicles measuring about 8 nm in diameter. They contain acid phosphatase and other hydrolytic enzymes. They serve as intracellular scavengers. (d) Membranous vesicles do not come under the above heading. Some contain engulfed substances that move through the cytoplasm until they fuse with a lysosome. Such vesicles are often termed phagosomes.

8. In 1949, Barr and Bertram noticed the presence of a small, stainable body of chromatin (Barr body) situated at the inner surface of the nuclear envelope in the female that could not be seen in the cells of the male. It is one of the two X chromosomes present in the female. The presence or absence of the Barr body enables one to readily determine the sex of the individual from whom the tissue was removed.

9. With the electron microscope it is possible to resolve within the cytoplasm of a neuron small tubules that measure about 20 to 30 nm in diameter; there are also microfilaments measuring about 7 nm in diameter. The possible role that these structures play in cell transport is discussed on page 56.

10. The central nervous system is made up of the following tissues: (a) neurons, (b) neuroglia, (c) blood vessels, and (d) meninges. The peripheral nervous system is composed of the following tissues: (a) neurons, (b) Schwann cells, (c) connective tissue, and (d) blood vessels.

11. The structure of the plasma membrane is described on page 58. When a neuron is excited, the permeability of the plasma membrane to Na^+ ions is increased and these diffuse from the tissue fluid into the neuron cytoplasm. Local analgesics act as membrane stabilizers and inhibit the increase in permeability to Na^+ ions

in response to stimulation. It is not exactly understood how this stabilization is brought about. One theory is that the analgesic agent becomes attached to receptor sites on the protein layer of the plasma membrane, reducing the permeability to Na^+ ions and preventing depolarization from taking place. Small-diameter nerve fibers are more readily blocked than large fibers, and nonmyelinated more readily blocked than myelinated. For these reasons, nerve fibers that conduct pain and temperature are most easily blocked and the large motor fibers are the least easily blocked. The small autonomic nerve fibers are blocked early and account for the rapid appearance of vasodilatation.

12. (a) *Synapse* is the name given to the site where two neurons come into close proximity and where functional interneuronal communication occurs. The term has come to include a myoneural junction. (b) *Synaptic spines* are extensions of the surface of a neuron, usually dendrites, and form receptive sites for synaptic contact with afferent boutons. (c) *Synaptic cleft* is the name given to the space that exists between the presynaptic and postsynaptic membrane at a synapse. It measures about 20 nm wide. (d) *Presynaptic vesicles* are small membrane-bound structures situated in the neuronal cytoplasm close to the presynaptic membrane. They store and are involved in the release of neurotransmitter substances. (e) Acetylcholine, norepinephrine, epinephrine, and dopamine are examples of neurotransmitter substances at synapses; other examples are given on page 68.

13. (a) Tetraethylammonium salts and (b) hexamethonium salts. These salts closely resemble acetylcholine in structure and compete with acetylcholine at the postsynaptic membrane. By this means they successfully block a ganglion, although the amount of acetylcholine released is unaffected.

14. A list of the different neurotransmitters discovered so far in the central nervous system is given on page 68.

15. The neuroblastoma is a tumor of primitive neuroblasts and arises either in the suprarenal medulla or upper abdominal sympathetic ganglia. It is very malignant and is confined to children. The tumor metastasizes early and the metas-

tasis may be the reason the child receives medical attention, as in this case. The bones of the orbit are a common site for a neuroblastoma to metastasize.

CHAPTER 3

1. Neuroglia composes about one-half the total volume of the central nervous system. Neuroglial cells outnumber neurons by 5 to 10 times.

2. *Macroglia* is the term commonly used collectively to name astrocytes and oligodendrocytes. Microglial cells are smaller than astrocytes and oligodendrocytes. They are scattered throughout the central nervous system and closely resemble connective tissue macrophages in function. Neuroglia consists of several varieties of nonexcitable cells found within the central nervous system. Neuroglial cells, which serve to support the neurons, are of four main types: (1) astrocytes, (2) oligodendrocytes, (3) microglia, and (4) ependyma.

3. The different functions of neuroglia are fully discussed on pages 79, 80, and 84. Researchers increasingly feel that neuroglial cells probably play a far greater role in the function of the central nervous system than has been determined so far.

4. The reaction of tissue of the central nervous system to injury is characterized by the hyperplasia and hypertrophy of the astrocytes. The proliferation of the astrocytes is often referred to as *astrocytosis* or *gliosis*. The degree of gliosis is much greater in the presence of residual damaged brain tissue than with a clean surgical incision. The resulting scar tissue, so-called *gliotic scar*, in the case of a penetrating gunshot wound, may be extensive and may give rise to focal or generalized epileptic attacks. The majority of such patients who become epileptic do so within two years (Miller and Stern, 1965). After careful examination of these patients, including the performance of radiography, CT brain scans, MRIs, and electroencephalography, the trauma site should be explored with a view to removing the gliotic scar. Such a scar will be replaced by a much smaller surgical scar. This operative intervention cures many of these patients.

5. A history of severe headaches and nausea and the finding of a choked optic disc (swelling of the optic disc, congestion of the retinal veins, and retinal hemorrhages) are not always diagnostic of a brain tumor. However, the finding of weakness of the lateral rectus muscle of the right eye owing to compression of the right sixth cranial nerve against the floor of the skull, together with the positive radiological and other laboratory tests, made the diagnosis certain. The glioma (tumor of neuroglia) is the most common type of tumor found in such a patient. Unfortunately, gliomas tend to infiltrate the brain tissue and can not be completely removed surgically. A biopsy is taken to establish the diagnosis, as much of the tumor is removed as is clinically feasible, and the area is treated by deep x-ray therapy postoperatively. Survival time may also be increased by the use of chemotherapy.

CHAPTER 4

1. The median nerve is a mixed peripheral nerve that contains motor, sensory, and autonomic nerve fibers. The nerve fibers are axons of nerve cells and the majority are myelinated. The nerve fibers are arranged in parallel bundles and each fiber is supported by delicate connective tissue called *endoneurium*. Bundles of nerve fibers are surrounded by a connective tissue sheath called the *perineurium*. Several bundles are surrounded by a dense connective tissue sheath called the *epineurium*.
2. Nervous tracts are bundles of nerve fibers found in the brain and spinal cord, most of which are myelinated. Some of the main structural differences between a myelinated nerve tract and a myelinated peripheral nerve fiber are as follows:

Nerve Tract
oligodendrocyte
mesaxon absent
Schmidt-Lanterman incisures present
nerve fibers supported by neuroglia

Peripheral Nerve Fiber
Schwann cell

mesaxon present
Schmidt-Lanterman incisures present
nerve fibers supported by connective tissue sheaths, endoneurium, perineurium, and epineurium

3. (a) The myelin sheath is not part of a neuron; it is formed by a supporting cell, the oligodendrocyte in the central nervous system, and the Schwann cell in the peripheral nervous system. The myelin sheath serves as an insulator and separates the axolemma from the surrounding tissue fluid except at the node of Ranvier; it thus plays an important role in nerve conduction (see p. 105). The sheath is formed from the plasma membrane of the supporting cell (oligodendrocyte or Schwann cell) and consists of a series of laminae of lipoprotein. (For further details, see p. 91) (b) The node of Ranvier is the gap that exists between two adjacent Schwann cells (or oligodendrocytes, in the central nervous system) in a myelinated nerve; nodes of Ranvier do not exist in a nonmyelinated nerve. A myelinated nerve can be stimulated only at a node of Ranvier. (c) Schmidt-Lanterman incisures are seen on longitudinal sections of myelinated nerve fibers. They represent areas of localized persistence of Schwann cell cytoplasm. They involve all the layers of the myelin and there is thus a continuous spiral of cytoplasm from the outermost region of the Schwann cell to the region of the axon. It may serve as a pathway for the conduction of metabolites from the surface region of the Schwann cell to the axon. Schmidt-Lanterman incisures also occur in myelinated nerve fibers of the central nervous system. (d) Satellite cells in sensory and autonomic ganglia envelop the neuron cell bodies. They should be regarded as modified Schwann cells and probably serve to insulate the neurons from adjacent nervous activity.
4. Myelination is fully described on page 91. Myelin sheaths begin to be formed during fetal development and during the first year postnatally.
5. In the central nervous system a single oligodendrocyte may be responsible for the formation of myelin for as many as 60 nerve fibers. Clearly, it would not be possible for an oligodendrocyte to rotate on each axon as did the Schwann cell in the peripheral nervous system.

It is believed that in the central nervous system the mesaxon grows in length and wraps itself around the axon.

6. (a) The smaller axons in the central nervous system, (b) postganglionic axons of the autonomic part of the nervous system, and (c) fine sensory pain fibers.

7. Peripheral nerve fibers may be classified into groups according to their size and speed of conduction. Group or type A fibers are 1 to 20 μm in diameter and they conduct at the rate of 5 to 120 meters per second. They are myelinated somatic efferent and afferent fibers. Group or type B fibers are 1 to 3 μm in diameter and they conduct at 3 to 15 meters per second. They are myelinated efferent preganglionic autonomic fibers.

The resting membrane potential is the potential difference across the axolemma when a nerve fiber is at rest. A typical resting potential is 80 mV.

The absolute refractory period is the short period of time that immediately follows the passage of a nerve impulse when a second stimulus, however strong, is unable to excite the nerve.

Conduction velocity and saltatory conduction are fully explained on page 107.

8. (a) The microscopic changes that occur in the proximal and distal segments of a divided peripheral nerve are fully described on page 109. Remember that in the proximal segment the changes occur only as far proximally as the next node of Ranvier, whereas the changes spread distally from the site of the lesion and include its terminations. (b) If one bears in mind the considerations outlined on pages 109–117 and that the surgeon has the experience to perform nerve suture, the following treatment should be instituted. If the knife was clean the nerve should be immediately sutured and any arterial damage repaired. On the other hand, if the knife was contaminated or the wound was more than 6 hours old, the wound should be treated and the nerve ignored. In the latter case, when the wound has healed and there is no sign of residual infection the nerve ends should be explored and sutured together without tension. In either case, the paralyzed muscles are protected with a suitable splint and the joints are gently exercised daily. (c) Once the regenerating axons have entered the distal segment, the nerve distal to the section becomes very sensitive to mechanical stimulation (Tinel's sign). (d) Sensory recovery occurs first. Deep pressure sensation is the first sign of recovery. This is followed by the return of superficial cutaneous pain and vasomotor control of blood vessels, later the sensations of heat and cold return, and later still light touch and tactile discrimination reappear. Sensory recovery occurs before there is return of voluntary movement. (e) For clinical purposes a figure of 1.5 mm per day is the average rate of regeneration. It is possible, using this figure, to determine approximately how long it will take for a regenerating nerve to reach its end-organs.

9. (a) *Wallerian degeneration* is the term used to describe the changes that occur in the distal segment of an axon following its section. The details are fully described on page 109. (b) The band fiber is the endoneurial sheath and the contained cords of Schwann cells that replace the degenerated peripheral nerve following nerve section. The band fiber will serve to guide regenerating axons to their end-organs. A band fiber is not formed in the central nervous system. (c) Transneuronal degeneration occurs in the central nervous system when one group of neurons is injured and a second group, farther along the pathway and serving the same function, undergoes degeneration.

10. Bell's palsy is produced by swelling of the seventh cranial nerve (facial nerve) in the facial nerve canal of the skull. Its cause is unknown, although it often follows exposure to cold. Since the facial canal is bony, the nerve cannot expand and consequently becomes compressed and ischemic. In severe cases the muscles of facial expression are paralyzed on one side of the face and there is loss of taste sensation in the anterior part of the tongue on the same side. Massage of the paralyzed muscles should be undertaken to preserve their integrity until nerve function returns. The majority recover completely. There existed in this patient a serious residual palsy after three years. A treatment that has been successful in many cases is to section the hypoglossal nerve below and behind the angle of the mandible and the anas-

tomosis of its proximal end to the distal end of the facial nerve. Although the right half of the tongue would be paralyzed, this causes little disability. A reasonable return of facial movement can be expected. The patient learns to move the face instead of the tongue by practicing in front of a mirror. Note that both the hypoglossal and facial nerves are peripheral nerves and therefore regeneration is possible. The prognosis is especially good since the hypoglossal nerve is purely a motor nerve.

11. Lead causes neuronal degeneration in the central nervous system and demyelination in the tracts of the spinal cord and peripheral nerves. The treatment is to remove the child from the source of the lead and to aid rapid excretion by administering a chelating agent, calcium disodium versenate. Nontoxic lead versenate is excreted in the urine.

12. The cauda equina consists of the anterior and posterior roots of the spinal nerves below the level of the first lumbar segment of the spinal cord. These are peripheral nerves with endoneurial sheaths and Schwann cells and therefore regeneration will take place if adequate treatment is promptly instituted.

13. As the result of experiments in which dyes have been injected into peripheral nerves, spaces have been demonstrated between individual nerve fibers in the endoneurium. These spaces are believed to provide the route for the ascent of the tetanus toxin to the spinal cord.

14. A benign fibroma or a malignant sarcoma may arise from fibroblasts in the connective tissue of the endoneurium, perineurium, or epineurium. Neurolemmomas are thought to arise from Schwann cells.

15. Xylocaine is a local anesthetic that, when applied to a nerve fiber, blocks nerve conduction. The anesthetic acts on the axolemma and interferes with the transient increase in permeability of the axolemma to Na^+ ions and in the resting axon reduces the permeability of the axolemma to Na^+, K^+, and other ions. The small diameter pain fibers are more susceptible to the action of this drug.

16. *Neuropraxia* is the term applied to a transient nerve block. Pressure is the most common cause and this case was due to the pressure of the upper edge of the chair back on the brachial

plexus in the axilla. The loss of function is probably caused by ischemia of the nerve fibers. There is no microscopic evidence of degeneration. Axonotmesis is the term applied to a nerve lesion where the axons are damaged but the surrounding connective tissue sheaths remain intact. Neurotmesis is the term applied to complete section of the nerve trunk.

The prognosis in this patient is excellent for rapid, complete recovery. It is important that the paralyzed muscles not be stretched by antagonist muscles or by gravity. Therefore, suitable splints should be applied and gentle passive movement of the joints should be performed once daily.

17. Degeneration occurs in the central nervous system in a manner similar to that found in the peripheral nervous sytem. The axon breaks up into small fragments and the debris is digested by the neighboring microglial cells. The myelin sheath is broken down into lipid droplets, which are also phagocytosed by the microglial cells.

There is an attempt at regeneration of the axons as evidenced by sprouting of the axons, but there is no evidence that restoration of function ever occurs. The reasons for the failure of regeneration are fully described on page 112.

CHAPTER 5

1. Syringomyelia is a chronic disease of the spinal cord and is due to a developmental abnormality in the formation of the central canal. It is characterized by the appearance of a fluid-filled cavity within the spinal cord that gradually enlarges, causing destruction of surrounding nervous tissue. In this patient, the cavity or syrinx was located in the lower cervical and upper thoracic segments of the cord, causing destruction of the ascending tracts that serve pain and temperature from the upper limbs. The cavity was encroaching on the motor anterior horn cells of both sides also, causing weakness of the small muscles of the hands.

It is now generally accepted that the type of sensation felt is determined not by a specific receptor but by the specific area of the central nervous system to which the afferent nerve fiber passes. Free nerve endings are commonly associated with axons serving pain and temperature. The examination of a patient to test different sensory modalities is discussed on page 140.

2. The only sensory receptors present in the cornea are free nerve endings. The cornea is sensitive to touch and temperature changes in addition to pain.

3. The pacinian corpuscles are the largest sensory receptors (excluding the eye and the ear). They measure about 2 mm long and about 100 to 500 μm wide.

4. Touch, including pressure, heat, cold, and pain are the four modalities of cutaneous sensation. With our present knowledge, we believe that sensory reception is not dependent upon specific histological receptors but rather on the delivery of nerve impulses to specific areas of the brain. This matter is discussed on page 128.

5. All hair follicles possess a rich innervation. Free nerve endings are found as a branching network that winds around the follicle below the entrance of the sebaceous duct. Merkel's discs also are found in the epidermis of the follicle. The hair shaft acts as a lever, so that the slightest movement of the hair readily stimulates the nerve endings in the hair follicle. In this patient, who was suffering from trigeminal neuralgia, the temporal region of the scalp was the trigger area, which on stimulation initiated the intense stabs of pain in the distribution of the maxillary division of the trigeminal nerve.

6. Numerous free nerve endings are found in the connective tissue of tendons and the testes. Normally, squeezing of these structures elicits an aching type of pain. In tabes dorsalis the disease process affects the sensory neurons in the posterior roots of the spinal nerves.

7. The intrafusal fibers are elongated when the entire muscle is stretched. The annulospiral and the flower spray endings are stimulated, and impulses reach the spinal cord through afferent neurons. The large alpha motor neurons situated in the anterior gray horns of the spinal cord are stimulated; nerve impulses reach the mass, and the muscle contracts.

Thus it is seen that the intrafusal fibers play an important role in the control of skeletal muscle activity. There are two types of intrafusal fibers: (a) nuclear bag fibers, which are associated with position and velocity of contraction, and (b) nuclear chain fibers, which are concerned with static, slow contractions. Nerve impulses traveling in the gamma efferent motor fibers reach the intrafusal fibers. They cause the polar regions of the intrafusal fibers to contract, thus stretching the equatorial region. If the stretching process is sufficiently great, the annulospiral and flower spray endings will be stimulated. This mechanism allows centers in the central nervous system, such as the reticular formation, the basal ganglia, and the cerebellum, to influence voluntary muscle activity.

8. Striking the ligamentum patellae with a reflex hammer causes elongation of the intrafusal fibers of the muscle spindles of the quadriceps muscle and stimulation of the annulospiral and flower spray endings. The nerve impulses reach the spinal cord in the afferent neurons within the femoral nerve and enter the cord at the level of L2, 3, and 4. The afferent neurons synapse with the large alpha motor neurons in the anterior gray horns of the spinal cord. Nerve impulses now pass via the efferent motor neurons in the femoral nerve and stimulate the extrafusal muscle fibers of the quadriceps muscle, which then contracts. The muscle spindle afferent impulses inhibit the motor neurons of the antagonist muscles (see reciprocal inhibition, p. 131).

9. (a) Annulospiral endings that are associated with the intrafusal muscle fibers of neuromuscular spindles in skeletal muscle; these are sensitive to stretch. (b) Flower spray endings that are associated with intrafusal muscle fibers of neuromuscular spindles in skeletal muscle; these are also sensitive to stretch. (c) Neurotendinous spindles with club-shaped nerve endings; these are sensitive to tension. (d) Free nerve endings found in the connective tissue of muscle; these are probably sensitive to pain.

10. (a) A motor unit consists of a single motor neuron and the group of muscle fibers that it supplies. (b) A neurovascular hilus is in a more or less constant position and is where the nerve supply and blood supply enter a skeletal muscle. (c) A sole plate is a slightly elevated site on a skeletal muscle fiber at the neuromuscular

junction; it constitutes the muscular element of the junction. The elevation is due to the local accumulation of sarcoplasm beneath the sarcolemma and the presence of numerous nuclei and mitochondria. (d) The junctional folds of a neuromuscular junction are folds of sarcolemma in the floor of the surface groove in which lies the naked axon of the motor nerve; they serve to increase the surface area of the sarcolemma that lies close to the axon. (e) The synaptic cleft of a neuromuscular junction is the space that is situated between the plasma membrane of the axon (axolemma) and the plasma membrane of the muscle fiber (sarcolemma); it measures about 20 to 50 nm.

11. To test position sense, the patient is placed in the supine position and asked to close his eyes. The big toe is grasped at the sides between the thumb and index finger and extended and flexed. The patient is asked, on completion of each movement, the position of the toe—is it pointing up or down? Another simple test is to ask the patient, again with the eyes closed, to place his right heel on his left shin and run it down the shin to the dorsum of the left foot. The patient is then asked to repeat the performance with the left heel on the right shin.

   Vibratory sense may be tested by placing the handle of a vibrating tuning fork on the tibial tuberosity, the anterior border of the tibia, and the medial or lateral malleoli. The patient is asked to indicate when he first feels the vibration and when it ceases. Symmetrical points on the two limbs may be compared and the physician can use his own limbs as a control. In the normal individual the sense of position depends on the central nervous system's receiving adequate information from the pressure receptors (pacinian corpuscles) in the joint capsules and ligaments; touch receptors (free nerve endings) in the tissues in and around joints; and the stretch receptors in the muscles and tendons (especially the neurotendinous spindles).

   Vibration sense is normally believed to be due to the stimulation of superficial and deep pressure receptors (pacinian corpuscles).

   The appreciation of the passive movements of joints, postural sensibility, and vibration sense are often lost in tabes dorsalis due to syphilitic destruction of the posterior columns

of the spinal cord and degeneration of the posterior roots.

12. D-Tubocurarine, dimethyl tubocurarine, gallamine, and benzoquinonium are examples of competitive blocking agents. These drugs compete with the neurotransmitter acetylcholine. The competitive blocking agents are believed to combine with the same sites at the postsynaptic membrane (sarcolemma) of the motor endplate normally used by acetylcholine.

13. Decamethonium and succinylcholine paralyze skeletal muscle by causing depolarization of the motor end-plate.

14. *C. botulinum* produces a toxin that inhibits the release of acetylcholine at the motor end-plate. Death results from paralysis of the respiratory muscles.

15. Skeletal muscles that are not used, for example in a limb fitted with a splint immobilizing a fracture, undergo disuse atrophy. The longer the muscles are not used, the greater the degree of atrophy, and in severe cases, it may amount to as much as a quarter of the muscle mass. The muscle fibers rapidly atrophy following section of a motor nerve, so that the total mass of the muscle may be reduced by as much as three-quarters in as little as three months. The precise reason for this severe atrophy is not understood, but apparently the maintenance of normal muscle depends on the continued reception of acetylcholine at the postsynaptic membrane at the neuromuscular junction. The latter mechanism would be impossible if the motor nerve were sectioned and the distal end had degenerated.

16. This patient is suffering from myasthenia gravis. The insidious onset of muscle fatigue, with early involvement of the extraocular muscles, the facial muscles, then the pharyngeal and palatal muscles, with acerbations and remissions is characteristic. The intramuscular injection of an anticholinesterase drug, such as neostigmine, results in prompt relief of the muscular weakness. The cause of myasthenia gravis is discussed on page 142.

17. The smooth muscle of the bladder wall (the detrusor muscle) receives its innervation from the postganglionic parasympathetic fibers of the inferior hypogastric plexus. Each nerve fiber branches extensively, so that a single neuron ex-

erts control over a large number of muscle fibers. The nerve fibers are nonmyelinated and terminate as varicosed branches. An interval of 10 to 100 nm may exist between the axon and the muscle fiber. The Schwann cell is retracted so that the axon lies within a shallow groove on its surface. Thus part of the axon is naked, permitting the free diffusion of acetylcholine from the axon to the muscle fiber. Acetylcholine is the neurotransmitter that brings about depolarization of the smooth muscle fiber and its contraction. Because acetylcholine is rapidly destroyed by the cholinesterases, it cannot be used clinically to bring about contraction of the detrusor muscle. Methylcholine chloride and carbechol chloride are less susceptible to destruction by the cholinesterases and could therefore be used in clinical practice.

CHAPTER 6

1. Your knowledge of the dermatomes of the lower limb will enable you to ascertain that the patient's pain was felt in the area of distribution of the fifth lumbar and first sacral nerve roots. The involvement of these roots is usually due to herniation of the fourth or fifth lumbar intervertebral disc.

2. Herpes zoster is a viral infection of the posterior root ganglia (or sensory ganglia of the cranial nerves), the posterior root, or the posterior gray horn of the spinal cord. This patient experienced pain and had a skin eruption in the area of distribution of the fifth left intercostal nerve. The virus was producing an acute inflammation at some point along the course of the sensory neurons of the fifth segment of the spinal cord on the left side.

3. The trigeminal (fifth cranial) nerve innervates the skin of the greater part of the face. The next dermatome that occurs inferior to this is that of the second cervical nerve. The sixth to the twelfth cranial nerves do not innervate the skin of the face. At the junction of the neck with the thorax, the fourth cervical dermatome is contiguous with the second thoracic dermatome; the anterior rami of the lower cervical and first thoracic spinal nerves have lost their cutaneous distribution on the neck and trunk during the development of the upper limb.

4. (a) The physical examination revealed weakness of the rhomboid, deltoid, and biceps brachii muscles, which are innervated by the fifth and sixth cervical segments of the spinal cord. These spinal cord segments lie within the vertebral foramina of the sixth and seventh cervical vertebrae, respectively. (b) The fifth and sixth cervical segments of the spinal cord are being pressed upon. (c) The biceps brachii reflex arc involves the fifth and sixth segments of the spinal cord. (d) The rhomboids and deltoid muscles showed diminished muscle tone because the reflex arcs upon which their tone depends travel through the compressed segments of the spinal cord, i.e., the reflex arcs were no longer functioning normally. Because of the pressure of the tumor on the cervical region of the spinal cord, the nervous pathways passing down to lower segments of the spinal cord were interrupted. This resulted in the motor anterior gray column cells of the segments of the cord below the level of compression receiving diminished information from the higher centers, with a consequent increase in muscle tone.

5. Any disease process that can interrupt the normal functioning of the basic spinal reflex arc upon which skeletal muscle tone is dependent will cause loss of muscle tone. Some examples are spinal shock following trauma to the spinal cord; section of or pressure upon a spinal nerve, a posterior root, or an anterior root; syringomyelia; and poliomyelitis.

6. Tabes dorsalis, which is a syphilitic infection of the brain and spinal cord, produces degeneration of the central processes of the posterior root ganglion cells and also, usually, the ganglion cells themselves. The lower thoracic and lumbar sacral segments of the cord are involved first, and the interruption of the proprioceptive fibers results in impairment of appreciation of posture, and the tendency to fall down if one closes the eyes while standing. Eyesight in this patient compensated for lack of proprioception.

7. In a normal individual standing and walking are largely automatic but, as you have read in this chapter, these activities are highly complex and require the proper integration of neural mechanisms at all levels of the spinal cord and brain. The basic mechanism underlying muscle

tone is the spinal segmental reflex. In order to maintain normal posture, these reflex arcs must receive adequate nervous input from higher levels of the nervous system. Diseases involving the corpus striatum (caudate and lentiform nuclei) or the substantia nigra result in an alteration in the pattern of nervous impulses impinging on the anterior horn cells of the spinal cord; hence the abnormal muscle tone. The increased tone is equal in extent in opposing muscle groups. The tremor of the parkinsonian syndrome is produced by the alternating movements of the agonist and antagonist muscles of a joint. The tremor is most prominent when the limb is at rest, ceases temporarily when voluntary movement is performed, and then starts again when the movement is completed. The tremor ceases when the patient is asleep. In Parkinson's disease there is a neuronal degeneration in the substantia nigra, resulting in the loss of inhibitory control of the substantia nigra over the lentiform nucleus, putamen, and caudate nucleus (see p. 399).

8. The syndrome of petit mal commonly has three sets of symptoms: (a) myoclonic jerks, in which the patient experiences sudden involuntary contraction of the muscles of the trunk and extremities; (b) akinetic seizures, in which there is a sudden loss of tone in all muscles of the body; and (c) brief losses of consciousness, in which the patient loses contact with his environment for a few seconds.

9. Destruction of the anterior gray column cells in the lumbar and sacral regions of the spinal cord resulted in paralysis and atrophy of the muscles of both legs. The twitching of groups of muscle fibers is referred to as muscular fasciculation and is commonly seen in patients with chronic disease affecting the anterior horn cells.

10. (a) Muscular hypotonia is present on the same side of the body as the lesion. Passively move the joints on the right side of the body and then on the left side and compare the resistance to these movements by the muscles on the two sides of the body. (b) Posture. The shoulder girdle on the affected side drops, because of loss of muscle tone. With the patient disrobed ask him to stand up straight with his back toward you. With a unilateral cerebellar lesion the shoulder on the affected side may be lower than that on the opposite, normal side. (c) Disorders of voluntary movement (ataxia) due to loss of muscle coordination. The finger–nose test and the heel–knee test are described on page 159. These tests will reveal ataxia on the side of the body in which the lesion is situated. (d) Nystagmus. This may be defined as an involuntary to-and-fro movement of the eyes. It is commonly demonstrated in cerebellar disease and is due to lack of muscle coordination. When the eyes are turned horizontally laterally there are quick, rhythmic jerks in the direction of gaze. In unilateral cerebellar lesions, the amplitude of nystagmus is greater and its rate slower when the eyes are rotated toward the side of the lesion than when they are displaced to the opposite side.

CHAPTER 7

1. This patient was suffering from cervical spondylosis with pressure on the anterior and posterior roots of the fifth and sixth spinal nerves. As the result of repeated trauma and of aging, degenerative changes occurred at the articulating surfaces of the fourth, fifth, and sixth cervical vertebrae. Extensive spur formation, owing to new bone growth, resulted in narrowing of the intervertebral foramina with pressure on the nerve roots. The burning pain, hyperesthesia, and partial analgesia were due to pressure on the posterior roots, and the weakness, wasting, and fasciculation of the deltoid and biceps brachii muscles were due to pressure on the anterior roots. Movements of the neck presumably intensified the symptoms by exerting further traction or pressure on the nerve roots. Coughing or sneezing raised the pressure within the vertebral canal and resulted in further pressure on the nerve roots.

2. The patient was operated on and a laminectomy of the third, fourth, and fifth thoracic vertebrae was carried out. At the level of the fourth thoracic vertebra a small swelling was seen on the posterior surface of the spinal cord; it was attached to the dura mater. Histological examination showed that it was a meningioma. The tumor was easily removed and the patient successfully recovered from the operation.

There was a progressive recovery in the power of the lower limbs, and the patient is now walking without a stick. This patient emphasizes the importance of making an early, accurate diagnosis, because benign extramedullary spinal tumors are readily treatable. The lateral spinal thalamic tracts are responsible for the conduction of pain impulses up the spinal cord. These tracts are situated in the lateral white columns of the spinal cord (see p. 170). Postural sense and vibration sense are conducted up the spinal cord in the posterior white column through the fasciculus cuneatus from the upper limbs and the upper part of the thorax, and in the fasciculus gracilis from the lower part of the trunk and the leg. The difficulty in walking was due to pressure on the corticospinal tracts in the lateral white column. The exaggeration in the tendon reflexes of the lower limbs and the bilateral extensor plantar responses were due to the pressure on the descending tracts in the spinal cord at the level of the tumor. This also resulted in spastic paralysis of the muscles of the lower limbs.

3. A detailed description of the procedures for performing a lumbar puncture are given on page 32. The pressure of fluid can be measured and this is raised in patients, for example, with intracranial tumor or hemorrhage, hydrocephalus, meningitis, and encephalitis. The normal pressure is between 60 and 150 mm of water with the patient lying on his side. A sample of cerebrospinal fluid may be obtained so that cytological and chemical analysis can be performed. For details of the normal composition of cerebrospinal fluid, see page 176. Normal cerebrospinal fluid is clear and colorless. Substances may be inserted into the subarachnoid space, e.g., antibiotics and anesthetics, and opaque media may be introduced in order to perform myelography.

4. Queckenstedt's sign is positive if the cerebrospinal fluid pressure, measured by means of the lumbar puncture, does not rise promptly following the application of pressure to the internal jugular veins in the neck. It indicates that the subarachnoid space is blocked. For details, see page 33.

5. The blood supply to the spinal cord is fully described on page 173. The anterior spinal artery supplies the anterior two-thirds of the spinal cord. The upper and lower thoracic segments of the spinal cord have a relatively poor supply of blood, because the anterior spinal artery in this region may be extermely small.

6. Compare your diagram with that shown in Figure 7–2. Also read the description of the gray matter of this region on page 165.

7. Compare your diagram with that shown in Figure 7–7. Also read the descriptions of the white matter and the arrangement of the major ascending and descending tracts on page 169. In syringomyelia, a long cavity or cavities surrounded by gliosis appear close to the central canal in the upper cervical region of the spinal cord. The patients exhibit, principally, pain and thermal sensory loss with muscular wasting, especially in the small muscles of the hand. Later, involvement of the lateral white column results in loss of function in the corticospinal and other descending tracts, with spastic paralysis of the lower limbs. Involvement of the descending fibers of the sympathetic part of the autonomic system may produce a Horner's syndrome. (See p. 510.)

8. The lack of filling with radiopaque material of the lateral extension of the subarachnoid space around the fourth left thoracic spinal nerve in the myelogram would indicate that this extension was being pressed upon by a space–occupying lesion in the lateral part of the vertebral canal or within the intervertebral foramen. The lesion may have been a tumor or a herniated intervertebral disc. The lateral extension of the subarachnoid space around each spinal nerve is due to the meninges being prolonged laterally around the anterior and posterior spinal nerve roots. Within the intervertebral foramen the meninges fuse with the epineurium around the spinal nerve. Today MRI would be used to make the diagnosis, and only in very difficult cases would the neurologist use myelography.

9. The statement is correct. Unfortunately, many students, on examining thin transverse sections of the spinal cord, forget that the sections enable them to see the cells in only two dimensions, while in fact these cell groups extend up and down the spinal cord as columns of cells.

10. (a) The ligamentum denticulatum is formed as a thickening of pia mater. The ligamenta den-

ticulata are situated on both sides of the spinal cord between the spinal nerve roots of adjacent segments of the spinal cord. They extend laterally, where they terminate as toothlike attachments to the dura. They suspend the spinal cord within the dural sheath. (b) The filum terminale is a fibrous cord that is a prolongation of the pia mater extending from the apex of the conus medullaris to be attached inferiorly to the posterior surface of the coccyx. Its function is to anchor the spinal cord inferiorly. (c) The substantia gelatinosa is a group of nerve cells situated at the apex of the posterior gray column throughout the length of the spinal cord. The nerve cells are concerned mainly with the conduction of the sensations of pain, temperature, and touch. (d) The nucleus proprius is a group of large nerve cells situated in the posterior gray horn anterior to the substantia gelatinosa throughout the length of the spinal cord. They are associated with the proprioception, tactile discrimination, and vibration senses. (e) The anterior gray commissure is that part of the gray matter located anterior to the central canal of the spinal cord. The anterior and posterior gray commissures together constitute what is known as the gray commissure of the spinal cord.

CHAPTER 8

1. Until involvement of one of the last four cranial nerves occurs, localization of a lesion to the medulla oblongata remains uncertain. For example, involvement of the main ascending sensory pathways or descending pathways may be caused by a lesion in the medulla, the pons, the midbrain, or the spinal cord. Involvement of the glossopharyngeal nerve can be detected by inadequacy of the gag reflex and loss of taste sensation on the posterior third of the tongue. Involvement of the vagus nerve can be assumed if the patient demonstrates some or all of the following symptoms: impairment of pharyngeal sensibility, difficulty in swallowing, nasal regurgitation of fluids with asymmetry of movement of the soft palate, and hoarseness of the voice with paralysis of the laryngeal muscles. The cranial part of the accessory nerve is distributed within the vagus nerve so that it is not possible to test for this nerve alone. The spinal part of the accessory nerve, which supplies the sternocleidomastoid and trapezius muscles, arises from the spinal cord (see p. 446) and is therefore unaffected by tumors of the medulla. The hypoglossal nerve involvement may be tested by looking for wasting, fasciculation, and paralysis of one-half of the tongue.

2. The malformation in which the cerebellum and the medulla oblongata are found in the cervical part of the vertebral canal is known as the Arnold–Chiari malformation. This condition is a common cause of infantile hydrocephalus. The hydrocephalus may be due to distortion or malformation of the openings in the roof of the fourth ventricle, which normally allow the cerebrospinal fluid to escape into the subarachnoid space. A myelocele is commonly associated with this malformation. The reason for this is not exactly known, although several investigators believe that the myelocele is the primary cause and that it tethers the lower part of the spinal cord to the surrounding tissues at the time when disproportionate growth of the spinal cord and the vertebral column occurs. This would serve to pull the medulla oblongata and the cerebellum inferiorly through the foramen magnum into the vertebral canal.

3. This patient is suffering from a thrombosis of the posterior inferior cerebellar artery or vertebral artery on the right side. The vertigo is caused by the involvement of the cerebellum or the vestibular nuclei, or both. The hot, painful skin sensations are due to the involvement of the spinal tract and nucleus of the trigeminal nerve on the right side. The abnormal movement of the soft palate and the fixation of the right vocal cord are due to involvement of the nucleus of the vagus and accessory nerve on the right side. The ptosis, enophthalmos, and myosis (Horner's syndrome) are due to involvement of the descending fibers of the sympathetic part of the autonomic nervous system. The pointing of the tongue to the right is caused by involvement of the right hypoglossal nucleus (the right genioglossus muscle is paralyzed). The loss of pain and temperature sensations on the opposite side of the body are due to involvement of the ascending lateral spinothalamic tracts. This characteristic clinical syndrome re-

sults from cutting off the arterial supply to a wedge-shaped area in the posterolateral part of the medulla oblongata and the inferior surface of the cerebellum.

4. The ninth, tenth, and cranial part of the eleventh cranial nerves emerge from the medulla oblongata in a groove between the olives and the inferior cerebellar peduncles.

CHAPTER 9

1. This 10-year-old girl later was found to have an astrocytoma of the pons. The right unilateral facial weakness, together with weakness of the right lateral rectus muscle of the eye, was due to involvement of the right facial and abducent nuclei by the tumor. The absence of paresthesia of the face indicated that the principal sensory nucleus of the trigeminal nerve was intact on both sides. The weakness in the movements of the left arm and left leg was due to the involvement of the corticospinal fibers in the pons. (Remember that the majority of these fibers cross over to the opposite side at the decussation of the pyramids in the medulla.)

2. "Pinpoint" pupils indicate that the constrictor pupillae muscles are strongly contracted and the dilator pupillae muscles are paralyzed. The dilator pupillae muscles are supplied by the sympathetic fibers, which descend through the pons (position not precisely known) to the lateral gray columns of the thoracic part of the spinal cord. Here the fibers synapse and the thoracolumbar sympathetic outflow occurs (see p. 486).

3. The deafness and vertigo were due to lesions in the cochlear and vestibular nuclei in the upper part of the pons. The double vision (diplopia) was produced by the involvement of the abducent nerve nucleus on the right side of the pons. The history of severe headaches and vomiting was due to a progressive rise in intracranial pressure caused by a tumor of the pons. The right unilateral facial palsy was due to the involvement of the right facial nerve nucleus. The sensory impairment of the skin of the middle and lower part of the right side of the face was due to the tumor involvement of the principal sensory nucleus of the right trigeminal nerve.

CHAPTER 10

1. This man, at operation, was found to have an astrocytoma of the right cerebellar hemisphere. This fact explains the occurrence of unilateral symptoms and signs. The lesion was on the right side and the clumsiness, tremor, muscle incoordination, and hypotonia occurred on the right side of the body. The progressive worsening of the clinical condition could be explained on the basis that more and more of the cerebellum was becoming destroyed as the tumor rapidly expanded. The flaccidity of the muscles of the right arm and leg was due to hypotonia, that is, a removal of the influence of the cerebellum on the simple stretch reflex involving the muscle spindles and tendon organs. The clumsiness, tremor, and overshooting on the finger–nose test were due to lack of cerebellar influence on the process of coordination between different groups of muscles. The falling to the right side, the tilting of the head, and the drooping of the right shoulder were due to loss of muscle tone and fatigue.

2. A diagnosis was made of medulloblastoma of the brain in the region of the roof of the fourth ventricle, with involvement of the vermis of the cerebellum. The child died 9 months later after extensive deep x-ray therapy. The sudden onset of vomiting, the increased size of the head beyond normal limits, the sutural separation, and the severe bilateral papilledema could all be accounted for by the rapid rise in intracranial pressure owing to the rapid increase in size of the tumor. The broad-based, unsteady gait and the tendency to fall backward (or forward), and not to one side, indicate a tumor involving the vermis. The presence of bilateral hypotonia, especially during the later stages, was due to involvement of both cerebellar hemispheres. At autopsy the tumor was found to have invaded the fourth ventricle extensively, and there was evidence of internal hydrocephalus because the cerebrospinal fluid had been unable to escape through the foramina in the roof of the fourth ventricle.

3. Nystagmus, an involuntary oscillation of the eyeball, may occur physiologically, as when a person watches rapidly moving objects, or by

rapid rotation of the body. It commonly occurs in diseases of the nervous system, eye, and inner ear. In cerebellar disease, nystagmus is due to ataxia of the muscles moving the eyeball. There is lack of coordination between the agonists and antagonists involved in the eyeball movement. For full understanding of the different forms of nystagmus, a textbook of neurology should be consulted.

4. The different types of neurons found in the cerebellar cortex are fully described on page 215. The functions of these different cells are fully discussed on page 219 under Cerebellar Cortical Mechanisms. Remember that a great deal more research is required into the fine structure and physiology of these cells before we shall fully understand the functions of this interesting, computerlike organ.

5. Acute lesions, such as those resulting from a thrombosis of a cerebellar artery or a rapidly growing tumor, produce sudden severe symptoms and signs owing to the sudden withdrawal of the influence of the cerebellum on muscular activity. Patients can recover quickly from large cerebellar injuries, and this can be explained on the basis that the cerebellum influences muscular activity not directly but indirectly through the vestibular nuclei, reticular formation, red nucleus, tectum, and corpus striatum and the cerebral cortex; it may well be that these other areas of the central nervous system take over this function. In chronic lesions, the symptoms and signs are much less severe and there is enough time to allow the other areas of the central nervous system to compensate for loss of cerebellar function.

6. The climbing fibers are one set of afferent fibers to the cerebellar cortex. They originate in the olives and pass into the cortex "climbing" through the granular and Purkinje layers to end by synapsing on the dendrites of a single Purkinje cell.

The mossy fibers are the second set of afferent fibers to the cerebellar cortex. They originate from many areas of the central nervous system (see p. 406) except the olives, and pass into the granular layer of the cortex. They terminate by synapsing with many granular cell processes. Their mode of termination closely resembles the branching of the small leafy plant called moss.

7. The cerebellar peduncles, of which there are three pairs, superior, middle, and inferior, are composed of bundles of nerve fibers that pass to and from the cerebellum, connecting it with the remainder of the nervous system. The fiber content of each is described on page 218.

The middle cerebellar peduncle is the largest of the peduncles and is made up entirely of the corticopontocerebellar fibers that originate in the neurons of the pontine nuclei. The fibers then cross the midline as the transverse fibers of the pons and pass through the middle cerebellar peduncle to reach the cortex of the neocerebellum of the contralateral hemisphere. These fibers constitute an important link between the cerebral cortex and the cerebellum.

8. The intracerebellar nuclei are situated in each cerebellar hemisphere. They are, from lateral to medial: the dentate, the emboliform, the globose, and the fastigial nuclei. The axons of the neurons of these nuclei form the main outflow from the cerebellum to the remainder of the central nervous system. It follows, therefore, that if these nuclei are destroyed, the cerebellum is totally cut off from influencing the rest of the nervous system (except connections that pass directly from the Purkinje cells to the vestibular nuclei). If the cortex and the nuclei both are destroyed, the cerebellum clearly is no longer functioning.

9. A person who has a unilateral lesion involving one cerebellar hemisphere demonstrates absence of coordination between different groups of muscles on the same side of the body. This disturbance affects not only agonists and antagonists in a single joint movement, but all associated muscle activity. For example, a normal person when walking swings his arms at both sides; in cerebellar disease this activity would be lost on the side of the lesion.

CHAPTER II

1. This man was operated on and found to have a large astrocytoma of the vermis of the cerebellum. The tumor had severely encroached upon the cavity of the fourth ventricle, producing in-

ternal hydrocephalus and pressure on the floor of the ventricle.

The symptoms of headache and persistent vomiting were produced by a raised intracranial pressure caused by the enlarging tumor. The tumor also blocked off the median and lateral apertures in the roof of the fourth ventricle, causing an internal hydrocephalus, which further raised the intracranial pressure. The bilateral papilledema was secondary to the raised intracranial pressure. The inability to sit up in bed (truncal ataxia) and the loss of equilibrium on standing were due to the tumor involvement of the vermis of the cerebellum. The loss of tone of the muscles of the right limbs indicated spread of the tumor to involve the right cerebellar hemisphere. Central deafness on the right side was due to involvement of the right eighth cranial nerve nuclei by the tumor mass. The patient died six months after neurosurgical exploration.

2. Steroid hormones (e.g., prednisone) inhibit the normal inflammatory reaction and thereby reduce the incidence of fibrous adhesions. Such adhesions may block the openings in the roof of the fourth ventricle, thus preventing the escape of cerebrospinal fluid into the subarachnoid space from within the ventricular system. Adhesions also may prevent the flow of cerebrospinal fluid over the cerebral hemispheres or reduce the absorption of the fluid into the arachnoid granulations. Thus it is seen that adhesions of the meninges may result in hydrocephalus.

3. (a) Central aperture in roof (foramen of Magendie), (b) two lateral apertures in roof (foramina of Luschka), (c) central canal of medulla oblongata and spinal cord (there is no opening into the subarachnoid space from this canal), and (d) cerebral aqueduct of midbrain (leads into the third and lateral ventricles but there is no opening into the subarachnoid space).

4. The superior medullary velum is a thin sheet of white matter connecting the two superior cerebellar peduncles. It is covered on the outside by pia mater and is lined on the inside by ependyma. It forms the superior part of the roof of the fourth ventricle. The function of the white matter is not known.

The inferior medullary velum has no nervous tissue within it and consists of a layer of pia mater lined with ependyma. It forms the lower part of the roof of the fourth ventricle and stretches between the inferior cerebellar peduncles. It has a large aperture in the midline, the median aperture, and the choroid plexus is suspended from the inferior medullary velum (see p. 343). The important function of the median aperture and the function of the choroid plexus are described on page 346.

5. The important structures that lie beneath the floor of the fourth ventricle are as follows:

Beneath the superior half and within the pons are the abducent nerve nucleus, part of the seventh cranial nerve, which loops around it to form the facial colliculus, and the vestibular nuclei.

Beneath the inferior half and within the medulla oblongata are the hypoglossal nucleus, the dorsal motor nucleus of the vagus, and the vestibular nuclei.

CHAPTER 12

1. The herniated uncus and the subdural hemorrhage caused pressure of the opposite crus cerebri of the midbrain against the sharp edge of the tentorium. The distortion of the midbrain caused narrowing of the cerebral aqueduct, further raising the supratentorial pressure by blocking the passage of cerebrospinal fluid from the third to the fourth ventricle. Under these circumstances, severe hemorrhage may occur within the midbrain and affect the third and fourth cranial nerve nuclei and various important descending and ascending tracts.

2. This child had hydrocephalus. The physical examination and the special tests showed that the third and lateral ventricles of the brain were grossly dilated owing to the accumulation of cerebrospinal fluid in these cavities. Mechanical obstruction to the flow of cerebrospinal fluid from the third into the fourth ventricle through the cerebral aqueduct was present. After the possibility of the presence of cysts or resectable tumors had been excluded, it was assumed that the cause of the obstruction was a congenital atresia or malformation of the cerebral aqueduct. If the condition were progress-

ing, that is, the block in the aqueduct was complete and the head continued to increase in size at an abnormal rate, some form of neurosurgical procedure should have been performed whereby the cerebrospinal fluid would be shunted from the third or lateral ventricles into the subarachnoid space, or into the venous system of the neck.

3. Two years later the patient died. At autopsy a large astrocytoma was found that involved the central part of the tegmentum at the level of the superior colliculi. The patient had exhibited all signs and symptoms associated with a raised intracranial pressure. The raised pressure was due in part to the expanding tumor, but the problem was compounded by the developing hydrocephalus resulting from blockage of the cerebral aqueduct.

    The symptoms and signs exhibited by the patient when he was first seen by the neurologist could be explained by the presence of the tumor in the central gray matter at the level of the superior colliculi, and involving the third cranial nerve nuclei on both sides. This resulted in bilateral ptosis, bilateral ophthalmoplegia, and bilateral fixed, dilated pupils. The resting position of the eyes in a downward and lateral position was due to the action of the superior oblique muscle (trochlear nerve) and lateral rectus muscle (abducent nerve).

4. The patient had a hemorrhage into the right side of the tegmentum of the midbrain that involved the right third cranial nerve. The ascending tracts of the left trigeminal nerve also were involved. After emerging from the sensory nuclei of the left trigeminal nerve, they cross the midline and ascend through the trigeminal lemniscus on the right side. The loss of sensation seen in the left upper and lower limbs was due to involvement of the right medial lemniscus. The athetoid movements of the left leg could be explained on the basis of the involvement of the right red nucleus. The absence of spasticity of the left arm and leg would indicate that the lesion did not involve the right descending tracts. For further clarification, consult the descriptions of the various tracts (see pp. 395 and 396).

5. Autopsy later revealed a vascular lesion involving a branch of the posterior cerebral artery.

Considerable brain softening was found in the region of the substantia nigra and crus cerebri on the left side of the midbrain. The left oculomotor nerve was involved as it passed through the infarcted area. The corticonuclear fibers that pass to the facial nerve nucleus and the hypoglossal nucleus were involved as they descended through the left crus cerebri (they cross the midline at the level of the nuclei). The corticospinal fibers on the left side were also involved (they cross in the medulla oblongata), hence the spastic paralysis of the right arm and leg. The left trigeminal and left medial lemnisci were untouched, which explains the absence of sensory changes on the right side of the body. This is a good example of Weber's syndrome.

CHAPTER 13

1. This man had a thrombosis of the thalamogeniculate branch of the right posterior cerebral artery. This resulted in a degenerative lesion within the right thalamus causing the impairment of superficial and deep sensations on the left side of the body. The contralateral hemiparesis, involving the left leg and left arm with increased muscle tone, was produced by edema in the nearby posterior limb of the right internal capsule causing blocking of the corticospinal fibers. As the edema resolved, the paralysis and spasticity improved. The choreoathetoid movements of the left leg and the intention tremor of the left arm were probably due to damage to the right thalamus or to the right dentatothalamic nerve fibers.

    The development of the agonizing pain of the left leg—characteristic of the thalamic syndrome—was due to the lesion in the right thalamus.

2. This woman exhibited continuous uncoordinated activity of the proximal musculature of the right arm and right leg, resulting in the limbs being flung violently about. The muscles of the right side of the face were also slightly affected. This condition is known as *hemiballismus*. It was caused by hemorrhage into the left subthalamic nucleus.

3. During the third decade of life, calcareous concretions appear in the neuroglia and connective tissue of the pineal gland. This provides a use-

ful midline landmark to the radiologist. A lateral displacement of such a landmark would indicate the presence of an intracranial mass. In this patient, the pineal gland shadow was in the midline and all the other investigations, including computed tomography (CT scan), showed no evidence of a cerebral tumor.

4. Melatonin has been shown to cause the aggregation of melanin granules within the melanophores of amphibian skin. It has no action on the melanocytes of mammalian skin. Melatonin is produced in large quantites in the pineal gland by the enzyme hydroxymethyltransferase; the gland also is capable of converting serotonin into melatonin.

5. Adiposity alone or associated with genital dystrophy can occur with disease of the hypothalamus.

CHAPTER 14

1. The right middle frontal gyrus is located on the lateral surface of the frontal lobe of the right cerebral hemisphere. It is bounded superiorly and inferiorly by the superior and inferior frontal sulci, respectively. The right middle frontal gyrus is overlaid by the frontal bone of the skull.

2. The important central sulcus is large and runs downward and forward across the lateral aspect of each hemisphere. Superiorly, it indents the superior medial border of the hemisphere about 1 cm behind the midpoint; it lies between two parallel gyri. It is the only sulcus of any length that indents the superior medial border. The arrangement of the sulci and gyri is very similar on both sides of the brain. There are, however, great individual variations in the details of their arrangement.

3. The lateral ventricle is a C-shaped cavity situated within each cerebral hemisphere. The lateral ventricle wraps itself around the thalamus, the lentiform nucleus, and the caudate nucleus. It is divided into a body that occupies the parietal lobe, an anterior horn that extends into the frontal lobe, a posterior horn that extends into the occipital lobe, and an inferior horn that runs forward and inferiorly into the temporal lobe. The cerebrospinal fluid is produced in the choroid plexus of the lateral ventricle and

drains through the small interventricular foramen into the third ventricle. In later life, the choroid plexus, especially in its posterior part, sometimes shows calcified deposits, which are occasionally revealed on radiographs, as in this case. This patient later was found to have a cerebral tumor that was compressing the left interventricular foramen, hence the enlarged left ventricle.

4. The corpus callosum occasionally fails to develop and in those patients no definite neurological signs and symptoms appear. If, however, the corpus callosum is divided during a surgical procedure in the adult, the loss of interconnections between the two hemispheres becomes apparent (see p. 280).

5. The *corpus striatum* is the collective term for the caudate nucleus and the lentiform nucleus. The name is derived from the gross appearance of the horizontal brain slice of this region, which shows strands of gray matter connecting the head of the caudate nucleus through the white matter of the internal capsule to the putamen of the lentiform nucleus.

The basal ganglia comprise the caudate nucleus, the lentiform nucleus, and the amygdaloid nucleus. The basal nuclei are the same structures as those that form the basal ganglia.

CHAPTER 15

1. The cerebral cortex is made up of six identifiable layers. In the motor cortex in the precentral gyrus, there is a lack of granular cells in the second and fourth layers, and in the somesthetic cortex in the postcentral gyrus, there is a lack of pyramidal cells in the third and fifth layers. The motor cortex is thicker than the sensory cortex.

2. This patient had a cerebral tumor involving the left parietal lobe with advanced destruction of the superior parietal lobule. This is the somesthetic association area, where the sensations of touch, pressure, and proprioception are integrated. It is essential that the patient be allowed to finger the object so that these different sensations can be appreciated.

3. This patient had a cerebrovascular lesion involving the left precentral gyrus. The damage to the pyramidal cells that give origin to the

corticospinal fibers was responsible for the right-sided paralysis. The increased tone of the paralyzed muscles was due to the loss of inhibition caused by involvement of the extrapyramidal fibers (see p. 305).

4. Destructive lesions of the frontal eye field of the left cerebral hemisphere caused the two eyes to deviate to the side of the lesion and an inability to turn the eyes to the opposite side. The frontal eye field is thought to control voluntary scanning movements of the eye and is independent of visual stimuli.

5. A small discrete lesion of the primary motor cortex results in little change in muscle tone. Larger lesions involving the primary and secondary motor areas, which are the most common, result in muscle spasm. The explanation for this is fully given on page 305.

6. This patient is suffering from Jacksonian epileptic seizures, in this case caused by cerebral scarring secondary to the automobile injury. The weakness of the right leg immediately after the accident was due to damage to the superior part of the left precentral gyrus. Her initial attacks of epilepsy were of the partial variety and were caused by irritation of the leg area of the left precentral gyrus. In her last attack, the epileptiform seizure spread to other areas of the left precentral gyrus, thus involving most of the right side of her body, and she lost consciousness.

7. As the result of the patient and extensive histological researches of Brodmann, Campbell, Economo, and the Vogts, it has been possible to divide the cerebral cortex into areas that have a different microscopic arrangement and different types of cells. These cortical maps are fundamentally similar and the one proposed by Brodmann is used widely. Because the functional significance of many areas of the human cerebral cortex is not known, it has not been possible to closely correlate structure with function. In general, it can be said that the motor cortices are thicker than the sensory cortices, and that the motor cortex has less prominent second and fourth granular layers and has large pyramidal cells in the fifth layer. Other areas with a different structure may have similar functional roles. More recent studies using electrophysiological techniques have indicated that it is more accurate to divide the cerebral cortex according to its thalamocortical projections. The vertical chain mechanism of the cerebral cortex is fully described on page 296.

8. In this patient, the persistence of coarse voluntary movements of the right shoulder, hip, and knee joints can be explained on the basis that coarse postural movements are controlled by the premotor area of the cortex and the basal ganglia and these areas were spared in this patient.

9. The professor's altered behavior was due to a severe lesion involving both frontal lobes of the cerebrum secondary to the depressed fracture of the frontal bone. While destruction of the prefrontal cortex does not cause a marked loss of intelligence, it does result in the individual's losing initiative and drive, and often the patient no longer conforms to the accepted modes of social behavior.

10. The understanding of spoken speech requires the normal functioning of the secondary auditory area, which is situated posterior to the primary auditory area in the lateral sulcus and in the superior temporal gyrus. This area is believed to be necessary for the interpretation of sounds, and the information is passed on to the sensory speech area of Wernicke.

11. The understanding of written speech requires the normal functioning of the secondary visual area of the cerebral cortex, which is situated in the walls of the posterior part of the calcarine sulcus on the medial and lateral surfaces of the cerebral hemisphere. The function of the secondary visual area is to relate visual information received by the primary visual area to past visual experiences. This information is then passed on to the dominant angular gyrus and relayed to the anterior part of Wernicke's speech area (see p. 301).

12. *Coma* is the term applied to an unconscious patient. The patient will not speak and will respond only reflexly to painful stimuli. In deeply comatose individuals, there will be no response. The eyes are closed and do not move.

Sleep is a changed state of consciousness; it is discussed on page 308.

An electroencephalogram (EEG) is a recording of the electrical activity of the cerebral cortex made by placing electrodes on the scalp. Detection of abnormalities of the alpha, beta, and delta rhythms may assist in the diagnosis of cerebral tumors, epilepsy, and cerebral abscesses.

CHAPTER 16

1. The Klüver-Bucy syndrome consists of the signs and symptoms found in monkeys following bilateral removal of the temporal lobe. The monkeys became docile and unresponsive and display no signs of fear or anger. They have an increased appetite and increased sexual activity, which is often perverse. They are unable to recognize objects seen. Human subjects in whom the amygdaloid area is destroyed do not usually demonstrate this syndrome. It has, however, been described in humans following the bilateral removal of large areas of the temporal lobes.
2. The olfactory aura that preceded the general convulsions of the epileptic attack would indicate that the temporal lobe of the cerebral cortex was intially involved.
3. An autopsy study revealed extensive invasion of the hippocampus, fornix, and mammillary bodies in both cerebral hemispheres. It appears that the hippocampus is involved in the storage and categorizing of afferent information related to recent memory.

CHAPTER 17

1. This child is suffering from Sydenham's chorea. This condition occurs, in the majority of cases, in female children between the ages of 5 and 15. It is characterized by the presence of rapid, irregular, involuntary movements that are purposeless. The disease is associated with rheumatic fever and complete recovery is the rule. The subthalamic nuclei and the caudate nuclei are involved.
2. Huntington's chorea is a progressive inherited disease that usually appears between 30 and 45. The involuntary movements arc usually more rapid and jerky than those seen in patients with Sydenham's chorea. Progressive mental changes lead to dementia and death. There is a progressive degeneration of the

GABA-secreting, substance P–secreting, and the acetylcholine-secreting neurons of the striatonigral pathway. This results in the dopamine-secreting neurons of the substantia nigra becoming overactive so that the nigrostriatal pathway inhibits the caudate nucleus and the putamen. This causes the involuntary movements. The involuntary movements can be reduced by blocking the dopamine receptors (perphenazine) or depleting the presynaptic dopamine production (reserpine). Atrophy of the caudate nucleus and putamen occurs.
3. The clinical sign is known as hemiballismus. The sudden onset is usually caused by vascular impairment due to hemorrhage or occlusion. Hemiballismus is the result of destruction of the contralateral subthalmic nucleus or its neuronal connections, causing the violent, uncoordinated movements of the axial and proximal limb muscles.

CHAPTER 18

1. The common sites for blockage of the flow of cerebrospinal fluid are where the passages are narrowest, namely, the interventricular foramina (foramina of Monro), the cerebral aqueduct, the median aperture in the roof of the fourth ventricle (foramen of Magendie), and the aperture in each lateral recess of the fourth ventricle (foramen of Luschka). It is possible for inflammatory exudate secondary to meningitis or a cerebral tumor to narrow down or even obliterate the opening in the tentorial notch so that the passage of the cerebrospinal fluid to the outer surface of the cerebral hemispheres is impeded or stopped. The flow may also be impeded by interference with the absorption of cerebrospinal fluid at the arachnoid granulations.
2. The cerebrospinal fluid serves as a cushion between the brain and the surrounding skull bones. It permits pressure applied at one point on the skull to be evenly distributed over the brain surface. Unfortunately, the brain is suspended in the fluid and is free to move, so that damage due to distortion, or as the result of momentum, can still occur. For a discussion of these problems, see page 529.

3. A magnetic resonance image (MRI) shows the outline of the ventricles very well. Occasionally, when these methods show insufficient detail a ventriculogram may be obtained. This procedure consists of the introduction of air or oxygen into the lateral ventricle through a needle inserted through a burr hole in the skull.

Since the left lateral ventricle was the only part of the ventricular system that showed distention and distortion, one can assume that the tumor had closed off the left interventricular foramen and therefore was in the vicinity of that foramen. This was confirmed on the CT scan.

4. Hydrocephalus is a condition in which there is an abnormal increase in the volume of cerebrospinal fluid within the skull. Congenital atresia of the cerebral aqueduct, meningitis, tumors, and blockage of the arachnoid granulations by subarachnoid bleeding or inflammatory exudate are common causes of this condition in young children.

5. There is an extension of the intracranial subarachnoid space forward around the optic nerve to the back of the eyeball. A rise in cerebrospinal fluid pressure caused by an intracranial tumor will compress the thin walls of the retinal vein as it crosses the extension of the subarachnoid space to enter the optic nerve. This will result in congestion of the retinal vein, bulging of the optic disc, and edema of the disc. Since both subarachnoid extensions are continuous with the intracranial subarachnoid space, both eyes will exhibit papilledema.

CHAPTER 19

1. The blood-brain barrier is a semipermeable barrier that exists between the blood and the extracellular spaces of the nervous tissue of the brain. It permits the passage of water, gases, glucose, electrolytes, and amino acids, but it is impermeable to substances with a large molecular weight.

The antibiotic penicillin, when injected intramuscularly into a normal individual, is found in much lower concentrations in the cerebrospinal fluid than in the blood; this is due to the existence of the blood-brain barrier and the

blood–cerebrospinal fluid barrier. Inflammation of the meninges results in an increased permeability of the meningeal blood vessels, and consequently the concentration of penicillin rises in the cerebrospinal fluid. It is important, however, for the treatment to be effective in patients with meningitis, to give very large doses of penicillin intravenously.

By contrast, chloramphenicol and the sulfonamides rapidly cross the blood–brain and blood-cerebrospinal fluid barriers, so that an adequate concentration in the cerebrospinal fluid can easily be maintained.

2. The blood-brain barrier in the newborn child is not fully developed and is more permeable than in the adult. Indirect bilirubin readily crosses the barrier in the newborn but does not do so in the adult. Once the bile pigment reaches the extracellular spaces of the brain tissue in the newborn it passes into the neurons and neuroglial cells. This results in abnormal cell function and eventually neuronal death.

3. The pineal gland, the posterior lobe of the pituitary, the tuber cinereum, the wall of the optic recess, and the vascular area postrema at the inferior end of the fourth ventricle are parts of the brain where the capillary endothelium contains open fenestrations across which proteins and small organic molecules may pass. It is in these areas that the blood-brain barrier appears to be absent.

The reason for the absence of the barrier in the pineal gland is not understood. It is possible that the pinealocytes, in order to function normally, require a close relationship with the blood plasma in order to sample the concentrations of hormones.

The absence of the blood-brain barrier in the region of the hypothalamus may allow this area of the brain to sample the chemical content of the plasma, so that appropriate modifications of metabolic activity may take place, thus protecting the nervous tissue as a whole.

CHAPTER 20

1. A fracture dislocation of the ninth thoracic vertebra would result in severe damage to the tenth thoracic segment of the spinal cord. The

unequal sensory and motor losses on the two sides indicate a left hemisection of the cord. The narrow band of hyperesthesia on the left side was due to the irritation of the cord immediately above the site of the lesion. The band of anesthesia and analgesia was due to the destruction of the cord on the left side at the level of the tenth thoracic segment—that is, all afferent fibers entering the cord at that point were interrupted. The loss of pain and thermal sensibilities and the loss of light touch below the level of the umbilicus on the right side were caused by the interruption of the lateral and anterior spinothalamic tracts on the left side of the cord.

2. This patient has the early signs and symptoms of syringomyelia. The gliosis and cavitation had resulted in interruption of the lateral and anterior spinothalamic tracts as they decussated in the anterior gray and white commissures of the spinal cord at the level of the eighth cervical and first thoracic segments of the spinal cord. Because of uneven growth of the cavitation, the condition was worse on the left than on the right side. Since tactile discrimination was normal in both upper limbs, the fasciculus cuneatus in both posterior white columns was unaffected. This dissociated sensory loss is characteristic of this disease.

3. The peculiar stamping gait and the swaying posture on closing the eyes are the characteristic signs of loss of appreciation of proprioceptive sensation from the lower limbs. These, together with the inability to detect the vibrations of a tuning fork placed on the medial malleoli of both legs, indicated that the patient had a lesion involving the fasciculus gracilis in both posterior white columns. Further questioning of this patient indicated that he had been treated for syphilis. The diagnosis was tabes dorsalis.

4. The treatment of intractable pain in terminal cancer is a difficult problem. The narcotic drugs with their strong analgesic action are generally used. The likelihood that these drugs will be habit-forming is accepted in a dying patient. An alternative treatment is surgical section of the nerve fibers carrying the sensations of pain into the nervous system. The techniques of posterior rhizotomy and cordotomy are described on page 377.

CHAPTER 21

1. The lower motor neuron in the spinal cord has its cell body and dendrites situated in the anterior gray column. The axon leaves the gray matter, crosses the white matter, and enters the anterior root of the spinal nerve. It then travels through the spinal nerve and peripheral nerve to innervate skeletal muscle.

    Internuncial neurons are sometimes referred to as interneurons, or connector neurons. Large numbers are found in the anterior gray columns of the spinal cord in close relation to the lower motor neurons. Their function is to receive the descending fibers of the many descending tracts and other afferent sensory fibers, and to relay the information to the lower motor neurons. The part that these cells play in the production of the prolonged asynchronous discharge is discussed on page 392. The Renshaw cell is a special member of this group and inhibits the activity of the lower motor neuron (see p. 392).

    The *final common pathway* is a term used to describe the lower motor neuron. It is the neuron that receives multiple impulses from different levels of the central nervous system and channels them along this common pathway to the muscle. The *upper motor neurons* have cell bodies situated at supraspinal levels. They give rise to nerve fibers that descend through the brainstem as corticonuclear fibers that end on cranial motor nerve nuclei, or as corticospinal fibers that descend in the spinal cord and influence the lower motor neurons in the cord.

2. Spinal shock is a temporary interruption of the physiological function of the spinal cord following injury. It may in part be a vascular phenomenon involving the gray matter of the spinal cord; on the other hand, some authorities believe it is due to the sudden interruption of the influence of the higher centers on the local segmental reflexes. Whatever the cause, it usually disappears after one to four weeks. The condition is characterized by a flaccid paralysis and

loss of sensation and reflex activity below the level of the lesion; this includes paralysis of the bladder and rectum.

Paraplegia in extension and paraplegia in flexion follow severe injury to the spinal cord. Paraplegia in extension indicates an increase in the extensor muscle tone owing to the overactivity of the gamma efferent nerve fibers to the muscle spindles as the result of the release of these neurons from the higher centers. However, some neurologists believe that the vestibulospinal tracts are intact in these cases. Should all the descending tracts be severed, the condition of paraplegia in flexion occurs where the reflex responses are flexor in nature when a noxious stimulus is applied. It should be emphasized that paraplegia in extension and paraplegia in flexion occur only after spinal shock has ceased. Paraplegia in extension may change to paraplegia in flexion if the damage to the spinal cord becomes more extensive and the vestibulospinal tracts are destroyed.

3. The term *pyramidal tract* simply means those corticospinal fibers that are grouped together in the medulla oblongata to form a visible swelling known as the pyramid. Clinicians often use the term too loosely and include the corticonuclear fibers (see p. 419) and even all the upper motor neurons under this term.

The term *extrapyramidal tracts* is used loosely by clinicians to include all descending pathways in the spinal cord other than those that are descending directly from the primary motor area of the cerebral cortex. The term is imprecise and should be dropped.

4. If it is assumed that this patient had a lesion in the left internal capsule following a cerebral hemorrhage, the corticospinal fibers would have been interrupted as they descended through the posterior limb of the internal capsule. Since most of these fibers crossed to the right side at the decussation of the pyramids, or lower down at the segmental level of the spinal cord, the muscles of the opposite side would have been affected. Interruption of these corticospinal fibers would have produced the following clinical signs: (a) Babinski sign positive, (b) loss of superficial abdominal and cremasteric reflexes, and (c) loss of performance of fine, skilled voluntary movements, especially at the distal ends of the limbs.

In patients with severe hemorrhage into the internal capsule, subcortical connections between the cerebral cortex and the caudate nucleus and the globus pallidus and other subcortical nuclei may be damaged. Moreover, some of the nuclei themselves may be destroyed. The interruption of other descending tracts from these subcortical centers would produce the following clinical signs: (a) severe paralysis on the opposite side of the body; (b) spasticity of the paralyzed muscles; (c) exaggerated deep muscle reflexes on the opposite side of the body to the lesion (clonus may be demonstrated); and (d) clasp-knife reaction, which may be felt in the paralyzed muscles.

5. A lateral radiograph of the thoracic part of the vertebral column showed a fracture dislocation involving the tenth thoracic vertebra. The first lumbar segment of the spinal cord is related to this vertebra. The first lumbar dermatome overlies the inguinal ligament and the total anesthesia over the right ligament would suggest a partial lesion of the spinal cord involving the total sensory input at that level. The loss of tactile discrimination and vibratory and proprioceptive sense in the right leg was caused by the interruption of the ascending tracts in the posterior white column on the right side of the spinal cord. The loss of pain and temperature sense in the skin of the left leg was due to destruction of the crossed lateral spinothalamic tracts on the right side at the level of the lesion. The loss of tactile sense in the skin of the left leg was caused by the destruction of the crossed anterior spinothalamic tracts on the right side. The spastic paralysis of the right leg and the right-sided ankle clonus were due to the interruption of the right-sided descending tracts other than the corticospinal tracts. The right-sided Babinski response was brought about by the interruption of the corticospinal fibers on the right side.

The complete motor and sensory loss of both legs and the absence of all deep tendon reflexes of both legs during the first 12 hours were due to spinal shock.

6. The spinal cord occupies the vertebral canal of

the vertebral column and under normal circumstances, therefore, is well protected. Unfortunately, once the integrity of the bony protection is destroyed by a fracture dislocation, especially in the thoracic region, where the canal is of small diameter, the bone can damage the cord and sever it just as a knife cuts through butter. It is essential that all patients suspected of having an injury to the spine be handled with great care to prevent the bones undergoing further dislocation and causing further injury to the cord. The patient should be carefully lifted by multiple supports under the feet, knees, pelvis, back, shoulders, and head and placed on a rigid stretcher or board for transportation to the nearest medical center.

7. Urinary infection secondary to bladder dysfunction is extremely common in paraplegic patients. The patient not only has lost control of the bladder but does not know when it is full. (For details on the autonomic control of the bladder, see p. 504.) An indwelling Foley catheter is placed in the bladder immediately for continuous drainage and antibiotic therapy is instituted.

Bedsores are very common in patients who have lost all sensory perception over their bony points, such as the ischial tuberosities and the sacrum. Bedsores are best prevented by (a) keeping the skin scrupulously clean, (b) frequently changing the position of the patient, and (c) keeping soft padding beneath the bony points.

Nutritional deficiency is common in active individuals who are suddenly confined to their beds and who are paralyzed. Loss of appetite must be combated by giving the patients a high-calorie diet that has all the required ingredients, especially vitamins.

Muscle spasms occur in paraplegia in extension or paraplegia in flexion and may follow only minor stimuli. Warm baths are helpful but occasionally, in extreme cases, nerve section may be necessary.

Pain occurs in the anesthetic areas in about a quarter of patients who have a complete section of the spinal cord. The pain may be burning or shooting and superficial, or deep visceral. Analgesics should be tried, but in some

individuals rhizotomy or even chordotomy may be necessary.

An accurate prognosis is not possible until the stage of spinal shock has ended and this may last as long as four weeks.

8. The characteristic coarse tremor of the right hand (pill rolling) and right arm, the unsmiling masklike face with unblinking eyes, and the cogwheel rigidity of the involved muscles make the diagnosis of early Parkinson's disease (paralysis agitans) certain. Degenerative lesions occur in the substantia nigra and other subcortical nuclei, including the lentiform nucleus. The loss of normal function of these subcortical areas and the absence of their influence on the lower motor neurons are responsible for the increased tone and tremor.

9. (a) Intention tremor occurs in cerebellar disease.

(b) Athetosis occurs in lesions of the corpus striatum.

(c) Chorea occurs in lesions of the corpus striatum.

(d) Dystonia occurs in disease of the lentiform nucleus.

(e) Hemiballismus occurs in disease of the opposite subthalamic nucleus.

CHAPTER 22

1. This 10-year-old girl had the symptoms and signs of Friedreich's ataxia, an inherited degenerative disease of the cerebellum and posterior and lateral parts of the spinal cord.

Degeneration of the cerebellum was revealed by the altered gait, clumsy movements of the right arm, tendency to fall to the right, intention tremor of the right arm and leg, hypotonocity of the right arm and right leg, and nystagmus of both eyes.

Involvement of the fasciculus gracilis was evidenced by loss of vibratory sense, loss of two-point discrimination, and loss of muscle joint sense of the lower limbs.

Corticospinal tract degeneration resulted in weakness of the legs and the presence of the Babinski plantar response. The exaggerated knee jerks were due to involvement of the upper motor neurons other than the corticospinal tract.

The loss of the ankle jerks was due to the interruption of the reflex arcs at spinal levels S1 and S2 by the degenerative process.

The clubfoot and scoliosis can be attributed to altered tone of the muscles of the leg and trunk over a period of many years.

CHAPTER 23

1. The medial strabismus of her right eye, the diplopia, and the inability to turn the right eye laterally were due to paralysis of the right lateral rectus muscle caused by a lesion of the abducent nerve. The glucosuria, high blood glucose, polyuria, polydipsia, and weight loss are the classic signs and symptoms of diabetes mellitus. The lesion of the abducent nerve was an example of diabetic neuropathy, a complication of untreated or poorly treated diabetes. Once the patient's diabetes was carefully controlled, the right lateral rectus palsy disappeared after three months.

2. This boy suffered from anosmia secondary to a lesion involving both olfactory tracts. The watery discharge from the nose was due to a leak of cerebrospinal fluid through the fractured cribriform plate of the ethmoid bone. It was the fracture and the associated hemorrhage that had damaged both olfactory tracts. Many normal persons with an acute sense of smell cannot name common scents. Since both olfactory tracts communicate with each other through the anterior commissure, it is unlikely that a lesion of one olfactory cortex can produce complete anosmia.

3. This patient has a paralysis of the right superior oblique muscle resulting from a lesion of the trochlear nerve. Since the trochlear nerves decussate on emergence from the midbrain, the left trochlear nucleus is the site of the lesion. This patient had a thrombosis of a small artery supplying the left trochlear nucleus. The difficulty in reading, the diplopia, and the difficulty in walking downstairs were due to the paralysis of the right superior oblique muscle.

4. As the result of the great increase in the thickness of the bones due to new bone formation in osteitis deformans, mental deterioration may occur owing to compression of the cerebral hemispheres. Those cranial nerves that pass through relatively small foramina in the skull are likely to be compressed by the new bone growth. The nerves commonly involved are the vestibulocochlear and facial nerves, following narrowing of the internal acoustic meatus. The olfactory and optic nerves also may be compressed as they pass through the cribriform plate and the optic canal, respectively.

5. Multiple sclerosis may affect white matter in widely disseminated areas of the central nervous system. Although remissions may occur, it is inevitably progressive. Thirty years later, when this patient died, numerous areas of sclerosis were found throughout the brainstem and white matter of the spinal cord. It was noted that the region of the vestibular nuclei beneath the floor of the fourth ventricle was involved in the disease process.

6. The trapezius muscle is supplied by the spinal part of the accessory nerve. The spinal nucleus of this nerve in the upper five cervical segments of the spinal cord receives cortical fibers from both cerebral hemispheres. This would account for the absence of muscular weakness in this patient with a left-sided hemiplegia. For a muscle to atrophy (except for disuse atrophy), the integrity of the monosynaptic reflex arc must be destroyed. This was not the case in this patient.

7. The severe pain over the forehead and the right eye was due to irritation of the ophthalmic division of the trigeminal nerve by the slowly expanding aneurysm of the internal carotid artery as it was lying in the cavernous sinus. The double vision (diplopia) and the lateral deviation of the right eye were due to the unopposed action of the lateral rectus muscle (supplied by the abducent nerve). The dilatation of the right pupil, with loss of direct and consensual light reflexes, paralysis of accommodation, and paralysis of all right-sided ocular movement except laterally, were due to pressure on the right oculomotor nerve by the aneurysm. The nerve at this point is situated in the lateral wall of the cavernous sinus. Note that the lateral move-

ment of the eyeball was accomplished by contracting the lateral rectus muscle (abducent nerve) and the inferolateral movement was due to the contraction of the superior oblique muscle (trochlear nerve).

8. The Argyll Robertson pupil is a common finding in neurosyphilis, although it may occur in other diseases. The lesion is believed to be located where the pretectal fibers pass to the parasympathetic oculomotor nuclei on both sides of the midbrain. This lesion effectively destroys the direct and consensual light reflexes of both eyes but leaves the pathway for the accommodation reflex intact. (For details of pathway, see p. 425.)

9. (a) Complete blindness of the right eye
    (b) Bitemporal hemianopia
    (c) Left homonymous hemianopia
    (d) Left homonymous hemianopia
    (e) Left homonymous hemianopia, usually with some macular sparing owing to the very large area of the cortex allotted to the macula

10. The glossopharyngeal nerve supplies the posterior one-third of the tongue with fibers that subserve common sensations and taste. This may be tested easily. The vagus nerve, by means of its pharyngeal branch, supplies many muscles of the soft palate and these may be tested by asking the patient to say "ah" and observing that normally the uvula is elevated in the midline. A lesion of the vagus nerve would result in the uvula being elevated to the opposite side. Additional tests may be carried out by observing the movements of the vocal cords through a laryngoscope.

    The spinal part of the accessory nerve may be tested by asking the patient to shrug her shoulders by using the trapezius muscles or to rotate her head so that she looks upward to the opposite side by contracting the sternocleidomastoid muscles. Both muscles are innervated by the spinal part of the accessory nerve.

11. It will be remembered that the afferent fibers entering the central nervous system through the trigeminal nerve pass either to the main sensory nucleus in the pons or to the spinal nucleus situated in the medulla oblongata and the first two cervical segments of the spinal cord. The sensations of touch and pressure are served by the main sensory nucleus, while those of pain and temperature are served by the more inferiorly placed spinal nucleus. In this patient, the lesion of syringomyelia was situated in the medulla oblongata and the cervical part of the spinal cord and the main sensory nucleus in the pons was intact.

12. The wrinkled, wasted right half of the tongue and the pointing of the protruded tongue to the right indicated a lesion of the right hypoglossal nerve at some point between its nucleus in the medulla oblongata and the tongue muscles supplied. This patient had advanced bronchogenic carcinoma of the right lung with numerous metastases in the deep cervical lymph nodes. One of the metastases had invaded the right hypoglossal nerve.

13. The physician grouped together the facial paralysis, the slurred speech, and the hypertension and, in the absence of other findings, made the erroneous diagnosis of cerebral hemorrhage. Unfortunately, the physician had forgotten his neuroanatomy. A lesion of the corticonuclear fibers on one side of the brain will cause paralysis only of the muscles of the lower part of the opposite side of the face. This patient had a complete paralysis of the entire right side of the face, which could be due only to a lesion of the lower motor neuron. The correct diagnosis was Bell's palsy, a condition in which the facial nerve swells in the bony canal; the paralysis usually recovers within two weeks in most patients.

14. The vagal nuclei are (a) main motor nucleus, (b) parasympathetic nucleus, and (c) sensory nucleus. The main motor and parasympathetic nuclei are controlled by both cerebral hemispheres, so that hemiplegia will have no effect on the movement of the vocal cords. The vagal nuclei are practically continuous with the nuclei of the glossopharyngeal and accessory nerves and these usually are involved together in lesions of the medulla oblongata.

CHAPTER 25

1. This boy was suffering from Fröhlich's syndrome secondary to a chromophobe adenoma of the anterior lobe of the hypophysis. This space-occupying lesion had gradually eroded the sella turcica of the skull and had com-

pressed the optic chiasma, producing bitemporal hemianopia. The size of the tumor was causing a raised intracranial pressure that was responsible for the headaches and attacks of vomiting. Pressure on the hypothalamus interfered with its function and resulted in the characteristic accumulation of fat in the trunk, especially the lower part of the abdomen. The hypogonadism and absence of secondary sex characteristics could have been due to pressure of the tumor on the hypothalamic nuclei and the consequent loss of control on the anterior lobe of the hypophysis, or it may have been due to the direct effect of the tumor pressing on the neighboring cells of the anterior lobe of the hypophysis.

2. This patient is now suffering from diabetes insipidus. The condition was caused either by traumatic damage to the posterior lobe of the hypophysis or to the supraoptic nucleus of the hypothalamus. In any event, production of vasopressin was inhibited. It should be pointed out that a lesion of the posterior lobe of the hypophysis is usually not followed by diabetes insipidus, since the vasopressin produced by the neurons of the supraoptic nucleus escapes directly into the bloodstream. The action of vasopressin on the distal convoluted tubules and collecting tubules of the kidney is fully explained on page 477.

3. Hydrocephalus, caused by blocking the three foramina in the roof of the fourth ventricle or by blocking the cerebral aqueduct, will result in a rise in pressure in the third ventricle, with pressure on the hypothalamus. This pressure on the hypothalamus, which is situated in the floor and lower part of the lateral walls of the third ventricle, if great enough, could easily cause malfunctioning of the hypothalamus.

4. The hypothalamus is the main subcortical center regulating the parasympathetic and sympathetic parts of the autonomic system. It exerts its influence through descending pathways in the reticular formation.

5. The hypothalamohypophyseal tract is described on page 477, and the hypophyseal portal system is described on page 478. Remember that the hypothalamus exerts its control over metabolic and visceral functions through the hypophysis cerebri and the autonomic system.

CHAPTER 26

1. As a result of holding onto the moving truck with the right hand, this man had sustained a severe traction injury of the eighth cervical and first thoracic roots of the brachial plexus. The various paralyzed forearm and hand muscles together with the sensory loss were characteristic of Klumpke's paralysis. In this case, the pull on the first thoracic nerve was so severe that the white ramus communicantes to the inferior cervical sympathetic ganglion was torn. This effectively cut off the preganglionic sympathetic fibers to the right side of the head and neck, causing a right-sided Horner's syndrome. This was exemplified by (a) constriction of the pupil, (b) drooping of the upper lid, and (c) enophthalmos. The arteriolar vasodilatation, due to loss of sympathetic vasonconstrictor fibers, was responsible for the red, hot cheek on the right side. The dryness of the skin of the right cheek also was due to the loss of the sympathetic secretomotor supply to the sweat glands.

2. This 3-year-old boy has Hirschsprung's disease, a congenital condition in which there is a failure of development of the myenteric plexus (Auerbach's plexus) in the distal part of the colon. The proximal part of the colon is normal but becomes greatly distended due to the accumulation of feces. In this patient, the lower sigmoid colon, later at operation, was shown to have no parasympathetic ganglion cells. Thus, this segment of the bowel had no peristalsis and effectively blocked the passage of feces. Once the diagnosis had been confirmed by taking a biopsy of the distal segment of the bowel, the treatment was to remove the aganglionic segment of the bowel by surgical resection.

3. This patient has given a classic history of Raynaud's disease. The disease is much more common in women than in men, especially those who have a nervous disposition. The initial pallor of the fingers is due to spasm of the digital arterioles. The cyanosis that follows is due to local capillary dilatation due to accumulation of metabolites. Since there is no blood flow through the capillaries, deoxygenated hemoglobin accumulates within them. It is during this period of prolonged cyanosis that the patient

experiences severe aching pain. On exposing the fingers to warmth, the vasospasm disappears and oxygenated blood flows back into the very dilated capillaries. There is now a reactive hyperemia and an increase in the formation of tissue fluid that is responsible for the swelling of the affected fingers. The sweating of the fingers during the attack probably is due to the excessive sympathetic activity, which may be responsible in part for the arteriolar vasospasm.

The arteries of the upper limb are innervated by sympathetic nerves. The preganglionic fibers originate from the cell bodies in the second to the eighth thoracic segments of the spinal cord. They ascend in the sympathetic trunk to synapse in the middle cervical, inferior cervical, and first thoracic or stellate ganglia. The postganglionic fibers join the nerves that form the brachial plexus and are distributed to the digital arteries within the branches of the brachial plexus.

In this patient the attacks were relatively mild. The patient should be reassured and told to keep her hands warm as much as possible. However, should the condition worsen the patient should be treated with drugs, such as reserpine, that inhibit sympathetic activity. This would result in arterial vasodilatation with consequent increase in blood flow to the fingers.

4. The patient was suffering from gallstone colic. The visceral pain originated from the cystic duct or bile duct and was due to stretching or spasm of the smooth muscle in its wall. The pain afferent fibers pass through the celiac ganglia and ascend in the greater splanchnic nerve to enter the fifth to the ninth thoracic segments of the spinal cord. The pain was referred to the fifth through the ninth thoracic dermatomes on the right side, that is, to the skin over and inferior to the right scapula.

Referred pain to the right shoulder in gallbladder disease can be explained by the fact that the right phrenic nerve (C3, 4, and 5) supplies the peritoneum under the diaphragm close to the gallbladder with sensory fibers. Afferent impulses ascend in the phrenic nerve to the spinal cord and the pain is referred to the skin over the right shoulder, which is innervated by the right supraclavicular nerves (C3 and 4). For a full discussion of referred pain, see page 512.

5. This patient has an Argyll Robertson pupil, which is a small fixed pupil that does not react to light, but contracts with accommodation. The condition usually is due to a syphilitic lesion. The innervation of the iris is described on page 497. The neurological lesion in this patient interrupted the fibers running from the pretectal nucleus to the parasympathetic nuclei of the oculomotor nerve on both sides.

6. The urinary bladder is innervated by sympathetic fibers from the first and second lumbar segments of the spinal cord and by parasympathetic fibers from the second, third, and fourth sacral segments of the spinal cord. In this patient, the cauda equina was sectioned at the level of the third lumbar vertebra. This meant that the preganglionic sympathetic fibers that descend in the anterior roots of the first and second lumbar nerves were left intact, since they leave the vertebral canal to form the appropriate spinal nerves above the level of the bullet. The preganglionic parasympathetic fibers were, however, sectioned as they descended in the vertebral canal within the anterior roots of the second, third, and fourth sacral nerves. The patient would, therefore, have an autonomous bladder and would be without any external reflex control. The bladder would fill to capacity and then overflow. Micturition could be activated by powerful contraction of the abdominal muscles by the patient, assisted by manual pressure on his anterior abdominal wall in the suprapubic region.

7. The sympathetic outflow refers to the origin of the preganglionic sympathetic fibers from the spinal cord from the first thoracic to the second lumbar segments. The parasympathetic outflow refers to the origin of the preganglionic parasympathetic fibers in the cranial nerves 3, 7, 9, and 10, and the gray matter of the spinal cord at the level of the second, third, and fourth sacral segments.

8. The precise cause of essential hypertension is unknown. Nevertheless, the objective of the treatment is to lower the blood pressure and keep it, if possible, within normal limits before the complications of cerebral hemorrhage, renal failure, or heart failure develop. The best

way to accomplish this in patients with mild hypertension is to reduce the plasma fluid volume by the use of diuretics. Beta-receptor blocking agents are now extensively used. These reduce the rate and force of contraction of the cardiac muscle and lower the cardiac output.

9. (a) Acetylcholine, (b) acetylcholine, (c) acetylcholine, (d) norepinephrine, and (e) acetylcholine.

10. Sympathetic endings that use norepinephrine as a transmitter substance are called *adrenergic endings*. There are two major kinds of receptors called *alpha* and *beta receptors* for adrenergic endings. For details, see page 492.

CHAPTER 27

1. Loss of function of the dominant hemisphere results in not only the loss of acquired skills of the dominant hand but also the loss of certain mental functions. The degree of disability depends on the degree of dominance of one hemisphere over the other. A child's brain possesses a degree of flexibility that is not present in the adult, so that good recoveries can be expected in the young child.

   The meninges and the cerebrospinal fluid afford a remarkable degree of protection to the delicate brain. The dural partitions limit the extent of brain movement within the skull.

   The thin-walled cerebral veins are liable to be damaged during excessive movements of the brain relative to the skull, especially at the point where the veins join the dural venous sinuses. The thick-walled cerebral arteries are rarely damaged.

   The small-diameter cranial nerves of long length are particularly prone to damage during head injuries. The trochlear, abducent, and oculomotor nerves are commonly injured.

2. Meningiomas arise from the arachnoid villi found along the dural venous sinuses. They are therefore most commonly found along the superior sagittal sinus and the sphenoparietal sinuses. They are rare below the tentorium cerebelli.

3. The anterior facial vein, the ophthalmic veins, and the cavernous sinus are in direct communication with one another. Infection of the skin of the face alongside the nose, ethmoidal sinus-

itis, and infection of the orbital contents may lead to thrombosis of the veins and ultimately cavernous sinus thrombosis. If untreated with antibiotics, this condition may be fatal, since the cavernous sinus drains many cerebral veins from the inferior surface of the brain.

4. The internal carotid artery passes forward on the lateral surface of the body of the sphenoid within the cavernous sinus. An aneurysm of the artery may press on the abducent nerve and cause paralysis of the lateral rectus muscle. Further expansion of the aneurysm may cause compression of the oculomotor nerve and the ophthalmic division of the trigeminal nerve as they lie in the lateral wall of the cavernous sinus. This patient had left lateral rectus paralysis and paralysis of the left pupillary constrictor muscle owing to involvement of the abducent and oculomotor nerves, respectively. The slight anesthesia of the skin over the left forehead was due to pressure on the ophthalmic division of the left trigeminal nerve.

5. The optic nerves are surrounded by sheaths derived from the pia mater, arachnoid mater, and dura mater. There is an extension of the intracranial subarachnoid space forward around the optic nerve to the back of the eyeball. A rise in cerebrospinal fluid pressure due to an intracranial tumor will compress the thin walls of the retinal vein as it crosses the extension of the subarachnoid space in the orbital cavity. This will result in congestion of the retinal vein and bulging of the optic disc, involving both eyes.

6. During the descent of the fetal head through the birth canal in labor, the bones of the calvarium overlap, a process known as molding. If this process is excessive or takes place too rapidly, as in malpresentations or in premature deliveries (when there is rapid birth of a small fetus), an abnormal strain is put on the falx cerebri. This stress involves the superior sagittal sinus, especially if the anteroposterior compression is excessive, and the sinus may tear where it joins the transverse sinus. The great cerebral vein may tear as well. The result is either a subarachnoid or subdural hemorrhage with accompanying brain damage.

7. The initial loss of consciousness was due to concussion or cerebral trauma. The swelling over the right temporalis and the radiographic find-

ing of a fracture over the right middle meningeal artery were due to hemorrhage from the artery into the overlying muscle and soft tissue. This patient had an extradural hemorrhage. The right homolateral hemiplegia was due to the compression of the left cerebral peduncle against the edge of the tentorium cerebelli. This is unusual. A left hemiplegia due to pressure on the right percentral gyrus is more common. The right-sided, fixed, dilated pupil was due to the pressure on the right oculomotor nerve by the hippocampal gyrus, which had herniated through the tentorial notch.

8. A subdural hematoma is an accumulation of blood clot in the interval between the meningeal layer of dura and the arachnoid mater. It results from tearing of the superior cerebral veins at their point of entrance into the superior sagittal sinus. The cause is usually a blow on the front or the back of the head, causing excessive anteroposterior displacement of the brain within the skull. A subdural hematoma can be easily identified by CT scan as a dense rim of blood extending along the inner table of the skull obliterating the cerebral fissures and displacing the cerebral structures to the opposite side.

CHAPTER 28

1. The circulus arteriosus lies within the subarachnoid space at the base of the brain and essentially is formed by the anastomosis of the two internal carotid and two vertebral arteries and their branches. The anterior communicating, the anterior cerebral, the internal carotid, the posterior communicating, the posterior cerebral, and the basilar arteries all contribute to the circle. The functional importance of the circle is that it provides a collateral circulation should one of the main arteries to the brain be temporarily or permanently occluded. (see Cerebral Circulation for more detail, on p. 542).

2. Once the terminal branches of the cerebral arteries enter the brain substance, no further anastomoses occur. Blockage of such end arteries by disease is quickly followed by neuronal death and necrosis. The surrounding neuroglia then usually proliferates and invades the area, producing a neuroglial scar or forming a cystic

cavity. The following important anastomoses exist between the cerebral arteries: (1) the circulus arteriosus of Willis, (2) anastomoses between the branches of the cerebral arteries on the surface of the cerebral hemispheres and the cerebellar hemispheres, and (3) anastomoses between the branches of the internal and external carotid arteries: (a) at their origin at the common carotid artery, (b) at the anastomosis between the branches of the ophthalmic artery within the orbit and the facial and maxillary arteries, and (c) between the meningeal branches of the internal carotid artery and the middle meningeal artery.

3. The work of McDonald and Potter in 1951 showed that the posterior communicating artery is the site at which the streams of blood from the internal carotid and vertebral arteries on the same side come together, and since their pressures at this point are equal, they do not mix. Nevertheless, in clinical practice, good filling of the posterior cerebral artery with radiopaque material with carotid angiography occurs in about 25 percent of patients. Slight filling also may be seen in other normal individuals. The variable results can be explained on the basis that the size of the arteries making up the arterial circle is subject to considerable variation and consequently the blood flow in different individuals may vary.

4. The sudden severe headache followed by loss of consciousness is a common clinical finding in patients with a blockage of a cerebral artery. Intraventricular hemorrhage associated with this condition is often responsible for the severe headache. The depth of coma is related to the extent of the arterial blockage. The following signs indicate that the cerebral lesion occurred on the left side of the brain: (a) paralysis of the lower part of the face on the right side, (b) the patient's head and eyes turned to the side of the lesion, that is, to the left, (c) the muscle tone in the limbs initially diminished on the right side and then increased above normal as the weeks pass, (d) the loss of the right abdominal reflexes and the presence of a positive Babinski response on the right side, and (e) the presence of right hemianesthesia.

The following physical signs strongly suggested involvement of the left middle cerebral artery or its branches: (a) paralysis of the right side of the face and the right arm that was more severe than that of the right leg, and (b) aphasia. It will be remembered that the middle cerebral artery supplies the entire lateral surface of the hemisphere, except for the narrow strip supplied by the anterior cerebral artery, the occipital pole, and the inferolateral surface of the hemisphere, which are supplied by the posterior cerebral artery. Central branches supply the lentiform and caudate nuclei and the internal capsule.

5. A history of a sudden collapse in an elderly woman, followed by coma and recovery of consciousness 24 hours later, with left-sided hemiplegia (mainly involving the leg) and left-sided hemianesthesia, is strongly suggestive of cerebrovascular disease with a lesion involving the right cerebral hemisphere. The paralysis mainly involving the leg would indicate that the right anterior cerebral artery or one of its branches was blocked by a thrombus or embolus.

6. The occlusion of the cortical branches of the left posterior cerebral artery will give rise to right-sided homonymous hemianopia because of the ischemia of the primary visual area in the calcarine fissure. The escape of the macular region could be accounted for by the overlapping of the arterial supply of this area of the occipital lobe by the left posterior and left middle cerebral arteries. The right-sided hemianesthesia and the severe burning pain in the right leg are referred to clinically as the thalamic syndrome and are due to occlusion of one of the central branches of the left posterior cerebral artery that supplies the sensory nuclei of the left thalamus. The presense of a mild fleeting right-sided hemiparesis could be explained by a temporary occlusion of a branch of the left posterior cerebral artery to the left cerebral peduncle.

7. Artheromatous plaques tend to occur at the following sites: (a) carotid sinus of the internal carotid artery at or just beyond the bifurcation of the common carotid artery, (b) the first main bifurcation of the middle cerebral artery, (c) where the vertebral arteries join to form the basilar artery, (d) where the anterior cerebral artery curves superiorly and posteriorly over the genu of the corpus callosum, (e) where the posterior cerebral artery passes around the lateral side of the cerebral peduncle.

8. A stroke may be defined as a sudden development of a neurological defect, usually associated with the development of some degree of hemiplegia and sometimes accompanied by unconsciousness; it is usually caused by a cerebrovascular accident. The symptoms and signs will depend on the cause of the interruption of cerebral blood flow and the size of the artery involved. For example, cerebral embolism or cerebral hemorrhage is a sudden event, whereas the development of atheroslerosis in a patient with hypertension is a slow process that suddenly may become worse when thrombosis occurs at the site of the atheromatous plaque. Hemiplegia is the most common sign, but many additional sensory defects may develop that will depend on the artery blocked, for example, hemianesthesia, hemianopia, dysphasia, and dysarthria.

9. Occlusion of the middle cerebral artery or its branches can produce, in addition to paralysis of the muscles of the opposite side of the body, contralateral hemianesthesia owing to ischemia of the postcentral gyrus and homonymous hemianopia owing to ischemia of the optic radiation.

   Occlusion of the anterior cerebral artery or its branches may produce contralateral sensory loss of the leg, feet, and toes owing to ischemia of the leg area of the cerebral cortex. Occlusion of the posterior cerebral artery or its branches may produce contralateral homonymous hemianopia owing to ischemia of the primary visual area in the region of the calcarine fissue. If the branches to the thalamus also are blocked, there will also be contralateral hemianesthia and possibly the development of severe pain in the same areas.

   The above sensory deficits are the main ones seen. The degree of sensory involvement will depend on the size and number of branches of the artery occluded.

10. The internal carotid and the basilar arteries are equally affected by disease. The internal carotid artery supplies predominantly one cerebral hemisphere through the anterior cerebral and middle cerebral branches and, therefore,

occlusion of the internal carotid artery will produce contralateral hemiplegia, hemianesthesia, hemianopia, and aphasia and agnosia, depending on whether the dominant hemisphere is involved. On the other hand, the basilar artery contributes to the blood supply of both sides of the brain through the two posterior cerebral arteries and the many branches to both sides of the brainstem. Consequently, occlusion of the basilar artery will result in bilateral motor and sensory losses and involvement of the cranial nerves and cerebellum on both sides of the body.

11. The dominant hemisphere possesses the language function. In right-handed individuals (and in some left-handed persons) language is a function of the left hemisphere. A cerebrovascular accident involving the middle cerebral artery on the left side will therefore be more serious than one on the right side, since it will involve the cortical speech area and cause a total sensory motor aphasia. In persons who have a dominant right hemisphere, the reverse occurs.

12. The middle cerebral artery, in addition to giving off cortical branches, gives off central branches that supply part of the posterior limb of the internal capsule and the optic radiation. Occlusion of these branches will cause contralateral homonymous hemianopia.

13. Since so many important ascending and descending tracts travel in the internal capsule, an occlusion of its blood supply would produce a widespread neurological deficit. The internal capsule is supplied by the medial and lateral striate central branches of the middle cerebral artery and by the central branches of the anterior cerebral artery.

14. This patient has the symptoms of the carotid sinus syndrome. For a full description of this syndrome, see page 543.

15. It has been estimated that irreversible changes start to occur in the cerebral nervous tissue about 4 minutes following the complete arrest of cerebral blood flow. (This figure may be larger if the patient's body has been cooled.)

16. The impairment of vision of the right eye with motor symptoms in the left leg strongly suggests partial occlusion of the right internal carotid artery. When these are coupled with impairment of memory and a systolic bruit over the right internal carotid artery, the diagnosis is almost certain. The right-sided headaches are also common symptoms in this condition. A right-sided carotid angiogram confirmed the presence of extreme narrowing of the internal carotid artery at its origin. Ophthalmodynamometric measurements showed diminished retinal arterial pressure on the right side owing to diminished pressure in the right ophthalmic artery.

17. This patient had a congenital aneurysm of the anterior communicating artery. The sudden onset of a severe headache, which is often so dramatic that the patient feels as though he has been hit on the head, is characteristic of rupture of a congenital aneurysm into the subarachnoid space. The stiff or rigid neck is due to meningeal irritation caused by the presence of blood in the subarachnoid space. This patient had no evidence of previous pressure on the optic nerve leading to unilateral visual defect, which sometimes occurs when the aneurysm is situated on the anterior part of the circle of Willis. The loss of tone in the left leg muscles is difficult to explain, although it may be due to the sudden hemorrhage into the subarachnoid space causing damage to the right cerebral hemisphere.

18. This patient had a right-sided extradural hemorrhage due to a fracture of the anterior part of the parietal bone, which tore the anterior division of the right middle meningeal artery. The history of the patient being found unconscious, then recovering consciousness for a period only to relapse into unconsciousness, is a characteristic finding. The initial trauma usually is responsible for the initial loss of consciousness. The relapse into an unconscious state is due to the accumulation of a large blood clot under arterial pressure outside the meningeal layer of dura. This is responsible for the dilated pupil on the right side due to indirect pressure on the right oculomotor nerve. The pressure on the right precentral gyrus causes the hemiplegia and weakness of the left leg; it also causes the positive Babinski sign on the left side. The presence of a large blood clot in the intracranial cavity was easily recognized on a CT scan. The presence of the clot was also responsible for the

raised cerebrospinal fluid pressure. The slight blood staining of the fluid obtained from a lumbar puncture was due to a small leakage of blood from the extradural space into the subarachnoid space at the fracture site.

19. This patient had a chronic subdural hematoma following trauma to the head three weeks previously. This resulted from one of the superior cerebral veins tearing at its point of entrance into the superior sagittal sinus. The blood accumulated under low pressure between the dura and the arachnoid. The headaches, drowsiness, and mental confusion were due to the raised intracranial pressure. The blood clot could be seen easily on the CT scan. The blood clot was successfully removed through a bur hole in the skull and the patient had no further symptoms.

20. The history of hypertension, sudden onset of severe headache, slurring of speech, right lower facial weakness, right-sided hemiplegia, right positive Babinski sign, right-sided hemianesthesia, and deviation of the eyes to the left side are all diagnostic of a cerebrovascular accident involving the left cerebral hemisphere. The perforating central branches of the left middle cerebral artery were found at autopsy to be extensively affected by atherosclerosis. One of these arteries had ruptured, resulting in a large hemorrhage into the left lentiform nucleus and left internal capsule. The combination of hypertension and atherosclerotic degeneration of the artery was responsible for the fatal hemorrhage. The dilated fixed pupils, the irregularity in breathing, and, finally, death were due to the raised pressure within the hemisphere causing downward pressure effects within the brainstem.

CHAPTER 29

1. This patient has spina bifida occulta involving the fifth lumbar vertebra. The condition is a result of failure of the mesenchyme to grow between the neural tube and the surface ectoderm and form the vertebral arch; the vertebral canal remains open posteriorly. The defect therefore has existed since before birth and could not be seen or felt on physical examination because it was covered by the postvertebral muscles. The spinal cord and spinal nerve roots usually are normal. No treatment is required.

2. This child has a myelocele. In addition to the failure of the formation of the vertebral arches of the fourth and fifth lumbar vertebrae, the neural tube failed to close in this region. The oval raw area seen in this patient is the neural groove whose lips have not united. The central canal is discharging clear cerebrospinal fluid onto the skin surface. The deformities of the knee joints and feet are the result of the maldevelopment of the spinal cord in the lumbar region, with consequent interference with the innervation of certain muscle groups in the legs.

3. This child has hydrocephalus. A postmortem examination performed 1 year later showed that the cerebral aqueduct was not normally developed and consisted of a number of small tubules. This had resulted in the excessive accumulation of cerebrospinal fluid within the lateral and third ventricles of the brain. The distention of the ventricles, with the consequent enlargement of the brain and increased intracranial pressure, forced apart the bones of the cranial vault so that the head became greatly enlarged. The optic atrophy probably was caused by the stretching of the optic nerve on each side. The increased muscle tone of the lower limbs was almost certainly the result of destruction of the corticospinal and other descending tracts by the expanding lateral ventricles. Although in some cases the head ceases to enlarge spontaneously, in most patients the hydrocephalus is progressive and death ultimately occurs. Surgical treatment of hydrocephalus may be attempted (see p. 578).

Answers to National Board Type Questions

CHAPTER I

1. (b)	8. (b)	14. (c)
2. (d)	9. (c)	15. (a)
3. (a)	10. (e)	16. (d)
4. (c)	11. (b)	17. (e)
5. (d)	12. (a)	
6. (b)	13. (b)	
7. (a)		

CHAPTER 2

1. (b)	6. (c)	11. (b)
2. (c)	7. (e)	12. (c)
3. (a)	8. (b)	13. (d)
4. (a)	9. (d)	14. (e)
5. (b)	10. (a)	15. (a)

CHAPTER 3

1. (a)	5. (e)	9. (b)
2. (b)	6. (b)	10. (c)
3. (c)	7. (a)	11. (d)
4. (e)	8. (c)	12. (a)

CHAPTER 4

1. (c)	7. (c)	13. (c)
2. (a)	8. (d)	14. (b)
3. (d)	9. (d)	15. (a)
4. (b)	10. (e)	16. (d)
5. (d)	11. (a)	17. (a)
6. (c)	12. (b)	

CHAPTER 5

1. (c)	7. (e)	12. (d)
2. (a)	8. (e)	13. (a)
3. (b)	9. (a)	14. (b)
4. (c)	10. (d)	15. (b)
5. (c)	11. (c)	
6. (d)		

CHAPTER 6

1. (d)	5. (c)	9. (b)
2. (d)	6. (b)	10. (e)
3. (a)	7. (c)	11. (e)
4. (a)	8. (a)	12. (c)

CHAPTER 7

1. (a)	9. (b)	17. (e)
2. (c)	10. (c)	18. (e)
3. (a)	11. (d)	19. (c)
4. (c)	12. (a)	20. (a)
5. (c)	13. (d)	21. (b)
6. (b)	14. (a)	22. (d)
7. (a)	15. (c)	23. (e)
8. (c)	16. (b)	

CHAPTER 8

1. (b)	8. (e)	15. (b)
2. (c)	9. (c)	16. (a)
3. (a)	10. (e)	17. (b)
4. (d)	11. (b)	18. (b)
5. (b)	12. (e)	19. (b)
6. (a)	13. (d)	20. (c)
7. (c)	14. (a)	

CHAPTER 9

1. (d)	7. (d)	13. (c)
2. (c)	8. (c)	14. (b)
3. (b)	9. (e)	15. (b)
4. (c)	10. (a)	16. (b)
5. (b)	11. (e)	17. (a)
6. (a)	12. (b)	

CHAPTER 10

1. (c)	5. (c)	9. (e)
2. (b)	6. (a)	10. (a)
3. (e)	7. (d)	11. (a)
4. (b)	8. (c)	12. (e)

CHAPTER 11

1. (b)	4. (b)	7. (c)
2. (b)	5. (a)	
3. (e)	6. (c)	

CHAPTER 12

1. (c)	6. (a)	11. (e)
2. (d)	7. (c)	12. (e)
3. (b)	8. (e)	13. (c)
4. (c)	9. (e)	14. (e)
5. (a)	10. (e)	

CHAPTER 13

1. (c)	6. (a)	11. (b)
2. (a)	7. (b)	12. (c)
3. (b)	8. (d)	13. (e)
4. (c)	9. (a)	14. (e)
5. (c)	10. (e)	

CHAPTER 14

1. (c)	8. (e)	15. (e)
2. (a)	9. (c)	16. (a)
3. (b)	10. (e)	17. (b)
4. (d)	11. (c)	18. (d)
5. (e)	12. (e)	19. (e)
6. (a)	13. (e)	20. (c)
7. (b)	14. (e)	

CHAPTER 15

1. (c)	7. (a)	13. (e)
2. (a)	8. (b)	14. (b)
3. (b)	9. (e)	15. (c)
4. (d)	10. (c)	16. (b)
5. (c)	11. (c)	17. (d)
6. (d)	12. (e)	18. (a)

CHAPTER 16

1. (d)	5. (e)	9. (b)
2. (c)	6. (b)	10. (d)
3. (a)	7. (e)	11. (c)
4. (a)	8. (b)	12. (a)

CHAPTER 17

1. (a)	6. (e)	11. (d)
2. (b)	7. (a)	12. (e)
3. (e)	8. (c)	13. (c)
4. (a)	9. (f)	14. (a)
5. (a)	10. (b)	

CHAPTER 18

1. (d)	5. (b)	9. (b)
2. (a)	6. (e)	10. (a)
3. (c)	7. (a)	11. (d)
4. (d)	8. (a)	12. (c)

CHAPTER 19

1. (c)	3. (d)	5. (b)
2. (a)	4. (c)	6. (a)

CHAPTER 20

1. (c)	8. (a)	15. (b)
2. (a)	9. (b)	16. (a)
3. (c)	10. (e)	17. (d)
4. (b)	11. (c)	18. (c)
5. (a)	12. (e)	19. (d)
6. (b)	13. (e)	20. (e)
7. (b)	14. (c)	

CHAPTER 21

1. (c)	8. (e)	15. (c)
2. (a)	9. (c)	16. (a)
3. (c)	10. (d)	17. (d)
4. (d)	11. (d)	18. (d)
5. (c)	12. (d)	19. (a)
6. (b)	13. (d)	20. (c)
7. (a)	14. (b)	

CHAPTER 22

1. (c)	6. (a)	11. (e)
2. (b)	7. (b)	12. (d)
3. (a)	8. (c)	13. (d)
4. (c)	9. (b)	14. (a)
5. (a)	10. (b)	

CHAPTER 23

1. (e)	10. (c)	19. (e)
2. (a)	11. (c)	20. (e)
3. (a)	12. (a)	21. (c)
4. (d)	13. (c)	22. (b)
5. (c)	14. (c)	23. (a)
6. (b)	15. (b)	24. (d)
7. (d)	16. (a)	25. (a)
8. (c)	17. (d)	
9. (a)	18. (e)	

CHAPTER 24

1. (a)	4. (c)	7. (e)
2. (c)	5. (a)	8. (a)
3. (d)	6. (c)	

CHAPTER 25

1. (b)	5. (c)	9. (a)
2. (c)	6. (b)	10. (c)
3. (b)	7. (e)	
4. (b)	8. (e)	

CHAPTER 26

1. (c)	13. (c)	25. (b)
2. (c)	14. (b)	26. (a)
3. (c)	15. (c)	27. (d)
4. (b)	16. (c)	28. (d)
5. (c)	17. (a)	29. (a)
6. (d)	18. (b)	30. (c)
7. (c)	19. (a)	31. (d)
8. (c)	20. (c)	32. (c)
9. (d)	21. (e)	33. (a)
10. (e)	22. (d)	34. (b)
11. (b)	23. (b)	
12. (d)	24. (c)	

CHAPTER 27

1. (d)	5. (d)	9. (a)
2. (c)	6. (c)	10. (c)
3. (a)	7. (d)	
4. (b)	8. (c)	

CHAPTER 28

1. (c)	9. (b)	17. (c)
2. (c)	10. (a)	18. (a)
3. (c)	11. (b)	19. (b)
4. (a)	12. (c)	20. (c)
5. (b)	13. (c)	21. (e)
6. (c)	14. (d)	22. (d)
7. (c)	15. (c)	23. (e)
8. (a)	16. (b)	24. (a)

CHAPTER 29

1. (c)	5. (c)	9. (a)
2. (b)	6. (a)	10. (b)
3. (c)	7. (e)	
4. (a)	8. (e)	

Index

623